T0325554

Advances in Malignant Hematology

Advances in Malignant Hematology

EDITED BY

Hussain I. Saba MD, PHD

James A. Haley Veterans' Hospital
H. Lee Moffitt Cancer Center and Research Institute
University of South Florida College of Medicine
Tampa, FL, USA

Ghulam J. Mufti MB, DM, FRCP, FRCPATH

Department of Haematological Medicine
Guy's and St Thomas' School of Medicine
King's College Hospital
London, UK

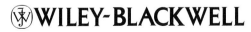

A John Wiley & Sons, Ltd., Publication

Library of Congress Cataloging-in-Publication Data

Advances in malignant hematology / edited by Hussain I. Saba, Ghulam Mufti.
      p. ; cm.
   Includes bibliographical references and index.
   ISBN 978-1-4051-9626-0 (hardcover : alk. paper) – ISBN 978-1-4443-9399-6 (ePDF) – ISBN 978-1-4443-9400-9 (ePub)
  1. Leukemia. 2. Lymphomas. 3. Myelodysplastic syndromes. I. Saba, Hussain I. II. Mufti, G. J.
   [DNLM: 1. Leukemia, Myeloid–metabolism. 2. Leukemia, Lymphoid. 3. Leukemia, Myeloid–therapy.
4. Myelodysplastic Syndromes–therapy. WH 250]
   RC643.A35 2011
   616.99'446–dc22

                                                                    2010047405

A catalogue record for this book is available from the British Library.

This book is published in the following electronic formats: ePDF 9781444393996; Wiley Online Library 9781444394016; ePub 9781444394009

Set in 9/12pt Meridien by Thomson Digital, Noida, India
Printed and bound in Singapore by Fabulous Printers Pte Ltd

1   2011

Contents

The colour plate section can be found facing p. 130

List of Contributors

Lionel Ades
Service d'hématologie clinique, Hôpital Avicenne (Assistance Publique –Hôpitaux de Paris) and Paris 13 University, Bobigny, France

Jessica K. Altman
Northwestern University Feinberg School of Medicine, and Robert H. Lurie Comprehensive Cancer Center, Chicago, Illinois, USA

Claudio Anasetti
Department of Blood and Marrow Transplantation, H. Lee Moffitt Cancer Center, University of South Florida, Tampa, Florida, USA

Jessica Clima
St. Vincent's Comprehensive Cancer Center, New York, New York, USA

Jorge Cortes
Department of Leukemia, University of Texas M.D. Anderson Cancer Center, Houston, Texas, USA

Nicholas C.P. Cross
Wessex Regional Genetics Laboratory, Salisbury and Human Genetics Division, University of Southampton, Southampton, UK

Michael Crump
University of Toronto and Division of Medical Oncology and Hematology, Princess Margaret Hospital, Toronto, Canada

Raymond Cruz
St. Vincent's Comprehensive Cancer Center, New York, New York, USA

Arshia A. Dangol
James A. Haley Veterans' Hospital, and H. Lee Moffitt Cancer Center and Research Institute, University of South Florida College of Medicine, Tampa, Florida, USA

Meletios Athanasios Dimopoulos
Department of Clinical Therapeutics, University of Athens School of Medicine, Athens, Greece

Donald C. Doll
James A. Haley Veterans' Hospital, and H. Lee Moffitt Cancer Center and Research Institute, University of South Florida College of Medicine, Tampa, Florida, USA

Stefan Faderl
Department of Leukemia, The University of Texas M.D. Anderson Cancer Center, Houston, Texas, USA

Pierre Fenaux
Service d'hématologie clinique, Hôpital Avicenne (Assistance Publique –Hôpitaux de Paris) and Paris 13 University, Bobigny, France

Nathan Fowler
Department of Lymphoma/Myeloma, University of Texas M.D. Anderson Cancer Center, Houston, Texas, USA

Naomi Galili
St. Vincent's Comprehensive Cancer Center, New York, New York, USA

Angela Hamblin
Department of Immunohaematology, Cancer Sciences Division, University of Southampton, Southampton, UK

Terry Hamblin
Department of Immunohaematology, Cancer Sciences Division, University of Southampton, Southampton, UK

Monique A. Hartley
Department of Medical Hematology and Oncology, University of South Florida, and Department of Malignant Hematology, H. Lee Moffitt Cancer Center and Research Institute, Tampa, Florida, USA

Suzanne Hayman
Laboratory Medicine and Pathology, Mayo Clinic College of Medicine, Rochester, Minnesota, USA

Lori A. Hazlehurst
Department of Malignant Hematology, H. Lee Moffitt Cancer Center and Research Institute, Tampa, Florida, USA

Elias Jabbour
Department of Leukemia, University of Texas M.D. Anderson Cancer Center, Houston, Texas, USA

Hagop M. Kantarjian
Department of Leukemia, University of Texas M.D. Anderson Cancer Center, Houston, Texas, USA

Efstathios Kastritis
Department of Clinical Therapeutics, University of Athens School of Medicine, Athens, Greece

Ghulam Sajjad Khan
St. Vincent's Comprehensive Cancer Center, New York, New York, USA

Kevin T. Kim
Division of Hematology/Oncology, Scripps Clinic, La Jolla, California, USA

Rami S. Komrokji
H. Lee Moffitt Cancer Center and Research Institute, Tampa, Florida, USA

Shaji Kumar
Mayo Clinic College of Medicine, Rochester, Minnesota, USA

Robert A. Kyle
Laboratory Medicine and Pathology, Mayo Clinic College of Medicine, Rochester, Minnesota, USA

Alan List
H. Lee Moffitt Cancer Center and Research Institute, Tampa, Florida, USA

Xin Liu
Penn State Hershey Cancer Institute, Penn State University, Hershey, Pennsylvania, USA

Thomas P. Loughran, Jr.
Penn State Hershey Cancer Institute, Penn State University, Hershey, Pennsylvania, USA

Peter McLaughlin
Department of Lymphoma/Myeloma, University of Texas M.D. Anderson Cancer Center, Houston, Texas, USA

Ruben A. Mesa
Division of Hematology/Oncology, Mayo Clinic, Scottsdale, Arizona, USA

Susan O'Brien
Department of Leukemia, University of Texas M.D. Anderson Cancer Center, Houston, Texas, USA

Eric Padron
Department of Malignant Hematology, H. Lee Moffitt Cancer Center and Research Institute, Tampa, Florida, USA

Ritesh Parajuli
Northwestern University Feinberg School of Medicine, and Robert H. Lurie Comprehensive Cancer Center, Chicago, Illinois, USA

Joseph Pidala
Department of Blood and Marrow Transplantation, H. Lee Moffitt Cancer Center, and University of South Florida, Tampa, Florida, USA

Javier Pinilla-Ibarz
Department of Malignant Hematology, H. Lee Moffitt Cancer Center and Research Institute, Tampa, Florida, USA

Jerald Radich
Fred Hutchinson Cancer Research Center, Seattle, Washington, USA

S. Vincent Rajkumar
Mayo Clinic College of Medicine, Rochester, Minnesota, USA

Azra Raza
Columbia University Medical Center, New York, New York, USA

Hussain I. Saba
James A. Haley Veterans' Hospital, and H. Lee Moffitt Cancer Center and Research Institute, University of South Florida College of Medicine, Tampa, Florida, USA

Elizabeth M. Sagatys
Department of Oncological Sciences and Experimental Therapeutics Program, and Department of Malignant Hematology, H. Lee Moffitt Cancer Center and Research Institute, Tampa, Florida, USA

Alan Saven
Division of Hematology/Oncology, Scripps Clinic, La Jolla, California, USA

Bijal D. Shah
University of South Florida, Tampa, Florida, USA

Kenneth H. Shain
Department of Malignant Hematology, H. Lee Moffitt Cancer Center, Tampa, Florida, USA

Darren S. Sigal
Division of Hematology/Oncology, Scripps Clinic, La Jolla, California, USA

Lubomir Sokol
University of South Florida College of Medicine and Moffitt Cancer Center and Research Institute, Tampa, Florida, USA

Mohamed Sorror
Fred Hutchinson Cancer Research Center and University of Washington, Seattle, Washington, USA

Eduardo M. Sotomayor
Department of Oncological Sciences and Experimental Therapeutics Program, and Department of Malignant Hematology, H. Lee Moffitt Cancer Center and Research Institute, Tampa, Florida, USA

Jamie Stratton
St. Vincent's Comprehensive Cancer Center, New York, New York, USA

Jonathan C. Strefford
Cancer Genomics Group, Cancer Sciences Division, University of Southampton, Southampton, UK

Martin S. Tallman
Northwestern University Feinberg School of Medicine, and Robert H. Lurie Comprehensive Cancer Center, Chicago, Illinois, USA

Jianguo Tao
Department of Oncological Sciences and Experimental Therapeutics Program, and Department of Malignant Hematology, H. Lee Moffitt Cancer Center and Research Institute, Tampa, Florida, USA

Ayalew Tefferi
Department of Hematology, Mayo Clinic College of Medicine, Rochester, Minnesota, USA

Sylvain Thépot
Service d'hématologie clinique, Hôpital Avicenne (Assistance Publique –Hôpitaux de Paris) and Paris 13 University, Bobigny, France

Deborah Thomas
University of Texas M.D. Anderson Cancer Center, Houston, Texas, USA

Kenneth S. Zuckerman
H. Lee Moffitt Cancer Center, and University of South Florida, Tampa, Florida, USA

Acknowledgement

The editors are grateful to Ms. Genevieve A. Morelli for her excellent help and energy in coordinating all the contributors in the development and assembly of this book. Her many organizational skills and tireless efforts in contacting, proofing and coordinating the work of the authors, editors, and publishers of the two subcontinents of Europe and America have been remarkable. The editors greatly appreciate her efforts.

Preface

In the last decade, there has been a remarkable explosion of scientific knowledge in many areas of hematological malignancies. This information has led to many new insights in the understanding of the pathobiology of malignant hematological diseases. New knowledge of cellular disease processes, molecular pathology, and cytogenetic, epigenetic, and genomic changes have impacted our current outlook toward hematological malignancies. There was a time when the practicing hematologist could not offer anything but a few symptomatic treatments for malignant disease states. Now, treatment attempts are being offered to attack and eradicate at their molecular level. This, in some instances, has led us to achieve a near cure and, perhaps a complete cure in the near future, for some of the malignant hematological malignancies.

The recent and ongoing expansion of knowledge in this area has become extensive and dynamic. Important aspects of this information are spread and scattered over the Internet and research publications. It is our belief that much of this important information is not utilized to its full capacity due to diffuse distribution. This has led to the need to capture and compile new and current information about hematologic malignancies in the form of a comprehensive book. *Advances in Malignant Hematology* is the result of our efforts to fulfill this need.

The editors have been able to involve the experts of the American and European continents, and have them share their current thoughts and knowledge about the pathobiology of malignant hematological diseases of the blood, as well as their view on current treatment strategies and future developments in the area of these hematological diseases. It is our hope that this book proves helpful in the battle against hematologic cancer.

We understand that current scientific knowledge is dynamic and constantly changing. What is new information today may well be obsolete tomorrow. This publication presents what is current in this area today. In order to keep up with the evolutionary changes and developing knowledge that will, hopefully, lead to future cures, the editors and publisher have agreed to consider updating this book every three years or sooner. The editors are indebted for the cooperation they have received from all of the expert contributors to this work, and wish to express their deepest appreciation for their dedication to the advancement of science in the area of hematological cancer.

Hussain I. Saba and Ghulam J. Mufti
Tampa and London

List of Main Abbreviations

Chapter 1

AML	acute myeloid leukemia
APC	adenomatous polyposis coli
AGM	aorta-gonad-mesonephros
BMPR1A	bone morphogenic protein receptor type 1A
BFU-Mk	burst forming unit-megakaryocytic
BFU-E	burst forming unit-erythroid
CFU	colony forming units
CFU-GEMM	colony forming unit-granulocyte, erythroid, macrophage, megakaryocyte
CFU-S	megakaryocytic cells
CLCF	cardiotrophin-like cytokine factor
CLP	common lymphoid progenitor
CMP	common myeloid progenitor
CNTF	ciliary neurotrophic factor
CSF	colony-stimulating factor
DC	dendritic cells
EBF	Early B-cell factor
ECM	extracellular matrix
EDCP	early DC progenitors
EHZF	early hematopoietic zinc finger
EPO	erythropoietin
FACS	fluorescence activated cell sorting
Flt3	FMS-like tyrosine kinase 3 receptor
G-CSF	granulocyte-CSF
GH	growth hormone
GM-CSF	granulocyte-macrophage-CSF
GMP	granulocyte-monocyte progenitors
HSC	hematopoietic stem cell
IFN	interferon
Ig	immunoglobulin
IL	interleukin
LEF	lymphocyte enhancer binding factor
LIC	leukemia initiating cells
LIF	leukemia inhibitory factor
LT-HSC	long-term hematopoietic stem cell
M-CSF; CSFS-1	macrophage-CSF
MDP	macrophage dendritic cell progenitor
MEP	megakaryocyte-erythroid progenitors
miRNA	microRNA
MPP	multipotent progenitor
mRNA	messenger RNA
NK	natural killer (cells)
PI3K	phosphatidylinositol-3 kinase
PRL	prolactin
RARα	retinoic acid receptor alpha
RBCs	red blood cells
SCF	stem cell factor
SCID	severe combined immunodeficiency
SF	steel factor
ST-HSC	short-term hematopoietic stem cell
TCFTPO	T-cell factor thrombopoietin
TGFβ	tumor growth factor-β
TNFα	tumor necrosis factor-α

Chapter 2

AID	activation-induced cytidine deaminase
ALL	acute lymphoblastic leukemia
ATRA	all-trans retinoic acid
CML	chronic myeloid leukemia

DNA	deoxyribonucleic acid		**AP**	accelerated phase
DSB	double-stranded breakage		**BP**	blast phase
FISH	fluorescence in situ hybridization		**CP**	chronic phase
PCG	protein coding genes		**EFS**	event-free survival
PDGFR	platelet-derived growth factor receptor		**EMA**	European Medicines Agency
			MMR	major molecular response
Ph	Philadelphia chromosome		**OS**	overall survival
RXR	retinoid X receptor		**PFS**	progression-free survival
UPD	uniparental disomy		**SCT**	stem cell transplantation
			START	SRC/ABL Tyrosine kinase inhibition Activity Research Trials of dasatinib (START)-C trial
Chapter 3			**TFS**	transformation-free survival
			TOPS	Tyrosine kinase inhibitor OPtimization and Selectivity trial
EMH	extramedullary hematopoiesis			
IFN-α	interferon-alpha			
IMiDs	immunomodulatory inhibitory drugs			
IWG-MRT	International Working Group for Myelofibrosis Research and Treatment		**Chapter 6**	
			ATRA	all-trans retinoic acid
MDS	myelodysplastic syndromes		**CBF**	xore binding factor
MPNs	myeloproliferative neoplasms		**CDKs**	cyclin-dependent kinases
Pegasys	pegylated interferon-2a		**CLC**	committed leukemia cell
PEG-IFN-α	pegylated interferon alpha		**FISH**	fluorescence in situ hybridization
PEG-Intron	pegylated (PEG)-IFN-α-2b		**GAP**	GTPase activating proteins
			GEP	gene expression profile
Chapter 4			**HATs**	histone acetylases
			HDAC	histone deacetylases
BCR	breakpoint cluster region		**HSC**	hematopoietic stem cell
(BP)-CML	blast phase CML		**ITD**	internal tandem duplication
CEBP-alpha	CCAAT/enhancer-binding protein-alpha		**JAK/STAT**	Janus kinase-signal transducer and activator of transcription
(CP)-CML	chronic phase CML		**LPC**	leukemia progenitor cells
FDA	(USA) Food and Drug Administration		**LSC**	leukemia stem cell
GMP	granulocyte-macrophage progenitor cells		**MAPK**	mitogen-activating protein kinases
IRIS	International Randomized Study of Interferon and STI571 trial		**MLL**	Mixed lineage leukemia gene
			NBs	nuclear bodies
LSCs	leukemic stem cells		**RING**	really interesting gene
NHEJ	non-homologous end joining			
ROS	reactive oxygen species		**Chapter 7**	
TKI	tyrosine kinase inhibitors		**APL**	acute promyelocytic leukemia
			ATO	arsenic trioxide
Chapter 5			**ALSG**	Australian Leukemia Study Group
AEs	adverse events		**ATRA**	all-trans retinoic acid

CALGB	Cancer and Leukemia Group B
CR	complete remission
CRp	all criteria for CR except incomplete recovery of platelets
ECOG	Eastern Cooperative Oncology Group
ENT1	equilibrative nucleoside transporter 1
GO	Gemtuzumab ozogamicin
GVHD	graft-versus-host disease
GVL	graft-versus-leukemic
HiDAC	high-dose cytarabine
HOVON	Dutch-Belgian Hemato-Oncology Cooperative Group
HSCT	hematopoietic stem cell transplantation
MDS	myelodysplastic syndrome
MPN	myeloproliferative neoplasm
(UK) MRC	Medical Research Council in the United Kingdom
MRD	minimal residual disease
MSD	matched sibling donor
MUD	matched unrelated donor
NCI	National Cancer Institute
SEER	Surveillance, Epidemiology, and End Results [Program of the NCI]
SWOG	Southwest Oncology Group
TRM	transplant-related mortality
WBC	white blood cell count

Chapter 8

ARDS	adult respiratory distress syndrome
ATRA	all-trans retinoic acid
BM	bone marrow
CoR	co-repressor complex
CIR	cumulative incidence of relapse
DIC	disseminated intravascular coagulation
FDP	fibrinogen-fibrin degradation products
GO	gemtuzumab ozogamycin
HAT	histone acetyltransferase
HDAC	histone deacetylase
LAS	leukocyte activation syndrome

MRD	minimal residual disease
NPM	nucleophosmin
NuMA	nuclear matrix associated
NUMA	nuclear mitotic apparatus
PB	peripheral blood
PML	promyelocytic leukemia gene
PLZF	promyelocytic leukemia zinc finger
RARE	response elements
RXR	retinoid X receptor
STAT5B	signal transducer and activator of transcription 5B
STC	stem cell transplantation
TNF	tumor necrosis factor

Chapter 9

SBDS	Shwachman-Bodian-Diamond syndrome gene
TNFα	tumor necrosis factor alpha

Chapter 10

AA	aplastic anemia
aCML	atypical chronic myelogenous leukemia
ANC	absolute neutophil count
AR	Auer rods
BSC	best supportive care
CMML	chronic myelomonocytic leukemia
ESA	erythroid stimulating agents
IPSS	International Prognostic Scoring System
ITP	immune thrombocytopenic purpura (or: idiopathic thrombocytopenic purpura c.11)
ITT	intention to treat
IWG	International Working Group
JMML	juvenile myelomonocytic leukemia
MGFs	myeloid growth factors
ORR	overall response rates
PNH	paroxysmal nocturnal hemaglobinuria
PR	partial remission
pRBCs	packed red blood cells

QOL	quality of life		**(J)**	joining
RA	refractory anemia		**KIRs**	killer-immunoglobulin-like receptors
RARS	RA with ringed sideroblasts			
RAEB	Refractory Anemia with Excess Blasts		**MAPK**	mitogen-activated protein kinase
RAEB-T	Refractory Anemia with Excess Blasts in Transformation		**PBMNC**	peripheral blood mononuclear cellS
RCUD	Refractory Anemia with Unilineage Dysplasia		**SNPs**	single nucleotide polymorphisms
RN	refractory neutropenia		**TFS**	treatment-free survival
RT	refractory thrombocytopenia		**(V)**	variable
shRNA	short hairpin RNA			
SPARC	secretion protein acidic cysteine-rich		**Chapter 13**	
TI	transfusion independence		**AHA**	autoimmune hemolytic anemia
t-MDS	treatment-related MDS		**BCR**	B-cell receptor
			CT	computerized tomography
Chapter 11			**del 11q**	deletion 11q (etc.)
			IWCLL	International Workshop on CLL
DNMT	DNA methyl-transferases		***IGHV***	immunoglobulin heavy chain variable (NB: italicized)
G-CSF	granulocyte colony-stimulating factor		**LDT**	lymphocyte doubling time
ITP	idiopathic thrombocytopenic purpura		**MBL**	monoclonal B-cell Lymphocytosis
PEG-rHuMGDF	pegylated recombinant megakaryocyte growth and development factor		***p53***	italicized gene
			QALY	quality-adjusted-life-year
rhEPO	recombinant erythropoietin		**SNP**	single nucleotide polymorphisms
rHuTPO	recombinant human thrombopoietin		**TK**	thymidine kinase
SQ	subcutaneous		**US**	ultrasound
TI	transfusion independent/ence			
			Chapter 14	
Chapter 12			**CSF**	cerebrospinal fluid
CDR3	complementarity determining region 3		**HAART**	highly active antiretroviral treatment
(D)	diversity		**GMALL**	German Multicenter Study Group for Adult Acute Lymphoblastic Leukemia
DISC	death-inducing signaling complex			
FCR	fludarabine, cyclophosphamide, and rituxumab		**GOELAMS**	Groupe Ouest-Est d'Etude des Leucémies et Autres Maladies du Sang
GC	germinal center		**PCR**	polymerase chain reaction
Ig	immunoglobulin		**sIg**	surface immunoglobulin
IgHV	immunoglobulin heavy chain variable		**TdT**	terminal deoxynucleotidyl transferase
ITAMs	immunoreceptor tyrosine-based activation motifs		**TCR**	T-cell receptor
			XRT	irradiation

Chapter 15

EBV	Epstein-Barr virus
HTLV-II	human T-cell leukemia virus
KIRs	killer cell immunoglobulin-like receptors
MHC	major histocompatibility complex
PAH	pulmonary artery hypertension
PCR	polymerase chain reaction
PRCA	pure red cell aplasia
PNH	paroxysmal nocturnal hemoglobinuria
XCIP	X-chromosome inactivation pattern

Chapter 16

ADA	adenosine deaminase
CR	complete remission
CHR	complete hematologic remission
FC	flow cytometry
IHC	immunohistochemistry
IFN	interferon alpha
PCA-1	plasma cell-associated antigen
PCR	polymerase chain reaction
PLL	prolymphocytic leukemia
SLVL	Sslenic lymphoma with villous lymphocytes
SCID	severe combined immunodeficiency disorder
TRAP	tartarate-resistant acid phosphatase

Chapter 17

AID	activation-induced cytosine deaminase
ATR	ataxia telangiectasia and Rad3-related genes
B-ALL	B-acute lymphoblastic leukemia
BLIMP1	B-lymphocyte-induced maturation protein 1
CDR	complementary-determining regions
DLBCL	diffuse large B-cell lymphomas
EBB	extrafollicular B-blast
Ig	immunoglobulin

IgH	immunoglobulin heavy chain
MCL	mantle cell lymphoma
SHM	somatic hypermutation
XBP1	X-box binding protein 1

Chapter 18

ABC	activated B-cell
AITL	angioimmunoblastic T-cell lymphoma
ALCL	anaplastic large cell lymphoma
ALK	anaplastic lymphoma kinase
ATLL	adult T-cell leukemia/lymphoma
BL	Burkitt's lymphoma
CLL	chronic lymphocytic leukemia
DLBCL	diffuse large B-cell lymphomas
EFS	event-free survival
FDC	follicular dendritic cells
FISH	fluorescence in situ hybridization
FL	follicular lymphoma
FLIPI	The Follicular Lymphoma International Prognostic Index
GEP	gene expression profiling
HAART	highly active antiretroviral therapy
HL	Hodgkin lymphoma
HSCT	hematopoietic stem cell transplant
IgH	immunoglobulin heavy chain
IMiDs	immunomodulatory drugs
IPI	International Prognostic Index
MCL	mantle cell lymphoma
MF	mycosis fungoides
MALT	mucosa-associated lymphoid tissue
MZL	marginal zone B-cell lymphomas
NHL	non-Hodgkin lymphoma
NOS	not otherwise specified
PCR	polymerase chain reaction
PKC	protein kinase C
PTCL	peripheral T-cell lymphoma
PMLBCL	primary mediastinal large B-cell lymphoma

REAL	Revised European-American Lymphoma (scheme)
RIT	radioimmunotherapy
RT	radiation therapy
SLL	small lymphocytic lymphoma
TBI	total body irradiation
T-LBL	T-lymphoblastic leukemia/ lymphoma
TTF	time to treatment failure
WF	Working Formulation

Chapter 19

CMT	combined modality therapy
EFRT	extended-field radiotherapy
EORTC	European Organization for Research and Treatment of Cancer
Esc	escalated
FDG-PET	fluorodeoxyglucose positron emission tomography
FFTF	freedom from treatment failure
FF2F	freedom from/free of second treatment failure
GELA	Groupe d'Etude des Lymphomes de l'Adulte
GHSG	German Hodgkin Study Group
GISL	Intergruppo Italiano Linfomi
IFRT	involved field radiotherapy
INRT	involved nodal radiation
MOPP	MOPP regimen (mechlorethamine, vincristine, procarbazine, prednisone
mTOR	mammalian target of rapamycin
PR	partial response
SEER	Surveillance Epidemiology and End Results (program)
STNI	subtotal nodal (or "extended field") radiation
TRM	treatment-related mortality

Chapter 20

BMT	bone marrow transplant
CCT	conventional chemotherapy
DVT	deep vein thrombosis
MGUS	monoclonal gammopathy of undetermined significance

MM	multiple myeloma
HGF	hepatocyte growth factor
IGF-1	insulin like growth factor
ONJ	osteonecrosis of the jaw
RIC	reduced-intensity conditioning
ROTI	related organ or tissue impairment
SDF	stromal dependent growth factor
SMM	smoldering myeloma
TBI	total body irradiation
TTP	time to progression
TWiST	time without symptoms, treatment, and toxicity
VEGF	vascular endothelial growth factor
VGPR	very good partial response

Chapter 21

AL amyloidosis	amyloidosis of AL type (primary)
anti-MAG	anti-myelin associated glycoprotein
CAP	cyclophosphamide, doxorubicin (adriamycin), and prednisone
CHOP	cyclophosphamide, doxorubicin, vincristine, and prednisone
CLL	chronic lymphocytic leukemia
IgM	immunoglobulin M
IPSS WM	International Prognostic Staging System for WM
LDH	lactate dehydrogenase
LPL	lymphoplasmacytic lymphoma
MGUS	monoclonal gammopathy of unknown significance
MM	multiple myeloma
SWM	smoldering WM
WM	Waldenström's macroglobulinemia

Chapter 22

AA	amyloid A
AL amyloidosis	primary systemic amyloidosis (AL)
CHF	congestive heart failure
ESRD	end-stage renal disease
FLC	free light chain

HDM-ASCT	high-dose melphalan with autologous stem cell transplantation
IFE	immunofixation electrophoresis
LCDD	light chain deposition disease
MDex	melphalan with dexamethasone
MP	melphalan with prednisone
SAP	serum amyloid P

Chapter 23

aGVHD	acute graft- versus.- host disease
AML	acute myelogenous leukemia
ATG	antithymocyte globulin
BMSC	bone marrow stem cells
BMT CTN	Blood and Marrow Transplant Clinical Trials Network
BU	busulfan
cGVHD	chronic graft-versus-host disease
CIBMTR	Center for International Blood and Marrow Transplant Research
CML	chronic myelogenous leukemia
CMV	cytomegalovirus
CR1	first complete remission
CSA	cyclosporine
CY	cyclophosphamide
DLI	donor lymphocyte infusion
FLU	fludarabine
HLA	human leukocyte antigen
IS	*immunosuppressive treatment*
MCL	*mantle cell lymphoma*
MDS	myelodysplastic syndrome
MEL	melphalan
MHC	major histocompatibility complex
MM	multiple myeloma
MMF	mycophenolate mofetil
MTX	methotrexate
NIH	National Institutes of Health (USA)
NMDP	National Marrow Donor Program (USA)

NRM	non-relapse mortality
PBSC	peripheral blood stem cells
PCR	polymerase chain reaction
QOL	quality of life
RIC	reduced-intensity conditioning
SIR	sirolimus
TAC	tacrolimus
TBI	total body irradiation
Tregs	regulatory T-cells
VGPR	very good partial response
ZAP-70	zeta-associated protein 70

Chapter 24

BSFI	Brief Sexual Function Inventory
CF	chronic fatigue
EF	executive function
EORTC	European Organization for Research and Treatment of Cancer
EWB	emotional well-being
FACIT	Functional Assessment of Chronic Illness Therapy
FLIC	Functional Living Index – Cancer
GELA	Groupe d'Études des Lymphomes de l'Adulte
IFN + LDAC	interferon alfa plus subcutaneous low-dose cytarabine
HM	hematological malignancies
LH	luteinizing hormone
MFI-20	Multidimensional Fatigue Inventory
NHP	Nottingham Health Profile
SF12	Medical Outcomes Study Short Form 12
SF-36	Short Form-36
SFWB	social and family well-being
SIP	Sickness Impact Profile
TF	total fatigue
TOI	trial outcome index

PART 1
Hematopoiesis

CHAPTER 1

Normal and Malignant Hematopoiesis

Bijal D. Shah[1] and Kenneth S. Zuckerman[1,2]
[1]University of South Florida, Tampa, Florida, USA
[2]H. Lee Moffitt Cancer Center, Tampa, FL, USA

Introduction

Hematopoiesis, simply stated, describes the regulated process of hematopoietic stem cell (HSC) self-renewal and differentiation into lineage committed progeny. Pluripotent HSC are rare cells (<1 of 10 000 bone marrow cells) specifically characterized by their proliferative capacity (though under steady state conditions >95% of HSC are quiescent, nondividing cells at any one time), pluripotency (they can regenerate the entire spectrum of mature blood derived cells), and self-renewal. The hierarchy of hematopoietic cell differentiation is depicted in Figure 1.1. HSC reside in close association with hematopoietic stromal cells within specific micro-environmental niches that function in concert with a variety of both multilineage and single lineage-specific hematopoietic growth factors, stromal cells, and extracellular matrix molecules to regulate their survival, cell cycle progression, proliferation, and differentiation. These processes of self-renewal, proliferation, differentiation, and cell death are tightly regulated under normal conditions throughout life. A normal individual maintains steady state numbers of blood cells within a very tight range with no more than a few percent variation from day-to-day, with constant production of the number of new cells required to replace the number of senescent cells that die. On average erythrocytes survive in the circulation for about 120 days, platelets for about 10 days, and neutrophils for about 6–12 hours. In order to replace senescent blood cells, the bone marrow of normal adult humans must produce about 180–250 billion erythrocytes, 60–100 billion neutrophils, and 80–150 billion platelets every day, or about 10^{16} (10 quadrillion) blood cells in a lifetime, with only minimal reduction in the bone marrow cell production capacity as a result of aging. The bone marrow can respond rapidly, in lineage-specific manner, to increase production of new blood cells by 6- to 8-fold over baseline under conditions of demand for each specific type of blood cells, such as *in vivo* destruction of erythrocytes, platelets, or neutrophils, infections requiring increased neutrophil production, and hemorrhage requiring increased erythrocyte production. Regulation of lymphocyte numbers is much less clearly understood, although it is known that some types of T and B lymphocytes may survive for many years. An understanding of these normal regulatory components in normal hematopoiesis is essential to unraveling the mechanisms that drive malignancy.

Isolation of hematopoietic progenitors

In 1961, Till and McCulloch isolated single cell-derived colonies of myeloid, erythroid, and mega-karyocytic cells (CFU-S) from the spleens of lethally irradiated mice 1–2 weeks after rescue by bone marrow transplantation [1]. These colonies were

Advances in Malignant Hematology, First Edition. Edited by Hussain I. Saba and Ghulam J. Mufti. © 2011 Blackwell Publishing Ltd.
Published 2011 by Blackwell Publishing Ltd.

(A)

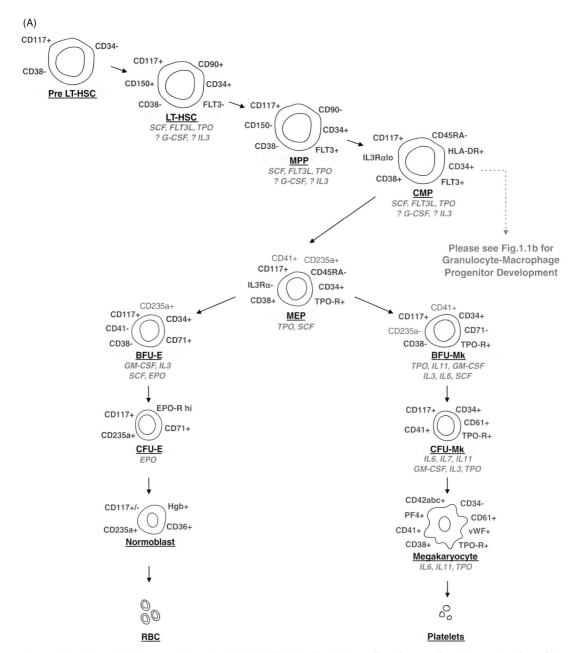

Figure 1.1 Schematic diagram of hematopoiesis highlighting identifying cell surface markers (in gray) and cytokines affecting each stage of hematopoietic differentiation (in italic). (A) Differentiation from hematopoietic stem cells through erythrocytes and megakaryocytes/platelets. (B) Differentiation from hematopoietic stem cells through granulocytes and monocytes/macrophages. (C) Differentiation from hematopoietic stem cells through lymphocytes.

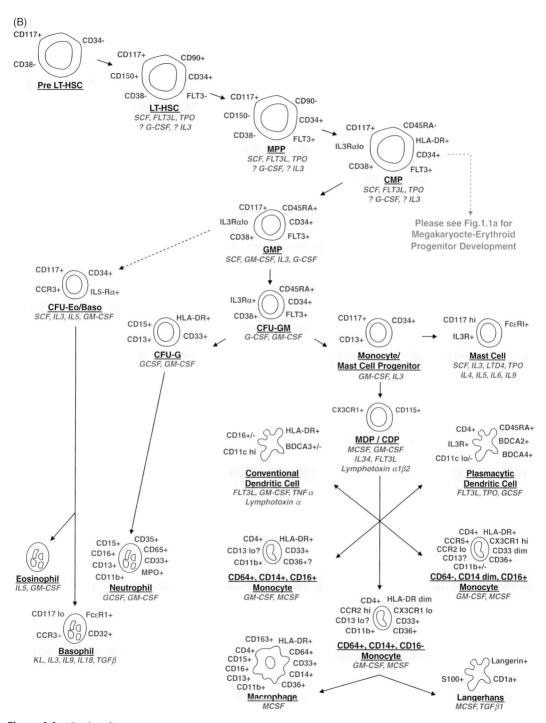

Figure 1.1   *(Continued)*

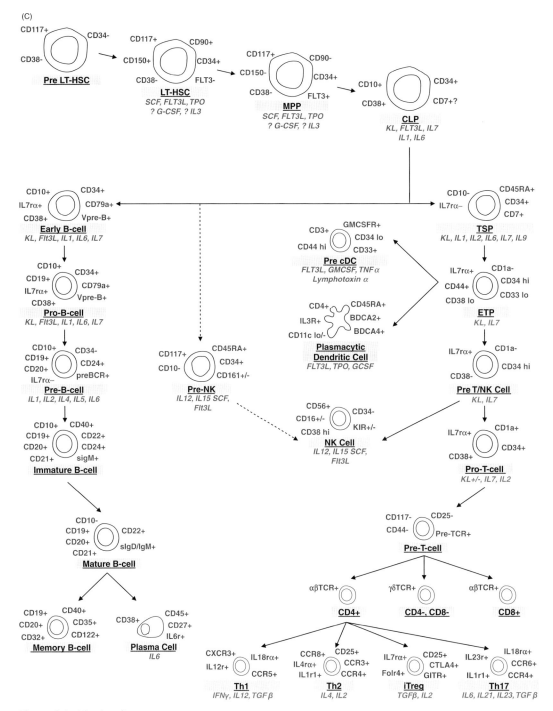

Figure 1.1 *(Continued)*

capable of extensive proliferation *in vivo*, exhibited some potential for self-renewal and, for the first time, conclusively demonstrated the presence of a multipotent hematopoietic progenitor cell. However, the lack of lymphoid colony development, as well as experiments in which 5-fluoruracil killed CFU-S without killing cells capable of replenishing CFU-S suggested that a more primitive "pre-CFU-S" must exist [2].

These data were further refined with the advent of flow cytometry, fluorescence activated cell sorting (FACS), *in vitro* hematopoietic progenitor cell systems, and xenotransplantation models, which revealed that long-term bone marrow repopulating HSCs were distinct from CFU cells, or multipotent progenitors (MPPs), and could be further subdivided into cells with short-term (ST-HSC) and long-term (LT-HSC) hematopoietic stem cell repopulation capacity. Specifically, LT-HSCs are defined by their extensive self-renewal capacity, allowing for full reconstitution of an irradiated host following transplantation of these cells. ST-HSCs, alternatively, have less capacity for self-renewal and instead more avidly differentiate into more committed MPPs. As such, ST-HSCs provide short-term hematopoietic cell reconstitution, but are incapable of permanently rescuing humans or other mammals with an aplastic bone marrow after lethal ionizing radiation.

Although some controversy exists, the most widely accepted model suggests that hematopoietic lineage commitment is both a stochastic and instructive process that occurs at specific branchpoints, manifested at the time of cell division. During cell division, HSCs can either divide asymmetrically (a maintenance event with the production of one identical immature daughter cell and one differentiating daughter cell), symmetrically (an expansion/self-renewal event which serves to generate two identically immature daughter cells (self-renewal)), or terminally differentiate (an extinction event, in which both daughter cells are committed to terminal differentiation). The hierarchy of differentiation from HSC to mature end-stage hematopoietic cells is shown in Figure 1.1. As cells progressively differentiate into functional components of the hematopoietic system, they lose proliferative and multilineage differentiation capacity. Regulation of self-renewal, cell cycling, terminal differentiation, and apoptosis is therefore critically important to maintaining the production of hematopoietic elements over a lifetime. It is now clear that extrinsic and intrinsic systems act in concert to generate a network of events that govern HSC fate.

Cytokine regulation

Cytokines/growth factors include interleukins, lymphokines, monokines, interferons, chemokines, colony-stimulating factors (CSFs), and other hematopoietic hormones. These secreted factors interact with receptors on both pluripotent stem cells and committed hematopoietic progenitor cells to affect their survival, proliferation, and differentiation. The stages of differentiation from pluripotent HSC to fully mature hematopoietic cells of all lineages and the growth factors that play roles in these differentiation events are shown in Figure 1.1. Kit-ligand (also known as stem cell factor (SCF), and Steel factor (SF)) and Flt3 ligand, which function to drive proliferation by binding to the Kit and Flt3 tyrosine kinase receptors, respectively, on $CD34^+CD38^-$ progenitors are important regulators of the early stages of hematopoietic differentiation from HSC. SCF, in particular, cooperates with multiple cytokines and cytokine receptors to influence differentiation, as well as upregulating BCL-2, BCL-X_L, and perhaps other antiapoptotic molecules to promote target cell survival. These receptors are downregulated during normal differentiation. Colony-stimulating factors, including erythropoietin (EPO), thrombopoietin (TPO), granulocyte-macrophage-CSF (GM-CSF), granulocyte-CSF (G-CSF), and macrophage-CSF (M-CSF; CSF-1), induce the differentiation and function of specific hematopoietic cell lineages. These factors accordingly are named for the lineages that they predominantly stimulate, although several also have effects on multipotent hematopoietic progenitors and perhaps even on pluripotent HSC. Alternatively, TGFβ (tumor growth factor-β), TNFα (tumor necrosis factor-α), and IFNs (interferons) all tend to negatively influence hematopoiesis.

Table 1.1 Cytokine receptor families

Type I Cytokine receptors	
Homodimerizing receptors	G-CSF-R, EPO-R, TPO-R
Heterodimerizing receptors	
gp130 receptor family	IL6-Rα, LIF-Rβ, IL11-Rα, Oncostatin M-Rα, CNTF-Rα, CLCF-R
β$_C$ (Common β receptor) receptor family	GM-CSFRα, IL3-Rα, IL5-Rα
IL2-R family (γ chain) receptor family	IL4-Rα, IL7-Rα, IL9-Rα, IL13-Rα, IL15-Rα, IL21-Rα
Type II Cytokine receptors (interferon family)	IFNα-R, IFNγ-R1/2, IL10-R1/2
Receptors with intrinsic tyrosine kinase activity	Flt3, c-Kit

G: granulocyte; CSF: colony-stimulating factor; R: receptor; EPO: erythropoietin; TPO: thrombopoietin; IL: interleukin; LIF: leukemia inhibitory factor; CNTF: ciliary neurotrophic factor; CLCF: cardiotrophin-like cytokine factor; GM: granulocyte-macrophage; IFN: interferon.

Although cytokine-receptor interactions would appear to generate a level of specificity with regards to transcriptional and genomic regulation and, hence, lineage-specific cell differentiation, the convergence of similar molecular pathways upon genomic targets makes it difficult to delineate this. What can be said, however, is that cytokine receptors appear to fall into specific families based upon their signal transducing subunits (see Table 1.1), and that these signaling subunits rely on three major pathways to ultimately influence transcription. These pathways include the JAK-STAT pathway, the MAPK pathway, and the PI3/AKT pathways, although other pathways involving NF-κB, TGF/ SMAD, and protein kinase C pathways also play roles in the regulation of hematopoiesis. Importantly, mutations that affect these pathways are well described in lymphomas, myeloproliferative neoplasms, and leukemias [3–6].

Mechanistically, growth factors and cytokines act as ligands for transmembrane receptors that are located on the surface of hematopoietic cells, with differing receptor expression on HSC, multipotent progenitors, single lineage precursors and mature hematopoietic cells of different lineages. Dimerization (or conformational change) of receptors occurs following ligand binding. This receptor dimerization and conformational change leads to autophosphorylation of the intracellular portion of the receptors and recruitment of signaling molecules to docking sites on the activated receptors. This leads, in turn, to recruitment, phosphorylation, and activation of a broad range of cytoplasmic effector signaling molecules, such as STATs, Src-kinases, protein phosphatases, Shc, Grb2, IRS1/2 and PI3K via binding at the conserved SH2 domains and phosphorylation sites on the receptors themselves. For example, phosphorylation of STATs leads to the generation of STAT homo- and heterodimers, which are then translocated to the nucleus, where they can bind specific nucleotide sequences in the regulatory regions of specific genes to influence transcription of those genes, which determines the proliferation, survival, differentiation, and function of those cells. Similarly, phosphorylation of Grb2 facilitates the activation of SOS, which in turn, influences transcription via activation of the Ras/Raf/Mek/Erk, and the Rho/Mlk-Mekk/Mek/ p38-JNK pathways. Activation of phosphatidylinositol-3 kinase (PI3K), either directly or indirectly via RAS or IRS 1 and 2, generates PIP3, which in turn activates PKC, SGK, RAC1/CDC42 and AKT. Activation of AKT is particularly relevant to both normal and malignant hematopoiesis, as it can phosphorylate multiple transcription factors, leading to activation of mTOR, MDM2, and NFκB and inhibition GSK3β, FKHR, and BAD. Notably, multiple related proteins and isoforms of many of the signal transduction molecules exist (including JAK, STAT, Mek, Mlk, Mekk, Erk, p38, JNK, PI3K, PIP3, and AKT), and appear to have different nuclear targets depending on the cell type in which activation occurs [3–5].

Transcriptional regulation

Transcription factors are proteins that interact with the regulatory region of genes, either alone or in protein complexes, to increase or decrease expression of genes that contain specific sequences of nucleotides in these regulatory regions, which are recognized by the specific transcription factors. Transcriptional networks play a central role in the intrinsic regulation of HSC and lineage-committed progenitor cell survival, proliferation, and differentiation. Accordingly, these pathways are commonly perturbed in hematopoietic malignancies. Unfortunately, our knowledge in many cases is limited to non-human and *in vitro* models, which may not accurately reflect human hematopoiesis. Nonetheless, these experimental approaches have helped to define several important concepts in transcriptional regulation, including timing, autonomous and antagonistic pathways, cofactor regulation, and cellular signaling-related changes to transcription factor activity/function. A summary of relevant transcription factors thought to be involved in varying steps in the hematopoietic differentiation pathways is provided in Figure 1.2 and the transcriptional regulatory factors involved in each of the specific lineages of hematopoietic differentiation are described in more detail in the sections below on each of those lineages.

MicroRNA regulation

MicroRNAs (miRNA) have been recently implicated in the control of gene expression in hematopoiesis (Figure 1.2). miRNAs are small non-coding RNAs that bind to the 3′-untranslated regions and destabilize messenger RNAs (mRNAs) leading to their rapid degradation or, less commonly, may bind to the coding region of targeted genes and inhibit transcription of those genes. To date over 700 miRNAs have been identified in humans, with over 33% of human genes identified as potential targets of these miRNAs, based on identification of sequences in those genes that are reverse complements of specific miRNAs. A thorough review of the involvement of miRNAs in hematopoiesis is beyond the scope of this review; however, interested readers are referred to several recent reviews highlighting the importance of miRNA in both normal and malignant hematopoiesis [7–11].

Hematopoietic microenvironment

HSCs are most likely generated independently in the yolk sac and aorta-gonad-mesonephros (AGM) region in the developing embryo, after which they migrate to the placenta, attaching via VE-cadherin, and subsequently to the liver and spleen via β1 integrin-dependent interactions with the extracellular matrix (ECM). Mesenchymal cell development in the liver and spleen creates a unique microenvironment that fosters HSC survival and expansion. During most of human fetal development the liver is the primary source of hematopoietic cell production, with erythrocyte production predominating, and the spleen contributes a small proportion of fetal hematopoiesis. Shortly before birth, HSCs migrate to the bone marrow, presumably under the influence of CXCL12/CXCR4, c-Kit/SCF, CD44/hyaluronic acid, and α4β1 integrin (VLA-4)/ECM and stromal cell interactions. At that point, hepatic and splenic hematopoiesis virtually ceases, and essentially all subsequent human hematopoietic cell production is restricted to the bone marrow. It is now well accepted that stem cells routinely circulate into and out of the bone marrow niche throughout life, although the purpose of circulating hematopoietic stem and progenitor cells is not known. The same molecules that are involved in movement of HSCs to the bone marrow during development appear to play similar roles in HSC homing and marrow engraftment throughout adulthood. Curiously, in adults, CD44 is fucosylated, converting it to an E-selectin ligand, and accordingly facilitates binding and retention by bone marrow endothelial cells [12, 13]. CD44/hyaluronic acid and CD44/E-selectin interactions, which serve redundant roles in normal stem cell homing and engraftment, also have been found to be required for both human CML and

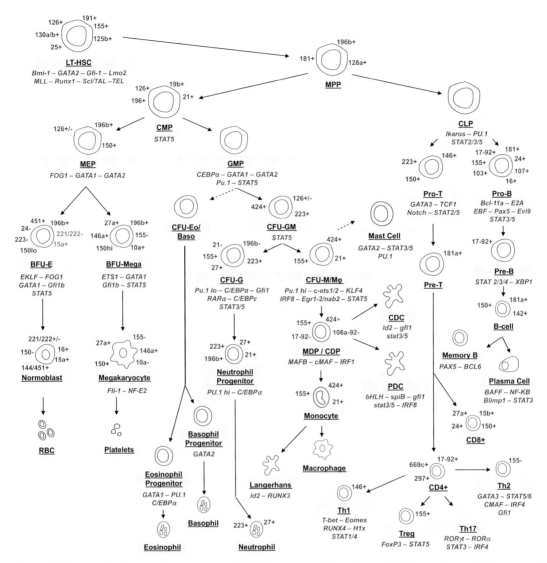

Figure 1.2 Schematic diagram of hematopoiesis highlighting transcription factors (in italic) and microRNAs (in gray) that are active at each of the stages of hematopoietic differentiation.

AML leukemia cell growth in mouse xenograft models [14, 15].

HSC and early hematopoietic progenitors tend to predominantly lodge into endosteal niches near N-cadherin-expressing osteoblasts, where they tend to remain quiescent, perhaps under the influence of osteoblast-secreted Angiopoietin-1, active at HSC TIE2 receptors. Increasing the osteoblast population via conditional inactivation of bone morphogenic protein receptor type 1A (BMPR1A)

or administration of PTH leads to an increase in the number of HSCs in the marrow. PTH also increases CXCL12 expression by osteoblasts, and indeed CXCR4 appears to retain its importance in HSC repopulation even after homing. SCF and extracellular calcium-ion concentration (sensed via the calcium receptor, CaR) also may play a role in localization to the endosteum (reviewed in [12]).

Interestingly, a separate population of HSCs is also found adjacent to endothelial cells, where

N-cadherin expression is lower. Endothelial inter-actions likely play a role in HSC retention and egress, and may also facilitate HSC expansion and differentiation. For example, Tie2 is also expressed on endothelial cells, and blocking of this receptor impairs neoangiogenesis and delays hematopoiesis following myelosuppression. Angiopoietin-1, conversely, can rescue hematopoiesis in TPO-defi-cient mice [16]. Together these data suggest that two pools of HSCs may exist, a quiescent fraction adjacent to osteoblasts in the endosteal niche, and a more rapidly proliferating and differentiating fraction adjacent to blood vessels.

Adhesive interactions via osteopontin/CD44 and β1 integrins, N-cadherin, c-Kit/SCF, CXCL12/CXCR4, Jagged1/Notch and TIE2/Angiopoietin-1 all play roles in maintenance of the bone marrow niche and in HSC quiescence. These adhesive inter-actions are commonly altered in hematologic malignancies. Increased expression appears to con-fer a more aggressive and more drug-resistant "stem cell" phenotype, while decreased expression, as seen with AML1/ETO translocations, appears to confer a more migratory phenotype (reviewed in [17]). CXCL12 is particularly important in HSC retention, and interestingly has been found to be expressed at a higher level among a subset of stromal reticular cells. These CXCL12-abundant reticular cells, or CAR cells, are found throughout the marrow, generally surrounding sinusoidal endothelial cells. Rhythmic noradrenaline secre-tion via local sympathetic nerves modulates CXCL12 expression via β3 adrenoreceptor-medi-ated regulation of Sp1 levels. HSC egress is com-monly provoked using high doses of G-CSF, which acts on neutrophils to facilitate proteolytic cleavage of these adhesive interactions, and may also regu-late CXCL12 expression via CSF receptors found on sympathetic nerves [12]. Importantly, the marrow niche also critically regulates more mature cells as well. Osteoblast and endothelial cell niches play a role in both myelopoiesis (via G-CSF secretion) and B-cell lymphopoiesis (via IL-7 secretion and VCAM-1/cannabinoid receptor 2 expression). On the other hand, erythroid maturation is critically dependent on specialized bone marrow macro-phage interactions [18].

Hematopoietic developmental pathways

Human HSCs with long-term repopulation potential were initially found in the $CD34^+CD38^-CD90^+$ bone marrow compartment. Later flow cytometry-based studies have disclosed a rare "side population" with a $CD34^-$ or $CD34^{lo}$ phenotype with 1000-fold greater repopulating potential [19]. It remains unclear whether $CD34^-$ cells serve as progenitors to $CD34^+$ cells, as expression of this protein does not appear to be a terminal event. In fact, HSCs likely cycle expression of CD34 depending on specific microen-vironmental niches, wherein CD34 expression may facilitate adhesion and decreased proliferation [20].

Pluripotent, self-renewing, long-term repopulat-ing HSCs appear to progress through several stages of MPPs, which probably have reduced self-renewal capacity, before beginning the process of what is recognizable as differentiation by proceeding down either a lymphoid (CLP, common lymphoid progen-itor) or myeloid (CMP, common myeloid progenitor) developmental pathway, after which they are inca-pable of self-renewal in xenotransplant models. The lymphoid pathway ultimately generates T-cells, B-cells, natural killer (NK) cells, and dendritic cells. The myeloid pathway generates all the remaining mature hematopoietic phenotypes, including red blood cells (RBCs), granulocytes (neutrophils, eosi-nophils, basophils), mast cells, monocyte-macro-phages, and megakaryocytes-platelets, and provides an additional mechanism for generating dendritic cells. This hierarchy of differentiation from HSC to the broad spectrum of mature hematopoietic cells, cell surface molecules that serve as markers of the various stages of differentiation, and the growth factors that impact the differentiation processes, are depicted in Figure 1.1.

The initial decision to pursue either a lymphoid or myeloid fate is understandably important and the product of extensive investigation. Although much remains unknown about the mechanisms of these cell fate determinations, changes in regulation of gene expression through transcription factors, miRNA expression, epigenetic changes such as his-tone methylation or acetylation, among others, are thought to be critical to such cell-fate decisions. An analysis of SCL and E2A expression suggests that SCL encourages myeloid differentiation, while high levels of E2A (a helix-loop-helix protein) may be required for lymphoid development [21, 22]. Graded expression of the Ets family member, PU.1, likewise impacts myeloid/lymphoid lineage decisions, with low and high levels specifying lymphoid and myeloid commitment, respectively [23]. RUNX1 may play an early role in CMP lineage commitment by increasing PU.1 expression [24].

Common lymphoid progenitors (CLP)

Galy et al. were the first to characterize human lymphoid committed progenitors ($CD34^+CD38^+$ $CD45RA^+CD10^+$) from the bone marrow using both xenotransplant and *in vitro* culture systems. Using limiting dilution assays, this population was found to contain B, NK, and DC progenitors. Additionally, injection of $CD34^+CD10^+$ cells into fetal thymic organs provided evidence that these cells could also develop into T-cells [25]. IL-7Rα, a critical marker for murine CLPs, has since been found among $CD34^+CD45RA^+CD10^+$ adult human marrow CLPs. In fact, these cells were found to express transcripts for both B-cells (including Pax-5 and Igβ) and T-cells (including GATA3 and pTα). Interestingly, however, *in vitro* studies suggest a bias towards B-cell development among this subset (though limited NK cell development was observed) [26]. Indeed, a bias towards T- and NK cell lineage commitment appears to be found among $CD34^+CD45RA^+CD7^+CD10^-IL-7R\alpha^-$ cells. Whether both populations derive from a $CD34^+CD45RA^+CD10^+CD7^+$ cell population remains unknown, largely due to the scarcity of this phenotype in adult marrow (0.3% of cells) [27, 28].

Low levels of PU.1, likely act in parallel with Ikaros to provide transcriptional control of the maturation of HSCs into lymphoid precursors. In this context, PU.1 promotes IL-7Rα and EBF1 expression, while Ikaros promotes Flt3 receptor expression, all important in B- and T-cell development (reviewed in [29]). Additional regulation via the Notch1 receptor appears to be critical in T lineage commitment from the CLP. Deletion or inhibition of Notch

receptor signaling in CLPs prevents T-cell formation and promotes development of B-cells [30].

In the absence of Notch, the transcription factors E2A and EBF1 (early B-cell factor) appear to work together to induce expression of Pax-5. Indirect data implicating EBF in B-cell lineage commitment comes from an analysis of the EBF inhibitor, EHZF (early hematopoietic zinc finger). EHZF is highly expressed in CD34+ cells, but absent following differentiation to CD19+ B-cells [31]. Furthermore, *in vitro* inhibition of E2A with Id3 inhibits B-cell formation, possibly by inhibiting development/survival of CD10+IL-7Rα+ expressing B-cell biased lymphoid progenitors [32]. Pax-5 also plays an important role in the activation of B-cell lineage-specific genes, and repression of lineage-inappropriate genes, such as Notch1, c-Fms (which encodes the macrophage colony-stimulating factor receptor, and accordingly supports myeloid development), and CCL3 (which promotes osteoclast formation) [33–35]. Finally, Bcl11a (a zinc finger transcription factor) is also critical to B-cell lineage commitment, as its absence blocks B lymphopoiesis from the CLP [36]. Translocations involving Bcl11a are particularly relevant in malignant transformation [37].

Common myeloid progenitors (CMP)

CMPs (also known as CFU-GEMM; colony-forming unit-granulocyte, erythroid, macrophage, megakaryocyte) give rise to all myeloid lineages. CMPs are thought to give rise to two or more intermediate differentiated multipotent progenitor cell types. Granulocyte-monocyte progenitors (GMP), give rise to neutrophils, eosinophils, basophils, and monocyte/macrophages. The other, called megakaryocyte-erythroid progenitors (MEP) subsequently give rise to two separate lineages of hematopoietic cells, erythroid and megakaryocytic. The CMP, GMP, and MEP have all been isolated within the $CD34^+CD38^+$ compartment in both human marrow and cord blood. These cells lack the lymphoid markers CD10, CD7, and IL-3Rα, and can be isolated according to CD45RA and IL-3Rα expression: CMPs are $CD45RA^-IL-3R\alpha^{lo}$; GMPs are $CD45RA^+IL-3R\alpha^{lo}$; and MEPs are $CD45RA^-IL-3R\alpha^-$. Importantly

CD33 is also expressed by CMPs but lost beyond the myelocyte stage and accordingly is a recognized target for the treatment of certain types of acute myeloid leukemia (AML) [38].

Another important marker in hematopoiesis is the FMS-like tyrosine kinase 3 receptor (Flt3). Interestingly, expression of Flt3 in human progenitor populations differs considerably from that of mice. Around 40–80% of human $CD34^+$ bone marrow and cord blood cells are $Flt3^+$, and its presence appears to correlate with a capacity for long-term repopulation. Specifically, a fraction of both $Flt3^+$ and $Flt3^-$ populations generate multilineage colonies containing all the myelo-erythroid components, with $Flt3^+$ populations forming more GM colonies, and $Flt3^-$ populations more erythroid colonies [39]. Further exploration using xenotransplant models has characterized the $Flt3^+CD34^+CD38^-$ as LT-HSCs, and has identified Flt3 on both GMPs and CLPs [40, 41]. In contrast, murine Flt3 expression is limited to MPPs with both granulocytic and lymphocytic (but not megakaryocytic-erythroid) potential. Cells with similar potential have not been isolated in humans. The specific role of Flt3 is still being delineated; however, persistent activation as a consequence of activating mutations is commonly seen in AML, and is associated with a worse prognosis.

Transcriptional control of lineage bifurcation between the MEP and GMP populations is at least driven by antagonism between PU.1 and GATA1, with the former driving GMP formation, and the latter encouraging MEP development. PU.1 in association with Rb, binds to the promoters of GATA1 target genes, inhibiting their transcription, and has specifically been shown to inhibit α-globin expression and erythroid differentiation. GATA1 also suppresses myeloid differentiation via binding to the Ets domain of PU.1, blocking binding of the coactivator c-Jun and, accordingly, inhibiting PU.1 DNA-binding [42, 43].

Megakaryocytopoiesis and erythropoiesis

Megakaryocytes and erythroid cells originate from the CMP/CFU-GEMM. The process begins with differentiation of the CMP into the MEP intermedi-

ate. Progression beyond the MEP stage is associated with lineage commitment to either the erythroid or megakaryocyte lineages. Specifically, the MEP initially differentiates into a highly proliferative burst forming unit-megakaryocytic or burst forming unit-erythroid (BFU-Mk or BFU-E), which is followed by further maturation to colony forming units (CFU-Mk or CFU-E, respectively), and ultimately either megakaryocyte/platelet formation or erythroid cell production. In fact, the existence of MEP cells was postulated prior to their isolation, given the numerous similarities in transcriptional regulation (SCL, GATA1, GATA2, NF-E2), cell surface molecules (TER119, CD235a/glycophorin A), and cytokine receptors (IL-3, SCF, EPO, and TPO). Additionally, several erythroid and megakaryocytic leukemia cell lines can be induced to display features of both lineages. Furthering this concept are the structural and downstream signaling similarities after binding of EPO and TPO to their respective cell surface receptors, which display a modest degree of synergy in stimulating the growth of progenitors of both lineages.

Although the mechanisms by which these differentiation decisions are made are not fully elucidated, it is known that specific transcription factors play roles in determining whether MEPs proceed down the differentiation pathway towards erythropoiesis or megakaryocytopoiesis. Here, Fli-1 and EKLF appear to play similarly antagonistic roles, with Fli-1 supporting the development of BFU-Mk, and EKLF the formation of BFU-E. EKLF expression relies on GATA1 and CP1. Cells committed to the megakaryocytic lineage express CD41 and CD61 (integrin αIIβ3), CD42 (glycoprotein I) and glycoprotein V, von Willebrand factor, platelet factor 4 and other platelet proteins. As MEP maturation along the erythroid pathway occurs, they lose CD41 expression, and express the transferrin receptor (CD71) at the BFU-E stage, and subsequently erythroid membrane proteins, erythroid enzymes, and hemoglobins.

Megakaryocytopoiesis

The mature megakaryocyte progenitor proceeds down a regimented pathway, forming promegakaryoblasts, which generate megakaryoblasts, and in turn produce megakaryocytes. Megakaryocytes are unique among hematopoietic cells, in that after the CFU-MK stage, DNA replication is not accompanied by cell division, resulting in production of progressively larger cells with complex nuclei containing 4N to as high as 128N chromosomes. Platelets are generated by fragmentation of the mature megakaryocyte cytoplasmic pseudopodial projections, called proplatelets. The sliding of microtubules over one another drives the elongation of proplatelet processes and organelle transportation (into the proplatelets) in a process that consumes the megakaryocyte and results in production of 2000–3000 platelets from each mature megakaryocyte (reviewed in [44]).

Although influenced by multiple cytokines (SCF, GM-CSF, IL-3, IL-6, IL-7, IL-11, EPO), TPO and IL-3 are particularly important in the generation and release of mature platelets [45]. Studies conducted following the purification of TPO have found that it is capable of stimulating the growth of 75% of all CFU-MKs, with the remainder proliferating with the addition of IL-3. Additionally, TPO and either IL-3 or SCF are required for the generation of more complex, larger hematopoietic colonies from earlier progenitor populations [46]. Consistent with these experimental data is the observation of amegakaryocytic thrombocytopenia among those with inactivating TPO receptor mutations. The relative contributions of elevated levels of TPO or increased TPO receptor expression to enhancement of megakaryocyte and platelet production remain unclear, though it is likely that both play roles *in vivo*.

Several megakaryocyte DNA promoter binding domains have been identified in mice, with some clinical homology demonstrated in humans with mutations involving associated proteins. It should be stressed that these proteins likely interact with one another, as well as with other transcriptional proteins to ultimately affect the generation of mature progeny.

GATA1 and GATA2 are the major GATA zinc finger DNA binding-proteins influencing differentiation in both the erythroid and megakaryocytic lineages. In both series, GATA1 levels increase while GATA2 levels decrease with progressive differentiation. Additionally, GATA proteins are co-regulated by FOG1 (friend of GATA), a large multifinger pro-

tein that influences transcription independent of DNA-binding. GATA1 and FOG1 knockout mice both demonstrate abnormalities in erythropoiesis and megakaryocytopoiesis. Interestingly, human mutations affecting the binding of GATA1 to FOG1 appear to have greater impact on megakaryocytopoiesis than erythropoiesis (reviewed in [47]). Indeed, GATA1-mediated expression of Gfi-1b and repression via interactions with Eto-2 are required for terminal differentiation of megakaryocytes [48, 49]. In fact, mutations involving both Gfi-1b and Eto-2 have been observed in leukemias [50, 51]. GATA2 instead contributes to proliferation of progenitor cells [52].

Another transcriptional regulator is the family of core binding factors, consisting of the DNA binding proteins RUNX1–3 and the non-DNA binding element, CBFβ. The complex of RUNX1 and CBFβ is particularly important in hematopoietic ontogeny. In fact mutations involving these proteins are commonly observed in human acute leukemias. Inactivation of either RUNX1 or CBFβ in murine models leads to a profound defect in megakaryocytic differentiation (with little impact on erythropoiesis). Clinically, RUNX1 mutations are associated with the autosomal dominant familial platelet disorder with predisposition to AML (FPD/AML), with these leukemias likely occurring as a direct consequence of perturbed HSC homeostasis [53].

Ets factor binding sites are also commonly observed among megakaryocytic promoters. The Ets family of transcription factors includes approximately 30 members, with both stimulatory and inhibitory consequences on gene expression. Four Ets factors are of particular consequence to murine megakaryocytopoiesis: Fli-1, GABPα, TEL1, and Ets-1. Selective deletion of TEL1 has been shown to increase CFU-MKs, yet produce a dramatic decrease in platelet production (with little impact on erythrocytes). Decreasing GABPα expression leads to decreased megakaryocyte formation, accompanied by decreased expression of GPIIb and the TPO receptor. Fli-1 deletion similarly decreases megakaryocyte formation with an accompanying decrease in gpIX expression. Ets-1 is normally upregulated in megakaryocytic differentiation, and, alternatively downregulated in erythroid development. Enforced expression of Ets-1 appears to enhance megakaryo-cyte development, and, likewise inhibit erythroid formation. Interestingly, knockout models of Ets-1 do not significantly impact murine megakaryocyte development (reviewed in [47]).

Erythropoiesis

Akin to megakaryocytopoiesis, the initial steps in erythropoiesis are driven by SCF, GM-CSF, IL-3, and TPO. Erythropoietin (EPO) receptors are not highly expressed until the CFU-E stage, where EPO functions to prevent apoptosis, induce hemoglobin synthesis, and drive maturation to proerythro-blasts, from which point erythroid maturation proceeds through nucleated normoblasts to enu-cleated red blood cells without further contribution by erythropoietin. Interestingly, EPO does not contribute significantly to lineage commitment among HSCs or MPPs [54].

The transition to lineage-committed erythroid cells requires both the downregulation of prolifer-ation associated genes, such as GATA2, c-Myb, c-Myc, and c-Kit, and the upregulation of terminal differentiation genes, including P4.2, glycophorin A, α and β globins. The transcriptional regulatory process is governed by the SCL complex. Prolifer-ation in this setting is driven by GATA1, which binds to the c-Myb promoter to enhance its expres-sion. However, FOG1 expression, which is also induced by GATA1, subsequently binds GATA1, generating a complex that inactivates c-Myb and similarly represses GATA2 activity. GATA1 also acts to transiently increase Gfi-1b, which likely acts in concert with the EPO/GM-CSF-driven JAK/STAT pathway to increase the proliferation of erythroid progenitors [55]. *In vitro* models suggest that Gfi-1b must be downregulated beyond the proerythro-blast stage to facilitate survival, though, interest-ingly, increased expression has been observed in erythroleukemia [50, 56]. GATA1 additionally downregulates c-Myc and indirectly maintains Rb expression, which downregulates c-Kit expres-sion via binding to the SCL complex. Finally, GATA1 also regulates EKLF expression in conjunc-tion with CP1; and EPO receptor genes in conjunc-tion with Sp1 (reviewed in [57]).

Granulocytopoiesis

Progression beyond the GMP stage along the granulocytic pathway facilitates the production of neutrophils, eosinophils, and basophils. This pro-gression occurs via similarly discrete intermediate steps in all three series, beginning with myeloblasts and progressing through promyelocytic, myelocytic, metamyelocytic, and band stages before culminat-ing in a mature granulocyte. Primary, secondary, and tertiary granules important to granulocyte func-tion are acquired at the promyelocyte, myelocyte, and band stages, respectively. CD11b, CD13, CD14, CD15, and CD16 are common markers of maturing and mature neutrophils and monocytes. Neutrophil elastase, myeloperoxidase, lactoferrin, and leuko-cyte alkaline phosphatase are markers of maturing and mature neutrophilic granulocytes. Muramidase and lysozyme are common markers of mature monocytes/macrophages. Not surprisingly, G-CSF, GM-CSF, and IL-3 are important cytokines in the generation of functional granulocytes.

Expression of the CCAAT/enhancer binding pro-tein (C/EBP)α and interaction with c-Jun increase the activity of PU.1, while also inhibiting Pax-5 (paired box gene 5), and likely other lymphoid transcriptional elements, to further commit cells to the GMP stage. Graded expression of PU.1 beyond this stage facilitates lineage bifurcation, with low and high levels specifying granulocytic and mono-cytic commitment, respectively. Downstream tar-gets of PU.1 include the EGR/Nab transcription factors. Antagonism between Egr-1/2 acting with its co-repressor Nab-2, and Gfi-1 function to drive lineage commitment down either a macrophage or neutrophil pathway. Specifically, the Egr-1/2/Nab2 complex drives macrophage-specific gene expres-sion, while repressing neutrophil-specific genes, including Gfi-1. Gfi-1, which is downstream of C/EBPα, does precisely the opposite, and similarly represses the Egr-1/2/Nab-2 complex (reviewed in [58]).

The paradoxical role of C/EBPα may be explained by M-CSF/PLCγ/ERK-mediated phosphorylation at serine 21, potentially weakening C/EBPα granu-locytic gene interactions by limiting C/EBPα homodimerization, while simultaneously fostering monocytic gene interactions via stabilization of c-Fos and subsequent phospho-C/EBPα(S21):c-Fos heterodimers. G-CSF, alternatively, acts via STAT3-mediated phosphorylation of SHP2, which may limit PU.1:IRF8 interactions, influence HoxA9/10 genomic interactions, and alter ERK activity to favor granulocytic development [59–62]. Interestingly, activating mutations in SHP2 have been found in MDS, AML, and JMML, wherein constitutive expression of SHP2 more potently activates ERK (akin to M-CSF) [63, 64].

In addition to Gfi-1, C/EBPα and RARα (retinoic acid receptor alpha) induce C/EBPε in the context of low PU.1 to ultimately influence granulocytic maturation. C/EBPα and C/EBPβ may serve somewhat redundant roles in myelopoiesis; however, only C/EBPα is capable of inhibiting cell cycle progression to facilitate terminal differentiation. C/EBPα interacts with E2F1 to bind to the c-myc promoter, and ultimately to repress its transcription (reviewed in [58]). Indeed, C/EBPα mutations reflect a recurring theme in both adult and pediatric AML [65, 66]. Terminal differentiation of granulocytes is also afforded by repression of CAAT displacement protein (CDP) and downmodulation of the retinoid x receptor, RXRα [67–69]. Alterations in RAR:RXR signaling are commonly seen in acute promyelocytic leukemia, in which treatment with all-trans retinoic acid is instead used to facilitate terminal granulocytic differentiation. Likewise, failure to downmodulate CDP in experimental models has been shown to generate a myeloproliferative phenotype with an excess of neutrophils in the bone marrow and spleen [70].

Eosinophil formation

Eosinophils are thought to be generated from an eosinophil-basophil progenitor derived from the GMP [71]. The cytokines IL-3, IL-5, and GM-CSF are important in the regulation of eosinophils, most likely by providing permissive proliferation/differentiation signals in concert with transcriptional signals (mediated by GATA1, PU.1, and C/EBPs, see below). Of these growth factors, IL-5 is most specific to the eosinophils, promoting selective differentiation of eosinophils as well as their release from

the marrow. Overproduction of these cytokines (particularly IL-5) is seen in a variety of malignancies, and has a known association with eosinophilia (reviewed in [72]).

The timing of expression, as well as interactions between GATA, PU.1, and C/EBP members influences eosinophil lineage commitment. Of these GATA1 appears to be most important, as deletion of the high affinity palindromic GATA binding site in the GATA1 promoter prevents eosinophil formation. This binding site appears to be specific to eosinophil development, as deletion does not appear to influence the development of other GATA1[+] lineages, including megakaryocyte, erythroid, and mast cell lineages. Similar binding sites exist outside of the promoter region in the regulatory regions of eosinophil specific genes, such as the eotaxin receptor, CCR3, MBP, and IL-5Rα. These palindromic binding sites may also facilitate synergy between the normally antagonistic functions of GATA1 and PU.1 (reviewed in [72]).

Basophil and mast cell formation

As indicated above, basophils likely derive from a bipotent precursor with both eosinophil and basophil differentiation capacity (although other differentiation pathways have been proposed, see [73]). The existence of this bipotent precursor has not been proven, but it is supported by *in vitro* clonogenic assays, as well as the presence of cells with a hybrid eosinophil/basophil phenotype in some patients with CML and AML [74]. Although murine mast cells appear to derive from a common basophil/mast cell progenitor, human mast cell development does not appear to conform to this pathway [75, 76]. Human mast cell progenitors, which are distinct from basophil progenitors, are marked by expression of CD34, c-Kit, and CD13, and they appear to have both monocytic and mast cell potential, which may explain why monocytosis (but not basophilia) is observed in patients with mast cell neoplasia [77, 78].

IL-3 plays a major role in basophil growth and differentiation, and basophilia (and eosinophilia) is seen shortly after exogenous administration [79].

Interestingly, IL-3-deficient mice have normal basophil counts, suggesting that the final steps in basophil maturation may occur without a growth factor requirement. In support of this theory, a 3–4 hour exposure of cord blood progenitors to IL-3 was sufficient to drive basophil differentiation for three weeks [80]. TGF-β and IL-18 work synergistically with IL-3 to inhibit eosinophil differentiation and increase IL-4/histamine production by basophils, respectively. Finally, GM-CSF and IL-5 also drive basophil (and eosinophil) production (reviewed in [73]).

Mast cell differentiation is primarily dependent on SCF and IL-3, although it is likely that other factors (TPO, leukotriene D4) and T helper type II (Th2) associated cytokines, such as IL-4, IL-5, IL-6, and IL-9, also play a role [76, 81–83]. Emphasizing the importance of SCF in mast cell development are the findings that exogenous SCF administration in humans produces mast cell proliferation and degranulation, and that there are activating mutations (D816V) of c-Kit in the majority of cases of mastocytosis [84].

Transcriptional regulation of human basophil differentiation is still being elucidated. Murine models suggest that increased GATA2 in conjunction with low levels of C/EBPα appear to be important in early basophil and mast cell lineage commitment. Failure to decrease C/EBPα at this early stage instead leads to eosinophil production. Following basophil lineage commitment, C/EBPα must again be upregulated to facilitate basophil development. Signaling via Notch2-Delta1-Hes1 may be important in repressing C/EBPα at this stage, which, alternatively, drives mast cell production [85–87]. Importantly, PU.1 and GATA2 do not appear to antagonize one another, and, indeed, elevated PU.1 is important in mast cell differentiation [88].

Monocyte/macrophage development

Monocytes derive from the GMP, proceeding through an intermediate, the macrophage dendritic cell progenitor (MDP). The MDP reflects the first committed stage of monocytic development, and is characterized by the expression of CSF-1 receptor (CD115, M-CSFR) and the chemokine receptor, CX3CR1. As the name suggests, MDPs give rise to monocytes, macrophages, and both lymphoid/non-lymphoid and plasmacytic types of dendritic cells (see below) [89].

Human monocytes are categorized into three distinct populations on the basis of CD64, CD14 and CD16 expression. Large $CD64^+CD14^+CD16^-$ monocytes comprise 80–90% of the circulating monocytes, and are characterized by high levels of the chemokine receptor CCR2, and low levels of CX3CR1. These cells possess higher phagocytic/myeloperoxidase activity, higher superoxide release, and secrete IL-10 on stimulation with lipopolysaccharide (LPS). The smaller $CD16^+$ monocytes, alternatively, express high levels of CX3CR1 and low levels of CCR2. This population is comprised of two subsets: a $CD64^+CD14^+CD16^+$ "proinflammatory" subtype and $CD64^-CD14^{dim}CD16^+$ subtype whose function remains largely unknown. $CD14^+CD16^+$ monocytes also express the Fc receptor CD32, produce TNF-α and IL-1 in response to LPS, and likely mediate antibody-dependent cytotoxicity (reviewed in [90]).

M-CSF and IL-34 are the two known ligands for CSF-1R (M-CSFR), and both are important in monocytic development. Other cytokines, including GM-CSF, Flt3 ligand, and lymphotoxin α1β2, play similar, but likely redundant roles.

PU.1 plays a dominant role in early monocytic lineage commitment, antagonizing GATA1 (to inhibit MEP formation), GATA2 (to inhibit mast cell formation), and C/EBPα (to inhibit granulocytic development) [88, 91]. Targets of PU.1 activity include the Egr transcription factors (and their cofactor Nab), KLF4 (Kruppel-like family 4), and, likely, ICSBP/IRF-8 (IFN consensus sequence binding protein/IFN regulatory factor 8) [58, 92, 93]. PU.1, c-Ets-1, and c-Ets-2 transactivate the M-CSFR promoter, although, M-CSFR expression cannot rescue monocytic differentiation in PU.1 knockout models [94, 95].

The MafB and c-Maf transcription factors also induce monocyte development. MafB and c-Maf are also thought to cooperate to decrease proliferation in the context of terminal differentiation and, in fact,

MafB must be downregulated to allow dendritic cell maturation [96]. These factors likely act by repressing the transcription factor Ets-1, which is important in transducing CSF-1 receptor associated proliferative signals (via c-Myc and c-Myb), as well as directly inhibiting c-Myb transactivation [97].

Dendritic cell formation

Dendritic cells (DC) are unique among human hematopoietic cells in that they are able to develop from both myeloid and lymphoid progenitors. Many DC progenitor candidates have been proposed, and these can be divided into highly proliferative early DC progenitors (EDCP), late DC progenitors (LDCP) with limited proliferative capacity, and non-proliferative Gr1^{hi} monocytic precursors with immediate DC precursor potential. Multiple subtypes exist within the EDCP and LDCP categories, and are beyond the scope of this review (interested readers are referred to [98]). EDCP are lineage-negative cells characterized by c-Kit, while LDCP are negative for c-Kit, but express CD11c.

Mature DCs can be divided into two major populations: (1) migratory (non-lymphoid) and lymphoid tissue resident DCs, and (2) plasmacytic DCs (pDCs, also called interferon-producing cells). DCs can also be classified as "conventional DCs" (cDCs), which has been used to oppose lymphoid organ resident DCs with pDCs. In this schema, non-lymphoid organ DCs are referred to as "tissue DCs." Nonetheless, it is important to note that non-lymphoid tissue DCs are also different from pDCs, and that primary non-lymphoid tissue DCs can be found in LNs while migrating (but are not cDCs). Specifically, cDCs are characterized as HLA-DR$^+$, CD11c^{hi}, with a major BDCA3$^-$ (also known as thrombomodulin) and minor BDCA3$^+$ population. BDCA3$^-$ CDC can be further subdivided into CD16$^+$ and CD16$^-$ populations. PDC express very low to no CD11c, and instead demonstrate CD4, CD45RA, BDCA2 (a c-type lectin receptor), BDCA4 (a neuronal receptor often used to isolate pDCs), and high levels of IL-3R (CD123).

Flt3L appears to be of primary importance in dendritic cell development and, in fact, Flt3L levels are actively adjusted to maintain DC homeostasis in the BM and peripheral lymphoid organs. Cytokines important in differentiation of circulating precursors include GM-CSF and TNF-α, which prime monocyte-to-cDC commitment in the context of inflammation; M-CSF and TGF-β1, which are both non-redundant cytokines important in facilitating Langerhans cell development; and TPO (in cooperation with Flt3L) and G-CSF, which enhance pDC development and mobilization, respectively (reviewed in [98]).

Flt3L appears to act via STAT3, and deletion of STAT3 has been shown to decrease DC numbers [99]. Gfi-1 regulates STAT3 activation, and deletion reduces lymphoid-derived DCs while increasing LC production [100]. GM-CSF instead promotes cDC development via STAT5, which in turn suppresses IRF-8 (ICSBP) and inhibits pDC development. In fact, in the absence of STAT5, GM-CSF stimulated cultures generate pDCs. GM-CSF also increases STAT3 activation and IRF-4 expression, a transcription factor important in DC development [101]. Among its many effects, STAT3 signaling has been shown to increase PU.1 expression, which is important in both cDC and pDC development [102]. Interestingly, constitutive signaling of Flt3 via internal tandem repeat mutations appear to repress PU.1 and c/EBPα and activate STAT5, which may explain why these mutations have not been associated with DC neoplasias [103].

The basic helix-loop-helix (bHLH) transcription factors (E2-2, E2A encoded E12/E47, and HEB) also play an important role in DC homeostasis, with ectopic expression favoring pDC development. In fact, Spi-B, an Ets family member important in pDC development, may act in part by increasing E2-2 activity [104]. Id-2, an inhibitor of the bHLH factors, is increased following GM-CSF, and appears to favor production of cDCs. Likewise, TGF-β1 appears to signal increases in Id-2 (via RUNX3), which has been shown to inhibit E2A to favor LC development in the context of low C/EBPα. Haplo-insufficiency of E2-2 in humans leads to a functional pDC defect (Pitt-Hopkins syndrome), further confirming the importance of bHLH in pDC development [105].

The role of Notch1 is gaining increasing attention in the differentiation and function of DCs, with both pro- and antagonistic effects occurring depending on the ligand interaction (Delta-1 vs. Jagged-1), and on the immature cell type studied (HSC vs. immature thymic progenitors). Accordingly, Notch1 has been shown to influence multiple downstream signaling factors, including Wnt, NFκB, GATA3, and Spi-B [106, 107].

B-cell lymphopoiesis

B-cells are derived from CD34$^+$CD19$^-$CD10$^+$ cells. The earliest lineage-committed B-cell is the pro-B-cell, which is characterized by a CD19$^+$ phenotype. The vast majority of these cells also express terminal deoxynucleotidyl transferase (TdT), and potentially VpreB (a component of the pre-B-cell receptor). It is interesting to note that commitment to B-cell differentiation may occur prior to this based on the presence of cytoplasmic Vpre-B in CD19 negative cells – though, the lineage commitment of this cell remains controversial [108]. The pro-B-cell stage is defined by immunoglobulin (Ig) heavy chain gene rearrangement, initiated via the recombinase activating genes RAG1 and RAG2. Importantly, oncogenes such as Bcl-2 lie in close proximity to immunoglobulin genes, which may partially underlie the mechanism for translocation seen in B-cell neoplasias (reviewed in [29] and [109]).

If heavy chain gene rearrangement is successful, an Ig heavy chain of μ class is expressed on the cell surface in association with ΨL (VpreB and λ5) and CD79a/b to form the pre-B-cell receptor, which signals several rounds of division and termination of rearrangement. This is accompanied by loss of CD34 and TdT expression, and marks the transition to the pre-B-cell stage of development, while a persistence of TdT positivity is commonly seen in pre-B-cell ALL. Internalization of the pre-B-cell receptor and rearrangement of the light chains occur next, defaulting to the kappa gene. Lambda gene rearrangement and expression generally occurs only if kappa gene rearrangement is unsuccessful. Successful light chain rearrangement is heralded by cell surface expression of IgM, composed of the μIg and either κ or λ light chain. Failure to rearrange either the heavy or light chains induces apoptosis. Similarly, reaction to self antigen

at IgM can induce either apoptosis or anergy as a mechanism of negative selection (reviewed in [110]).

Secondary B-cell development is characterized by the migration of immature B-cells to the spleen where they differentiate into mature antigenically naïve B-cells, now characterized by surface IgD (in addition to IgM), CD21, and CD22, as well as a loss of CD10. Positive selection subsequently commences, with cells failing to react succumbing to cell death. Following this process, these cells migrate to secondary lymphoid tissue in anticipation of antigenic challenge, whereupon they can further differentiate into short-lived antibody secreting plasma cells or establish a germinal center. Within germinal centers, these antigen primed B-cells undergo rapid proliferation and a process of somatic hypermutation to increase antigen affinity. Somatic hypermutation is mediated by the enzyme activation-induced cytidine deaminase (AID). Akin to RAG1/2, AID can also generate neoplastic chromosomal translocations involving c-Myc and the IgH locus, as seen in Burkitt's lymphoma. Centrally proliferating B-cells are referred to as centroblasts, which divide to form smaller centrocytes that migrate to the periphery of the germinal center. Centrocytes with differing antigen affinity compete for antigen-binding sites on dendritic cells. Successful interaction is marked by expression of the antiapoptotic protein Bcl-XL, while unsuccessful interaction leads to apoptosis. Those surviving centrocytes subsequently depend on CD40-based interaction with T-cells to facilitate differentiation into long-lived plasma and memory-type B-cells. Secondary immune responses ultimately produce long-lived plasma cells in the spleen, which migrate back to the bone marrow where they can persist for a lifetime without need for self-renewal. However, if depleted, memory B-cells are capable of regenerating new marrow plasma cells [111].

We still have much to learn about cytokine regulation in B-cell development. Certainly, c-Kit and Flt3 are likely to play a role in the proliferation and survival of early pro-B-cells. However, the role of IL-7 in the survival and proliferation remains controversial. *In vitro* data supports a role for IL-7 in promoting Pax-5 and CD19 expression [112]. Yet, mutations of the IL-7 receptor complex in humans do not appear to significantly affect B-cell numbers (though their function is impaired) [113].

Pax-5 is perhaps the most important transcriptional regulator in B-cell development. As described above, Pax-5 is critical to early B-cell lineage commitment, where it likely represses Flt3 expression to enable the differentiation program that results in production of the mature phenotype. Pax-5 continues to retain its importance throughout the maturation of the B-cell by facilitating VH-DJH recombination and enhancing numerous B-cell specific genes, including Ebf1, ΨL, CD79a, CD19, CD21, CD23, adhesion/migration proteins, N-myc, LEF-1, and the central adaptor protein, BLNK. Together, these suggest Pax-5-mediated maintenance of the B-cell phenotype prior to plasma cell differentiation (which requires BLIMP1 associated Pax-5 inhibition) (reviewed in [114]). Indeed, conditional inactivation of Pax-5 in mature B-cells leads to de-differentiation to a pro-B-cell stage, wherein T-cell developmental potential can be induced [115]. Additionally, inactivation/mutation of Pax-5 in committed B-cells is also associated with transformation to B-cell ALL, as well as Ki+ B-cell lymphomas [116, 117].

The transcription factors FoxP1, E2A/E47, and EBF also play roles in B-cell development, acting to control DH-JH rearrangement by activating expression of RAG1/2 and promoting accessibility of the DH-JH region. Aberrant expression of B-cell transcription factors have known associations with malignant phenotypes, including E2A in pre- and pro-B cell ALL [118, 119].

The proto-oncogene Bcl6 encodes a nuclear transcriptional repressor, which appears to be necessary in germinal center formation. Bcl6 likely plays a role in suppression of apoptosis during the process of low-level physiologic DNA breaks that occur during somatic hypermutation, and mutations of Bcl6 are commonly observed in diffuse large B-cell lymphomas and follicular lymphomas.

T-cell lymphopoiesis

Immature T-cell progenitors are likely guided to the thymus via chemokine receptor/ligand CCR9/

CCL25 interactions [120]. Subsequent T-cell formation is analogous to B-cell formation, with maturation progressing through pro-T- and pre-T-cell stages marked by TCR gene rearrangement. T-cells begin their developmental paradigm by migrating to the thymus, initially as $CD34^+CD1a^-$ early thymic progenitors (ETP). The transition to CD1a positivity marks an irreversible commitment to the T-cell lineage, at which time they are referred to as pro-T-cells. Importantly, these cells are negative for both CD4 and CD8, and as such, are heralded as "double-negative" T-cells. These double-negative T-cells proceed through four discrete stages of maturation, DN1–4. The DN1 stage is marked by expression of c-Kit and CD44 (an adhesion molecule), but an absence of CD25 (the α-chain of the IL-2 receptor). Within approximately one day, these thymic lymphoid progenitors begin to express CD25, which marks the transition to the DN2 stage. Progression through the DN2 and DN3 stages, is accompanied by Sox13-mediated $\gamma\delta$ TCR expression or TCR β chain rearrangement, and is accompanied by a loss of c-Kit and CD44. Akin to B-cell gene rearrangement, this process is prone to anomalous chromosomal translocations that can drive neoplastic transformation. Successful rearrangement of the TCR β chain is followed by its expression on the cell membrane in conjunction with CD3 and pTα, to form the pre-T-cell receptor (pre-TCR), which, as in B-cells, is thought to inhibit further rearrangement and stimulate proliferation. The expression of the pre-T-cell receptor also demarcates the transition from pro-T-cells to pre-T-cells. Finally, CD25 expression is lost at the DN4 stage (reviewed in [121]).

T-cells subsequently mature by first proceeding through an immature single positive CD4 phase. Early double-positive T-cells then emerge ($CD4^+CD8\alpha^+\beta^-$), followed soon thereafter by precursor double-positive T-cells ($CD4^+CD8\alpha^+\beta^+$), which ultimately form the double-positive $TCR\alpha\beta^+$ cells. Pre-T-cells are subsequently induced to express either $CD4^+$ or $CD8^+$ cells via interaction of their TCR with MHC/peptide complexes expressed by thymic epithelial cells in a process referred to as positive selection. Successful interaction with MHC Class I molecules is associated with differentiation towards a CD8$^+$ cytotoxic T-cell phenotype, while successful interactions with MHC Class II molecules drive formation of CD4$^+$ helper T-cells. Following the process of positive selection, T-cells migrate to the thymic medulla under the influence of CCR7 (and likely other chemokines), where they are tested against self antigens on thymic dendritic cells – with those reacting strongly being induced to undergo apoptosis [122]. This latter process is commonly referred to as "negative selection" (reviewed in [121]).

Interestingly, while IL-7Rα$^+$ immature CLPs more avidly develop into B-cells, the absence of critical components of the IL-7R receptor appears to influence T-cell maturation more significantly [123]. The IL-7 receptor consists of two components, an IL-7Rα and gamma common (γc) chain (which also forms the IL-2, IL-4, IL-9, IL-15, and IL-21 receptors), and signals via the JAK1, JAK3/STAT5, and the PI3K (phosphatidylinositol-3 kinase)/Akt transduction pathways. Inactivating mutations in the γc, IL-7Rα, or JAK3 genes all produce severe combined immunodeficiency (SCID), with a marked reduction in T-cells. Specifically, in patients with γc mutations, there is an absence of T- and NK cells, while B-cell development appears to be preserved. Additionally, those with IL-7Rα mutations have significantly reduced T-cell numbers, with near normal B-cell and normal NK cell numbers [123–125].

However, given the role of IL-7 in B-cell development and the absence of IL-7Rα on ETPs, it is difficult to conclude that this interleukin drives αβ T-cell lineage commitment – rather, its effect is likely mediated at a later stage where it promotes T-cell maturation and/or survival. In fact, additional data demonstrate dependence of CD34$^+$CD1a$^+$ cells on IL-7 for transition to the CD4$^+$ immature single-positive phase, perhaps via expression of the anti-apoptotic Bcl-2-related protein Mcl-1 [126]. Interestingly, IL-7 is a prerequisite for TCR γδ formation via direct regulation of TCRγ locus accessibility and rearrangement [113].

SCF, Flt3, and BMP are also important, though they appear to be active during earlier stages of T-cell development. Neutralization of SCF both inhibits T-cell proliferation and accelerates T lineage maturation from lymphoid progenitors [127]. Likewise, knockout of c-Kit leads to a dramatic reduction in DN1 cellularity, suggesting SCF may play a role in maintenance of the undifferentiated lymphoid precursors [128]. BMP signaling appears to play a similar role, with increased levels corresponding to enhanced survival of immature thymocyte progenitors, and inhibition of differentiation through the DN stages [129, 130]. Flt3 ligand likely plays many roles in T-cell development, and has recently been shown in mice to enhance expression of CCR9, allowing for enhanced thymic migration [131].

Notch1 signaling retains its importance following T-cell lineage commitment, in which it regulates the survival and maturation of CD4-/CD8- (double-negative) T-cells. Notch1 activity at the DN1 stage likely functions to maintain T-cell lineage specification, as inhibition of Notch at this stage drives production of NK cells, monocytic/DC cells and plasmacytoid dendritic cells. Notch activity at the DN2 and DN3 stages of T-cell development facilitates expression of pTα, as well as β-chain rearrangement and β selection. During β selection, Notch functions in a trophic manner, supporting Akt activation and c-Myc expression. T-cell development beyond DN4 is accompanied by decreased Notch activity, and an increase in antagonistic proteins such as Ikaros (reviewed in [121]. This transition is tightly regulated, as persistent Notch activity in double-positive T-cells is highly oncogenic. In fact, activating mutations of Notch1 have been found in over 50% of T-cell acute lymphoblastic lymphomas (T-ALL) [132].

A second regulatory system is the Wnt-β-catenin pathway. Wnt drives the release of active β-catenin, which, in double-negative T-cells, forms a bipartite transcription factor complex with the HMG-box T-cell factor (TCF)/lymphocyte enhancer binding factor (LEF) family of proteins, ultimately promoting expression of TCF1, as well as c-Fos, c-Jun, and integrins. Inhibition of Wnt signaling leads to a maturation arrest at the DN2 stage. Similarly, unsuccessful TCRβ rearrangement at the DN3 stage leads to expression of β-catenin degrading proteins, including adenomatous polyposis coli (APC) and the E3 ubiquitin ligase, SIP [133, 134]. Wnt/TCF retains importance in double-positive T-cells as well, in which it functions to promote expression of CD4 and the antiapoptotic protein BCL-XL reviewed in [121]).

The bHLH subfamily of E-box binding (E) proteins (E12, E47, HEB, and E2-2) also play a critical role in T-cell development. These proteins are naturally antagonized by Id (inhibitors of DNA binding) proteins, specifically Id2 and Id3. Ectopic expression of these Id proteins in CD34$^+$ cells drives NK formation at the expense of T-cell formation [135]. Later introduction of Id3 into immature single-positive CD4 T-cells inhibited TCRαβ development, but allowed TCRγδ development – which could be reversed by the E-protein HEB, likely via an influence on pTα expression [29, 136].

Thymocyte progenitors are dependent on hedgehog (Hh) signals for survival, expansion, and differentiation prior to pre-TCR signaling. Knockout of sonic hedgehog (Shh) in mouse embryos leads to diminished thymic cellularity, likely due to defects in DN1 and DN2 progenitor expansion [137]. Additionally, the transition from double-negative to double-positive T-cells may also be regulated by concentration-dependent effects of Shh, as high concentrations of this protein appear to antagonize this progression [138]. New data are emerging on the role of dysregulation of the Shh pathway in leukemias and lymphomas. In particular, abnormally increased Shh and cyclopamine (a Shh inhibitor) mediated apoptosis have been observed in Alk + anaplastic large cell lymphoma, mantle cell lymphoma, and cytarabine-resistant leukemic cell lines [139, 140].

The role of GATA3 in T-cell development is still being delineated. Early experiments suggested that GATA3 overexpression in CD34$^+$ thymic progenitors stimulated development of CD4$^+$CD8$^+$ cells. However, the absolute numbers of TCRαβ cells were markedly reduced at later time-points, suggesting an inhibition of further development [141]. Murine GATA3-deficient models add further confusion, since GATA3 appears to be necessary for TCRβ expression and pre-TCR signaling [142]. Together, this information may suggest as yet unknown cooperative factors that mediate the activation/inhibition of GATA3.

Natural killer (NK) cell development

The formation and characterization of NK cells are still being elucidated. A bipotent T/NK progenitor

(TKNP) has been found in the human fetal thymus, and is characterized by being CD34$^+$CD7$^+$CD1a$^-$. Within the thymus, these TNKP are found in close relation to NK progenitors (NKP) as well as T-cells, suggesting that the TNKP are their immediate precursor. However, inducible deletion of murine notch, a membrane receptor critical for T-cell formation, does not appear to influence NK cell numbers, suggesting that NK cell formation may be a default program for cells failing to develop into T-cells.

NKP in humans have been difficult to characterize phenotypically. NK formation following IL15 signaling via CD122 is an essential feature of the NKP in mice; however, CD122 has been difficult to demonstrate in humans (despite IL-15 sensitivity). A more recent study isolated mature/functional CD56^{hi} NK cells from a novel hematopoietic precursor expressing CD34^{dim}CD45RA$^+$ α4β7^{hi} in a stromal cell culture system following the addition of IL-2 or IL-15. These precursors were found in the bone marrow and peripheral blood, but appeared to be highly enriched in lymph nodes, suggesting migration to these sites. In fact, further characterization of these cells revealed expression of the lymph node-homing ligand CCR7 and CD62L.

Following activation by APC surface-bound IL-15, circulating CD34$^+$/CD45RA$^+$ pro-NK mature through pre-NK and immature-NK intermediates before forming the CD56^{bright}NK (characterized as NKp46$^+$, CD94/NKG2A$^+$, cd117$^{+/-}$, KIR$^{+/-}$). The LN resident CD56^{bright}NK cell can produce significant amount of cytokines/chemokines on activation, but only poorly eliminate tumor cells. CD56^{dim}NK cells, alternatively, are more adept at cancer cell killing and less so at cytokine/chemokine release. These cells are characterized as NKp46$^+$CD94/NKG2A$^{+/-}$ CD16$^+$ (the low-affinity F$_C$ receptor IIIA), and KIR$^+$, and comprise the majority of circulating NK cells. F$_C$ binding to CD16 leads to NK cell degranulation and perforin-dependent cellular killing. In fact, NK cells harboring a CD16 polymorphism that increased affinity for Rituximab demonstrated an improved response to the drug. It is not yet clear whether CD56^{dim}NK cells mature from the CD56^{bright}NK cells, or whether these reflect two different maturation pathways.

The cytokines and transcriptional events involved in NK maturation are still being elucidated. NKP numbers are not clearly affected by mutations of c-Kit, and are only slightly reduced in the absence of Flt3, again suggesting that NK cell formation may be a default pathway. Alternatively, NK cell formation and function appear to be critically dependent on the transcription factors Ets-1 and Ikaros.

Leukemia stem cells

Leukemias appear to depend on a small population of leukemia stem cells (LSC), which also are called leukemia initiating cells (LIC), for their continued growth and propagation [143, 144]. The LSC/LIC is likely to be a crucial cellular target in the treatment of leukemias and, therefore, it is critical to understand the difference of cellular properties between LSCs and normal HSCs, and between LSCs and other proliferating leukemia cells.

Evidence for LSC/LIC was initially suggested by Buick and McCulloch, who found that AML-CFUs had a heterogeneous capacity for serial replating efficiency [145]. Dick et al. ultimately demonstrated this concept *in vivo* in 1994. In this now classic experiment, the transplantation of $CD34^+CD38^-$, but not $CD34^+CD38^+$ leukemia cells into lethally irradiated, immunodeficient NOD-SCID mice successfully repopulated the bone marrow and transmitted AML. These data suggest that, akin to normal hematopoiesis, leukemias may be maintained by a small minority of stem-like leukemia cells [146]. Furthering this concept has been the identification of LT-LSC and ST-LSC by Morrison and Weissman, and by Dick et al. [147, 148]. As was the case for LT-HSC, LT-LSC proved capable of long-term persistence in xenotransplanted mice, while ST-LSC demonstrated only an abbreviated capacity for repopulation.

It is not clear that mutational events must occur in HSCs. Transfection of MLL-GAS7, a chromosomal translocation known to produce mixed-lineage leukemias, was only able to do so in HSCs and MPPs, but not in lineage-restricted progenitors [149]. However, transfection with other leukemia encoding translocations (MOZ-TIF2, MLL-AF9, MLL-ENL) produced a leukemic phenotype regardless of the stage of differentiation of the transduced cells [150–152]. This concept is further refined by studies involving humans with leukemia arising out of the AML1-ETO translocation. In this setting, more primitive MPP cells ($CD34^+CD90^-CD38^-$) chimeric for this mutation produced normally differentiating multilineage clonogenic precursors, while more mature cells ($CD34^+CD90^-CD38^+$) produced leukemic blast colonies, suggesting that while the initial translocation may occur in a primitive stem cell, subsequent events must occur in the committed progenitor pool to enable development of LSC/LIC [153]. This notion of a "pre-leukemic" stem cell is supported by twin studies in which both share a compromising genotype (e.g., MLL, Tel-AML1), yet develop leukemia at different times [154]. In fact, Hong et al. have identified and xenotransplanted these unique preleukemic cells from the non-affected twin, and found them to be clonally related to LSC/LIC from the affected twin [155].

Alternatively, while normal hematopoiesis is thought to proceed in unidirectional manner, the genetic and epigenetic instability inherent to "committed" leukemic cells may allow for dedifferentiation to a LSC/LIC phenotype, as proposed in breast cancer [156]. Phenotypic analysis of LSC/LIC in AML suggests that they are significantly different from normal HSCs. For example, $CD34^+CD38^-$ LSCs in AML lack CD90 expression, and instead express IL-3Rα, similar to what is seen in GMPs. This phenotype could suggest evolution to an LSC/LIC from a mutated GMP via a loss of CD38. More importantly, its aberrant expression may allow targeted therapy without affecting non-leukemic resident HSCs [157]. Indeed, a clinical trial testing this hypothesis has recently completed accrual [158]. Similarly in ALL, LSC/LIC express a $CD34^+CD38^-$ phenotype while retaining CD19 expression [52].

Although stem cells have a high proliferative capacity, they spend most of their time in the G_0 phase of the cell cycle, limiting the efficacy of cell-cycle-specific chemotherapeutic agents or any treatment that requires cell replication in order to be cytotoxic. This may explain the high rate of relapse seen in acute myelogenous leukemias, even after seemingly near-complete eradication of detectable leukemia cells with conventional regimens. Additionally, the commonly observed decreases in progression-free survival and increases in chemotherapy resistance with successive chemotherapy regimens also may be a consequence of expansion of the LSCs, which are resistant to therapy.

Little is known about the LSC/LIC niche or microenvironment in the bone marrow, although in certain situations, the niche may even promote a malignant phenotype, as seen in Rb inactivation studies [159]. Presence of the $\alpha 4\beta 1$ integrin, VLA-4, on AML blast cells has been found to be associated with resistance to chemotherapy. It has been postulated that the VLA-4 induces resistance of the AML blasts to chemotherapy by mediating binding of the VLA-4$^+$ blasts (which may be LSC/LIC) to stromal fibronectin [160]. Emerging preclinical data are beginning to accumulate suggesting that targeted inhibition of specific chemokines (CXCR4) and cell surface molecules (e.g., CD44, CD123) may impair the ability of LSCs to interact with their niche, and allow for more successful therapeutic outcomes [15, 161, 162]. What is still unknown is whether LSC/LIC inhabit specific areas of the bone marrow microenvironment, particularly the endosteal region, which appears to protect normal LT-HSC that remain in the non-dividing G_0 state, and whether the normal niche functions to protect LSC/LIC by mechanisms similar to the effects of the niche on normal LT-HSC, or whether LSC/LIC are capable of interacting with distinct protective microenvironments of their own.

Summary

Malignancy in the hematopoietic system can be traced to multiple steps along respective developmental paradigms, reflecting distinct changes in factors that govern differentiation, survival, and proliferation. As described herein and in subsequent chapters, such stimuli are diverse, and often require perturbations in both intrinsic and extrinsic mechanisms before ultimately culminating in a neoplastic phenotype.

References

1 Till JE, McCulloch EA. (1961) A direct measurement of the radiation sensitivity of normal mouse bone marrow cells. *Radiat Res* **14**:213–22.

2 Rosendaal M, Dixon R, Panayi M. (1981) Haemopoietic stem cells: possibility of toxic effects of 5-fluorouracil on spleen colony formation. *Blood Cells* **7**:561–74.

3 Ward AC, Touw I, Yoshimura A. (2000) The Jak-Stat pathway in normal and perturbed hematopoiesis. *Blood* **95**:19–29.

4 Vivanco I, Sawyers CL. (2002) The phosphatidylinositol 3-Kinase AKT pathway in human cancer. *Nat Rev Cancer* **2**:489–501.

5 Platanias LC. (2003) Map kinase signaling pathways and hematologic malignancies. *Blood* **101**:4667–79.

6 McCubrey JA, Steelman LS, Abrams SL, et al. (2008) Targeting survival cascades induced by activation of Ras/Raf/MEK/ERK, PI3K/PTEN/Akt/mTOR and Jak/STAT pathways for effective leukemia therapy. *Leukemia* **22**:708–22.

7 Spizzo R, Nicoloso MS, Croce CM, Calin GA. (2009) SnapShot: MicroRNAs in Cancer. *Cell* **137**:586–586 e1.

8 Pelosi E, Labbaye C, Testa U. (2009) MicroRNAs in normal and malignant myelopoiesis. *Leuk Res* **33**:1584–93.

9 Fabbri M, Croce CM, Calin GA. (2009) MicroRNAs in the ontogeny of leukemias and lymphomas. *Leuk Lymphoma* **50**:160–70.

10 Zhang J, Jima DD, Jacobs C, et al. (2009) Patterns of microRNA expression characterize stages of human B-cell differentiation. *Blood* **113**:4586–94.

11 Hashimi ST, Fulcher JA, Chang MH, et al. (2009) MicroRNA profiling identifies miR-34a and miR-21 and their target genes JAG1 and WNT1 in the coordinate regulation of dendritic cell differentiation. *Blood* **114**:404–14.

12 Magnon C, Frenette, PS. (July 14, 2008) Hematopoietic stem cell trafficking. In The Stem Cell Research Community (eds.), *StemBook*, doi/10.3824/stembook.1.8.1, http://www.stembook.org (accessed September 23, 2010).

13 Xia L, McDaniel JM, Yago T, Doeden A, McEver RP. (2004) Surface fucosylation of human cord blood cells augments binding to P-selectin and E-selectin and enhances engraftment in bone marrow. *Blood* **104**:3091–6.

14 Krause DS, Lazarides K, von Andrian UH, Van Etten RA. (2006) Requirement for CD44 in homing and engraftment of BCR-ABL-expressing leukemic stem cells. *Nat Med* **12**:1175–80.

15 Jin L, Hope KJ, Zhai Q, Smadja-Joffe F, Dick JE. (2006) Targeting of CD44 eradicates human acute myeloid leukemic stem cells. *Nat Med* **12**:1167–74.

16 Kopp HG, Avecilla ST, Hooper AT, et al. (2005) Tie2 activation contributes to hemangiogenic regeneration after myelosuppression. *Blood* **106**:505–13.

17 Papayannopoulou T, Scadden DT. (2008) Stem-cell ecology and stem cells in motion. *Blood* **111**:3923–30.

18 Chasis JA, Mohandas N. (2008) Erythroblastic islands: niches for erythropoiesis. *Blood* **112**:470–8.

19 Goodell MA, Rosenzweig M, Kim H, et al. (1997) Dye efflux studies suggest that hematopoietic stem cells expressing low or undetectable levels of CD34 antigen exist in multiple species. *Nat Med* **3**:1337–45.

20 Gangenahalli GU, Singh VK, Verma YK, et al. (2006) Hematopoietic stem cell antigen CD34: role in adhesion or homing. *Stem Cells Dev* **15**:305–13.

21 Kunisato A, Chiba S, Saito T, et al. (2004) Stem cell leukemia protein directs hematopoietic stem cell fate. *Blood* **103**:3336–41.

22 Hoang T. (2004) The origin of hematopoietic cell type diversity. *Oncogene* **23**:7188–98.

23 Laslo P, Spooner CJ, Warmflash A, et al. (2006) Multilineage transcriptional priming and determination of alternate hematopoietic cell fates. *Cell* **126**:755–66.

24 Huang G, Zhang P, Hirai H, et al. (2008) PU.1 is a major downstream target of AML1 (RUNX1) in adult mouse hematopoiesis. *Nat Genet* **40**:51–60.

25 Galy A, Travis M, Cen D, Chen B. (1995) Human T, B, natural killer, and dendritic cells arise from a common bone marrow progenitor cell subset. *Immunity* **3**:459–73.

26 Ryan DH, Nuccie BL, Ritterman I, et al. (1997) Expression of interleukin-7 receptor by lineage-negative human bone marrow progenitors with enhanced lymphoid proliferative potential and B-lineage differentiation capacity. *Blood* **89**:929–40.

27 Haddad R, Guardiola P, Izac B, et al. (2004) Molecular characterization of early human T/NK and B-lymphoid progenitor cells in umbilical cord blood. *Blood* **104**:3918–26.

28 Rossi MI, Yokota T, Medina KL, et al. (2003) B lymphopoiesis is active throughout human life, but there are developmental age-related changes. *Blood* **101**:576–84.

29 Blom B, Spits H. (2006) Development of human lymphoid cells. *Annu Rev Immunol* **24**:287–320.

30 Radtke F, Wilson A, Stark G, et al. (1999) Deficient T cell fate specification in mice with an induced inactivation of Notch1. *Immunity* **10**:547–58.

31 Bond HM, Mesuraca M, Carbone E, et al. (2004) Early hematopoietic zinc finger protein (EHZF), the human homolog to mouse Evi3, is highly expressed in primitive human hematopoietic cells. *Blood* **103**:2062–70.

32 Jaleco AC, Stegmann AP, Heemskerk MH, et al. (1999) Genetic modification of human B-cell development: B-cell development is inhibited by the dominant negative helix loop helix factor Id3. *Blood* **94**:2637–46.

33 Souabni A, Cobaleda C, Schebesta M, Busslinger M. (2002) Pax5 promotes B lymphopoiesis and blocks T cell development by repressing Notch1. *Immunity* **17**:781–93.

34 Tagoh H, Ingram R, Wilson N, et al. (2006) The mechanism of repression of the myeloid-specific c-fms gene by Pax5 during B lineage restriction. *EMBO J* **25**:1070–80.

35 Delogu A, Schebesta A, Sun Q, et al. (2006) Gene repression by Pax5 in B cells is essential for blood cell homeostasis and is reversed in plasma cells. *Immunity* **24**:269–81.

36 Liu P, Keller JR, Ortiz M, et al. (2003) Bcl11a is essential for normal lymphoid development. *Nat Immunol* **4**:525–32.

37 Ferreira BI, Garcia JF, Suela J, et al. (2008) Comparative genome profiling across subtypes of low-grade B-cell lymphoma identifies type-specific and common aberrations that target genes with a role in B-cell neoplasia. *Haematologica*. **93**:670–9.

38 Manz MG, Miyamoto T, Akashi K, Weissman IL. (2002) Prospective isolation of human clonogenic common myeloid progenitors. *Proc Natl Acad Sci U S A* **99**:11872–7.

39 Rappold I, Ziegler BL, Kohler I, et al. (1997) Functional and phenotypic characterization of cord blood and bone marrow subsets expressing FLT3 (CD135) receptor tyrosine kinase. *Blood* **90**:111–25.

40 Sitnicka E, Buza-Vidas N, Larsson S, et al. (2003) Human CD34 + hematopoietic stem cells capable of multilineage engrafting NOD/SCID mice express flt3: distinct flt3 and c-kit expression and response patterns

on mouse and candidate human hematopoietic stem cells. *Blood* **102**:881–6.

41 Iwasaki H, Akashi K. (2007) Hematopoietic developmental pathways: on cellular basis. *Oncogene* **26**:6687–96.

42 Stopka T, Amanatullah DF, Papetti M, Skoultchi AI. (2005) PU.1 inhibits the erythroid program by binding to GATA-1 on DNA and creating a repressive chromatin structure. *EMBO J* **24**:3712–23.

43 Zhang P, Behre G, Pan J, et al. (1999) Negative between hematopoietic regulators: GATA proteins repress PU.1. *Proc Natl Acad Sci U S A* **96**:8705–10.

44 Battinelli EM, Hartwig JH, Italiano JE, Jr., (2007) Delivering new insight into the biology of megakaryopoiesis and thrombopoiesis. *Curr Opin Hematol* **14**:419–26.

45 Kaushansky K. (2008) Historical review: megakaryopoiesis and thrombopoiesis. *Blood* **111**:981–6.

46 Broudy VC, Lin NL, Kaushansky K. (1995) Thrombopoietin (c-mpl ligand) acts synergistically with erythropoietin, stem cell factor, and interleukin-11 to enhance murine megakaryocyte colony growth and increases megakaryocyte ploidy in vitro. *Blood* **85**:1719–26.

47 Goldfarb AN. (2007) Transcriptional control of megakaryocyte development. *Oncogene* **26**:6795–802.

48 Saleque S, Cameron S, Orkin SH. (2002) The zinc-finger proto-oncogene Gfi-1b is essential for development of the erythroid and megakaryocytic lineages. *Genes Dev* **16**:301–6.

49 Hamlett I, Draper J, Strouboulis J, et al. (2008) Characterization of megakaryocyte GATA1-interacting proteins: the corepressor ETO2 and GATA1 interact to regulate terminal megakaryocyte maturation. *Blood* **112**:2738–49.

50 Elmaagacli AH, Koldehoff M, Zakrzewski JL, et al. (2007) Growth factor-independent 1B gene (GFI1B) is overexpressed in erythropoietic and megakaryocytic malignancies and increases their proliferation rate. *Br J Haematol* **136**:212–9.

51 Gamou T, Kitamura E, Hosoda F, et al. (1998) The partner gene of AML1 in t(16;21) myeloid malignancies is a novel member of the MTG8(ETO) family. *Blood* **91**:4028–37.

52 Castor A, Nilsson L, Astrand-Grundstrom I, et al. (2005) Distinct patterns of hematopoietic stem cell involvement in acute lymphoblastic leukemia. *Nat Med* **11**:630–7.

53 Sun W, DowningJr., (2004) Haploinsufficiency of AML1 results in a decrease in the number of LTR-HSCs while simultaneously inducing an increase in more mature progenitors. *Blood* **104**:3565–72.

54 Wu H, Liu X, Jaenisch R, Lodish HF. (1995) Generation of committed erythroid BFU-E and CFU-E progenitors does not require erythropoietin or the erythropoietin receptor. *Cell* **83**:59–67.

55 Osawa M, Yamaguchi T, Nakamura Y, et al. (2002) Erythroid expansion mediated by the Gfi-1B zinc finger protein: role in normal hematopoiesis. *Blood* **100**:2769–77.

56 Kuo YY, Chang ZF. (2007) GATA-1 and Gfi-1B interplay to regulate Bcl-xL transcription. *Mol Cell Biol* **27**:4261–72.

57 Loose M, Swiers G, Patient R. (2007) Transcriptional networks regulating hematopoietic cell fate decisions. *Curr Opin Hematol* **14**:307–14.

58 Friedman AD. (2007) Transcriptional control of granulocyte and monocyte development. *Oncogene* **26**:6816–28.

59 Jack GD, Zhang L, Friedman AD. (2009) M-CSF elevates c-Fos and phospho-C/EBP{alpha}(S21) via ERK whereas G-CSF stimulates SHP2 phosphorylation in marrow progenitors to contribute to myeloid lineage specification. *Blood* **114**:2172–80.

60 Bei L, Lu Y, Eklund EA. (2005) HOXA9 activates transcription of the gene encoding gp91Phox during myeloid differentiation. *J Biol Chem* **280**:12359–70.

61 Eklund EA, Jalava A, Kakar R. (2000) Tyrosine phosphorylation of HoxA10 decreases DNA binding and transcriptional repression during interferon gamma-induced differentiation of myeloid leukemia cell lines. *J Biol Chem* **275**:20117–26.

62 Lindsey S, Huang W, Wang H, et al. (2007) Activation of SHP2 protein-tyrosine phosphatase increases HoxA10-induced repression of the genes encoding gp91(PHOX) and p67(PHOX). *J Biol Chem* **282**:2237–49.

63 Tartaglia M, Niemeyer CM, Fragale A, et al. (2003) Somatic mutations in PTPN11 in juvenile myelomonocytic leukemia, myelodysplastic syndromes and acute myeloid leukemia. *Nat Gene* **34**:148–50.

64 Loh ML, Vattikuti S, Schubbert S, et al. (2004) Mutations in PTPN11 implicate the SHP-2 phosphatase in leukemogenesis. *Blood* **103**:2325–31.

65 Wouters BJ, Lowenberg B, Erpelinck-Verschueren CA, et al. (2009) Double CEBPA mutations, but not

single CEBPA mutations, define a subgroup of acute myeloid leukemia with a distinctive gene expression profile that is uniquely associated with a favorable outcome. *Blood* **113**:3088–91.

66 Ho PA, Alonzo TA, Gerbing RB, et al. (2009) Prevalence and prognostic implications of CEBPA mutations in pediatric acute myeloid leukemia (AML): a report from the Children's Oncology Group. *Blood* **113**:6558–66.

67 Taschner S, Koesters C, Platzer B, et al. (2007) Down-regulation of RXRalpha expression is essential for neutrophil development from granulocyte/monocyte progenitors. *Blood* **109**:971–9.

68 Lawson ND, Khanna-Gupta A, Berliner N. (1998) Isolation and characterization of the cDNA for mouse neutrophil collagenase: demonstration of shared negative regulatory pathways for neutrophil secondary granule protein gene expression. *Blood* **91**:2517–24.

69 Khanna-Gupta A, Zibello T, Sun H, et al. (2001) C/EBP epsilon mediates myeloid differentiation and is regulated by the CCAAT displacement protein (CDP/cut). *Proc Natl Acad Sci U S A* **98**:8000–5.

70 Cadieux C, Fournier S, Peterson AC, et al. (2006) Transgenic mice expressing the p75 CCAAT-displacement protein/Cut homeobox isoform develop a myeloproliferative disease-like myeloid leukemia. *Cancer Res* **66**:9492–501.

71 Boyce JA, Friend D, Matsumoto R, Austen KF, Owen WF. (1995) Differentiation in vitro of hybrid eosinophil/basophil granulocytes: autocrine function of an eosinophil developmental intermediate. *J Exp Med* **182**:49–57.

72 Rothenberg ME, Hogan SP. (2006) The eosinophil. *Ann Rev Immunol* **24**:147–74.

73 Arock M, Schneider E, Boissan M, Tricottet V, Dy M. (2002) Differentiation of human basophils: an overview of recent advances and pending questions. *J Leukoc Biol* **71**:557–64.

74 Mlynek ML, Leder LD. (1986) Lineage infidelity in chronic myeloid leukemia. Demonstration and significance of hybridoid leukocytes. *Virchows Arch B Cell Pathol Incl Mol Pathol* **51**:107–14.

75 Kocabas CN, Yavuz AS, Lipsky PE, Metcalfe DD, Akin C. (2005) Analysis of the lineage relationship between mast cells and basophils using the c-kit D816V mutation as a biologic signature. *J Allergy Clin Immunol* **115**:1155–61.

76 Kirshenbaum AS, Goff JP, Semere T, et al. (1999) Demonstration that human mast cells arise from

a progenitor cell population that is CD34(+), c-kit (+), and expresses aminopeptidase N (CD13). *Blood* **94**:2333–42.

77 Lawrence JB, Friedman BS, Travis WD, et al. (1991) Hematologic manifestations of systemic mast cell disease: a prospective study of laboratory and morphologic features and their relation to prognosis. *Am J Med* **91**:612–24.

78 Horny HP, Parwaresch MR, Lennert K. (1985) Bone marrow findings in systemic mastocytosis. *Hum Pathol* **16**:808–14.

79 Lindemann A, Ganser A, Herrmann F, et al. (1991) Biologic effects of recombinant human interleukin-3 in vivo. *J Clin Oncol* **9**:2120–7.

80 Kepley CL, Pfeiffer JR, Schwartz LB, Wilson BS, Oliver JM. (1998) The identification and characterization of umbilical cord blood-derived human basophils. *J Leukoc Biol* **64**:474–83.

81 Galli SJ, Nakae S, Tsai M. (2005) Mast cells in the development of adaptive immune responses. *Nat Immunol* **6**:135–42.

82 Jiang Y, Kanaoka Y, Feng C, et al. (2006) Cutting edge: Interleukin 4-dependent mast cell proliferation requires autocrine/intracrine cysteinyl leukotriene-induced signaling. *J Immunol* **177**:2755–9.

83 Kirshenbaum AS, Akin C, Goff JP, Metcalfe DD. (2005) Thrombopoietin alone or in the presence of stem cell factor supports the growth of KIT(CD117) low/MPL(CD110)+ human mast cells from hematopoietic progenitor cells. *Exp Hematol* **33**:413–21.

84 Metcalfe DD. (2008) Mast cells and mastocytosis. *Blood* **112**:946–56.

85 Iwasaki H, Mizuno S, Arinobu Y, et al. (2006) The order of expression of transcription factors directs hierarchical specification of hematopoietic lineages. *Genes Dev* **20**:3010–21.

86 Arinobu Y, Iwasaki H, Gurish MF, et al. (2005) Developmental checkpoints of the basophil/mast cell lineages in adult murine hematopoiesis. *Proc Natl Acad Sci U S A* **102**:18105–10.

87 Sakata-Yanagimoto M, Nakagami-Yamaguchi E, Saito T, et al. (2008) Coordinated regulation of transcription factors through Notch2 is an important mediator of mast cell fate. *Proc Natl Acad Sci U S A* **105**: 7839–44.

88 Walsh JC, DeKoter RP, Lee HJ, et al. (2002) Cooperative and antagonistic interplay between PU.1 and GATA-2 in the specification of myeloid cell fates. *Immunity* **17**:665–76.

89 Auffray C, Fogg DK, Narni-Mancinelli E, et al. (2009) CX3CR1+ CD115+ CD135+ common macrophage/DC precursors and the role of CX3CR1 in their response to inflammation. *J Exp Med* **206**:595–606.

90 Auffray C, Sieweke MH, Geissmann F. (2009) Blood monocytes: development, heterogeneity, and relationship with dendritic cells. *Annu Rev Immunol* **27**:669–92.

91 Dahl R, Walsh JC, Lancki D, et al. (2003) Regulation of macrophage and neutrophil cell fates by the PU.1:C/EBPalpha ratio and granulocyte colony-stimulating factor. *Nat Immunol* **4**:1029–36.

92 Feinberg MW, Wara AK, Cao Z, et al. (2007) The Kruppel-like factor KLF4 is a critical regulator of monocyte differentiation. *EMBO J* **26**:4138–48.

93 Tamura T, Nagamura-Inoue T, Shmeltzer Z, Kuwata T, Ozato K. (2000) ICSBP directs bipotential myeloid progenitor cells to differentiate into mature macrophages. *Immunity* **13**:155–65.

94 Reddy MA, Yang BS, Yue X, et al. (1994) Opposing actions of c-ets/PU.1 and c-myb protooncogene products in regulating the macrophage-specific promoters of the human and mouse colony-stimulating factor-1 receptor (c-fms) genes. *J Exp Med* **180**:2309–19.

95 DeKoter RP, Walsh JC, Singh H. (1998) PU.1 regulates both cytokine-dependent proliferation and differentiation of granulocyte/macrophage progenitors. *EMBO J* **17**:4456–68.

96 Bakri Y, Sarrazin S, Mayer UP, et al. (2005) Balance of MafB and PU.1 specifies alternative macrophage or dendritic cell fate. *Blood* **105**:2707–16.

97 Sieweke MH, Tekotte H, Frampton J, Graf T. (1996) MafB is an interaction partner and repressor of Ets-1 that inhibits erythroid differentiation. *Cell* **85**:49–60.

98 Merad M, Manz MG. (2009) Dendritic cell homeostasis. *Blood* **113**:3418–27.

99 Laouar Y, Welte T, Fu XY, Flavell RA. (2003) STAT3 is required for Flt3L-dependent dendritic cell differentiation. *Immunity* **19**:903–12.

100 Rathinam C, Geffers R, Yucel R, et al. (2005) The transcriptional repressor Gfi1 controls STAT3-dependent dendritic cell development and function. *Immunity* **22**:717–28.

101 Esashi E, Wang YH, Perng O, et al. (2008) The signal transducer STAT5 inhibits plasmacytoid dendritic cell development by suppressing transcription factor IRF8. *Immunity* **28**:509–20.

102 Onai N, Obata-Onai A, Tussiwand R, Lanzavecchia A, Manz MG. (2006) Activation of the Flt3 signal transduction cascade rescues and enhances type I interferon-producing and dendritic cell development. *J Exp Med* **203**:227–38.

103 Choudhary C, Brandts C, Schwable J, et al. (2007) Activation mechanisms of STAT5 by oncogenic Flt3-ITD. *Blood* **110**:370–4.

104 Nagasawa M, Schmidlin H, Hazekamp MG, Schotte R, Blom B. (2008) Development of human plasmacytoid dendritic cells depends on the combined action of the basic helix-loop-helix factor E2-2 and the Ets factor Spi-B. *Eur J Immunol* **38**:2386–8.

105 Cisse B, Caton ML, Lehner M, et al. (2008) Transcription factor E2-2 is an essential and specific regulator of plasmacytoid dendritic cell development. *Cell* **135**:37–48.

106 Zhou J, Cheng P, Youn JI, Cotter MJ, Gabrilovich DI. (2009) Notch and wingless signaling cooperate in regulation of dendritic cell differentiation. *Immunity* **30**:845–59.

107 Cheng P, Gabrilovich D. (2008) Notch signaling in differentiation and function of dendritic cells. *Immunol Res* **41**:1–14.

108 Wang YH, Nomura J, Faye-Petersen OM, Cooper MD. (1998) Surrogate light chain production during B cell differentiation: differential intracellular versus cell surface expression. *J Immunol* **161**:1132–9.

109 LeBien TW, Tedder TF. (2008) B lymphocytes: how they develop and function. *Blood* **112**:1570–80.

110 LeBien TW. (2000) Fates of human B-cell precursors. *Blood* **96**:9–23.

111 DiLillo DJ, Hamaguchi Y, Ueda Y, et al. (2008) Maintenance of long-lived plasma cells and serological memory despite mature and memory B cell depletion during CD20 immunotherapy in mice. *J Immunol* **180**:361–71.

112 Goetz CA, Harmon IR, O'Neil JJ, et al. (2005) Restricted STAT5 activation dictates appropriate thymic B versus T cell lineage commitment. *J Immunol* **174**:7753–63.

113 Durum SK, Candeias S, Nakajima H, et al. (1998) Interleukin 7 receptor control of T cell receptor gamma gene rearrangement: role of receptor-associated chains and locus accessibility. *J Exp Med* **188**:2233–41.

114 Holmes ML, Pridans C, Nutt SL. (2008) The regulation of the B-cell gene expression programme by Pax5. *Immunol Cell Biol* **86**:47–53.

115 Cobaleda C, Jochum W, Busslinger M. (2007) Conversion of mature B cells into T cells by dedifferentiation to uncommitted progenitors. *Nature* **449**:473–7.

116 Mullighan CG, Goorha S, Radtke I, et al. (2007) Genome-wide analysis of genetic alterations in acute lymphoblastic leukaemia. *Nature* **446**:758–64.

117 Iida S, Rao PH, Nallasivam P, et al. (1996) The t(9;14)(p13;q32) chromosomal translocation associated with lymphoplasmacytoid lymphoma involves the PAX-5 gene. *Blood* **88**:4110–7.

118 Nourse J, Mellentin JD, Galili N, et al. (1990) Chromosomal translocation t(1;19) results in synthesis of a homeobox fusion mRNA that codes for a potential chimeric transcription factor. *Cell* **60**:535–45.

119 Inaba T, Roberts WM, Shapiro LH, et al. (1992) Fusion of the leucine zipper gene HLF to the E2A gene in human acute B-lineage leukemia. *Science* **257**:531–4.

120 Wurbel MA, Philippe JM, Nguyen C, et al. (2000) The chemokine TECK is expressed by thymic and intestinal epithelial cells and attracts double- and single-positive thymocytes expressing the TECK receptor CCR9. *Eur J Immunol* **30**:262–71.

121 Ciofani M, Zuniga-Pflucker JC. (2007) The thymus as an inductive site for T lymphopoiesis. *Annu Rev Cell Dev Biol* **23**:463–93.

122 Ueno T, Saito F, Gray DH, et al. (2004) CCR7 signals are essential for cortex-medulla migration of developing thymocytes. *J Exp Med* **200**:493–505.

123 Giliani S, Mori L, de Saint Basile G, et al. (2005) Interleukin-7 receptor alpha (IL-7Ralpha) deficiency: cellular and molecular bases. Analysis of clinical, immunological, and molecular features in 16 novel patients. *Immunol Rev* **203**:110–26.

124 Macchi P, Villa A, Giliani S, et al. (1995) Mutations of Jak-3 gene in patients with autosomal severe combined immune deficiency (SCID). *Nature* **377**:65–8.

125 Fischer A, Le Deist F, Hacein-Bey-Abina S, et al. (2005) Severe combined immunodeficiency. A model disease for molecular immunology and therapy. *Immunol Rev* **203**:98–109.

126 Opferman JT, Letai A, Beard C, et al. (2003) Development and maintenance of B and T lymphocytes requires antiapoptotic MCL-1. *Nature* **426**:671–6.

127 Wang H, Pierce LJ, Spangrude GJ. (2006) Distinct roles of IL-7 and stem cell factor in the OP9-DL1 T-cell differentiation culture system. *Exp Hematol* **34**:1730–40.

128 Rodewald HR, Kretzschmar K, Swat W, Takeda S. (1995) Intrathymically expressed c-kit ligand (stem cell factor) is a major factor driving expansion of very immature thymocytes in vivo. *Immunity* **3**:313–9.

129 Graf D, Nethisinghe S, Palmer DB, Fisher AG, Merkenschlager M. (2002) The developmentally regulated expression of Twisted gastrulation reveals a role for bone morphogenetic proteins in the control of T cell development. *J Exp Med* **196**:163–71.

130 Hager-Theodorides AL, Outram SV, Shah DK, et al. (2002) Bone morphogenetic protein 2/4 signaling regulates early thymocyte differentiation. *J Immunol* **169**:5496–504.

131 Schwarz BA, Sambandam A, Maillard I, et al. (2007) Selective thymus settling regulated by cytokine and chemokine receptors. *J Immunol* **178**:2008–17.

132 Weng AP, Ferrando AA, Lee W, et al. (2004) Activating mutations of NOTCH1 in human T cell acute lymphoblastic leukemia. *Science* **306**:269–71.

133 Gounari F, Chang R, Cowan J, et al. (2005) Loss of adenomatous polyposis coli gene function disrupts thymic development. *Nat Immunol* **6**:800–9.

134 Fukushima T, Zapata JM, Singha NC, et al. (2006) Critical function for SIP, a ubiquitin E3 ligase component of the beta-catenin degradation pathway, for thymocyte development and G1 checkpoint. *Immunity* **24**:29–39.

135 Yokota Y, Mansouri A, Mori S, et al. (1999) Development of peripheral lymphoid organs and natural killer cells depends on the helix-loop-helix inhibitor Id2. *Nature* **397**:702–6.

136 Blom B, Heemskerk MH, Verschuren MC, et al. (1999) Disruption of alpha beta but not of gamma delta T cell development by overexpression of the helix-loop-helix protein Id3 in committed T cell progenitors. *EMBO J* **18**:2793–802.

137 Shah DK, Hager-Theodorides AL, Outram SV, et al. (2004) Reduced thymocyte development in sonic hedgehog knockout embryos. *J Immunol* **172**:2296–306.

138 Outram SV, Varas A, Pepicelli CV, Crompton T. (2000) Hedgehog signaling regulates differentiation from double-negative to double-positive thymocyte. *Immunity* **13**:187–97.

139 Singh RR, Cho-Vega JH, Davuluri Y, et al. (2009) Sonic hedgehog signaling pathway is activated in ALK-positive anaplastic large cell lymphoma. *Cancer Res* **69**:2550–8.

140 Kobune M, Takimoto R, Murase K, et al. (2009) Drug resistance is dramatically restored by hedgehog inhibitors in CD34+ leukemic cells. *Cancer Sci* **100**:948–55.

141 Taghon T, De Smedt M, Stolz F, et al. (2001) Enforced expression of GATA-3 severely reduces human thymic cellularity. *J Immunol* **167**:4468–75.

142 Pai SY, Truitt ML, Ting CN, et al. (2003) Critical roles for transcription factor GATA-3 in thymocyte development. *Immunity* **19**:863–75.

143 Passegue E, Jamieson CH, Ailles LE, Weissman IL. (2003) Normal and leukemic hematopoiesis: are leukemias a stem cell disorder or a reacquisition of stem cell characteristics? *Proc Natl Acad Sci U S A* **100**:11842–9.

144 Huntly BJ, Gilliland DG. (2005) Leukaemia stem cells and the evolution of cancer-stem-cell research. *Nat Rev Cancer* **5**:311–21.

145 Buick RN, Minden MD, McCulloch EA. (1979) Self-renewal in culture of proliferative blast progenitor cells in acute myeloblastic leukemia. *Blood* **54**:95–104.

146 Lapidot T, Sirard C, Vormoor J, et al. (1994) A cell initiating human acute myeloid leukaemia after transplantation into SCID mice. *Nature* **367**:645–8.

147 Morrison SJ, Weissman IL. (1994) The long-term repopulating subset of hematopoietic stem cells is deterministic and isolatable by phenotype. *Immunity* **1**:661–73.

148 Hope KJ, Jin L, Dick JE. (2004) Acute myeloid leukemia originates from a hierarchy of leukemic stem cell classes that differ in self-renewal capacity. *Nat Immunol* **5**:738–43.

149 So CW, Karsunky H, Passegue E, et al. (2003) MLL-GAS7 transforms multipotent hematopoietic progenitors and induces mixed lineage leukemias in mice. *Cancer Cell* **3**:161–71.

150 Huntly BJ, Shigematsu H, Deguchi K, et al. (2004) MOZ-TIF2, but not BCR-ABL, confers properties of leukemic stem cells to committed murine hematopoietic progenitors. *Cancer Cell* **6**:587–96.

151 Krivtsov AV, Twomey D, Feng Z, et al. (2006) Transformation from committed progenitor to leukaemia stem cell initiated by MLL-AF9. *Nature* **442**:818–22.

152 Cozzio A, Passegue E, Ayton PM, et al. (2003) Similar MLL-associated leukemias arising from self-renewing stem cells and short-lived myeloid progenitors. *Genes Dev* **17**:3029–35.

153 Miyamoto T, Weissman IL, Akashi K. (2000) AML1/ETO-expressing nonleukemic stem cells in acute myelogenous leukemia with 8;21 chromosomal translocation. *Proc Natl Acad Sci U S A* **97**:7521–6.

154 Greaves MF, Wiemels J. (2003) Origins of chromosome translocations in childhood leukaemia. *Nat Rev Cancer* **3**:639–49.

155 Hong D, Gupta R, Ancliff P, et al. (2008) Initiating and cancer-propagating cells in TEL-AML1-associated childhood leukemia. *Science* **319**:336–9.

156 Mani SA, Guo W, Liao MJ, et al. (2008) The epithelial-mesenchymal transition generates cells with properties of stem cells. *Cell* **133**:704–15.

157 Jin L, Lee EM, Ramshaw HS, et al. (2009) Monoclonal antibody-mediated targeting of CD123, IL-3 receptor alpha chain, eliminates human acute myeloid leukemic stem cells. *Cell Stem Cell* **5**:31–42.

158 Phase I study of **CSL360** in patients with relapsed, refractory or high-risk acute myeloid leukemia, at http://clinicaltrials.gov/ct2/show/NCT00401739?term=CSL360&rank=1 (last accessed September 24, 2010).

159 Walkley CR, Shea JM, Sims NA, Purton LE, Orkin SH. (2007) Rb regulates interactions between hematopoietic stem cells and their bone marrow microenvironment. *Cell* **129**:1081–95.

160 Matsunaga T, Takemoto N, Sato T, et al. (2003) Interaction between leukemic-cell VLA-4 and stromal fibronectin is a decisive factor for minimal residual disease of acute myelogenous leukemia. *Nat Med* **9**:1158–65.

161 Nervi B, Ramirez P, Rettig MP, et al. (2009) Chemosensitization of acute myeloid leukemia (AML) following mobilization by the CXCR4 antagonist AMD3100. *Blood* **113**:6206–14.

162 Zeng Z, Shi YX, Samudio IJ, et al. (2009) Targeting the leukemia microenvironment by CXCR4 inhibition overcomes resistance to kinase inhibitors and chemotherapy in AML. *Blood* **113**:6215–24.

CHAPTER 2

The Leukemia Genome

Jonathan C. Strefford[1] and Nicholas C.P. Cross[2]
[1]Cancer Genomics Group, Cancer Sciences Division, University of Southampton, Southampton , UK
[2]Wessex Regional Genetics Laboratory, Salisbury and Human Genetics Division, University of Southampton, Southampton, UK

Introduction

The human genome is a blueprint of the genetic information required for human development and function, and is annotated by just over three billion base pairs of deoxyribonucleic acid (DNA). In the form of chromatin, DNA and bound proteins are super coiled and packed into 23 chromosome pairs, which have historically been identified by their size, centromeric position, and banding pattern (Figure 2.1(A)). Approximately 25 000 protein coding genes (PCG) are unevenly distributed between these chromosomes; a proportion of the remaining sequence has a regulatory function or encodes diverse RNA species. A further layer of control is provided by epigenetic changes, in the form of differential methylation and chromatin modifications. Early insights into the pivotal role of the genome in carcinogenesis emerged in the latter half of the nineteenth and early in the twentieth centuries. These studies analyzed cancer cells under the microscope, and showed the presence of complex aberrant mitoses, providing the first evidence that cancer is characterized by and caused by abnormalities at the DNA levels [1]. Later, the demonstration of chemically induced carcinogenesis by the use of DNA damaging agents, the identification of recurrent chromosomal abnormalities in cancer cells, and the induction of cancer in a phenotypically normal cell by the introduction of DNA from a cancer cell all supported a key role for genetic alterations in carcinogenic processes. Isolation of DNA sequences responsible for transformation led to the identification of the first naturally occurring sequence mutation, the single base-pair substitution in codon 12 of the *HRAS* gene [2]. As a consequence of a recent explosion of information, it is now well established that errors in the genetic code and dysfunction of a variety of DNA sequence regulatory mechanisms are the hallmark of human cancer. Due to the ease by which suitable material could be acquired, much of the genetic research relating to cancer has been in the context of hematological disease. Here we review our current understanding of the genetic alterations that occur in the leukemia genome, their role in disease pathophysiology and the application of this information to the clinical setting.

The leukemic cell

Although a leukemic cell is derived from embryonic tissue, and hence carries a diploid genome, it has acquired additional somatic alterations that include chromosomal rearrangements, large-scale copy number alterations, small insertions and deletions and single base-pair changes (Table 2.1). In addition, foreign DNA sequences can be acquired from external sources such as viruses. Epigenetic changes that alter chromatin structure and gene expression can also occur during cancer development and progression, while somatically acquired mitochondrial mutations have also been reported. DNA sequence changes present in a cancer cell are a reflection of the

Advances in Malignant Hematology, First Edition. Edited by Hussain I. Saba and Ghulam J. Mufti. © 2011 Blackwell Publishing Ltd.
Published 2011 by Blackwell Publishing Ltd.

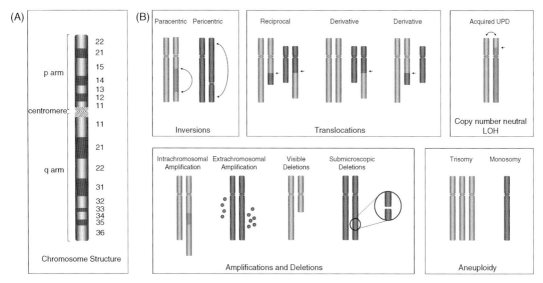

Figure 2.1 Cytogenetic nomenclature and chromosomal abnormalities in hematological malignancy. (A) Shows an idiogram for the human normal chromosome 7. The 46 chromosomes in a normal cell are divided into autosomes, numbered from 1 to 22 and sex chromosomes, referred to as X and Y. Each chromosome contains a centromere and two telomeres. The centromere divides the chromosome into a long (q) and short (p) arm. Chromosomes are captured during metaphase and chemically modified (generally an enzymatic digestion followed by staining the DNA) to produce a specific banding pattern when viewed using a microscope. The bands are numbered from the centromere outwards. Analysis of the resulting banding pattern can allow the identification of normal and structurally rearranged chromosomes. (B) Chromosomal alterations in human malignancy. These abnormalities can be subdivided based on whether the alteration results in no change in chromo-somal dosage (balanced) or a genomic imbalance (unbalanced). Balanced rearrangements include inversions, where the involvement of the centromere in the inversion event is termed a pericentric inversion, and translocation, where this is a reciprocal exchange of material between two chromosomes. Acquired uniparental disomy describes an LOH event with no corresponding copy number change, resulting from the duplication of a single ancestrally derived chromosome or genomic region. Genomic imbalances can be categorized into gains and loss. Genomic imbalances can be the result of numerical and structural rearrangements. Numerical alterations include loss (monosomy) and gain (trisomy) of entire chromosome. Structural imbalances include intrachromosomal or extrachromosomal amplification, cytogenetically visible and submicroscopic deletions, and imbalances that are the result of unbalanced translocations.

cell's evolutionary history. Under normal circumstances, DNA is continually damaged by external mutagens and as a consequence of normal cellular processes, such as DNA replication. The majority of these changes will be correctly repaired or the cell will undergo controlled cell death (apoptosis) to ensure that the alteration is not propagated into daughter cells. However, a small fraction of this continual DNA damage will be fixed into the genome and replicated through future mitotic cell divisions. The rate at which these mutations occur is still unclear, but it is well established that exposure to substantial exogenous mutagens, such as tobacco carcinogens, increase the mutation rate and is associated with increased frequency of certain epithelial cancer types. The rate of certain somatic alterations is also increased in several rare inherited diseases, each of which is associated with increased risk of malignancy. Certain fixed sequence changes can provide carcinogenic potential, and additional alterations can be acquired that contribute further to the cancer phenotype. Indeed, early mutational events can increase the rate at which cells acquire further damage by compromising key regulatory pathways, such as cell cycle checkpoints and DNA repair. Each somatic mutation in a cancer genome can be categorized based on the phenotypic effect. "Driver"

Table 2.1 Examples of somatically acquired genetic alterations in hematological neoplasia

Gene(s)	Frequency and disease type	Biological consequences	Reference
Gene mutations			
NOTCH1[1]	~50% of T ALL	Constitutive activation of this transmembrane receptor, regulates T-cell development	[71]
NPM1[2]	~35% of AML	Relocalize nucleocytoplasmic shuttling protein to the cytoplasm, regulates the TP53 pathway	[72]
FLT3	~20% of AML	Constitutive activation of this receptor tyrosine kinase, regulates hematopoiesis	[73]
WT1[3]	~13% of CN-AML[4]	Disruption is thought to promote proliferation and inhibit differentiation	[74]
Balanced translocations			
ETV6[5]-RUNX1	~25% of BCP ALL	Fusion converts RUNX1 to a negative transcriptional regulator impeding differentiation	[75]
TCF3[6]-PBX1[7]	~5% of ALL	Fusion contributes to deregulation of HOX genes	[76]
IGH@-CRLF2[8]	U[9]	Induces deregulation of CRLF2 drives cell proliferation	[77]
Unbalanced translocations			
PAX5-ETV6[5]	1% of ALL	Fusion acts as a dominant negative regulator of wild-type PAX5	[78]
Copy number gains			
NUP214-ABL1	~6% of T ALL	Amplified episomal fusion acts as a constitutively activated tyrosine kinase	[22]
MYB	~8% of T ALL	Duplication results in overexpression and blocks differentiation	[26]
Copy number losses			
CDKN2A	~20% B ALL	Loss of proliferative control and cell cycle regulation	
	~50% of T ALL		[79]
Copy number neutral LOH			
TET2[10]	~14% of MPN[11]	Inactivation mutation has proposed role in hematopoietic stem cell development	[80]

[1]Notch homolog 1, translocation-associated (Drosophila);
[2]Nucleophosmin (nucleolar phosphoprotein B23, numatrin);
[3]Wilms tumor 1;
[4]Cytogenetically normal acute myeloid leukemia;
[5]Ets variant 6;
[6]Transcription factor 3 (E2A immunoglobulin enhancer binding factors E12/E47);
[7]Pre-B-cell leukemia homeobox 1;
[8]Cytokine receptor-like factor 2;
[9]Unknown;
[10]Tet oncogene family member 2;
[11]Myeloproliferative neoplasms

mutations are causally implicated in oncogenesis, confer some type of cellular advantage, and are selected for during cancer evolution, while "passenger" mutations are unselected and provide no growth advantage; instead they are the consequence of co-selection with driver mutations. The number of driver mutations required for carcinogenesis is pivotal to understanding the genetic basis of cancer development and progression. Although the precise number has not been established, it is likely that multiple events are required and that epithelial cancers require more "hits" than hematological malignancies. Historically, the most productive route for identification of cancer genes has been through the analysis of cytogenetically visible chromosomal rearrangements in leukemia and lymphoma.

Chromosomal rearrangements

Although the presence of chromosomal abnormalities in cancer was initially described in the nineteenth century, it was only much later that the recurrent nature of these changes was recognized. In 1960, Nowell and Hungerford discovered the Philadelphia chromosome (Ph), a small abnormal chromosome in patients with chronic myeloid leukemia (CML) [3]. This landmark observation represented the identification of the first recurrent genetic aberration in cancer. With the advent of chromosomal banding techniques in the early 1970s [4], the Ph chromosome was shown to be the smaller derivative of a balanced translocation between chromosomes 9 and 22, the t(9;22)(q34;q11.2). Later, other rearrangements were identified in acute myeloid leukemia (AML) such as the t(15;17)(q22;q11) in acute promyelocytic leukemia, inversion of chromosome 16, inv(16)(p13q22) in acute myelomonocytic leukemia, and t(8;21)(q22;q22) in acute myeloblastic leukemia (reviewed in [5]). These three chromosomal rearrangements are associated with a relatively favorable clinical outcome. In acute lymphoblastic leukemia (ALL), the independent prognostic association of specific chromosomal changes has been known for some time. For example, high hyperdiploidy (51–65 chromosomes) is linked to a good outcome in childhood ALL [6]. Cancer cells exhibit a variety of chromosomal rearrangements, the majority of which are shown in Figure 2.1(B). The advent of molecular cytogenetic techniques, such as fluorescence in situ hybridization (FISH), multicolor FISH and array-based comparative genomic hybridization (aCGH) have added a further level of detail to our understanding of the relationship between changes at the chromosomal level and cancer pathophysiology (reviewed in [7]).

With regard to their functional consequences, recurrent chromosomal rearrangements are of two general types: alterations that result in the formation of a novel, functionally distinct chimeric fusion gene, and those that deregulate the expression of a structurally normal gene. There is now clear evidence that these rearrangements are early or initiating events in leukemogenesis. For instance, in children who develop acute leukemia, certain translocations occur in utero years before the appearance of overt disease [8]. The ability of these chromosomal abnormalities to act as leukemia-initiating events is further demonstrated by: (1) their ability to induce specific neoplastic disorders in experimental animal models [9], (2) reversal of the leukemic phenotype by in vitro silencing of the fusion gene transcript by the use of small non-coding RNA molecules [10], (3) the association of certain rearrangements with specific tumor phenotypes [11], (4) successful disease treatment is linked to a decrease or eradication of the disease-related fusion gene [12], and finally, (5) the clinical success of therapies targeted at specific acquired abnormalities.

Chimeric fusions can be categorized by the genes that are involved in these rearrangements, most commonly those that encode tyrosine kinases and transcription factors. The most notable example of the former remains the Ph chromosome, present in virtually all patients with CML, approximately 20–40% of patients with ALL, and in rare cases of AML. The t(9;22) that gives rise to the Ph chromosome fuses the *BCR* (breakpoint cluster region) gene on band 22q11.2 to part of the gene encoding the cytoplasmic *ABL1* (c-abl oncogene 1) tyrosine kinase on band 9q34.1. The resulting chimeric protein, BCR-ABL1, contains the catalytic domain of ABL1 fused to a domain of BCR that mediates constitutive oligomerization of the fusion protein in the absence of physiological activating signals, thereby promoting aberrant kinase activity. The discovery of BCR-ABL1 and the further understanding of the role of this fusion in leukemogenesis represented a huge step forward that has culminated in the use of a selective tyrosine kinase inhibitor, imatinib mesylate, to successfully treat patients with CML [13]. Mutations in the kinase domain of *ABL1* have been linked to relapse after imatinib therapy, which has in part prompted the development of second generation *BCR-ABL1* inhibitors, such as dasatinib, nilotinib and bosutinib [14]. In addition to *BCR-ABL1*, several other tyrosine kinase fusion proteins are also sensitive to tyrosine kinase inhibitors, such as those with *PDGFR* (platelet-derived growth factor receptor) rearrangements in myeloid neoplasm-associated eosinophilia [15]. Chromosomal rearrangements that interfere with transcription factor genes can generate fusion proteins with aberrant transcriptional activity that may result in under-expression or over-expression of target genes. A chromosomal translocation that represses transcriptional activity is the t(15;17)(q22;q21) resulting in the *PML* (*promyelocytic leukemia*)-*RARA* (*retinoic acid receptor, alpha*) fusion gene. The PML-RARA fusion protein contains the DNA-binding motif from RARA, the function of which is inhibited by the PML partner. This leukemic fusion sequence has been successfully targeted in the clinic. The use of all-*trans* retinoic acid (ATRA) or arsenic therapy reverses the repression caused by the fusion protein, and can induce complete remission with or without chemotherapy.

Chromosomal translocations that deregulate the expression of normal genes include those that juxtapose regulatory elements, such as gene promoters or enhancer sequences to proto-oncogenes resulting in increased expression of the oncogene. The most well-known example is the juxtapositioning of the immunoglobulin (Ig) heavy chain locus, *IGH@* (14q32), driving constitutive expression of the *MYC* (*v-myc myelocytomatosis viral oncogene homolog*) oncogene (8q24) in Burkitt's lymphoma [16]. *MYC* can also be juxtaposed to the immunoglobulin kappa (*IGK@*) and lambda (*IGL@*) light chains. The study of Ig translocations has provided useful insight into the

mechanism by which these translocations occur. It is well established that normal rearrangements of immunoglobulin loci are controlled by RAG-mediated site-specific recombination, and that aberrations in this process may give rise to leukemia-associated translocations. In addition, rearranged immunoglobulins are subject to double-stranded breakage (DSB) during antibody gene diversification by class switch recombination and somatic hypermutation. Recently it has become clear that activation-induced cytidine deaminase (AID), the enzymes required for antibody gene diversification, is also required for the formation of some somatically acquired Ig translocations. AID is also responsible for breakage within the *MYC* locus, and hence may play a more general role in the formation of acquired chromosomal rearrangements in lymphoid disorders [17]. A wide variety of Ig translocations and different partner genes have been reported in lymphoma. Recently, a number of novel *IGH@* partner genes have been identified in BCP ALL, including *IGH@* driving constitutive expression of *ID4* (*inhibitor of DNA binding 4*) and several members of the *CEBP* (*CCAAT/enhancer binding proteins*) gene family [18]. An analogous scenario is seen in T-cell ALL and lymphoma in which regulatory elements of the T-cell receptor (TCR) genes deregulate a variety of partner genes. Approximately 35% of T-cell ALL patients have a translocation of this nature, where TCR genes partner transcription factor genes, such as *TAL1* (*T-cell acute lymphocytic leukemia 1*), *LYL1* (*lymphoblastic leukemia derived sequence 1*) and *HOX11* (*homeobox-11*, also known as *TLX1*) [19].

Given the high frequency of chromosomal alterations in cancer and the heterogeneity of the regions involved, the Catalog of Chromosome Aberration in Cancer, now entitled the Mitelman Database of Chromosome Aberrations and Gene Fusions in Cancer, has become an important resource [20]. The first edition was welcomed in 1983 and contained karyotype data on 3144 tumors. In 2009, the database now holds information on more than 56 000 malignant karyotypes, providing a vital description of those recurrent chromosomal abnormalities and the tumors in which they occur. This resource has contributed to the identification of more than 350 fusion genes, 75% of which have been identified in hematological malignancies. Until recently the prevailing view was that gene fusions were restricted to hematological malignancies and some soft tissue tumors; however, it is now clear that fusions are also seen in epithelial tumors. These abnormalities had evaded detection because of the difficulty in performing cytogenetic analysis in solid malignancies, along with the genomic complexity that characterizes these disorders.

The frequency of most fusion genes in hematological malignancies is relatively low, with the exception of a few well-characterized changes that are seen in virtually all patients with a particular disease subtype. These include *BCR-ABL1* in CML, *IGH@-CCND1* (*cyclin D1*) in mantle cell lymphoma, *MYC* deregulation in Burkitt's lymphoma and *PML-RARA* in APL. Although more than 100 fusion genes have been identified in AML, a disease which represents 33% of all hematological malignancies, these are seen in only 20% of cases. It is clear, therefore, that although chromosomal rearrangements and gene fusions are an important feature of leukemogenesis, the concept that they cause hematological disorders is an oversimplification.

Copy number changes

Genomic copy number changes are gains or losses of chromosomal material and can arise from large-scale chromosomal aneuploidies or unbalanced rearrangements to intragenic, submicroscopic duplication and deletion events. Several examples of copy number changes are shown in Figure 2.2. The target or targets of many of these abnormalities are beginning to be elucidated, such as unbalanced translocations that target *PAX5* (*paired box 5*) in ALL [21], an interstitial deletion causing the *SIL-TAL1* fusion in T-cell ALL and episomal amplification resulting in the *NUP214-ABL1* fusion, also in T-cell ALL [22, 23]. The combination of high-resolution genome-wide approaches to copy number and expression analysis, integrated with functional genomics screens, are beginning to unravel the basis of well-established recurrent chromosomal imbalances. For example, 5q- syndrome, a subtype of myelodysplastic syn-

drome (MDS) characterized by a defect in erythroid differentiation has been studied for many years with screens for biallelic deletions, mutations, or epigenetic silencing being unsuccessful. Recently the use of an RNA-mediated interference-based approach demonstrated that knockdown of *RPS14* expression recapitulates the disease, while forced expression of *RPS14* rescues the phenotype in patient-derived bone marrow cells [24].

It has been assumed that most copy number gains contribute to leukemogenesis by affecting the expression of genes with the affected genomic regions. Large chromosomal gains, arising from non-dysjunction or unbalanced translocations, occur in a variety of leukemic conditions. Amongst the most common chromosomal gains include trisomies for chromosome 8 and 12, which are recurrent cytogenetic features of MDS and chronic lymphocytic leukemia (CLL) respectively. It has been difficult to identify the functionally relevant target on these chromosomes because the aberration involves many hundreds of genes. With recent technological advances, such as array-based comparative genomic hybridization (CGH), it may be possible to identify partial gains of these chromosomes that pinpoint relevant genes for further study. Furthermore, high-throughput functional genomic studies and those incorporating DNA, RNA, and protein analysis should help determine the important functional elements targeted by these chromosomal gains. Genomic profiling is beginning to identify key genes in other patient subgroups with poor clinical outcome, including ALL patients with intrachromosomal amplification of chromosome 21 (iAMP21) [25]. Previously thought to be an amplification of the *RUNX1* (*runt-related transcription factor 1*) gene locus, we now know that iAMP21 is highly complex, with multiple inversion, duplication, and deletion events affecting chromosome 21, probably the result of a series of break-fusion-bridge cycles. Copy number gains that target small genomic regions are beginning to emerge, as a result of the development of array-based CGH and SNP (aSNP) genotyping. These alterations will be easier to investigate, as a smaller number of genes will be involved. One such example occurs in approximately 8% of individuals with T-cell ALL, targets the *MYB* (*v-myb*

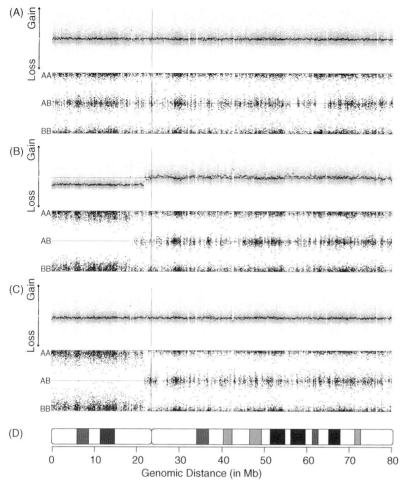

Figure 2.2 Genomic profiling of 17p deletions and cnnLOH events in patients with chronic lymphoblastic leukemia using the Affymetrix SNP6.0 platform. (A), (B), and (C) show copy number (upper track) and allele ratio (lower track) data for chromosome 17 from three CLL patients. The chromosome is positioned according to (D), running from the p telomere (right), through the centromere to the q telomere (left). The genomic distance is also shown (in megabases, Mb). For each copy number track (upper), the raw data is shown by the gray dots, while a moving average (black dots) of 50 consecutive array features has been used to calculate the segmental copy number changes. The allele ratio track (lower) shows the LOH data positioned as in (D). The SNP genotypes are shown from top to bottom as AA (homozygous for A), AB (heterozygous) and BB (homozygous for B). (A) Shows a patient with no 17p copy number changes. As expected the presence of the AB allele ratio shows both chromosomes (maternal and paternal) are present. (B) Shows a 17p deletion, with reduced copy number along 17p and the expected allele ratio. 17p deletions occur in 7–10% of CLL patients and are associated with an unfavorable prognosis and poor response to standard chemotherapy. Identification of a 17p deletion can direct sequencing of the retained *TP53* allele and in patient (B) identified a missense mutation. (C) Shows no copy number change on 17p, but an allele ratio suggestive of cnnLOH. Interestingly this patient responded poorly to chlorambucil chemotherapy. As there was no 17p deletion by FISH analysis, sequencing of the retained *TP53* allele was not performed at presentation. However, subsequent to the SNP profiling, sequence analysis revealed a missense codon 245 mutation in exon 7 of *TP53* and the patient responded well to the lymphocyte-depleting monoclonal antibody, alemtuzumab, and high-dose steroids.

myeloblastosis viral oncogene homolog) transcription factor and results in deregulated T-cell differentiation [26]. Focal amplifications in hematological malignancies could be exploited therapeutically, as exemplified by tyrosine kinase amplifications in certain epithelial cancers that are associated with responsiveness to kinase inhibitors.

The variety of copy number losses range from whole chromosome monosomies to single gene or intragenic deletions. It seems likely that many deletions contribute to pathogenesis by abrogating or reducing the expression of specific genes although, as indicated above, occasional deletions can produce fusion genes. In general, deletions pose more challenging therapeutic targets as they are less amenable to pharmacological intervention. However, it is likely that increased understanding of these deletion events may provide indirect targets for therapeutic intervention. Extensive genomic deletions, encompassing multiple genes are frequent in all types of hematological malignancy. The classical approach to the identification of tumor suppressor genes has had some success, where multiple deletion events are compared and a common region of deletion (CDR) is defined in all cases. These CDRs are then screened for deletions, mutations, and epigenetic modifications that inactivate the retained allele. These types of approach have identified key regulatory genes in a variety of leukemia types, including *TP53* (*tumor protein p53*, 17p13.1), *ATM* (*ataxia telangiectasia mutated*, 11q22-23) and *RB1* (*retinoblastoma 1*, 13q14.2), and are contributing to the identification of less tractable targets such as *RPS14* in 5q- syndrome. However, for many of the remaining recurrent deletions, such as the 6q and 7q deletions in lymphoid and myeloid disorders respectively, the targets remain unknown [27]. Novel genomic profiling methodologies have considerably improved the identification of microdeletions within larger, recurrent regions of deletion. This approach has been successfully applied to the study of the ALL genome, where the disruption of B-cell differentiation genes is apparent in 40% of B progenitor ALL cases, either by copy number change, mutation, or chromosomal rearrangements. Interestingly, the specific B-cell differentiation genes are related to cytogenetically defined subgroups: *PAX5* is fre-

quently targeted across ALL subtypes, while *IKZF1* (which encodes the lymphoid transcription factor, Ikaros) is deleted in more than 80% of *BCR-ABL1* positive patients. More recently, *IKZF1* deletions have been associated with a very poor outcome in B-cell progenitor ALL (reviewed in [28]). Recurrent copy number changes have also been identified in T-cell ALL, including cryptic deletions resulting in activation of *LMO2* (*LIM domains only 2*) and a *SET* (*SET nuclear oncogene*)-*NUP214* in-frame fusion gene [29]. Furthermore, these approaches are beginning to unravel karyotypic complexity in AML and have recently demonstrated that genomic complexity defined by microarray analysis is linked to a poor prognosis in patients with CLL [30, 31]. Genome-wide SNP profiling studies of leukemia subtypes have also identified extended regions of homozygosity in the absence of genomic copy number changes. If constitutional or remission material is available, it can be determined if these regions are inherited or acquired. If they are inherited they are then most likely to be regions that are identical by descent (i.e., inherited from both parents), although in rare instances they might result from constitutional uniparental disomy (UPD). These possibilities can only be distinguished by analyzing the corresponding regions from both parents. If the stretches of homozygosity are acquired, they can be legitimately termed copy number neutral LOH (cnnLOH) or acquired uniparental disomy (aUPD) arising from mitotic recombination and subsequent selection for one of the reciprocal products. It is likely that many of the genomic regions in the literature that have been described as malignancy-associated regions of UPD are, in fact, simply normal inherited regions of homozygosity. Genuine cnnLOH was first characterized in detail in polycythemia vera (PV) [32] but was subsequently found in a range of hematological malignancies, including 20% of AML with a normal karyotype [33]. During mitosis, a recombination event between chromosome homologs will generate daughter cells containing the reciprocal products. If one of these products confers a selective proliferative advantage, for example by duplication of a parentally inherited imprinted allele or a pre-existing heterozygous oncogenic mutation, then the new clone will be characterized by cnnLOH [34]. The identification of these events has been particularly productive in the identification of new cancer genes, most notably the identification of 9p cnnLOH and the JAK2V617F mutation in PV [35]. More recent examples include cnnLOH affecting 11q in patients with myeloid neoplasms and missense mutations of *CBL* (*Cas-Br-M ecotropic retroviral transforming sequence*) [36], multiple regions of cnnLOH containing mutations of *RUNX1*, *CEBPA*, *WT1* (*Wilms tumor 1*) and *FLT3* (*fms-related tyrosine kinase 3*) in patients with AML [34] and the presence of cnnLOH linked to clinical outcome in follicular lymphoma [37].

DNA methylation, histone modification, and non-coding RNAs

Modifications of DNA and chromatin proteins play a central role in transcriptional control, chromosome stability, DNA repair, and DNA replication. The complex interaction between DNA and chromatin modifications encodes a layer of information that acts in addition to the native nucleotide sequence. Once established, this "epigenetic" information is preserved during cellular replication and can be transferred in three principle ways: DNA methylation, histone modifications (acetylation, methylation, phosphorylation, ubiquitinylation and other changes), and non-coding RNA molecules. Because epigenetic changes are potentially reversible, they make attractive targets for therapeutic intervention with the use of demethylating agents and histone deacetylase inhibitors. Like chromosomal changes, altered methylation patterns can also be used as biomarkers for monitoring treatment and minimal residual disease.

DNA methylation
DNA methyltransferase catalyzes the addition of a methyl group to the carbon 5 position of the cytosine ring in the CpG dinucleotide and results in the formation of methylcytosine [38]. These CG dinucleotides are often located in repetitive elements and heterochromatin, but are also enriched in so-called "CpG islands," stretches of DNA that are typically 200–2000 base pairs long within the promoter regions of approximately 40–50% of human

genes [39]. In normal cells, many CpG islands display low levels of methylation, consistent with active transcription of associated genes in the setting of normal hemopoiesis. In leukemic cells, on the other hand, abnormal methylation of CpG islands has been widely described and is believed to play a central role in tumorigenesis [40]. The frequency of abnormal methylation, the variety of genes that are involved and the diversity of affected malignancies all point towards a critical role of epigenetic mechanisms in leukemia initiation and progression. Large numbers of genes have been studied for methylation changes in hematopoietic neoplasms, either by targeted approaches or, more recently, by global analyses. Investigations of single gene loci have mainly focused on genes involved in key regulatory processes, such as methylation of the cell cycle regulation genes *CDKN2B* (*cyclin-dependent kinase inhibitor 2B*, also known as *p15*) and *CDKN2A* (*cyclin-dependent kinase inhibitor 2A*, also known as *p16*), in AML, MDS, ALL, and non-Hodgkin lymphomas [41]. Genes disrupted by genetic mechanisms can also be inactivated by DNA methylation, for example *CEBPA* in AML [42]. A significant finding in patients with CLL was the promoter methylation of the death-associated protein kinase 1 (*DAPK1*) gene resulting in loss or reduction in gene expression [43]. Microarray analysis of gene methylation identified tumor type-specific DNA methylation events suggesting that these events could be utilized as diagnostic and prognostic markers [44]. Profound global hypermethylation has been associated with myelodysplastic syndromes (MDS) in particular but more recent analysis of ALL and AML showed surprisingly high levels of global promoter methylation, suggesting that gene silencing is also a significant feature of acute leukemia initiation [45, 46] and relapse [47]. Studies of patients with CLL have also shown CpG island promoter methylation effecting a wide number of loci, including the secreted frizzled-related protein, *SFRP4*, and the transcription factor, *TWIST2* [48].

Histone modifications
The four core histone proteins (H2A, H2B, H3 and H4) along with 147 bp of DNA comprise the nucleosome, the repeated structural unit of chromatin.

The N-terminal histone tails are subject to an array of covalent modifications that make up the "histone code." Generally, these modifications function by altering the net electrical charge of histone tails, resulting in changes in the interactions between histones, DNA, and accessory proteins in a manner that impacts on gene expression. The role of chromatin modification in leukemogenesis was first identified as the result of chromosomal translocations. *MLL* (*mixed-lineage leukemia*) encodes a trithorax gene family member that is targeted by diverse translocations in both AML and ALL. Many of the resulting chimeric proteins impact on the epigenetic regulations of homeobox genes, particularly *HOXA9* (*homeobox A9*) [49]. The PML-RARA fusion protein also acts by recruiting a chromatin modifying protein complex to its target genes [50]. The oligomerization capacity of the fusion protein generates a complex that includes PML, RARA, and the retinoid X receptor (RXR). This stabilizes the recruitment of a number of co-repressor complexes, including N-CoR (nuclear receptor co-repressor), SMRT (silencing mediator of retinoid and thyroid hormone), histone deacetylases, and histone methyltransferases, which in turn modify the histone code to repress transcription. Further evidence of epigenetic disruption was shown by the capacity of the PML-RARA oncogenic complex to compromise DNA-methyltransferases and methyl-CpG binding activities [51]. This mechanistic model highlights the importance of altered gene regulation mediating the pathogenesis of leukemia. More evidence is provided by the capacity of the RUNX1-RUNX1T1 (*runt-related transcription factor 1; translocated to 1*, also called *ETO*) fusion protein to regulate gene expression through direct interactions with co-repressor complexes [52]. As a consequence of the fusion protein, the compressor properties of the ETO protein influence RUNX1-mediated gene expression, by providing docking sites for recruitment of further nuclear repressor complexes and by providing a protein dimerization domain. Thus, RUNX1-RUNX1T1 can function as a transcriptional repressor of *RUNX1*-mediated genes. However, the role of the fusion protein is likely to be more complex, based on further protein:protein interactions. As therapeutic targets, both gene hypermethylation and hypoace-

tylation of histones are models for which therapeutic interventions are being developed. Initial approaches with demethylating agents have shown *in vitro* and *in vivo* utility, while HDAC inhibition has been shown to have therapeutic utility in patients with the PML-RARA fusion [53].

MicroRNAs

Recent evidence clearly implicates microRNA (miRNA) genes in the initiation and maintenance of leukemia. miRNAs are non-coding RNA molecules of 19–24 nucleotides encoded by phylogenetically conserved genes [54]. miRNAs derive from long, capped, and polyadenylated stem-loop precursor (primary micro RNAs (pri-miRNAs) and pre-miRNAs) processed by the RNase II endonuclease Drosha and Dicer. miRNAs inhibit protein translation or induce mRNA degradation, respectively, through an imperfect or perfect base pair binding to the 3'-untranslated (UTR) sequences of target miRNA molecules [55]. To date, more than 500 miRNAs have been identified in humans, and are involved in diverse biological processes including development, cell differentiation, proliferation, and apoptosis. Distinct miRNA expression signatures are apparent for different classes of leukemia [56] and are relevant for the pathogenesis, diagnosis and prognosis of both myeloid and lymphoid malignancies. In AML, the high expression of has-mir-191 and has-mir199a-1 was associated with a reduced overall and event-free survival [57], while a subset of 12 miRNAs was associated with event-free survival in patients with a normal karyotype [58]. In CLL, an expression signature of 13 miRNA genes differentiated patients based on ZAP-70 expression, IgV(H) mutation status, and disease progression. Interestingly, miRNAs expressed in hematopoietic cells have been found mutated or altered by chromosomal breakpoints in diverse leukemia types. The proposed link between an acquired copy number change and the deregulated expression of a miRNA was first described in CLL patients harboring a deletion of 13q14.3. This deletion constitutes the most frequent chromosomal change in CLL, occurring in more than half of all cases, and is associated with a favorable prognosis as a sole abnormality. A somatic cell hybrid model between mouse and human CLL cells carrying 13q14.3 deletions identified a minimal region of deletion between exons 2 and 5 of the *DLEU2* gene, a region which is also involved in translocations in CLL. Analysis of this region highlighted a cluster of two miRNA genes, *miR-15a* and *miR-16-1*, which were shown to be deleted in approximately 68% of CLL cases and rarely inactivated by mutation. A role of *miR-15a* and *miR-16-1* in the 13q14.3 deletion was further supported by the inverse correlation between their expression and that of the BCL2 protein, and the capacity for *miR-15a* and *miR-16-1* to induce apoptosis in leukemic cells through repression of BCL2. This association may also explain the high frequency of BCL2 protein overexpression seen in CLL which, in most cases, is not associated with traditional mechanisms such as juxtaposing with the *IGH@* locus [59]. miRNAs frequently reside in genomic regions targeted by acquired chromosomal aberrations, providing further support of their key role in carcinogenesis. Leukemia subtypes, defined by genetic characteristics cluster with miRNA expression profiles in an unsupervised manner. Further support is provided by the insertion of *miR-125b-1* into the immunoglobulin heavy chain locus in a patient with pre-B ALL, the juxtaposing of *C-MYC* with *miR-142* in a patient with aggressive APL and the inclusion of *miR-122a* in the minimal amplicon region around *MALT1* in aggressive marginal zone lymphoma (reviewed in [60]).

Of additional interest is the indirect interplay between chromosomal rearrangements and miRNA genes. For example, it is now clear that the RUNX1-RUNX1T1 fusion protein can directly regulate the transcriptional activity of a has-mir-223. This is achieved by the RUNX1-RUNX1T1-mediated heterochromatic silencing of the genomic region containing miRNA-223 [61]. Several miRNAs are transcriptionally repressed by the APL-associated PML-RARA oncoprotein and are released after treatment with all-trans retinoic acid [62]. Recently, an important link has been made between genetic and epigenetic silencing of *miR-203* and activation of the BCR-ABL1 fusion protein [63]. Preliminary data suggests that the MLL-AF4 and MLL-AF9 fusion proteins can target Drosha-mediated miRNA processing [64]. In addition, emerging evidence suggests that miRNA molecules and well-characterized transcription factors can regulate each other's function via negative feedback mechanisms, including miRNA interactions with *NFIA* (nuclear factor I/A), *CEBPA*, *TCL1* (T-cell leukemia/lymphoma 1), *MYC* and *CDKN2B* [65–67]. Moreover, a potential link between miRNA activities and DNA methylation has been reported, either by downregulation of miRNA expression through genomic DNA methylation or the reverse; miRNA mediated epigenetic control, thus implicating epigenetic modulation in the regulation of miRNA molecules [61]. Therefore, emerging evidence clearly demonstrates a pivotal role of miRNAs in the initiation and maintenance of the leukemic phenotype. Preliminary data suggests that these genes are linked to prognosis in AML and CLL [58], and represent attractive therapeutic targets.

Dissecting the leukemia genome with second generation sequencing technologies

The availability of the reference human genome sequence and recent developments in sequencing technologies means that it is now possible to characterize entire cancer genomes making a full catalogue of all somatically acquired mutations in human cancer a reality in the next few years. These sequencing approaches can be adapted to include mitochondrial DNA alterations, epigenetic modifications, and the transcriptome. This has all been made possible by the development of "second generation" sequencing technologies, which can produce billions of bases of DNA sequence per week, a rate which may further increase dramatically over the next few years. Recent, proof-of-principle studies confirm this potential, including the first complete genome sequence of a cancer specimen, a patient with AML [68]. In a landmark study, Ley et al. sequenced a normal karyotype AML genome, and its constitutional counterpart from the same patient's skin. On analysis of coding regions they reported 10 genes with acquired mutations, two of which had been previously described. None of the novel loci were mutated in a large cohort of other

AML cases, raising the possibility that they may be passenger mutations, or perhaps hinting at an extreme heterogeneity of acquired abnormalities in this disease. Overall, the number of sequence changes was surprisingly small given the prevailing view that many malignancies are considered to be driven by genomic instability; however, it remains to be seen if this genome is typical of AML and whether significant pathogenetic changes are present outside of coding regions.

Although not yet applied to hematological malignancies, other studies have used second generation sequencing technologies to very efficiently screen for chromosomal rearrangements and copy number changes, as well as to characterize the cancer cell transcriptome [69, 70]. Campbell et al. employed second generation sequencing to generate sequence reads from both ends of short DNA fragments derived from the genomes of individuals with lung cancer [69]. The sequences reads were then mapped onto the normal genome sequence to identify fragments that did not align correctly and therefore represented structural variants. This approach identified a large number of somatic rearrangements at base-pair resolution, demonstrating the feasibility of this approach in cancer gene identification. As we are entering a new era in the genomic analysis of the malignant genome, the International Cancer Genome Consortium (http://www.icgc.org/) has been established to catalogue the acquired sequence alterations in a least 50 cancer classes, which will probably require at least 20-fold sequence coverage of more than 20 000 cancer genomes. This enormous undertaking will include a number of hematological malignancies, for example the recently launched CLL genome project. The data generated will require enormous bioinformatic resources, but will provide a definitive description of the genetic changes in cancer.

Conclusions and future directions

Our knowledge of the leukemia genome has expanded exponentially over the past 50 years. Cytogenetic analysis remains an important, albeit low resolution whole genome scanning technique and it is striking that, even today, the majority of known cancer genes have been identified though the characterization of cytogenetically visible aberrations. Further advances in our understanding have gone hand-in-hand with technological improvements. In the 1980s, the gap between molecular genetics and cytogenetics was bridged with the advent of FISH and other molecular cytogenetic approaches, which for the first time provided a truly integrated approach to genomic analysis. In the late 1990s and into the new millennium, developments in microarray technology have further bridged this gap, allowing the causative gene loci targeted by chromosomal abnormalities to be accurately and rapidly identified. The completion of the Human Genome Project has facilitated our improved understanding of the genomic architecture of normal cells. One outcome was the validation of the polymorphic nature of significant regions of the genome, including copy number variation and single nucleotide polymorphisms, allowing the development of novel technologies, and providing a more rapid means of validating the pathogenic nature of sequence changes detected in leukemia cells. We are now entering an exciting phase of genomic research that will be driven forward by second generation sequencing technologies and efforts to sequence a large number of cancer genomes. Whole genome sequencing currently requires enormous technical and bioinformatic infrastructure facilities that are probably only available in the main sequencing centers. However, more targeted sequencing approaches aimed at specific chromosomal regions, or at genes encoding components of certain pathways, will provide valuable data in a cost-effective way. For example, sequences within recurrent regions of copy number change or cnnLOH can now be acquired using a DNA capture microarray and then sequenced, and thus high-throughput sequencing represents a complementary tool, which can be used in unison with traditional cytogenetics, molecular cytogenetics, molecular biology, and microarray analysis to address key scientific questions. Functional validation of mutated genes, however, still remains a significant challenge but is essential to prove causation and also as a means to develop novel abnormalities as drug targets.

References

1 Von Hansemann D. (1890) Ueber asymmetrische Zelltheilung in Epithelkrebsen und deren biologische Bedeutung. *Virchows Arch A Pathol Anat Histopathol* **119**:299–326.

2 Reddy EP, Reynolds RK, Santos E, et al. (1982) A point mutation is responsible for the acquisition of transforming properties by the T24 human bladder carcinoma oncogene. *Nature* **300**:149–52.

3 Nowell PC, Hungerford DA. (1960) A minute chromosome in human chronic granulocytic leukemia. *Science* **132**:1497.

4 Caspersson T, Zech L, Johansson C. (1970) Analysis of human metaphase chromosome set by aid of DNA-binding fluorescent agents. *Exp Cell Res* **62**:490–2.

5 Rowley JD. (2008) Chromosomal translocations: revisited yet again. *Blood* **112**:2183–9.

6 Moorman AV, Richards SM, Martineau M, et al. (2003) Outcome heterogeneity in childhood high-hyperdiploid acute lymphoblastic leukemia. *Blood* **102**:2756–62.

7 Strefford JC, Harrison CJ. (2007) Advances in molecular cytogenetics to study the leukaemia genome. *Laboratory Medicine* **38**:1–8.

8 Ford AM, Ridge SA, Cabrera ME, et al. (1993) In utero rearrangements in the trithorax-related oncogene in infant leukaemias. *Nature* **363**:358–60.

9 Daley GQ, Van Etten RA, Baltimore D. (1990) Induction of chronic myelogenous leukemia in mice by the P210bcr/abl gene of the Philadelphia chromosome. *Science* **247**:824–30.

10 Thomas M, Greil J, Heidenreich O. (2006) Targeting leukemic fusion proteins with small interfering RNAs: recent advances and therapeutic potentials. *Acta Pharmacol Sin* **27**:273–81.

11 Mitelman F, Mertens F, Johansson B. (2005) Prevalence estimates of recurrent balanced cytogenetic aberrations and gene fusions in unselected patients with neoplastic disorders. *Genes Chromosomes Cancer* **43**:350–66.

12 Deininger M, Buchdunger E, Druker BJ. (2005) The development of imatinib as a therapeutic agent for chronic myeloid leukemia. *Blood* **105**:2640–53.

13 O'Brien SG. Guilhot F. Larson RA, et al. (2003) Imatinib compared with interferon and low-dose cytarabine for newly diagnosed chronic-phase chronic myeloid leukemia. *N Eng J Med* **348**:994–1004.

14 Chu SC, Tang JL, Li CC. (2006) Dasatinib in chronic myelogenous leukemia. *N Engl J Med* **355**:1062–3.

15 Apperley JF, Gardembas M, Melo JV, et al. (2002) Response to imatinib mesylate in patients with chronic myeloproliferative diseases with rearrangements of the platelet-derived growth factor receptor beta. *N Engl J Med* **347**:481–7.

16 Dalla-Favera R, Martinotti S, Gallo RC, et al. (1983) Translocation and rearrangements of the c-myc oncogene locus in human undifferentiated B-cell lymphomas. *Science* **219**:963–7.

17 Robbiani DF, Bothmer A, Callen E, et al. (2008) AID is required for the chromosomal breaks in c-myc that lead to c-myc/IgH translocations. *Cell* **135**:1028–38.

18 Russell LJ, Akasaka T, Majid A, et al. (2008) t(6;14)(p22;q32): a new recurrent IGH@ translocation involving ID4 in B-cell precursor acute lymphoblastic leukemia (BCP-ALL). *Blood* **111**:387–91.

19 Aifantis I, Raetz E, Buonamici S. (2008) Molecular pathogenesis of T-cell leukaemia and lymphoma. *Nat Rev Immunol* **8**:380–90.

20 Mitelman F, Johansson B, Mertens FE. (eds.) Mitelman Database of Chromosome Aberrations and Gene Fusions in Cancer. 2009. Available from: http://cgap.nci.nih.gov/Chromosomes/Mitelman (last accessed October 4, 2010).

21 An Q, Wright SL, Konn ZJ, et al. (2008) Variable breakpoints target PAX5 in patients with dicentric chromosomes: A model for the basis of unbalanced translocations in cancer. *Proc Natl Acad Sci USA* **105**:17050–4.

22 Graux C, Cools J, Melotte C, et al. (2004) Fusion of NUP214 to ABL1 on amplified episomes in T-cell acute lymphoblastic leukemia. *Nat Genet* **36**:1084–9.

23 Bernard O, Lecointe N, Jonveaux P, et al. (1991) Two site-specific deletions and t(1;14) translocation restricted to human T-cell acute leukemias disrupt the 5′ part of the tal-1 gene. *Oncogene* **6**:1477–88.

24 Ebert BL, Pretz J, Bosco J, et al. (2008) Identification of RPS14 as a 5q- syndrome gene by RNA interference screen. *Nature* **451**:335–9.

25 Strefford JC, Van Delft FW, Robinson HM, et al. (2006) Complex genomic alterations and gene expression in acute lymphoblastic leukemia with intrachromosomal amplification of chromosome 21. *Proc Natl Acad Sci U S A* **103**:8167–72.

26 Lahortiga I, De Keersmaecker K, Van Vlierberghe P, et al. (2007) Duplication of the MYB oncogene in T-cell acute lymphoblastic leukemia. *Nat Genet* **39**:593–5.

27 Döhner K, Brown J, Hehmann U, et al. (1998) Molecular cytogenetic characterization of a critical region in bands 7q35-q36 commonly deleted in malignant myeloid disorders. *Blood* **92**:4031–5.

28 Mullighan CG, Downing JR. (2009) Genome-wide profiling of genetic alterations in acute lymphoblastic leukemia: recent insights and future directions. *Leukemia* **23**:1209–18.

29 Van Vlierberghe P, van Grotel M, Tchinda J, et al. (2008) The recurrent SET-NUP214 fusion as a new HOXA activation mechanism in pediatric T-cell lymphoblastic leukemia. *Blood* **111**:4668–80.

30 Rucker FG, Bullinger L, Schwaenen C, et al. (2006) Disclosure of candidate genes in acute myeloid leukemia with complex karyotypes using microarray-based molecular characterization. *J Clin Oncol* **24**:3887–94.

31 Saddler C, Ouillette P, Kujawski L, et al. (2008) Comprehensive biomarker and genomic analysis identifies p53 status as the major determinant of response to MDM2 inhibitors in chronic lymphocytic leukemia. *Blood* **111**:1584–93.

32 Kralovics R, Guan Y, Prchal JT. (2002) Acquired uniparental disomy of chromosome 9p is a frequent stem cell defect in polycythemia vera. *Exp Hematol* **30**:229–36.

33 Raghavan M, Lillington DM, Skoulakis S, et al. (2005) Genome-wide single nucleotide polymorphism analysis reveals frequent partial uniparental disomy due to somatic recombination in acute myeloid leukemias. *Cancer Res* **65**:375–8.

34 Fitzgibbon J, Smith LL, Raghavan M, et al. (2005) Association between acquired uniparental disomy and homozygous gene mutation in acute myeloid leukemias. *Cancer Res* **65**:9152–4.

35 Kralovics R, Passamonti F, Buser AS, et al. (2005) A gain-of-function mutation of JAK2 in myeloproliferative disorders. *N Engl J Med* **352**:1779–90.

36 Grand FH, Hidalgo-Curtis CE, Ernst T, et al. (2009) Frequent CBL mutations associated with 11q acquired uniparental disomy in myeloproliferative neoplasms. *Blood* **113**:6182–92.

37 O'Shea D, O'Riain C, Gupta M, et al. (2009) Regions of acquired uniparental disomy at diagnosis of follicular lymphoma are associated with both overall survival and risk of transformation. *Blood* **113**:2298–301.

38 Holliday R, Grigg GW. (1993) DNA methylation and mutation. *Mutation Research* **285**:61–7.

39 Gardiner-Garden M, Frommer M. (1987) CpG islands in vertebrate genomes. *J Mol Biol* **196**:261–82.

40 Herman JG, Baylin SB. (2003) Gene silencing in cancer in association with promotor hypermethylation. *N Engl J Med* **349**:2042–54.

41 Drexler HG. (1998) Review of alterations of the cyclin-dependent kinase inhibitor INK4 family genes p15, p16, p18 and p19 in human leukemia-lymphoma cells. *Leukemia* **12**:845–59.

42 Hackanson B, Bennett KL, Brena RM, et al. (2008) Epigenetic modification of CCAAT/enhancer binding protein alpha expression in acute myeloid leukemia. *Cancer Res* **68**:3142–51.

43 Raval A, Tanner SM, Byrd JC, et al. (2007) Down-regulation of death-associated protein kinase 1 (DAPK1) in chronic lymphocytic leukemia. *Cell* **129**:879–90.

44 Costello JF, Frühwald MC, Smiraglia DJ, et al. (2000) Aberrant CpG-island methylation has non-random and tumour-type-specific patterns. *Nat Genet* **24**:132–8.

45 Kuang SQ, Tong WG, Yang H, et al. (2008) Genome-wide identification of aberrantly methylated promoter associated CpG islands in acute lymphocytic leukemia. *Leukemia* **22**:1529–38.

46 Rush LJ, Dai Z, Smiraglia DJ, et al. (2001) Novel methylation targets in de novo acute myeloid leukemia with prevalence of chromosome 11 loci. *Blood* **97**:3226–33.

47 Kroeger H, Jelinek J, Estécio MR, et al. (2008) Aberrant CpG island methylation in acute myeloid leukemia is accentuated at relapse. *Blood* **112**:1366–73.

48 Rush LJ, Raval A, Funchain P, et al. (2004) Epigenetic profiling in chronic lymphocytic leukemia reveals novel methylation targets. *Cancer Res* **64**:2424–33.

49 Erfurth FE, Popovic R, Grembecka J, et al. (2008) MLL protects CpG clusters from methylation within the Hoxa9 gene, maintaining transcript expression. *Proc Natl Acad Sci U S A* **105**:7517–22.

50 Grignani F, De Matteis S, Nervi C, et al. (1998) Fusion proteins of the retinoic acid receptor-alpha recruit histone deacetylase in promyelocytic leukaemia. *Nature* **391**:815–8.

51 Di Croce L, Raker VA, Corsaro M, et al. (2002) Methyltransferase recruitment and DNA hypermethylation of target promoters by an oncogenic transcription factor. *Science* **295**:1079–82.

52 Fazi F, Zardo G, Gelmetti V, et al. (2007) Heterochromatic gene repression of the retinoic acid pathway in acute myeloid leukemia. *Blood* **109**:4432–40.

53 Warrell RP Jr., He LZ, Richon V, et al. (1998) Therapeutic targeting of transcription in acute promyelocytic leukemia by use of an inhibitor of histone deacetylase. *J Natl Cancer Inst* **90**:1621–5.

54 Lee RC, Feinbaum RL, Ambros V. (1993) The C. elegans heterochronic gene lin-4 encodes small RNAs with antisense complementarity to lin-14. *Cell* **75**:843–54.

55 Ambros V. (2004) The functions of animal microRNAs. *Nature* **431**:350–5.

56 Mi S, Lu J, Sun M, et al. (2007) MicroRNA expression signatures accurately discriminate acute lymphoblastic leukemia from acute myeloid leukemia. *Proc Natl Acad Sci U S A* **104**:19971–6.

57 Garzon R, Volinia S, Liu CG, et al. (2008) MicroRNA signatures associated with cytogenetics and prognosis in acute myeloid leukemia. *Blood* **111**:3183–9.

58 Marcucci G, Radmacher MD, Maharry K, et al. (2008) MicroRNA expression in cytogenetically normal acute myeloid leukemia. *N Engl J Med* **358**:1919–28.

59 Adachi M, Tefferi A, Greipp PR, et al. (1990) Preferential linkage of bcl-2 to immunoglobulin light chain gene in chronic lymphocytic leukemia. *J Exp Med* **171**:559–64.

60 Nicoloso MS, Kipps TJ, Croce CM, et al. (2007) MicroRNAs in the pathogeny of chronic lymphocytic leukaemia. *Br J Haematol* **139**:709–16.

61 Fazi F, Racanicchi S, Zardo G, et al. (2007) Epigenetic silencing of the myelopoiesis regulator microRNA-223 by the AML1/ETO oncoprotein. *Cancer Cell* **12**:457–66.

62 Saumet A, Vetter G, Bouttier M, et al. (2008) Transcriptional repression of microRNA genes by PML-RARA increases expression of key cancer proteins in acute promyelocytic leukemia. *Blood* **113**:412–21.

63 Bueno MJ, Pérez de Castro I, Gómez de Cedrón M, et al. (2008) Genetic and epigenetic silencing of microRNA-203 enhances ABL1 and BCR-ABL1 oncogene expression. *Cancer Cell* **13**:496–506.

64 Nakamura T, Canaani E, Croce CM. (2007) Oncogenic All1 fusion proteins target Drosha-mediated microRNA processing. *Proc Natl Acad Sci U S A* **104**:10980–5.

65 O'Donnell KA, Wentzel EA, Zeller KI, et al. (2005) c-Myc-regulated microRNAs modulate E2F1 expression. *Nature* **435**:839–43.

66 Yu W, Gius D, Onyango P, et al. (2008) Epigenetic silencing of tumour suppressor gene p15 by its antisense RNA. *Nature* **451**:202–6.

67 Pekarsky Y, Santanam U, Cimmino A, et al. (2006) Tcl1 expression in chronic lymphocytic leukemia is regulated by miR-29 and miR-181. *Cancer Res* **66**:11590–3.

68 Ley TJ, Mardis ER, Ding L, et al. (2008) DNA sequencing of a cytogenetically normal acute myeloid leukaemia genome. *Nature* **456**:66–72.

69 Campbell PJ, Stephens PJ, Pleasance ED, et al. (2008) Identification of somatically acquired rearrangements in cancer using genome-wide massively parallel paired-end sequencing. *Nat Genet* **40**:722–9.

70 Jones S, Zhang X, Parsons DW, et al. (2008) Core signaling pathways in human pancreatic cancers revealed by global genomic analyses. *Science* **321**:1801–6.

71 Weng AP, Ferrando AA, Lee W, et al. (2004) Activating mutations of NOTCH1 in human T cell acute lymphoblastic leukemia. *Science* **306**:269–71.

72 Falini B, Mecucci C, Tiacci E, et al. (2005) Cytoplasmic nucleophosmin in acute myelogenous leukemia with a normal karyotype. *N Engl J Med* **352**:254–66.

73 Nakao M, Yokota S, Iwai T, et al. (1996) Internal tandem duplication of the flt3 gene found in acute myeloid leukemia. *Leukemia* **10**:1911–8.

74 Virappane P, Gale R, Hills R, et al. (2008) Mutation of the Wilms' tumor 1 gene is a poor prognostic factor associated with chemotherapy resistance in normal karyotype acute myeloid leukemia: the United Kingdom Medical Research Council Adult Leukaemia Working Party. *J Clin Oncol* **26**:5429–35.

75 Romana SP, Mauchauffe M, Le Coniat M, et al. (1995) The t(12;21) of acute lymphoblastic leukemia results in a tel-AML1 gene fusion. *Blood* **85**:3662–70.

76 Carroll AJ, Crist WM, Parmley RT, et al. (1984) Pre-B cell leukemia associated with chromosome translocation 1;19. *Blood* **63**:721–4.

77 Russell LJ, Capasso M, Vater I, et al. (2009) Deregulated expression of cytokine receptor gene, CRLF2, is involved in lymphoid transformation in B cell precursor acute lymphoblastic leukemia. *Blood (ASH Annual Meeting Abstracts)* **112**:Abstract No. 787.

78 Fazio G, Palmi C, Rolink A, et al. (2008) PAX5/TEL acts as a transcriptional repressor causing down-modulation of CD19, enhances migration to CXCL12, and confers survival advantage in pre-BI cells. *Cancer Res* **68**:181–9.

79 Sulong S, Moorman AV, Irving JA, et al. (2008) A comprehensive analysis of the CDKN2A gene in childhood acute lymphoblastic leukaemia reveals genomic deletion, copy number neutral loss of heterozygosity and association with specific cytogenetic subgroups. *Blood* **113**:100–7.

80 Delhommeau F, Dupont S, Della Valle V, et al. (2009) Mutation in TET2 in myeloid cancers. *N Engl J Med* **360**:2289–301.

PART 2
Myeloid Malignancies

CHAPTER 3
Myeloproliferative Neoplasms

Ruben A. Mesa[1] and Ayalew Tefferi[2]
[1]Division of Hematology/Oncology, Mayo Clinic, Scottsdale, AZ, USA
[2]Department of Hematology, Mayo Clinic, Scottsdale, AZ, USA

Background on the myeloproliferative neoplasms

Historical and clinical origins

Williams Damashek is credited with the observation that a group of diseases with shared phenotypic features of myeloproliferation shared a potential pathogenetic origin and overlapping natural history [1], and entitled these disorders the myeloproliferative diseases. The WHO in 2008 recognized the shared clonal and neoplastic origin of these disorders, and identified them as the myeloproliferative neoplasms (MPNs) [2]. The MPNs have classically included the disorders of polycythemia vera (PV), essential thrombocythemia (ET), and primary myelofibrosis (PMF), with a cumulative incidence of approximately 8 cases/100 000 persons/year, and a median age of onset of approximately 60 years (however, patients <50 years of age are still commonly seen) [3]. Clinically, MPN patients are at risk of thrombohemorrhagic complications early in the disease course and, with progression, can develop profound cytopenias and hepatosplenomegaly, eventually culminating in leukemic transformation. MPN can lead to premature death, with the most aggressive entity, myelofibrosis having a median survival of 69 months [4]. Patients may have PMF or may develop myelofibrosis in the advanced phases of both PV and ET; the latter complication is known as post-polycythemia vera myelofibrosis (post-PV MF) and post-essential thrombocythemia myelofibrosis (post-ET MF), respectively. Even in the absence of myelofibrosis, patients with PV and ET have compromised survivals compared to age-matched controls [5]. The sources of mortality in ET and PV are the short-term risk of thrombohemorrhagic complications and long-term risk of leukemic transformation, as well as development of post-ET/PV MF with their attendant cytopenias [5].

MPN patients suffer from a full range of disease-associated symptoms, some of which are shared with patients with other chronic leukemias and other malignancies, and some which are unique to the disorders themselves. Symptoms that are particularly and sometimes uniquely associated with the myeloproliferative disorders include a risk of both thrombosis and/or bleeding, especially in patients with ET and PV. These symptoms have a range of manifestations. In the setting of acute venous thrombosis, one can be left with deep venous thrombosis or post-phlebitic symptoms of the legs including pain, chronic peripheral edema, and difficulties of that nature. Chronic pulmonary emboli, which can arise in these patients, can lead to short-term morbidity from arrhythmia as well as long-term problems, such as pulmonary hypertension, chronic dyspnea, and general compromise in cardiac or lung function. Vascular events can also be more subtle. Individuals with extremes of either erythrocytosis or thrombocytosis can have compromised microvascular circulation even in the absence of frank thrombosis and have periods that are self-described by

Advances in Malignant Hematology, First Edition. Edited by Hussain I. Saba and Ghulam J. Mufti. © 2011 Blackwell Publishing Ltd.
Published 2011 by Blackwell Publishing Ltd.

patients as confusion, lack of ability to concentrate, migraine headaches, and visual disturbances. Hemorrhagic symptoms can range from acute gastrointestinal bleeding to more chronic bleeding events from esophageal varices or gastrointestinal sources. This can lead to or exacerbate chronic anemia and all of the challenges with dyspnea and fatigue that the anemia can bring.

The presence of itching or pruritus is very common across the spectrum of myeloproliferative disorders, and particularly amongst those individuals with PV. These individuals classically have aquagenic pruritus meaning that, after exposure to water and drying, the itching in the skin is most prominent. The itching can also occur in the absence of exposure to water. It is believed that this could potentially be associated with histamine release and other cytokine mediators in the skin. Other skin mass sensations can include painful microvascular circulation, difficulties known as erythromelalgia. Patients with MPNs can suffer from significant constitutional symptoms including a loss of lean muscle mass (cachexia) that is believed to be potentially associated with underlying disease manifestations that have a selective predisposition for the consumption of lean muscle mass. Additionally, patients can have fevers and night sweats that are likely cytokine-driven in association with the underlying myeloid process. MPNs are characterized by increases in circulating white blood cells and, in the case of PMF, a variety of immature myeloid cells. This can lead to the development of sequestration of these cells or extramedullary hematopoiesis (EMH). This can particularly lead to significant splenomegaly and/or hepatomegaly. The splenomegaly can be sufficient to cause significant early satiety, pain, abdominal bloating, difficulty with finding a comfortable position, difficulties with bending over, portal hypertension, worsening of peripheral edema, and a whole constellation of symptoms including painful splenic infarcts. EMH can develop in a variety of organs, and has been found everywhere, including the pericardium (causing pericardial effusions), the spinal canal (causing cord compression) and the lungs (causing pulmonary hypertension), all of which can lead to very significant symptomatic burden in these groups of patients (Table 3.1).

Table 3.1 Self-reported constitutional symptoms in 1179 patients with MPN

Symptom	PV (N = 405)	ET (N = 304)	MF (N = 456)	Total (N = 1179)
Fatigue	85%	72%	84%	81%
Bone pain	65%	40%	50%	53%
Fever	49%	41%	56%	50%
Pruritus	43%	41%	47%	44%
Night sweats	13%	9%	18%	14%
Symptomatic splenomegaly	10%	7%	20%	13%
Weight loss (>10%)	4%	9%	7%	6%

MF: Includes primary and post-ET and post-PV myelofibrosis.

Pathogenetic insights

The watershed moment for MPNs occurred in 2005, with the heavily publicized discovery of the $JAK2^{V617F}$ mutation [6–9]. This latter point mutation, in the pseudo-kinase domain of JAK2 (a key component of the cell growth and differentiation JAK-STAT pathway), leads to constitutive activation of the pathway. This mutation joined the pantheon of constitutively active tyrosine kinases identified as playing a role in myeloid neoplasms, including BCR-ABL in chronic myeloid leukemia, FIP1L1-PDGFRA for chronic eosinophilic leukemia and systemic mastocytosis, KIT^{D816V} for systemic mastocytosis amongst many others [10]. Subsequently, several additional genetic mutations with potential pathogenetic implications were discovered, including the c-MPL$^{W515L/K}$ (in 5% of PMF and 1% of ET) [11] and alternative mutations in exon 12 of JAK2 in some PV patients previously identified as wild type for JAK2 [12]. All of these mutations seem to feed into a final common pathway of cellular activation through the PI3 kinase, the STAT, and the MAP kinase pathways [13].

Very recently, somatic mutations in TET2 were identified in about 15% of myeloid neoplasms, and an event preceding the JAK2 mutation in MPN patients [14]; however the clinical relevance or true impact on the pathogenesis of MPNs remains unclear [15]. Additional insights recently suggest that variability in other genes through SNP analysis [16], or perhaps inherited haplotypes may play a role in MPN pathogenesis [17, 18]. Although the last five years have seen significant advances in the understanding of MPN pathophysiology, many questions remain regarding the initiating genetic event, the phenotypic diversity amongst the diseases, and the mechanisms of disease progression.

Diagnosis of MPNs in 2009

The diagnosis of the BCR-ABL negative MPNs had always been limited by the absence of a gold standard, an absolute molecular marker. This latter deficiency has led to a series of clinico-pathological diagnostic criteria relying upon features helpful in distinguishing an MPN from: (1) a reactive state, (2) an alternative myeloid malignancy, and (3) an alternative MPN diagnosis. These criteria were usually the easiest to apply to overt MPN cases, but not uncommonly would leave others with uncertainty. The World Health Organization (WHO) has taken a lead role in diagnostic criteria for MPNs and the current WHO criteria [2] attempt to incorporate the diagnostic implications of the new wave of mutations (such as the JAK2^{V617F}) into the criteria.

Polycythemia vera (PV)

PV is the MPN in which the presence of the JAK2^{V617F} is of greatest diagnostic importance, as it is seen in well in excess of 90% of afflicted individuals [6–9]. Many of those whom clinically have PV, yet have wild-type JAK2, may have an alternative mutation that similarly activates the JAK-STAT pathway such as mutations in the exon 12 of the JAK2 gene. In aggregate, these described mutations are present in 98% of PV, and not in secondary forms of erythrocytosis. The current WHO diagnostic criteria for PV have been updated to establish the diagnosis of PV by both the presence of (1) clear erythrocytosis or increased red cell mass, and (2) the presence of known PV molecular lesions (JAK2^{V617F} or JAK2 exon 12 mutation). If both of the latter features are present, a diagnosis of PV is highly likely and confirmed with the presence of one

of the minor criteria including bone marrow biopsy consistent with PV (hypercellularity and panmyelosis with prominent trilineage proliferation). In the rare circumstance of PV patients lacking the known PV molecular lesion, the diagnosis can still be established if two of the minor criteria are reached. The updated WHO criteria have the practical advantage of greatly simplifying the diagnosis of those with erythrocytosis who are JAK2^{V167F} positive who are highly likely to have PV.

Essential thrombocythaemia (ET)

The negative predictive value of a wild-type JAK2^{V617F} mutation is significantly more limited in ET, given that only about 50% of afflicted individuals express the mutation [6, 7, 9]. When present, however, it is diagnostically helpful. In the revised WHO criteria for ET [19], sustained unexplained thrombocytosis has been lowered from 600×10^9/L to any sustained value greater than normal ($>450 \times 10^9$/L) given the fact that many patients with ET, even with thrombosis, can present with platelet counts between 450 and 600×10^9/L. Secondly, if the JAK2^{V617F} is present (or another marker of clonality by karyotype is met), the burden of clinical investigations to exclude secondary causes is diminished. The need to carefully examine the marrow to make a diagnosis of essential thrombocythemia (by excluding other myeloid disorders) remains.

Primary myelofibrosis (PMF)

PMF has been known by a wide range of synonyms, including chronic idiopathic myelofibrosis, agnogenic myeloid metaplasia, and myelofibrosis with myeloid metaplasia. Given that the disorder is neither idiopathic, nor always accompanied by myeloid metaplasia, the International Working Group for Myelofibrosis Research and Treatment (IWG-MRT; an international ad hoc collaborative group of over 40 dedicated myelofibrosis and MPN experts) reached the consensus that PMF would be the most accurate and appropriate diagnostic term [20]. PMF designates those patients who present with *de novo* disease, distinguished from patients who progress to a myelofibrotic stage from previous PV or ET, designated post-PV myelofibrosis (post-PV MF) and post-ET myelofibrosis (post-ET MF) respectively [20].

The WHO criteria for MF attempt to bridge the spectrum across the phenotypic variability in the disorder by requiring that three main features must be present to diagnose PMF. The first: bone marrow histologic changes consistent with the disorder, specifically the presence of megakaryocyte proliferation and atypia (small to large megakaryocytes with an aberrant nuclear/cytoplasmic ratio and hyperchromatic, bulbous or irregularly folded nuclei, and dense clustering) that are usually accompanied by either reticulin and/or collagen fibrosis. However, in the absence of significant reticulin fibrosis, the megakaryocyte changes must be accompanied by an increased bone marrow cellularity characterized by granulocytic proliferation and, often, decreased erythropoiesis (this substitutes for the previous pre-fibrotic/cellular-phase disease). The second required characteristic is the absence of criteria suggesting an alternative myeloid disorder. The third is either a marker of clonality (such as the JAK2^{V617F}, c-MPL$^{W515L/K}$, or other clonal marker) or, if such a clonal marker is absent, no evidence of the fibrosis being related to an inflammatory or reactive state. Two out of four minor criteria are required to secure the diagnosis of PMF including peripheral blood manifestations (anemia, leukoerythroblastosis, or increased lactate dehydrogenase) or splenomegaly (presumably from extramedullary hematopoiesis).

Post-ET/PV MF

The distinction of the point at which a patient with PV or ET transforms to post-PV MF or post-ET MF (respectively) remains a clinical one, given the lack of clear molecular changes to define this form of progression in ET and PV. Currently used criteria for diagnosing disease progression were developed by the IWG-MRT [21] and rely upon (1) a clear WHO diagnosis of ET or PV, (2) a clear grade 2 increase in reticulin fibrosis, and (3) the development of at least two clinical features to support disease progression.

Current therapy of MPNs: an overview of currently available therapies

The natural history of MPNs includes a variable period of risk of vascular events, and a long-term risk of transformation to either an overt myelo-fibrotic phase or death. Current available therapies have rarely been able to impact this natural history beyond palliating symptoms or decreasing the risk of vascular events. Given these challenges, how should MPN patients be optimally managed? Currently, incorporation of the results from the modest numbers of randomized clinical trials, larger number of non-randomized phase II trials, and clinical judgment should all be considered in the development of a therapeutic algorithm for the MPNs. Therapeutic algorithms for the MPNs will hopefully continue to evolve as therapeutic modalities improve and are vetted by appropriate clinical trials.

After the appropriate diagnosis of an MPN is established, or sometimes even suspected, patients should be stabilized for immediate problems if present, such as coagulopathies from severe erythrocytosis, thrombocytosis, or concurrent or pre-existing thrombotic events. Management decisions will then flow partially from the clinician's estimation of overall disease prognosis, and the separate estimation of the risk of vascular events. In ET and PV, high-risk patients are defined as either having a prior vascular event or older than 60 years of age, low-risk patients lack either of these features and do not have a platelet count in excess of 1000×10^9/L. Intermediate-risk ET and PV lack these prior features but have cardiovascular risk factors. Newly identified potential vascular risk factors include leukocytosis at diagnosis (at least in PV; $>15 \times 10^9$/L [22]) or high JAK2^{V617F} mutation allele burden [23]. If and how these new factors should be included in modeling MPN vascular risk is not yet known, and requires further study. Overall prognostic models for survival are best established in PMF, in which the IWG-MRT criteria [4] differentiate patients into low, intermediate 1 and 2, and high risk with a range of survival from 27 months to 135 months. The IWG-MRT include five features of independent significance: age >60, anemia, leukocytosis, constitutional symptoms, and circulating blasts.

Short-term plan

The immediate therapeutic concerns for MPN patients at presentation are both adequate prophylaxis against vascular events and palliation, when possible, for MPN symptomatology. Available therapies for both ET and PV, at this juncture, have only been successful in decreasing the risks of thrombotic or hemorrhagic (i.e., vascular) events. Management of PV patients includes control of erythrocytosis (by phlebotomy) and, when no contraindication exists, the use of low-dose aspirin as validated by the ECLAP study (European Collaborative Low-Dose Aspirin Trial) [24]. The degree to which a patient needs to be phlebotomized has been questioned, with traditional dogma suggesting a goal hematocrit of <42% for women and 45% for men. Recent retrospective analysis of vascular events of patients on the ECLAP trial has suggested that modestly higher targets (perhaps up to hematocrits of 55%) may not increase the risk of vascular events [25]. Whether goal hematocrits should be changed for PV is a question that should be addressed by appropriately designed trials.

What about myelosuppressive therapy for managing the MPNs? Hydroxyurea was shown in a randomized fashion to aid in the prevention of thrombotic events in patients with high-risk ET [26]. The UK MRC (United Kingdom Medical Research Council) PT-1 (primary thrombocythemia-1) trial randomized hydroxyurea and anagrelide (both along with low-dose aspirin) for ET patients and found hydroxyurea plus aspirin to be superior in regards to preventing arterial events, hemorrhage, and transformation to post-ET MF [27]. Similar randomized data for the use of hydroxyurea or other myelosuppressive agent in high-risk PV does not yet exist. In the absence of such data, it still remains the most commonly used agent in practice [28]. Therefore, hydroxyurea is standard front-line therapy based on clinical experience for high-risk ET and PV patients who require platelet-lowering therapy. Although concerns linger as to whether hydroxyurea accelerates an MPN towards leukemic transformation, this has never been proven when used as a single agent [29]. The use of pegylated interferon-2 alpha has shown intriguing activity, and potentially improved tolerability, over traditional interferon for PV [30, 31]. An upcoming phase III clinical trial in high-risk ET and PV patients is planned to compare interferon to hydroxyurea.

Palliating symptoms in MPN patients can include therapies for pruritus (antihistamines, and selective serotonin reuptake inhibitors), erythromelalgia (aspirin), and fatigue (no clear therapy has been proven efficacious, but exercise may help as it has in other malignancies [32]). Cytopenias have improved in subsets of patients with erythropoietin supplementation [33], androgens [34], and/or corticosteroids. Similarly, the use of non-specific myelosuppressive regimens such as oral hydroxyurea [35] and cladribine [36] have all been reported to provide palliative reduction in painful splenomegaly.

Long-term therapeutic plan
Currently, no therapy has been shown to be curative, alter natural history, or to prolong survival in MPN patients except allogeneic stem cell transplantation. The long-term therapeutic plan for MPN patients, and particularly those with PMF (and post-ET/PV MF), can be divided into: (1) observation, (2) proceeding directly to an allogeneic stem cell transplant, and (3) enrollment in an appropriate clinical trial. Observation as a medical plan implies continued vigilance and therapy for the prevention of vascular events and appropriate therapy for palliation of MPN symptoms. Observation is most appropriate for those patients with low-risk PMF, and controlled ET and PV. Additionally, observation requires continued vigilance of the patient's disease status for disease progression to a point where (1) a clinical trial would be appropriate or (2) a stem cell transplant would be considered.

The choice and role of allogeneic stem cell transplant for MPN patients remains an evolving question. Amongst the MPNs allogeneic stem cell transplantation is most attractive for high-risk PMF, given this MPN is the most likely to decrease survival amongst those afflicted. Recent reports describe a 58% three-year survival in a group of 56 PMF (and post-ET/PV MF) patients (age 10–66), with a 32% non-relapse mortality rate [37]. The significant toxicity of full allogeneic transplant in PMF led to exploration of the use of reduced intensity conditioning trials [38, 39]. The latter trials have been encouraging in terms of decreased non-relapse mortality, and increasing ages of those successfully transplanted. However, allogeneic transplant still carries a significant risk of graft versus host disease (at least 33%) and the exact role and benefit depends on the long-term prognosis of the patient. The significant risks of any of the stem cell transplantation procedures make it difficult to justify this therapy for ET and PV given the overall good prognosis of these patients.

Observation is most appropriate for those patients with low-risk PMF. Observation requires continued vigilance of the patient's disease status for disease progression to a point where (1) a standard medical therapy or clinical trial would be appropriate, or (2) a stem cell transplant would be considered. When considering current medical therapies for MF (Table 3.2) there are two main groups. Tier 1 consists predominantly of oral agents with (usually) modest toxicities. Cytopenias have improved in subsets of patients with erythropoietin supplementation [33], androgens [34], and/or corticosteroids. Similarly, the use of non-specific myelosuppressive regimens such as oral hydroxyurea [35] and cladribine [36] have all been reported to provide palliative reduction in painful splenomegaly. Tier 2 includes more aggressive approaches, suitable for patients with severe splenomegaly or involvement of other organs by EMH (i.e., lungs, ascites, etc.). In those patients, a more intensive, intravenous, and myelosuppressive approach may be warranted. The choice of both initial and subsequent therapies should be based on the ability to tolerate myelosuppression.

Hydroxyurea

Hydroxyurea is an oral myelosuppressive agent that is active in decreasing splenomegaly in MF [40], and is the most common initial medical therapy used in these patients (estimated response rate of <50% for splenomegaly, although very little prospective clinical trial data exists). However, there are several limitations to the use of this agent for this indication in MF. First, hydroxyurea rarely induces a complete resolution of splenomegaly or even an IWG-MRT clinical improvement for splenomegaly (i.e., >50% improvement sustained for at least two months) [41]. Nevertheless, more modest reductions in splenomegaly may benefit some patients with MF. A second limitation is that splenomegaly is not as responsive to hydroxyurea (compared to thrombocytosis) and might require a higher dose (i.e., 2–3 grams/day).

Thirdly, particularly at higher doses, hydroxyurea therapy may potentially exacerbate cytopenias

Oral alkylators

Alkylators such as melphalan and busulfan can alleviate splenomegaly in some MF patients. However, this occurs with both potential myelosuppression and increased risk of blastic transformation. In one study, melphalan (e.g., 2.5 mg of oral melphalan three times-a-week) reduced spleen size in 66% of patients; however, 26% of the study cohort developed acute leukemia [42]. Busulfan may also be utilized [43], and was classically used in the related myeloproliferative disorder of chronic myeloid leukemia in the pre-imatinib era.

Interferon-alpha (IFN-α)

Therapy with IFN-α has been utilized in patients with MF based on its cytoreductive properties, and this agent has been active in patients with PV [31]. However, clinical trials of IFN-α MF with standard preparations [44] and pegylated interferon alpha (PEG-IFN-α) [45] have demonstrated poor patient tolerance and negligible response rates. In one study, subcutaneous pegylated (PEG)-IFN-α-2b (PEG-Intron) was administered weekly to 36 patients with Ph-negative MPNs, and none of the patients with MF responded [45].

Cladribine

Palliative benefit from the purine nucleoside analog, 2-chlorodeoxyadenosine (2-CdA), has been reported in MF patients [36]. 2-CdA has been administered as four to six once-monthly cycles of treatment with either 0.1 mg/kg/day intravenously by continuous infusion for seven days, or 5 mg/m^2 intravenously over two hours for five consecutive days. In the Mayo Clinic, we have observed responses in 55%, 50%, 55%, and 40% of patients for organomegaly, thrombocytosis, leukocytosis, and anemia, respectively. Responses were frequently durable and lasted for a median of six months after discontinuation of treatment.

Therapeutic splenectomy in MF

The experience with splenectomy in MF dates back to the beginning of the twentieth century [46]. Progressive surgical series demonstrated a signifi-

Table 3.2 Medical therapy for myelofibrosis (available medications)

Agent	Administration route	Dose/Schedule	Response rate[a]	Additional efficacy	Toxicities	Reference
Tier 1						
Hydroxyurea	Oral	500–3000 mg (Daily)	40–50%	None	• Myelosuppression Skin ulcers	[40]
Busulfan	Oral	2–4 mg Daily	Variable	None	• Myelosuppression Leukemia	[69]
Melphalan	Oral	2.5 mg 3x/Week	67%	None	• Myelosuppression • Leukemia	[42]
Interferon 2-alpha	Subcutaneous	$0.5 - 1.0 \times 10^6$ Units 3x/Weekly	Limited data: 75% with small spleens. Less with larger	None	• Myelosuppression • Depression	[70]
Thalidomide +/- Prednisone Taper	Oral	50 mg (Daily)	19%	Anemia / Thrombocytopenia	• Neuropathy • Sedation • Myeloproliferation	[52]
Lenalidomide +/- Prednisone Taper	Oral	5–10 mg (Daily)	33%	Anemia / Thrombocytopenia	• Myelosuppression • Rash • Diarrhea	[68]
Tier 2						
Cladribine (2-CdA)	Intravenous	5 mg/m²/Day x 5 days Monthly	56%	None	• Myelosuppression	[36]
Daunorubicin	Intravenous	60 mg/m²/Days 1–3	N/A	None	• Myelosuppression • Cardiotoxicity	None
5-Azacytidine	Subcutaneous	75 mg/m²/Days 1–7 (Monthly)	21%	Anemia	• Myelosuppression • Gastrointestinal	[58, 59]
Decitabine	Subcutaneous	20 mg/m²/Days 1–5 (Monthly)	N/A	None	• Myelosuppression	None

cant, but slowly decreasing, peri-operative mortality rate due to improvements in surgical technique, antimicrobials, and patient selection. Although splenectomy can be helpful for improving MF patient symptoms, it seems to have no clear outcome on patient survival, nor any impact on the disease course or intramedullary manifestations of the disease. We recently analyzed three decades of Mayo Clinic experience with palliative splenectomy in MF to see if better control of post-splenectomy thrombocytosis, and modern operative techniques and supportive care, have diminished morbidity and mortality [47]. Although meaningful improvements in symptoms can be observed in 30–50% of patients, complication rates (27.7% and 6.7% fatal) are sobering and require close peri-operative management and careful choice of candidates.

Radiation for MF

Extramedullary hematopoiesis (EMH) in patients with MF, regardless of location, is exquisitely sensitive to external beam radiotherapy. Sites frequently irradiated in patients with MF include the lungs [48] (where EMH can contribute to pulmonary hypertension), para-spinal masses [49], or the spleen. Splenomegaly can be palliated by external beam radiotherapy, but benefit is typically transient and myelosuppression can be severe. Several reports have described the palliative benefit to external beam radiation in improving symptomatic splenomegaly in MF [50, 51]. The Mayo Clinic experience [50] included a group of 23 MF patients who received a median radiation course of 277 cGy in a median of eight fractions. An objective decrease in spleen size was noted in 94% of patients; however, 44% of patients experienced post-treatment cytopenias (26% were severe; 13% fatal). Splenic radiation also seemed to increase morbidity and mortality of subsequent splenectomy when undertaken. This latter effect seems related to the development of splenic adhesions to the abdominal wall and surrounding viscera, leading to greater complexity with subsequent attempts at surgical extirpation. Additionally, delayed hemorrhage in irradiated areas in which the spleen had to be bluntly dissected away from other structures was common.

Experimental therapies for MPNs (Table 3.3)

Immunomodulatory inhibitory drugs (IMiDs)

The group of immunomodulatory, cytokine inhibitory, and anti-angiogenic agents collectively known as IMiDs have primarily been able to palliate cytopenias (anemia and thrombocytopenia) in MF, but may also reduce splenomegaly.

Low-dose (i.e., 50 mg/day) thalidomide with a prednisone taper (THAL-PRED regimen) achieves significant responses in MF for anemia (67%), thrombocytopenia (75%), and splenomegaly (33%) [52]. Subsequently, lenalidomide (LEN) (a second generation IMiD) was evaluated in 68 patients with symptomatic MF, with overall response rates of 22% for anemia, 33% for splenomegaly, and 50% for thrombocytopenia [53]. Mirroring the activity of lenalidomide in del(5q) myelodysplastic syndromes, MF patients with an abnormality of chromosome 5 seem to respond best to this agent [54].

Another promising IMiD, pomalidomide, is 20 000-fold more potent than thalidomide in inhibiting TNF-α, although cross-resistance with the latter does not appear to occur [55]. Due to its excellent oral absorption and adequate pharmacokinetics, pomalidomide is suitable for once-daily administration. In phase I trials in patients with multiple myeloma, the main side effects associated with pomalidomide therapy were related to myelosuppression and deep vein thrombosis [56]. Given the promising results obtained with lenalidomide, a randomized, placebo controlled, international clinical study was done in order to determine the activity of pomalidomide (with or without a prednisone taper) in MF and post-ET/PV MF. This treatment regimen has shown improvements for MF-associated anemia in over 30% of patients, with a favorable toxicity profile [57]. Future studies to optimize the dose, determine the effect on splenomegaly and marrow manifestations are ongoing. Additionally, analysis of the net impact of these agents on anemia-related symptoms such as fatigue are ongoing.

Hypomethylating agents

The two hypomethylating agents approved for myelodysplastic syndromes (MDS), azacitidine (AZA)

Table 3.3 Experimental agents for MPNs

Compound	Company	Indication	Stage of development	Mechanism of action
INCB018424	Incyte	MF, PV	III	Selective JAK2 Inhibitor
TG101348	Targen	MF	I	Selective JAK2 Inhibitor
XL019	Exelexis	MF	I	Selective JAK2 Inhibitor
CEP-701	Cephalon	MF, ET, PV	II	FLT3 and JAK2 Inhibitor
ITF2357	Italfarmaco	MF, ET, PV	II	HDAC and JAK2 Inhibitor
LBH539	Novartis	MF	II	HDAC and JAK2 Inhibitor
Pomalidomide	Celgene	MF	III	IMID
Azacitidine	Celgene	MF	II	Hypomethylation
Decitabine	Eisai	MF	II	Hypomethylation

and decitabine, have both been tested in MF in order to improve cytopenias, splenomegaly, or delay blastic transformation. Recent trials of AZA ($75\,\mathrm{mg/m^2/}$ day administered for either five or seven days) showed a 21% response rate for splenomegaly in MF, exclusively in the seven-day regimen [58, 59]. Decitabine, and trials in MF are ongoing. Limitation in the use of these therapies in MF include the frequent visits required for administration, and the myelosuppression that is their most common adverse effect.

JAK2 inhibition (Figure 3.1)

Various therapeutic strategies are being developed to try to block the proliferative stimulus associated with these MPN-associated mutations. Current testing of therapeutic inhibition of these inhibitors can be divided into three groups, specifically pre-clinical (based on *in vitro* activity against JAK2^{V617F} containing cells), those with ongoing testing in murine models, and those undergoing testing in clinical trials. Although there is a pipeline of 10–20 agents with reported *in vitro* or murine model activity, we will focus on those agents in which clinical activity has already been reported in the public forum. JAK2 inhibition clinical results can be divided into two categories of agents. The first category involves novel small molecules designed and tested for spec- ificity and selectivity against JAK2 (INCB 018424, XL019, TG101348). The second includes agents that inhibit a variety of kinases including JAK2 (ITF2357, CEP-701).

PV (with 99% of patients having a mutation somewhere in their JAK2) could well be the most straightforward target of JAK2 inhibition, and preliminary results of trials with XL019 [60], CEP-701 (Cephalon, Frazer, PA, USA) [61], and ITF2347 [62] show preliminary activity in decreasing erythrocytosis. However, these trials are too early in their accrual and analysis to make a conclusion on their efficacy at this time. Interestingly, in PV, the agent that has shown an ability to lead to significant reductions in JAK2^{V617F} allele burden in 30–40% of patients (including complete molecular remissions) is pegylated interferon-2a (Pegasys). Recently, reported outcomes from trials in Europe [31] and the US [30] have both confirmed these observations. Intriguingly, even patients on hydroxyurea (who have had an excellent clinical response) may have significant reductions in mutant allele burden [63].

The most mature clinical experience (Table 3.2) for a JAK2 inhibitor is for myelofibrosis. The first is INCB018424 (Incyte Co., Wilmington, DE) (selective against JAK1 and JAK2) with the largest MF trial in history (>120 patients), where the agent

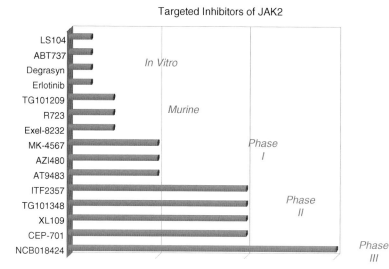

Figure 3.1 Pipeline of JAK2 inhibitors in MPNs.

leads to significant reduction in splenomegaly and dramatic improvement in constitutional symptoms [64]. Although a well-tolerated drug, the suppression of the JAK-STAT pathway (including normal hematopoiesis which signals through this pathway) can lead to treatment-related thrombocytopenia and anemia [64]. Additional drugs being tested are early in their results with the most promising being TG101348 – selective JAK2 inhibitor (TarGen, San Francisco, CA) now in the expanded second phase of the trial [65]. XL019 – selective JAK2 inhibitor (Exelexis, San Francisco, CA) [66] was associated with the development of neurologic toxicities, which have derailed development of this agent. Studies of CEP-701 (Cephalon, Frazer, PA, USA) [67] and ITF2357 (Italfarmaco, Italy) [62] also suggest improvements in splenomegaly and symptoms in MF patients, and are the subject of ongoing trials. No JAK2 inhibitor has yet reported a significant ability to improve cytopenias, fibrosis, or histologic changes associated with MF.

Conclusions

The pathogenetic understanding, diagnosis, and therapy of MPNs is currently at an exciting crossroad, where the significant pathogenetic observation of the role of the JAK2^{V617F} mutation and association of MPD mutations has led to the development of the largest number of potential drugs for the therapy of this disease that has ever existed. These trials show preliminary results that are encouraging, although largely represent partial responses for patients who have been treated. That latter effect being said, many of these agents in development have yet to undergo clinical testing and those agents in testing still are undergoing further delineation as to optimized dose and schedule. Finally, further discoveries in the pathogenesis of MF may yield additional insights in agents, including agents that work against this stromal reaction in the marrow, the cytokine storm, and the evolving story regarding the molecular genetics of myeloproliferation.

References

1 Damashek W. (1951) Some speculations on the myeloproliferative syndrome. *Blood* **6**:372–5.

2 Vardiman JW, Thiele J, Arber DA, et al. 2008. The revision of the WHO classification of myeloid neoplasms and acute leukemia: rationale and important changes. At http://bloodjournal.hematologylibrary.org/cgi/content/short/blood-2009-03-209262v1 (last accessed October 4, 2010)

3 Mesa RA, Silverstein MN, Jacobsen SJ, Wollan PC, Tefferi A. (1999) Population-based incidence and survival figures in essential thrombocythemia and agnogenic myeloid metaplasia: an Olmsted County Study, 1976–1995. *Am J Hematol* **61**:10–15.

4 Cervantes F, Dupriez B, Pereira A, et al. (2009) New prognostic scoring system for primary myelofibrosis based on a study of the International Working Group for Myelofibrosis Research and Treatment. *Blood* **113**:2895–901.

5 Passamonti F, Rumi E, Pungolino E, et al. (2004) Life expectancy and prognostic factors for survival in patients with polycythemia vera and essential thrombocythemia. *Am J Med* **117**:755–61.

6 Baxter EJ, Scott LM, Campbell PJ, *et al.* (2005) Acquired mutation of the tyrosine kinase JAK2 in human myeloproliferative disorders. *Lancet* **365**:1054–61.

7 Kralovics R, Passamonti F, Buser AS, et al. (2005) A gain-of-function mutation of JAK2 in myeloproliferative disorders. *N Engl J Med* **352**:1779–90.

8 James C, Ugo V, Le Couedic JP, et al. (2005) A unique clonal JAK2 mutation leading to constitutive signalling causes polycythaemia vera. *Nature* **434**:1144–8.

9 Levine RL, Wadleigh M, Cools J, et al. (2005) Activating mutation in the tyrosine kinase JAK2 in polycythemia vera, essential thrombocythemia, and myelofibrosis with myeloid metaplasia. *Cancer Cell* **7**:387–97.

10 Tefferi A, Gilliland DG. (2007) Oncogenes in myeloproliferative disorders. *Cell Cycle* **6**:550–66.

11 Pardanani AD, Levine RL, Lasho T, et al. (2006) MPL515 mutations in myeloproliferative and other myeloid disorders: a study of 1182 patients. *Blood* **108**:3472–76.

12 Scott LM, Tong W, Levine RL, et al. (2007) JAK2 exon 12 mutations in polycythemia vera and idiopathic erythrocytosis. *N Engl J Med* **356**:459–68.

13 Pardanani A. (2008) JAK2 inhibitor therapy in myeloproliferative disorders: rationale, preclinical studies and ongoing clinical trials. *Leukemia* **22**:23–30.

14 Delhommeau F, Dupont S, Della Valle V, et al. (2009) Mutation in TET2 in myeloid cancers. *N Engl J Med* **360**:2289–301.

15 Tefferi A, Pardanani A, Lim KH, et al. (2009) TET2 mutations and their clinical correlates in polycythemia vera, essential thrombocythemia and myelofibrosis. *Leukemia* **23**:905–11.

16 Pardanani A, Fridley BL, Lasho TL, Gilliland DG, Tefferi A. (2008) Host genetic variation contributes to phenotypic diversity in myeloproliferative disorders. *Blood* **111**:2785–9.

17 Jones AV, Chase A, Silver RT, et al. (2009) JAK2 haplotype is a major risk factor for the development of myeloproliferative neoplasms. *Nat Genet* **41**:446–9.

18 Olcaydu D, Harutyunyan A, Jager R, et al. (2009) A common JAK2 haplotype confers susceptibility to myeloproliferative neoplasms. *Nat Genet* **41**:450–4.

19 Tefferi A, Thiele J, Orazi A, et al. (2007) Proposals and rationale for revision of the World Health Organization diagnostic criteria for polycythemia vera, essential thrombocythemia, and primary myelofibrosis: recommendations from an ad hoc international expert panel. *Blood* **110**:1092–97.

20 Mesa RA, Verstovsek S, Cervantes F, et al. (2007) Primary myelofibrosis (PMF), post-polycythemia vera myelofibrosis (post-PV MF), post-essential thrombocythemia myelofibrosis (post-ET MF), blast phase PMF (PMF-BP): Consensus on terminology by the International Working Group for Myelofibrosis Research and Treatment (IWG-MRT). *Leuk Res* **31**:737–740.

21 Barosi G, Mesa RA, Thiele J, et al. (2008) Proposed criteria for the diagnosis of post-polycythemia vera and post-essential thrombocythemia myelofibrosis: a consensus statement from the International Working Group for Myelofibrosis Research and Treatment. *Leukemia* **22**:437–8.

22 Landolfi R, Di Gennaro L, Barbui T, et al. (2007) Leukocytosis as a major thrombotic risk factor in patients with polycythemia vera. *Blood* **109**:2446–52.

23 Vannucchi AM, Antonioli E, Guglielmelli P, et al. (2007) Clinical profile of homozygous JAK2 617V>F mutation in patients with polycythemia vera or essential thrombocythemia. *Blood* **110**:840–6.

24 Landolfi R, Marchioli R, Kutti J, et al. (2004) Efficacy and safety of low-dose aspirin in polycythemia vera. *N Engl J Med* **350**:114–24.

25 Di Nisio M, Barbui T, Di Gennaro L, et al. (2007) The haematocrit and platelet target in polycythemia vera. *Br J Haematol* **136**:249–59.

26 Cortelazzo S, Finazzi G, Ruggeri M, et al. (1995) Hydroxyurea for patients with essential thrombocythemia and a high risk of thrombosis. *N Engl J Med* **332**:1132–6.

27 Harrison CN, Campbell PJ, Buck G, et al. (2005) Hydroxyurea compared with anagrelide in high-risk essential thrombocythemia. *N Engl J Med* **353**:33–45.

28 Finazzi G, Barbui T. (2005) Risk-adapted therapy in essential thrombocythemia and polycythemia vera. *Blood Rev* **19**:243–52.

29 Finazzi G, Caruso V, Marchioli R, et al. (2005) Acute leukemia in polycythemia vera: an analysis of 1638 patients enrolled in a prospective observational study. *Blood* **105**:2664–70.

30 Quintas-Cardama A, Kantarjian HM, Garcia-Manero G, et al. (2008) Pegylated interferon-alpha-2A (PEG-IFN-α-2A; PEGASYS) therapy renders high clinical and molecular response rates in patients with essential thrombocythemia (ET) and polycythemia vera (PV). *Blood* **112**:658.

31 Kiladjian JJ, Cassinat B, Chevret S, et al. (2008) Pegylated interferon-alpha-2a induces complete hematologic and molecular responses with low toxicity in polycythemia vera. *Blood* **112**:3065–72.

32 Dimeo F, Schwartz S, Fietz T, et al. (2003) Effects of endurance training on the physical performance of patients with hematological malignancies during chemotherapy. *Support Care Cancer* **11**:623–8.

33 Cervantes F, Alvarez-Larran A, Hernandez-Boluda JC, et al. (2004) Erythropoietin treatment of the anaemia of myelofibrosis with myeloid metaplasia: results in 20 patients and review of the literature. *Br J Haematol* **127**:399–403.

34 Cervantes F, Hernandez-Boluda JC, Alvarez A, Nadal E, Montserrat E. (2000) Danazol treatment of idiopathic myelofibrosis with severe anemia. *Haematologica* **85**:595–9.

35 Lofvenberg E, Wahlin A, Roos G, Ost A. (1990) Reversal of myelofibrosis by hydroxyurea. *Euro J Haematol* **44**:33–8.

36 Faoro LN, Tefferi A, Mesa RA. (2005) Long-term analysis of the palliative benefit of 2-chlorodeoxyadenosine for myelofibrosis with myeloid metaplasia. *Eur J Haematol* **74**:117–20.

37 Deeg HJ, Gooley TA, Flowers ME, et al. (2003) Allogeneic hematopoietic stem cell transplantation for myelofibrosis. *Blood* **102**:3912–8.

38 Rondelli D, Barosi G, Bacigalupo A, et al. (2005) Allogeneic hematopoietic stem cell transplantation with reduced intensity conditioning in intermediate- or high-risk patients with myelofibrosis with myeloid metaplasia. *Blood* **105**:4115–9.

39 Kroger N, Thiele J, Zander A, et al. (2007) Rapid regression of bone marrow fibrosis after dose-reduced allogeneic stem cell transplantation in patients with primary myelofibrosis. *Exp Hematol* **35**:1719–22.

40 Lofvenberg E, Wahlin A. (1988) Management of polycythaemia vera, essential thrombocythaemia and myelofibrosis with hydroxyurea. *Eur J Haematol* **41**:375–81.

41 Tefferi A, Barosi G, Mesa RA, et al. (2006) International Working Group (IWG) consensus criteria for treatment response in myelofibrosis with myeloid metaplasia, for the IWG for Myelofibrosis Research and Treatment (IWG-MRT). *Blood* **108**:1497–503.

42 Petti MC, Latagliata R, Spadea T, et al. (2002) Melphalan treatment in patients with myelofibrosis with myeloid metaplasia. *Br J Haematol* **116**:576–81.

43 Silver RT, Jenkins DE, Jr., Engle RL, Jr., (1964) Use of testosterone and busulfan in the treatment of myelofibrosis with myeloid metaplasia. *Blood* **23**:341–53.

44 Tefferi A, Elliot MA, Yoon SY, et al. (2001) Clinical and bone marrow effects of interferon alfa therapy in myelofibrosis with myeloid metaplasia. *Blood* **97**:1896.

45 Verstovsek S, Lawhorn, K, Giles, F, et al. (2004) PEG-Intron for myeloproliferative diseases: an update of ongoing phase II study. *Blood* **104**:11 [Abstract 633].

46 Hickling RA. (1937) Splenectomy in myeloid metaplasia. *Quart J Med* **30**:253.

47 Mesa RA, Nagorney DS, Schwager S, Allred J, Tefferi A. (2006) Palliative goals, patient selection, and perioperative platelet management: outcomes and lessons from three decades of splenectomy for myelofibrosis with myeloid metaplasia at the Mayo Clinic. *Cancer* **107**:361–70.

48 Steensma DP, Hook CC, Stafford SL, Tefferi A. (2002) Low-dose, single-fraction, whole-lung radiotherapy for pulmonary hypertension associated with myelofibrosis with myeloid metaplasia. *Br J Haematol* **118**:813–6.

49 Koch CA, Li CY, Mesa RA, Tefferi A. (2003) Nonhepatosplenic extramedullary hematopoiesis: associated diseases, pathology, clinical course, and treatment. *Mayo Clin Proc* **78**:1223–33.

50 Elliott MA, Chen MG, Silverstein MN, Tefferi A. (1998) Splenic irradiation for symptomatic splenomegaly associated with myelofibrosis with myeloid metaplasia. *Br J Haematol* **103**:505–11.

51 Bouabdallah R, Coso D, Gonzague-Casabianca L, et al. (2000) Safety and efficacy of splenic irradiation in the treatment of patients with idiopathic myelofibrosis: a report on 15 patients. *Leuk Res* **24**:491–5.

52 Mesa RA, Steensma DP, Pardanani A, et al. (2003) A phase 2 trial of combination low-dose thalidomide and prednisone for the treatment of myelofibrosis with myeloid metaplasia. *Blood* **101**:2534–41.

53 Tefferi A, Cortes J, Verstovsek S, et al. (2006) Lenalidomide therapy in myelofibrosis with myeloid metaplasia. *Blood* **108**:1158–64.

54 Tefferi A, Lasho TL, Mesa RA, et al. (2007) Lenalidomide therapy in del(5)(q31)-associated myelofibrosis: cytogenetic and JAK2V617F molecular remissions. *Leukemia* **21**:1827–8.

55 Muller GW, Chen R, Huang SY, et al. (1999) Aminosubstituted thalidomide analogs: potent inhibitors of TNF-alpha production. *Bioorg Med Chem Lett* **9**:1625–30.

56 Schey SA, Fields P, Bartlett JB, et al. (2004) Phase I study of an immunomodulatory thalidomide analog, CC-4047, in relapsed or refractory multiple myeloma. *J Clin Oncol* **22**:3269–76.

57 Tefferi A, Verstovsek S, Barosi G, et al. (2008) Pomalidomide therapy in anemic patients with myelofibrosis: results from a Phase-2 randomized multicenter study. *Blood* **112**:663.

58 Quintás-Cardama A, Tong W, Kantarjian H, et al. (2008) A Phase II study of 5-azacitidine for patients with primary and post-essential thrombocythemia/polcythemia vera myelofibrosis. *Leukemia* **22**:965–70.

59 Mesa RA, Verstovsek S, Rivera C, et al. (2009) 5-Azacitidine has limited therapeutic activity in myelofibrosis. *Leukemia* **23**:180–2.

60 Paquette R, Sokol L, Shah NP, et al. (2008) A Phase I study of XL019, a selective JAK2 inhibitor, in patients with polycythemia vera. *Blood* **112**:2810.

61 Moliterno AR, Roboz GJ, Carroll M, et al. (2008) An open-label study of CEP-701 in patients with JAK2 V617F-positive polycythemia vera and essential thrombocytosis. *Blood* **112**:99.

62 Rambaldi A, Dellacasa CM, Salmoiraghi S, et al. (2008) A Phase 2A study of the histone-deacetylase inhibitor ITF2357 in patients with Jak2V617F positive chronic myeloproliferative neoplasms. *Blood* **112**:100.

63 Besses C, Alvarez-Larran A, Martinez-Aviles L, et al. (2008) Major hematological response is the main factor for achieving a major molecular response in JAK2V617F-positive essential thrombocythemia and polycythemia vera patients treated with hydroxyurea. *Blood* **112**:660.

64 Verstovsek S, Kantarjian HM, Pardanani AD, et al. (2008) The JAK inhibitor, INCB018424, demonstrates durable and marked clinical responses in primary myelofibrosis (PMF) and post-polycythemia/essential thrombocythemia myelofibrosis (post-PV/ET MF). *Blood* **112**:1762.

65 Pardanani AD, Gotlib J, Jamieson C, et al. (2008) A Phase I study of TG101348, an orally bioavailable JAK2-selective inhibitor, in patients with myelofibrosis. *Blood* **112**:97.

66 Shah NP, Olszynski P, Sokol L, et al. (2008) A Phase I study of XL019, a selective JAK2 inhibitor, in patients with primary myelofibrosis, post-polycythemia vera, or post-essential thrombocythemia myelofibrosis. *Blood* **112**:98.

67 Verstovsek S, Tefferi A, Kornblau S, et al. (2007) Phase II study of CEP701, an orally available JAK2 inhibitor, in patients with primary myelofibrosis and post-polycythemia vera/essential thrombocythemia myelofibrosis. *Blood* **110**:3543.

68 Tefferi A, Cortes J, Verstovsek S, et al. (2006) Lenalidomide therapy in myelofibrosis with myeloid metaplasia. *Blood* **108**:1158–64.

69 Chang JC, Gross HM. (1988) Remission of chronic idiopathic myelofibrosis to busulfan treatment. *Am J Med Sci* **295**:472–6.

70 Levy B, Vandris K, Adriano F, Goldman J, Silver RT. (2008) Recombinant interferon alpha (rIFN{alpha}) may retard progression of early primary myelofibrosis (PM) by reducing splenomegaly and by changing marrow morphology. *Blood* **112**:1758.

CHAPTER 4

Molecular Pathogenesis of BCR-ABL in Chronic Myeloid Leukemia

Eric Padron, Lori A. Hazlehurst and Javier Pinilla-Ibarz

Department of Malignant Hematology, H. Lee Moffitt Cancer Center and Research Institute, Tampa, FL, USA

Introduction

When Nowell and Hungerford made an astute observation approximately 50 years ago, it would drastically change the landscape of research in chronic myeloid leukemia (CML). Nowell and Hungerford described a minute chromosome in a series of seven patients with chronic granulocytic leukemia [1]. After colleagues confirmed the presence of this chromosome in roughly 97% of CML cases, the chromosome was designated the "Philadelphia chromosome" as suggested by the Committee for the Standardization of Chromosomes who deemed abnormal chromosomes be named after the city in which they were discovered [2].

With improved cytogenetic banding techniques in the years to come, it was discovered that the Philadelphia chromosome was a result of a reciprocal translocation between chromosomes 9 and 22 [t(9:22)]. Molecular techniques later found that this translocation resulted in a fusion of the breakpoint cluster region (BCR) gene on chromosome 22 and the c-Abl gene on chromosome 9 [3, 4].

The BCR gene product is a 1271 amino acid phosphoprotein that has multiple catalytic functions including serine kinase activity, GTPase activating protein (GAP), and guanine nucleotide exchange factor activity [5–7]. Although the normal function of the c-Abl gene product is unknown, this protein has significant structural homology to the Src family

of tyrosine kinases and is thought to be part of a unique family of kinases (Figure 4.1). Nonetheless, the end product of this fusion is a promiscuous and constitutively active tyrosine kinase known as BCR-ABL, which resides in the cytoplasm and is responsible for activating numerous pathways important in aberrant cell survival [8].

Three predominant isoforms of BCR-ABL have been described. These result in distinct breakpoints within the BCR gene when fused to c-Abl. The corresponding fusion products will encode a p190, p210, or p230 molecular weight protein each associated with a phenotypically distinct leukemia (Figure 4.2). In the majority of cases, the breakpoint encoding p210 is known as the major breakpoint cluster region (M-BCR) and is responsible for its BCR-ABL isoform in CML. The minor breakpoint cluster region (m-BCR) encodes the p190 protein and is responsible for the BCR-ABL isoform in the majority of Philadelphia chromosome positive acute lymphoblastic leukemias (ALL) and a small minority of CMLs [9]. The breakpoint for p230 is located downstream of exon 19 in BCR and is responsible for the isoform in Philadelphia chromosome positive chronic neutrophilic leukemia (CNL) [10]. These isoforms also exhibit unique characteristics in pre-clinical mouse studies that seem congruent with their clinical phenotype [11]. In particular, p190 has the shortest latency period, and mice develop B-cell origin leukemia exclusively. In contrast, p210 transgenic mice typically develop leukemia of

Advances in Malignant Hematology, First Edition. Edited by Hussain I. Saba and Ghulam J. Mufti. © 2011 Blackwell Publishing Ltd. Published 2011 by Blackwell Publishing Ltd.

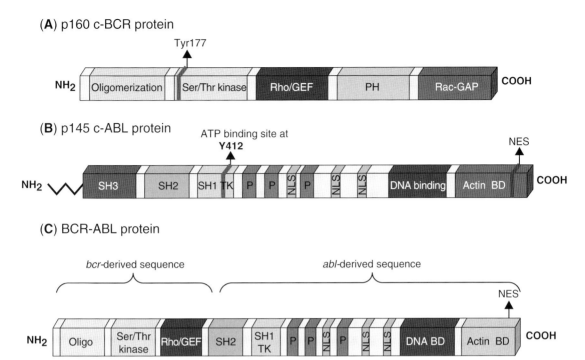

Figure 4.1 (A) A schematic highlighting the protein domains within the wild-type Bcr protein. The oligomerization domain is important for the autophosphorylation of the BCR-ABL fusion protein. The Tyr177 residue serves as the docking station for a protein complex that includes GRB2, responsible for RAS activation. (B) A schematic of the wild-type Abl protein whose homeostatic function is carried out in the nucleus. (C) A schematic of the BCR-ABL fusion partner whose abnormal localization in the cytoplasm and constitutive tyrosine phosphorylation results in novel downstream binding partners. Reproduced from Hazlehurst et al. [75] with permission.

B-, T-lymphoid, or myeloid origin. Finally, p230 transgenic mice showed the longest latency period and exhibited a less aggressive tumor, a finding that is consistent with CNL [12, 13].

BCR-ABL as an oncogene in CML

The importance of the BCR-ABL fusion kinase in the tumorogenesis of CML has been studied in the mouse model. Zhang and colleagues used a retroviral vector to transduce the p210 BCR-ABL isoform into mouse bone marrow cells [14]. Even at the most dilute concentrations of retrovirus, transfected mice developed a massive expansion of myeloid elements at the expense of normal hematopoiesis resulting in a myeloproliferative disorder akin to CML. Other mouse studies have yielded similar results when the

BCR-ABL fusion protein was placed under the control of the tetracycline response element [12, 13]. Inducible expression of BCR-ABL resulted in mice demonstrating splenomegaly, myeloid bone marrow hyperplasia, and extra medullary myeloid cell infiltration [13, 15]. It has been shown that it is the aberrant kinase activity of BCR-ABL that is tumorigenic. When mice were transfected with the aforementioned retroviral vector containing a BCR-ABL transcript that encoded a non-functional kinase domain, no myeloproliferative syndrome occurred. Thus, BCR-ABL kinase activity is sufficient for tumorigenesis [13].

This kinase activity responsible for leukemic transformation activates numerous downstream signaling pathways that are implicated in cell survival. A portion of the BCR moiety, (Tyr177) for instance [16], serves as a docking station for a pro-

1 *bcr-abl* oncogene, 3 BCR-ABL proteins

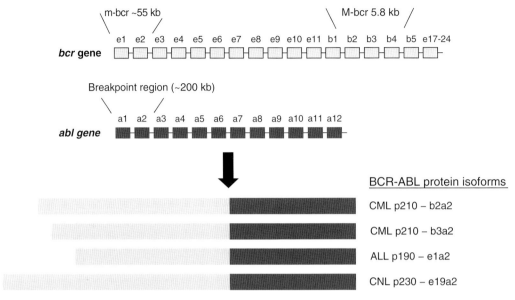

Figure 4.2 A schematic of the distinct BCR-ABL breakpoints and their resultant malignant phenotype. Reproduced from Hazlehurst et al. [75] with permission.

tein complex that includes growth factor receptor bound protein2 (GRB2) [17], SOS, and GAB2 [18]. This results in activation of RAS as well as constitutive activation of the phosphatidylinositol 3-kinase (PI3K)/AKT and ERK pathways that are thought to be critical to aberrant cell survival and leukemogenesis [19]. Indeed, GAB2 knockout mice fail to transform in spite of transfection of BCR-ABL [18]. Although controversial, BCR-ABL also upregulates transcription of STAT5 via phosphophorylation of HCK, an src kinase, and JAK2 [20–22]. The abnormal activation of these pathways leads to downstream upregulation of c-Myc, cyclin-D1, and JUN B which are all required for tumorigenesis in mouse models [23–25]. The RAC subfamily of guanosine triphosphatases is also aberrantly activated in CML and their experimental inhibition results in an increased latency period for CML-like syndromes in murine systems [26, 27] (Figure 4.3).

BCR-ABL also exhibits effects outside of increased myeloid proliferation. BCR-ABL binds to F-actin causing downstream activation and dysfunction of many proteins critical in cell adhesion, motility, and chemotaxis [28]. As alluded to previously, antiapoptotic agents are upregulated as well. The Bcl-xL deamidation pathway is altered in CML such that sequestration of Bcl-2, a pro-apoptotic factor, is inhibited and thus promotes cell survival [20]. In summary, BCR-ABL kinase activity promotes widespread phosphorylation of proteins whose net effect is an increased proliferative index, decreased apoptic rate, and altered cytoskeletal function, making it an excellent target for treatment.

BCR-ABL in the treatment of CML

BCR-ABL inhibitors

Early compounds directed toward inhibiting the kinase activity of BCR-ABL provided great promise *in vitro* following reports of impressive cytotoxicity in BCR-ABL-containing cells, but unfortunately *in vivo*, non-specificity and unacceptable toxicity limited their use. However, a novel 2-phenylaminopyrimidine compound was found that selectively inhibited the BCR-ABL kinase *in vitro* with minimal toxicity *in vivo*. In fact, this compound, later named imatinib mesylate (Gleevec™) was found to reverse

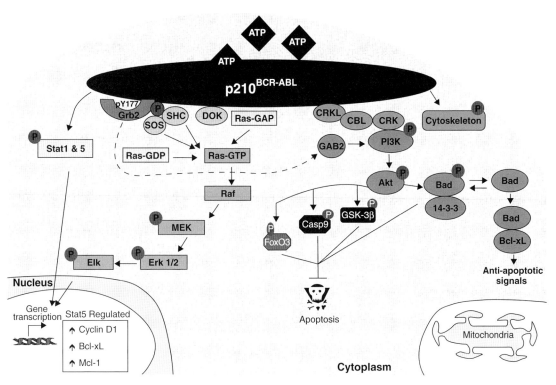

Figure 4.3 BCR-ABL is a constitutive and promiscuous tyrosine kinase. This is an abbreviated schematic of the known downstream pathways. Reproduced from Hazlehurst et al. [75] with permission.

the CML-like phenotype expressed by a BCR-ABL transfected mouse system in the vast majority of cases. Ultimately, a randomized phase III trial, the IRIS (International Randomized Study of Interferon and STI571) trial, compared imatinib mesylate to interferon [29, 30]. This trial showed imatinib to have improved cytogenetic and hematologic responses, less toxicity, and longer, deeper durable remissions. A later trial at M.D. Anderson provided imatinib with an overall survival advantage when compared to interferon [31].

Despite high response rates, there still remain a percentage of CML patients who become resistant to imatinib or, less common, refractory to imatinib on initial therapy [32]. More recently, second generation BCR-ABL kinase inhibitors have been developed and approved by the FDA (US Food and Drug Administration) for use in the second-line setting and more recently as front line. In fact, two recent randomized phase II trials demonstrated nilotinib and dasatinib, two more potent inhibitors of the BCR-ABL kinase, to be more effective in the front-line setting [33, 34].

BCR-ABL inhibitor resistance

Despite high response and low relapse rates with BCR-ABL kinase inhibitors, discontinuation of compounds like imatinib uniformly result in disease recurrence. Furthermore, primary or secondary resistance to tyrosine kinase (TK) inhibition, particularly imatinib, can occur in as many as 25% of cases [35]. The majority of these cases, particularly relating to secondary resistance, are due to mutations in the kinase domain of BCR-ABL [36–38]. The kinase domain consists of four relevant sites that include the ATP docking site (P-loop), the ATP binding site, the catalytic site, and activation loop (A-loop). Mutations in the kinase domain have been isolated in all four regions of the kinase domain [39].

Imatinib and nilotinib bind in close proximity to both the P- and A- loops and force the kinase to remain in its conformationally inactive state [40, 41].

Dasatinib, however, binds and inactivates the ABL kinase in its active conformation and has little interaction with the docking or activating loops [39, 42]. All three TKIs do have critical interactions with threonine 315. Indeed, T315I mutations are seen in 15% of CML cases and are associated with resistance to all known TKIs. This is because Thr315 forms a critical H-bond with all known TKIs to stabilize the drug in its pocket. T315I-sensitive BCR-ABL kinases are now under investigation [43, 44]. For instance, the aurora kinase inhibitor has been shown, *in vitro* and *in vivo*, to have off-target effects on BCR-ABL that are Thr315-independent [45, 46].

Genomic instability and BCR-ABL

The BCR-ABL kinase has been implicated in a mutator phenotype that is, in part, responsible for the clonal evolution seen in CML. Compared to cytokine-mediated cell growth in non-transformed cell lines, BCR-ABL-transformed cells exhibit relative increased production of reactive oxygen species (ROS) [47–49]. The ROS are responsible for a broad array of DNA damage including single and double strand breaks.

The DNA repair machinery exhibits decreased fidelity when attempting to repair this damage, perhaps due to the increased expression of DNA polymerase fl and the selective increase in the single strand annealing repair mechanisms, known to be particularly mutogenic [50]. Further, RAD3 and ataxia-telangectasia nuclear signaling is inhibited in BCR-ABL-transformed cells decreasing S-phase cell cycle checkpoints [51].

Under normal DNA homeostasis, non-homologous end joining (NHEJ) and homologous recombination (HR) are responsible for the majority of double-stranded break repair. A complex of proteins, including DNA-PK, thought to be responsible for the repair machinery in NHEJ is recruited by Ku70 and Ku80. Ku70 and Ku80 are sensitive too and bind double-stranded breaks in DNA. Deutsch et al. [52] showed that BCR-ABL expression results in decreased levels of DNA-PK, a critical component in NHEJ, ultimately reversed by treatment with a proteasome inhibitor. Investigators also showed that expression of BCR-ABL attenuates the levels of BRCA1 and that inhibition of the BCR-ABL kinase activity with imatinib restored the levels of BRCA1 [53]. BRCA1 is thought to localize to DNA damage foci containing FANCD2 and RD51 and facilitates HR-mediated DNA repair [54]. By modulating DNA-PK expression and attenuating the effects of BRCA1, BCR-ABL is able to disturb the function of the two sentinel mechanisms in double-strand break repair, NJEM and HR respectively.

Crossover events are also perturbed by BCR-ABL. Ectopic expression of BCR-ABL in UT-7 cells increased the frequency of sister chromatid exchange following gamma radiation [53, 55]. Taken together, BCR-ABL expression has properties that both damage DNA directly and affect the cells' ability to repair that damage by altering NJEM, HR, and promoting single strand annealing.

Transformation to blast-stage crisis

The pathogenesis of blast phase (BP)-CML is incompletely understood. It is known that expression and translation of BCR-ABL mRNA is increased in granulocyte-macrophage progenitor cells (GMP) of BP-CML compared to chronic phase (CP)-CML. GMPs are a subpopulation of cells that are expanded in BP-CML and will be discussed further below [56]. As mentioned previously, BCR-ABL has been implicated in proliferation and antiapoptosis but mounting evidence suggests it may play a role in promoting a more primitive, de-differentiated myeloid progenitor. Specifically, BCR-ABL modulates the activity of CCAAT/enhancer-binding protein-alpha (CEBP-alpha), a transcription required for normal myeloid differentiation. CEBP-alpha is downregulated in BP-CML and, in fact, is necessary for CP-CML tumorgenesis in a BCR-ABL-expressing xenograft murine model. In this experiment, BCR-ABL-expressing fetal liver +/- CEBP-alpha cells were transplanted in nude mice [57, 58]. Those CEBP-alpha -/- mice developed an erythroleukemia-like disease while those with CEBP-alpha +/+ developed a CML-like disease.

A recent study by Ito et al. has demonstrated that CML progression may be regulated by the Musashi-Numb axis. NUP98-HOXA9, an oncogene overexpressed in BP-CML, upregulates Musashi, an RNA-binding protein. Musashi, in turn, inhibits the expression of Numb. Murine models have shown that Numb expression inhibits BP-CML formation. Furthermore, microarray analysis of human BP-CML cells shows that Musashi, the inhibitor of Numb, is overexpressed [59]. The hedgehog-signaling pathway, important in adult hematopoiesis, is also important in CML progression. This pathway begins with a series of hedgehog ligands binding to Ptch, its transmembrane receptor. This releases Ptch and allows it to bind to Smo, another transmembrane protein, resulting in a conformational change that propagates downstream transcription of target genes like Gli1, Ptch1, cyclin D1, and Bcl2. BCR-ABL cells enjoy relative increase of this hedgehog-signaling pathway. Furthermore, transfection experiments have recently shown that Smo –/–, BCR-ABL-expressing cells lose the ability for re-transfection in a murine model suggesting depletion of the leukemic stem cell pool [60, 61]. Inhibitors to this pathway are currently under clinical investigation.

Despite the critical importance of BCR-ABL in BP-CML progression, BCR-ABL-independent mechanisms have also been implicated in the transition to blast phase. Although beyond the scope of this review, HCK, LYN, SFKs, FYN, and autocrine production of GM-CSF have all been implicated in the transition to BP-CML and TKI resistance [62–65].

CML stem cells

Leukemic stem cells (LSCs) are canonically defined as an abnormal cell population that retains the ability to both self-renew and differentiate into terminal leukemic cells. In CML, these cells are said to account for less than 5% of overall tumor bulk and are inherently resistant to conventional systemic therapy, in part, by upregulation of the MDR1 efflux pump [66]. Oct-1, a protein whose function is critical for imatinib influx, is also downregulated in CML progenitors. Through natural selection pressures, the fraction of LSCs may increase during imatinib treatment ultimately establishing clinically relevant residual disease.

It is thought that leukemogenesis begins with the acquisition of aberrant BCR-ABL kinase in an otherwise normal hematopoietic stem cell (HSC) causing transformation. Over time, critical genomic events occur during the expansion and differentiation of these cells to include activation of antiapoptotic pathways like BCL2 and inhibition of several pro-apoptotic molecules, such as Bim and TRAIL [67, 68]. Members of the telomerase complex as well as important signals in differentiation are also altered culminating in a small population of LSCs [69, 70]. These, in turn, expand and differentiate and are thought to cause full-blown CP-CML. Of note, although BCR-ABL kinase is sufficient for leukemogenesis in HSCs, it alone cannot transform a more differentiated cell [71].

In fact, it is thought that HSCs and LSCs are not primary players in the transition to BP-CML. Observations by Neering et al. [72] in a murine model of BP-CML reveal that while the HSC population remains stable, a more differentiated population of cells known as granulocyte-monocyte progenitors (GMP) enjoy more than a five-fold expansion. It is also known that the Wnt1/ß-catenin cascade, required for self-renewal [73], becomes "re-activated" in GMPs from patients with BP-CML [56]. *In vitro* this allows these GMP cells to exhibit properties including self-renewal, immortality, and differentiation.

Summary

The unprecedented advances in the treatment of chronic myeloid leukemia can be traced back to the astute observation made by Dr. Nowell nearly 50 years ago. This observation led to the development of imatinib, the first "targeted" therapy in oncology. Despite its impressive track record, the hope of a cure for CML remains elusive. However, with our increasing understanding of the molecular underpinnings of this disease, future therapies will undoubtedly make this hope a reality. Combining potent second generation TKIs or targeting pathways like that of Wnt1 or hedge-hog may make strides to this end in the near future.

References

1 Nowell PC, Hungerford DA. (1961) Chromosome studies in human leukemia. II. Chronic granulocytic leukemia. *J Natl Cancer Inst* **27**:1013–35.

2 Nowell PC. (2007) Discovery of the Philadelphia chromosome: a personal perspective. *J Clin Invest* **117**:2033–5.

3 Bartram CR, de Klein A, Hagemeijer A, et al. (1983) Translocation of c-ab1 oncogene correlates with the presence of a Philadelphia chromosome in chronic myelocytic leukaemia. *Nature* **306**:277–80.

4 Groffen J, Stephenson JR, Heisterkamp N, et al. (1984) Philadelphia chromosomal breakpoints are clustered within a limited region, bcr, on chromosome 22. *Cell* **36**:93–9.

5 Chuang TH, Xu X, Kaartinen V, et al. (1995) Abr and Bcr are multifunctional regulators of the Rho GTP-binding protein family. *Proc Natl Acad Sci U S A* **92**:10282–6.

6 Diekmann D, Brill S, Garrett MD, et al. (1991) Bcr encodes a GTPase-activating protein for p21rac. *Nature* **351**:400–2.

7 Maru Y, Witte ON. (1991) The BCR gene encodes a novel serine/threonine kinase activity within a single exon. *Cell* **67**:459–68.

8 Van Etten RA, Jackson P, Baltimore D. (1989) The mouse type IV c-abl gene product is a nuclear protein, and activation of transforming ability is associated with cytoplasmic localization. *Cell* **58**:669–78.

9 Voncken JW, Kaartinen V, Pattengale PK, et al. (1995) BCR/ABL P210 and P190 cause distinct leukemia in transgenic mice. *Blood* **86**:4603–11.

10 Pane F, Frigeri F, Sindona M, et al. (1996) Neutrophilic-chronic myeloid leukemia: a distinct disease with a specific molecular marker (BCR/ABL with C3/A2 junction). *Blood* **8**:2410–4.

11 Melo JV. (1996) The diversity of BCR-ABL fusion proteins and their relationship to leukemia phenotype. *Blood* **88**:2375–84.

12 Inokuchi K, Dan K, Takatori M, et al. (2003) Myelo-proliferative disease in transgenic mice expressing P230 Bcr/Abl: longer disease latency, thrombocytosis, and mild leukocytosis. *Blood* **102**:320–3.

13 Koschmieder S, Gottgens B, Zhang P, et al. (2005) Inducible chronic phase of myeloid leukemia with expansion of hematopoietic stem cells in a transgenic model of BCR-ABL leukemogenesis. *Blood* **105**:324–34.

14 Zhang X, Ren R. (1998) Bcr-Abl efficiently induces a myeloproliferative disease and production of excess interleukin-3 and granulocyte-macrophage colony-stimulating factor in mice: a novel model for chronic myelogenous leukemia. *Blood* **92**:3829–40.

15 Daley GQ, Van Etten RA, Baltimore D. (1990) Induction of chronic myelogenous leukemia in mice by the P210bcr/abl gene of the Philadelphia chromosome. *Science* **247**:824–30.

16 Zhang X, Subrahmanyam R, Wong R, et al. (2001) The NH(2)-terminal coiled-coil domain and tyrosine 177 play important roles in induction of a myeloproliferative disease in mice by Bcr-Abl. *Mol Cell Biol* **21**:840–53.

17 Pendergast AM, Quilliam LA, Cripe LD, et al. (1993) BCR-ABL-induced oncogenesis is mediated by direct interaction with the SH2 domain of the GRB-2 adaptor protein. *Cell* **75**:175–85.

18 Sattler M, Mohi MG, Pride YB, et al. (2002) Critical role for Gab2 in transformation by BCR/ABL. *Cancer Cell* **1**:479–92.

19 Skorski T, Kanakaraj P, Nieborowska-Skorska M, et al. (1995) Phosphatidylinositol-3 kinase activity is regulated by BCR/ABL and is required for the growth of Philadelphia chromosome-positive cells. *Blood* **86**:726–36.

20 Gesbert F, Griffin JD. (2000) Bcr/Abl activates transcription of the Bcl-X gene through STAT5. *Blood* **96**:2269–76.

21 Hoelbl A, Kovacic B, Kerenyi MA, et al. (2006) Clarifying the role of Stat5 in lymphoid development and Abelson-induced transformation. *Blood* **107**:4898–906.

22 Sillaber C, Gesbert F, Frank DA, et al. (2000) STAT5 activation contributes to growth and viability in Bcr/Abl-transformed cells. *Blood* **95**:2118–25.

23 Cortez D, Reuther G, Pendergast AM. (1997) The Bcr-Abl tyrosine kinase activates mitogenic signaling pathways and stimulates G1-to-S phase transition in hematopoietic cells. *Oncogene* **15**:2333–42.

24 Xie S, Wang Y, Liu J, et al. (2001) Involvement of Jak2 tyrosine phosphorylation in Bcr-Abl transformation. *Oncogene* **20**:6188–95.

25 Magne S, Caron S, Charon M, et al. (2003) STAT5 and Oct-1 form a stable complex that modulates cyclin D1 expression. *Mol Cell Bio* **23**:8934–45.

26 Cancelas JA, Lee AW, Prabhakar R, et al. (2005) Rac GTPases differentially integrate signals regulating hematopoietic stem cell localization. *Nat Med* **11**:886–91.

27 Thomas EK, Cancelas JA, Chae HD, et al. (2007) Rac guanosine triphosphatases represent integrating molecular therapeutic targets for BCR-ABL-induced myeloproliferative disease. *Cancer Cell* **12**:467–78.

28 Van Etten RA, Jackson PK, Baltimore D, et al. (1994) The COOH terminus of the c-Abl tyrosine kinase contains distinct F- and G-actin binding domains with bundling activity. *J Cell Biol* **124**:325–40.

29 Druker BJ, Guilhot F, O'Brien SG, et al. (2006) Five-year follow-up of patients receiving imatinib for chronic myeloid leukemia. *N Engl J Med* **355**:2408–17.

30 Kantarjian HM, Cortes JE, O'Brien S, et al. (2003) Imatinib mesylate therapy in newly diagnosed patients with Philadelphia chromosome-positive chronic myelogenous leukemia: high incidence of early complete and major cytogenetic responses. *Blood* **101**:97–100.

31 Kantarjian HM, Talpaz M, O'Brien S, et al. (2006) Survival benefit with imatinib mesylate versus interferon-alpha-based regimens in newly diagnosed chronic-phase chronic myelogenous leukemia. *Blood* **108**:1835–40.

32 Druker BJ. (2006) Circumventing resistance to kinase-inhibitor therapy. *N Engl J Med* **354**:2594–6.

33 Cortes JE, Jones D, O'Brien S, et al. (2010) Nilotinib as front-line treatment for patients with chronic myeloid leukemia in early chronic phase. *J Clin Oncol* **28**:392–7.

34 Kantarjian H, Shah NP, Hochhaus A, et al. (2010) Dasatinib versus imatinib in newly diagnosed chronic-phase chronic myeloid leukemia. *N Engl J Med* **362**:2260–70.

35 Hochhaus A, O'Brien SG, Guilhot F, et al. (2009) Six-year follow-up of patients receiving imatinib for the first-line treatment of chronic myeloid leukemia. *Leukemia* **23**:1054–61.

36 Shah NP, Nicoll JM, Nagar B, et al. (2002) Multiple BCR-ABL kinase domain mutations confer polyclonal resistance to the tyrosine kinase inhibitor imatinib (STI571) in chronic phase and blast crisis chronic myeloid leukemia. *Cancer Cell* **2**:117–25.

37 Corbin AS, La Rosee P, Stoffregen EP, et al. (2003) Several Bcr-Abl kinase domain mutants associated with imatinib mesylate resistance remain sensitive to imatinib. *Blood* **101**:4611–4.

38 Soverini S, Colarossi S, Gnani A, et al. (2006) Contribution of ABL kinase domain mutations to imatinib resistance in different subsets of Philadelphia-positive patients: by the GIMEMA Working Party on Chronic Myeloid Leukemia. *Clin Cancer Res* **12**:7374–9.

39 Nagar B, Bornmann WG, Pellicena P, et al. (2002) Crystal structures of the kinase domain of c-Abl in complex with the small molecule inhibitors PD173955 and imatinib (STI-571). *Cancer Res* **62**:4236–43.

40 Schindler T, Bornmann W, Pellicena P, et al. (2000) Structural mechanism for STI-571 inhibition of Abelson tyrosine kinase. *Science* **289**:1938–42.

41 Vajpai N, Strauss A, Fendrich G, et al. (2008) Solution conformations and dynamics of ABL kinase-inhibitor complexes determined by NMR substantiate the different binding modes of imatinib/nilotinib and dasatinib. *J Biol Chem* **283**:18292–302.

42 Tokarski JS, Newitt JA, Chang CY, et al. (2006) The structure of Dasatinib (BMS-354825) bound to activated ABL kinase domain elucidates its inhibitory activity against imatinib-resistant ABL mutants. *Cancer Res* **66**:5790–7.

43 O'Hare T, Eide CA, Deininger MW. (2007) Bcr-Abl kinase domain mutations, drug resistance, and the road to a cure for chronic myeloid leukemia. *Blood* **110**:2242–9.

44 Quintas-Cardama A, Cortes J. (2009) Molecular biology of bcr-abl1-positive chronic myeloid leukemia. *Blood* **113**:1619–30.

45 Weisberg E, Manley PW, Cowan-Jacob SW, et al. (2007) Second generation inhibitors of BCR-ABL for the treatment of imatinib-resistant chronic myeloid leukaemia. *Nat Rev Cancer* **7**:345–56.

46 Andrews PD. (2005) Aurora kinases: shining lights on the therapeutic horizon? *Oncogene* **24**:5005–15.

47 Nowicki MO, Falinski R, Koptyra M, et al. (2004) BCR/ABL oncogenic kinase promotes unfaithful repair of the reactive oxygen species-dependent DNA double-strand breaks. *Blood* **104**:3746–53.

48 Slupianek A, Nowicki MO, Koptyra M, Skorski T. (2006) BCR/ABL modifies the kinetics and fidelity of DNA double-strand breaks repair in hematopoietic cells. *DNA Repair (Amst)* **5**:243–50.

49 Koptyra M, Falinski R, Nowicki MO, et al. (2006) BCR/ABL kinase induces self-mutagenesis via reactive oxygen species to encode imatinib resistance. *Blood* **108**:319–27.

50 Canitrot Y, Lautier D, Laurent G, et al. (1999) Mutator phenotype of BCR-ABL transfected Ba/F3 cell lines and its association with enhanced expression of DNA polymerase beta. *Oncogene* **18**:2676–80.

51 Melo JV, Barnes DJ. (2007) Chronic myeloid leukaemia as a model of disease evolution in human cancer. *Nat Rev Cancer* **7**:441–53.

52 Deutsch E, Dugray A, AbdulKarim B, et al. (2001) BCR-ABL down-regulates the DNA repair protein DNA-PKcs. *Blood* **97**:2084–90.

53 Deutsch E, Jarrousse S, Buet D, et al. (2003) Down-regulation of BRCA1 in BCR-ABL-expressing hemato-poietic cells. *Blood* **101**:4583–8.

54 Kennedy RD, D'Andrea AD. (2005) The Fanconi Ane-mia/BRCA pathway: new faces in the crowd. *Genes Dev* **19**:2925–40.

55 Dierov J, Dierova R, Carroll M. (2004) BCR/ABL trans-locates to the nucleus and disrupts an ATR-dependent intra-S phase checkpoint. *Cancer Cell* **5**:275–85.

56 Jamieson CH, Ailles LE, Dylla SJ, et al. (2004) Granulocyte-macrophage progenitors as candidate leu-kemic stem cells in blast-crisis CML. *N Engl J Med* **351**:657–67.

57 Perrotti D, Cesi V, Trotta R, et al. (2002) BCR-ABL suppresses C/EBPalpha expression through inhibitory action of hnRNP E2. *Nat Genet* **30**:48–58.

58 Wagner K, Zhang P, Rosenbauer F, et al. (2006) Absence of the transcription factor CCAAT enhancer binding protein alpha results in loss of myeloid identity in bcr/abl-induced malignancy. *Proc Natl Acad Sci U S A* **103**:6338–43.

59 Ito T, Kwon HY, Zimdahl B, et al. (2010) Regulation of myeloid leukaemia by the cell-fate determinant Musashi. *Nature* **466**:765–8.

60 Zhao C, Chen A, Jamieson CH, et al. (2009) Hedgehog signaling is essential for maintenance of cancer stem cells in myeloid leukaemia. *Nature* **458**:776–9.

61 Dierks C, Beigi R, Guo GR, et al. (2008) Expansion of Bcr-Abl-positive leukemic stem cells is dependent on Hedgehog pathway activation. *Cancer Cell* **14**:238–49.

62 Donato NJ, Wu JY, Stapley J, et al. (2003) BCR-ABL independence and LYN kinase overexpression in chronic myelogenous leukemia cells selected for resis-tance to STI571. *Blood* **101**:690–8.

63 Ban K, Gao Y, Amin HM, et al. (2008) BCR-ABL1 mediates up-regulation of Fyn in chronic myelogenous leukemia. *Blood* **111**:2904–8.

64 Dai Y, Rahmani M, Corey SJ, et al. (2004) A Bcr/Abl-independent, Lyn-dependent form of imatinib mesylate (STI-571) resistance is associated with altered expres-sion of Bcl-2. *J Biol Chem* **279**:34227–39.

65 Wang Y, Cai D, Brendel C, et al. (2007) Adaptive secretion of granulocyte-macrophage colony-stimulat-ing factor (GM-CSF) mediates imatinib and nilotinib resistance in BCR/ABL + progenitors via JAK-2/STAT-5 pathway activation. *Blood* **109**:2147–55.

66 Jiang X, Zhao Y, Smith C, et al. (2007) Chronic myeloid leukemia stem cells possess multiple unique features of resistance to BCR-ABL targeted therapies. *Leukemia* **21**,926–35.

67 Essafi A, Fernandez de Mattos S, Hassen YA, et al. (2005) Direct transcriptional regulation of Bim by FoxO3a mediates STI571-induced apoptosis in -express-ing cells. *Oncogene* **24**:2317–29.

68 Stahl M, Dijkers PF, Kops GJ, et al. (2002) The forkhead transcription factor FoxO regulates transcription of p27Kip1 and Bim in response to IL-2. *J Immunol* **168**:5024–31.

69 Zheng C, Li L, Haak M, et al. (2006) Gene expression profiling of CD34 + cells identifies a molecular signa-ture of chronic myeloid leukemia blast crisis. *Leukemia* **20**:1028–34.

70 Radich JP, Dai H, Mao M, et al. (2006) Gene expression changes associated with progression and response in chronic myeloid leukemia. *Proc Natl Acad Sci U S A* **103**:2794–9.

71 Huntly BJ, Shigematsu H, Deguchi K, et al. (2004) MOZ-TIF2, but not BCR-ABL, confers properties of leukemic stem cells to committed murine hematopoi-etic progenitors. *Cancer Cell* **6**:587–96.

72 Neering SJ, Bushnell T, Sozer S, et al. (2007) Leukemia stem cells in a genetically defined murine model of blast-crisis CML. *Blood* **110**:2578–85.

73 Hu Y, Chen Y, Douglas L, Li S. (2009) Beta-catenin is essential for survival of leukemic stem cells insensitive to kinase inhibition in mice with BCR-ABL-induced chronic myeloid leukemia. *Leukemia* **23**:109–16.

74 Jiang X, Forrest D, Nicolini F. (2010) Properties of CD34 + CML stem/progenitor cells that correlate with different clinical responses to imatinib mesylate. *Blood* 2010, June 23 [Epub ahead of print].

75 Hazlehurst LA, Bewry NN, Nair RR, Pinilla-Ibarz J. (2009) Signaling networks associated with BCR-ABL-dependent transformation. *Cancer Control.* **16**:100–107.

CHAPTER 5

Standard Management of Patients with Chronic Myeloid Leukemia

Elias Jabbour, Jorge Cortes and Hagop Kantarjian
Department of Leukemia, University of Texas M.D. Anderson Cancer Center, Houston, TX, USA

Introduction

Chronic myeloid leukemia (CML) is a rare disease, but is one of the most extensively studied and best understood neoplasms for which a direct gene link has been found [1–3]. CML is characterized by a balanced genetic translocation, involving a fusion of the Abelson oncogene (ABL) from chromosome 9q34 with the breakpoint cluster region (BCR) on chromosome 22q11.2, t(9;22)(q34;q11.2), the Philadelphia chromosome (Ph). The molecular consequence of this translocation is the generation of a BCR-ABL fusion oncogene, which in turn translates into a Bcr-Abl oncoprotein [4, 5]. Bcr-Abl displays transforming activity owing to its constitutive kinase activity, which results in multiple signal transduction pathways leading to uncontrolled cell proliferation and reduced apoptosis, and resulting in the malignant expansion of pluripotent stem cells in bone marrow [6, 7].

CML is usually diagnosed in chronic phase (CP) and, if not treated, progresses through accelerated phase (AP) and a terminal blast phase (BP).

Treatment with imatinib

Historically, CML was treated with busulfan or hydroxyurea, and was associated with a poor prognosis [8]. These agents controlled the hematologic manifestations of the disease, but did not delay disease progression. Treatment with interferon-α (IFN-α) produced complete cytogenetic responses in 5–25% of patients with CML in CP, and improved survival compared with previous treatments [9]. Combining IFN-α with cytarabine produced additional benefits [10]. Allogeneic stem cell transplantation (SCT) may be curative in CML, but it is applicable to only a fraction of CML patients and carries a significant risk of morbidity and mortality.

Imatinib mesylate, a small molecule tyrosine kinase inhibitor (TKI), was the first drug that targets Bcr-Abl to be developed [11] and it has become the standard frontline therapy for all CML patients in early CP on the basis of the response rates and good tolerability shown in numerous clinical trials. This conclusion has been mainly reached through the results of the IRIS trial. A recent seven-year update of the phase III IRIS trial confirmed the long-term efficacy and safety of imatinib [12]. After seven years, the cumulative complete cytogenetic response rate for first-line imatinib-treated patients was 82%. The event-free survival (EFS) was 81%, and the estimated rate of freedom from progression to AP or BP was 93%. The estimated overall survival (OS) rate for patients treated with imatinib was 86%. At seven years, 332 patients (60%) randomized to imatinib remained on treatment [12, 13]. Imatinib was also found to be tolerable in the study, with the highest

Advances in Malignant Hematology, First Edition. Edited by Hussain I. Saba and Ghulam J. Mufti. © 2011 Blackwell Publishing Ltd.
Published 2011 by Blackwell Publishing Ltd.

grade adverse events (AEs) reported as cytopenias, elevated serum alanine or aspartate aminotransferase levels, pain, and nausea.

Although 400 mg/day is the recommended imatinib dose, early phase I dose-finding trials in patients who had previously received IFN-α demonstrated no dose-limiting toxicities at imatinib doses up to 1000 mg/day [14], and a dose–response relationship was observed. Based on these data, recent studies have assessed the efficacy of first-line therapy with high-dose imatinib, up to 800 mg/day. A single-arm study involving 114 patients with newly diagnosed CP-CML showed a complete hematologic response rate of 98% and a complete cytogenetic response rate of 90% in patients who received an imatinib dose of 800 mg/day [15]. These data compared favorably with historical controls from the same institution, with significantly higher complete cytogenetic response rates observed in patients who received 800 mg/day compared with those who received 400 mg/day (90% vs. 74%, respectively; $P = 0.01$). Transformation-free survival (TFS) was also significantly improved with the higher imatinib dose.

Two large, prospective, randomized trials are ongoing to assess the optimal imatinib starting dose in previously untreated patients with CML-CP. The Tyrosine kinase inhibitor OPtimization and Selectivity trial (TOPS) is a phase III study involving 476 patients randomized in a 2:1 ratio to receive 800 or 400 mg/day imatinib [16]. Recent reports from this trial indicate that imatinib (800 mg/day) showed a rapid response and trend of improved major molecular response (MMR) rates at 3, 6, 9, and 12 months compared with standard dose imatinib therapy, although the improvement was not statistically significant at 12 months. The European LeukemiaNet study [17] compared 400 versus 800 mg/day imatinib in 215 high Sokal-risk patients, with a primary endpoint of complete cytogenetic response at 12 months [35]. Results were similar to those in the TOPS trial. A trend toward higher rates of MMR with 800 mg/day compared with 400 mg/day was observed; however, the differences were not statistically significant.

For patients who started with 800 mg front line, the TOPS trial demonstrated that the majority of patients could tolerate higher imatinib doses, with only approximately 20% of patients unable to tolerate more than the standard dose by 12 months [16]. The most common grade 3–4 non-hematologic toxicities were rash, diarrhea, and myalgia occurring slightly more frequently in the 800 mg/day arm. Grade 3–4 hematologic toxicity occurred more frequently in patients receiving 800 mg/day. In the European LeukemiaNet study comparing 400 mg and 800 mg in patients with high Sokal-risk, the number of dropouts and the number of patients who went off treatment for AEs and serious AEs was not significantly different in the two arms, although it was slightly higher in the high-dose arm (18% or 16.6% vs. 10% or 9.2%; $P < 0.156$) [17].

Optimizing responses through careful monitoring

Following initial therapy with imatinib, patients should be routinely assessed for response, and therapy should be adjusted to maximize the chance of response for patients with lack of response or suboptimal response. While response rates to first-line therapy with standard-dose imatinib are high, with a best observed complete cytogenetic response rate of 82% by 60 months' follow-up [21], 18% of patients will not achieve an optimal response and others may lose an initial response. These patients may require dose adjustments or alternative therapy to optimize their treatment. In order to proactively identify patients with suboptimal responses or resistance to imatinib, several important levels of monitoring are recommended (Table 5.1) [18, 19].

Monitoring of the bone marrow for cytogenetic response is recommended at 3, 6, and 12 months. If a patient demonstrates a complete cytogenetic response, then bone marrow testing can be done annually. Peripheral blood should be collected and analyzed for BCR-ABL1 transcript levels every three months within the first 12 months of treatment. If a major molecular response is observed, the frequency of monitoring can occur every six months. In the event of increases in transcript levels, the level at which the change occurs should be considered, since accuracy of the test does depend on the amount

Table 5.1 Recommended frequencies of response assessment in patients with chronic myeloid leukemia [18, 19]

Assessment method	Initial monitoring (for suboptimal response)	Subsequent monitoring (for loss of response)
Hematologic	Every 2 weeks	Every 3 months once CHR is achieved
Cytogenetic	Every 6 months	Every 12 months once CCyR achieved
Molecular	Every 3 months	Every 3 months, increasing to monthly if a rising *BCR-ABL1* transcript level is detected
Mutational assessment	Immediately following detection of a suboptimal response	Immediately following detection of imatinib failure or rising *BCR-ABL1* transcript level

CHR: complete hematologic response; CCyR: complete cytogenetic response.

of residual BCR-ABL transcripts. The NCCN recommends the following monitoring schedule: any 1-log increase in BCR-ABL1 transcripts should be repeated in one month; if the increase is confirmed on subsequent sampling, the frequency of monitoring should be increased from every three months to every month, and mutation assays can be considered in case of elevations in BCR-ABL transcripts. Monitoring of mutations is becoming an increasingly important area of research, entering clinical practice and investigation to potentially determine the best therapeutic approach to treat patients in the second-line setting and will be discussed in more detail below.

Resistence to imatinib

The molecular mechanisms responsible for resistance are only partly understood. Most of the mechanisms involve BCR-ABL kinase domain mutations, with resulting impairment of the ability of imatinib to bind the ATP binding pocket of the Bcr-Abl tyrosine kinase domain. Up to now, more than 100 different mutants of BCR-ABL have been described, but some of them show a higher frequency than others [20]. Most of the clinically relevant mutations develop at just a few residues in the P-loop (G250E, Y253F/H, and E255K/V), contact site (T315I), and catalytic domain (M351T and F359V) [21].

Some of the resistant patients with mutations appear to bear more than one mutation at the same time. Another possible cause of resistance is overexpression of BCR-ABL. Although this was the most frequent cause of resistance identified in cell lines, and case reports have described clinical resistance to imatinib in association with BCR-ABL amplification or multiple copies of the Ph-chromosome, the percentage of patients whose primary or acquired resistance to imatinib appears to be due to this mechanism is probably low.

The acquisition of additional chromosomal abnormalities in the Ph-chromosome-positive cell population, generally referred as clonal evolution, appears to be one of the main mechanisms leading to both disease progression and imatinib resistance. Activation of members of the Src-kinase family or of other pathways downstream of BCR-ABL (like the PI3K-AKT pathway) has been reported and it is increasingly becoming evident that multiple mechanisms and events can be involved in the development of imatinib-resistant subclones [22]. All types of resistance can be ascribed to the high degree of genomic instability characterizing the Ph-positive clone [23]. So far the molecular mechanisms leading to this instability are only partly understood. Although it is proved that BCR-ABL activation is able to induce some degree of genomic instability, at least in some cases, a stem cell disease causing genomic instability and pre-existing the acquisition of the Ph-chromosome cannot be excluded.

Imatinib dose escalation

Dose escalation can improve the response in some of the patients with resistance to standard dose imatinib, and was the main option for managing suboptimal responses and treatment failures before the introduction of second-generation TKIs.

In an analysis of patients enrolled in the IRIS trial, in whom imatinib dose was escalated due to resistance to standard dose therapy, freedom-from-progression and OS rates were 89% and 84%, respectively, at three years [24]. In another study, 84 CML-CP patients were dose escalated to imatinib (600–800 mg/day) after developing hematologic failure (n = 21), or cytogenetic failure (resistance: n = 30; relapse: n = 33) to imatinib (400 mg/day). Among patients that met the criteria for cytogenetic failure, 75% (47/63) responded to imatinib dose escalation. Patients achieving major cytogenetic response after imatinib dose escalation had durable responses, with a sustained major cytogenetic response in 88% and 74% of patients at two and three years, respectively. In contrast, in patients where imatinib was dose escalated because of hematologic failure, 48% achieved a complete hematologic response and 14% (3/21) only attained a cytogenetic response [25]. Although dose escalation after failure to standard dose imatinib is an important option for patients with imatinib resistance, it is likely to be useful only in a subset of patients with previous cytogenetic response to standard imatinib therapy.

Second-generation TKIs

Strategies to overcome imatinib resistance are a logical progression for improving the prognosis of patients with CML. These include novel and more potent multi-tyrosine kinase inhibitors such as dasatinib (Sprycel; BMS-354825, Bristol-Myers Squibb), an orally bioavailable dual BCR-ABL and Src inhibitor, and potent selective Bcr-Abl inhibitors such as nilotinib (Tasigna; AMN-107). Both nilotinib and dasatinib induced significant clinical responses and have been approved by the FDA and EMA.

Dasatinib

Dasatinib is an orally available ABL kinase inhibitor with 325-fold greater *in vitro* selectivity for wild-type BCR-ABL compared with imatinib [26, 27]. It differs from imatinib in that it can bind to both the active and inactive conformations of the ABL kinase domain and also inhibits a distinct spectrum of kinases that overlaps with the array of kinases that imatinib inhibits. Targets of dasatinib include SFKs, c-Kit, PDGFR-β, and ephrin A. Dasatinib has activity against many imatinib-resistant kinase domain mutations of Bcr-Abl. BCR-ABL mutations associated with resistance to dasatinib have been characterized. In an *in vitro* mutagenesis study, mutations at six residues were found to form nine dasatinib-resistant BCR-ABL mutants. However, only two (F317V and T315I) were isolated at intermediate drug concentrations, and T315l was the only mutant to be isolated at maximal achievable plasma concentrations [28]. Dasatinib was approved by the FDA on the basis of its efficacy and safety profiles shown in a series of phase II trials in patients who failed or were intolerant to first-line imatinib therapy (Table 5.2) [29–31]. Dasatinib was initially approved at a dosage of 70 mg twice daily for all indications. The label has recently been changed and 100 mg once daily is now the recommended starting dose for patients with CML-CP, on the basis of a phase III dose-optimization study designed to evaluate the efficacy and safety of four different dasatinib doses in patients who had previously experienced imatinib failure. This study showed that the 100 mg, once daily dosage was efficaciously equivalent to 70 mg twice daily, with decreased rates of thrombocytopenia and pleural effusion [32, 33]. Dasatinib was registered for the treatment of CML-CP based on results from the SRC/ABL Tyrosine kinase inhibition Activity Research Trials of dasatinib (START)-C trial, a phase II international study of dasatinib (70 mg twice daily), which included 387 CML-CP patients with resistance or intolerance to imatinib [30]. Recent 24-month follow-up data demonstrated a

Table 5.2 Phase II data for dasatinib second line to imatinib failure

Disease	N	% Response			
			Cytogenetic response		
		MHR	Major	Complete	Overall survival
CML chronic	387	91	59	49	96% at 15 months
CML accelerated	107	81	64	39	76% at 10 months
CML myelo-blastic	109	34	33	26	11.8 months
CML lympho-blastic	48	35	52	46	5.3 months

MHR: major hematologic response.

two-year major cytogenetic response rate of 62% and a complete cytogenetic response rate of 53% [34]. The EFS at two years was 80% and the OS rate was 94%. Responses to dasatinib in patients with imatinib-resistant CML-CP enrolled in phase II studies of dasatinib have been assessed by baseline mutational status [28]. Complete cytogenetic response rates were similar among patients with un-mutated BCR-ABL and those harboring mutations. Importantly, responses to dasatinib did not appear to be diminished among patients harboring the P-loop mutations. However, the activity was somewhat reduced in patients with F317L mutations. As expected, no complete cytogenetic responses were achieved in patients harboring the T315I mutation. The most frequently detected mutations in patients exhibiting resistance to dasatinib are T315A/I, F317I/L, and V299L [28, 35–40].

Grade 3–4 toxicities included thrombocytopenia (49%) and neutropenia (50%), pleural effusion (9%), dyspnea (6%), bleeding (4%), diarrhea (3%), and fatigue (3%). Three percent of imatinib-intolerant patients developed similar grade 3–4 toxicities. The appearance of new higher grade toxicity between 12 and 24 months was uncommon [34].

Nilotinib

Nilotinib is an analog of imatinib with 10–50-fold greater potency against wild-type BCR-ABL than its parent compound imatinib, and has activity against all imatinib-resistant Bcr-Abl mutations except T315l [41]. It is approved at a schedule of 400 mg twice daily without food for two hours prior to and one hour after administration. Nilotinib was approved following an open-label phase II study in patients with CML who failed or who were intolerant to imatinib therapy [42, 43]. Follow-up data confirm the effectiveness of this compound in CP, AP and BP CML (Table 5.3) [44–46].

Ten nilotinib-insensitive BCR-ABL mutations have been isolated. In a mutagenesis study, the P-loop mutations Y253H and E255V persisted at intermediate drug concentrations, and T315I was isolated at maximum achievable plasma concentrations [28]. In the key phase II study, a total of 321 CML-CP patients (71% imatinib-resistant; 29% imatinib-intolerant) were evaluated. Imatinib-intolerant patients could not have achieved prior major cytogenetic response on imatinib therapy. Overall, complete hematologic response was reported in 94% of patients and in 76% among those with no baseline CHR at the start of nilotinib. Of all imatinib-resistant and -intolerant patients, 58% achieved major cytogenetic response, with 72% of patients having a baseline complete hematologic response achieving major cytogenetic response. The major cytogenetic response rate was 63% in imatinib-intolerant and 56% in imatinib-resistant patients, respectively. Overall, 42% of

Table 5.3 Phase II data for nilotinib second line to imatinib failure

Disease	N	% Response			
			Cytogenetic response		
		CHR	Major	Complete	Overall survival
CML chronic	321	76[a]	58	42	91% (18 months)
CML accelerated	138	30	32	19	82% (12 months)
CML blastic	136	11	40	29	42% (12 months)

[a] 76% of patients achieved a CHR among those with active disease. Overall 94% of patients achieved a CHR.
CHR: complete hematologic response.

patients achieved a complete cytogenetic response (50% in imatinib-intolerant and 39% in imatinib-resistant patients, respectively). The median time to complete hematologic response and major cytogenetic response was 1.0 and 2.8 months, respectively. Responses were durable, with 84% of patients maintaining their major cytogenetic response at 18 months. Estimated OS rates at 12 and 18 months were 95% and 91%, respectively. Median duration of exposure was 465 days (15.5 months) [44].

Of 321 CML-CP patients, 281 (88%) had baseline mutation data available, 41% had detectable BCR-ABL mutations prior to nilotinib therapy. Fourteen percent of imatinib-resistant patients had three mutations that were less sensitive to nilotinib *in vitro* ($IC_{50} > 150$ nM; Y253H, E255K/V, and F359C/V) and another 15% had a total of 16 mutations with unknown sensitivity to nilotinib. Cytogenetic response rates in patients harboring mutations sensitive to nilotinib (major cytogenetic response 59%; complete cytogenetic response 41%) or mutations with unknown sensitivity to nilotinib (major cytogenetic response 63%; complete cytogenetic response 50%) were comparable to those for patients without baseline mutations (major cytogenetic response 60%; complete cytogenetic response 40%). Patients with mutations less sensitive to nilotinib *in vitro* had a less favorable response after 12 months of therapy (23% major cytogenetic

response). No complete cytogenetic responses were observed in patients harboring L248V, Y253H, or E255K/V mutations [47]. Mutations most frequently associated with progression were E255K/V (6/7) and F359C/V (9/11).

Bosutinib (SKI-606)

Bosutinib (SKI606), an orally available dual Src/Abl inhibitor, is 30 to 50 times more potent than imatinib, with minimal inhibitory activity against c-Kit and PDGFR, therefore expected to produce less myelosuppression and fluid retention. The phase I study identified a treatment dose of 500 mg daily and showed evidence of clinical efficacy. The phase II study in patients with CP Ph + CML who have failed imatinib and second-generation TKI therapy is ongoing. Preliminary data for 302 treated patients have been reported. Among 69 patients with imatinib resistance only, 81% had complete hematological response, 45% achieved a major cytogenetic response, including 32% with a complete cytogenetic response. Treatment was generally well tolerated [48].

The most common adverse events were gastrointestinal (nausea, vomiting, diarrhea). These were usually grade 1–2, manageable and transient, diminishing in frequency and severity after the first three to four weeks of treatment [48].

Multikinase inhibitors

Imatinib, dasatinib, nilotinib, and bosutinib are ATP-competitive inhibitors and not active against the T315I mutant. Compounds that target binding sites unrelated to the ATP kinase domain may overcome this problem.

XL228 (Exelixis Inc., San Francisco, CA, USA) is a potent, multitargeted kinase inhibitor with potent activity against wild-type and T315I isoforms of BCR-ABL (wild-type ABL kinase, $IC_{50} =$ 5 nM; ABL T315I, 1.4 nM), Aurora A (3.1 nM), IGF-1R (1.6 nM), SRC (6.1 nM), and LYN (2 nM) kinases. A phase I dose escalation clinical trial in patients with CML or Ph+ ALL who are resistant or intolerant to at least two prior standard TKIs (including imatinib, dasatinib, and nilotinib) or have a known BCR-ABL T315I mutation is ongoing. XL228 was administered as a one-hour IV infusion either once weekly or twice weekly. XL228 has been generally well tolerated. Dose-limiting toxicities observed with once-weekly dosing, included grade 3 syncope and hyperglycemia in two patients. Preliminary evidence of clinical activity has been observed in patients treated at doses of 3.6 mg/kg and higher, including stable or decreasing white blood cell count and/or platelet count within two months (14 patients, 5 with T315I), and/or >1 log reduction in BCR-ABL levels by QPCR within three months (3 patients, 2 with T315I) [49].

PHA-739538 (Nerviano Medical Sciences, Nerviano, Italy) is an aurora kinase inhibitor with potent activity against native and mutated BCR-ABL, including T315I [50]. Strong antiproliferative effects of PHA-739358 have been observed in CD34+ cells harvested from untreated CML patients and from imatinib-resistant individuals, including those with the T315I mutation [50, 51]. Simultaneous short-term treatment with PHA-739358 in association with imatinib resulted in pronounced apoptosis of wild-type or low-grade imatinib-resistant BCR-ABL expressing cells while no such effects were observed in BCR-ABL negative or highly imatinib-resistant T315I mutants. In primary CD34+ cells of CML patients including non-dividing quiescent leukemic stem cells combination therapy with imatinib and PHA-739358 revealed a synergistic antiproliferative activity which also affected immature CD34+38- cells. However, neither mono- nor combination therapy led to a significant induction of apoptosis in this population of cells. PHA-739358 did not affect quiescent stem cells, but resistance emerged less frequently after incubation with PHA-739358 than with imatinib [51]. Preliminary results of a multicenter phase II study have been reported. Among seven patients treated (1 CP, 1 AP, 5 BP; 6 with T315I mutations), one patient with a T315I mutation achieved a CCyR and a second patient achieved a minor cytogenetic response [52].

Several other multikinase inhibitors have been progressed into clinical trials. MK-0457 a potent aurora kinase inhibitor, was the first agent to demonstrate clinical activity against the T315I phenotype and in a study of 14 evaluable patients with CML, 11 had an objective (hematologic, cytogenetic, and/or molecular) response, including nine patients with T315I [53]. However, clinical development of MK-0457 was recently halted over toxicity concerns. AP24534 is an oral, multitargeted kinase inhibitor with activity against native and kinase domain-mutant BCR-ABL, including T315I. Mutagenesis screening revealed that single-agent AP24534 (40 nM) completely suppressed outgrowth of most BCR-ABL mutants. This agent is being explored in patients with TKI failure [54]. DCC-2036 is highly selective for ABL, FLT3, TIE2, and Src family kinases and, when dosed at 100 mg/kg/day by oral gavage, significantly prolonged the survival of mice with CML-like myeloproliferative disease induced by retroviral expression of BCR-ABL WT and T315I in bone marrow [55]. This agent is being explored in a phase I clinical trial.

Other drugs

Other approaches are being developed for patients with TKI failure.

Panobinostat (*LBH589B*; Novartis Pharmaceuticals, Basle, Switzerland) is a histone deacetylase inhibitor that is being investigated in a number of hematologic malignancies [56]. Clinical trials of panobinostat (single drug or in combination with imatinib), are currently ongoing in patients with all phases of CML. Another histone deacetylase inhibitor, *vorinostat* (*Zolinza®*; Merck & Co., New Jersey, NJ, USA), induced expression of pro-apoptotic BH3-only protein in a variety of CML cell lines, including those expressing T315I and showed synergistic interactions with dasatinib or sorafenib in imatinib-sensitive and -insensitive cell lines [57]. This compound is also in phase I development in combination with decitabine in CML and ALL patients.

Two orally administered farnesyl transferase inhibitors (*tipifarnib, R115777*; and *lonafarnib, SCH66336*) have shown clinical activity both as single agents and in combinations with imatinib in heavily pre-treated patients with advanced phase disease [58–61]. Decitabine (5-aza-2'-deoxycytidine), administered to 35 patients with imatinib-resistant CML, induced hematologic response in 23 patients (66%; 34% complete hematologic response) and cytogenetic response in 16 (46%) [62, 63].

Omacetaxine mepesuccinate (*Omacetaxine®; homoharringtonine; HHT*; ChemGenex Pharmaceuticals, Victoria, Australia), a cephalotaxine ester, is a multitargeted protein synthase inhibitor that has been in clinical development for several years. Omacetaxine showed clinical activity against Ph + CML [64, 65], with a mechanism of action independent of tyrosine kinase inhibition. Omacetaxine in currently in phase II/III development in patients with CML (all phases) who are resistant or intolerant to at least two prior TKIs (including imatinib, dasatinib, and nilotinib) or who carry T315I-mutated BCR-ABL. Sixty-six patients with T315I have been treated, including 40 in CP, 16 in AP, and 10 in BP. A complete hematologic response has been reported in 85%, 31%, and 20% of patients in CP, AP, and BP, respectively. Major cytogenetic response has been reported in 15% of patients in CP, and 6% in AP. In addition, the T315I mutated clone became undetectable in 39% of all patients treated. The most frequently occurring grade 3–4 toxicities associated with omacetaxine therapy were thrombocytopenia (58%), neutropenia (41%), and anemia (36%) [66]. Recent reports suggest that omacetaxine is able to affect the leukemic stem cell compartment, which would make it attractive for the potential of total elimination of the leukemic cells and potential cure.

Vaccines

There is consolidated evidence that the immune system plays an important role in eliminating minimal residual disease in CML patients. Because the Bcr-Abl fusion protein represents a unique tumor-specific antigen, vaccination using peptides based on the BCR-ABL junction point may be useful. Native junction peptides have induced a specific immune response. To increase the immunogenicity of native peptides, synthetic peptides can be generated through selective mutations in their HLA-binding sequences (heteroclitic peptides). In a recent study at M.D. Anderson Cancer Center, 10 patients with CML were treated with imatinib using a heteroclitic junction peptide vaccine [67]. Only three patients who were treated achieved the primary endpoint of a 1-log reduction in BCR-ABL transcript levels, and all three responses were transient. These results were in contrast to the more favorable results from previous trials. In the study by Maslak et al., two of three patients who had low levels of FISH positivity assessed before the start of vaccination with an heterolitic junction peptide had negative FISH results during the vaccinations [68]. Bocchia et al. used native junction peptides to treat 16 patients, including nine patients who were not in complete cytogenetic response at the start of vaccinations [69]. Five of these patients achieved a complete cytogenetic response, and three of them achieved a complete molecular response. The only patient who was treated in complete cytogenetic response achieved a half-log reduction in BCR-ABL transcripts. Rojas et al. reported on 19 patients who received native junction peptide [70]. None of the five patients who entered that study without a major cytogenetic response to imatinib responded to the peptide vaccine, whereas 13 of 14 patients who had a major cytogenetic response at the start of vaccinations achieved a 1-log reduction in transcript levels. Differences in the combinations of peptides, schedules of administration, and adjuvant may be responsible for the different results of these studies. Other vaccines have also shown promising results. These include PR1, a non-peptide derived from proteinase 3 and able to induce immunologic and in some instances clinical responses [71].

Combination therapy

An important issue in the management of human malignancies relates to the timing of therapies. The current strategy, best exemplified in CML, is sequential treatment. Molecularly targeted kinase inhibitor therapies are currently administered sequentially rather than simultaneously. Newly diagnosed patients receive imatinib, followed by ABL-second-generation inhibitors at time of resistance or intolerance. The rationale for this approach is partly historical, since imatinib was approved for CML therapy prior to others on the basis of a very high single-agent response rate, and partly based on a molecular understanding of resistance mechanisms that led to the evaluation of other TKIs in imatinib-resistant CML.

There is growing interest in testing the hypothesis that administration of multiple Abl kinase inhibitors in early-phase patients, such as nilotinib, dasatinib, and imatinib, could be used to delay or prevent the emergence of drug-resistant clones [34, 72, 73]. Both nilotinib and dasatinib hold promise for treating patients with imatinib-resistant CML. Cross resistance between nilotinib and dasatinib is limited to T315I, which is also the only mutant isolated at drug concentrations equivalent to maximal achievable plasma trough levels [27]. Since the T315I mutation of BCR-ABL is highly resistant to imatinib, nilotinib, and dasatinib, this approach needs to be extended to include inhibitors of T315I BCR-ABL to prevent this mutation from becoming more prevalent. Alternatively, it is also important to explore the potential for synergy between TKI and other classes of inhibitors that work through mechanisms not involving inhibition of ABL tyrosine kinase activity [74–76].

Novel approaches to prevent resistance

Second-generation TKIs as first-line therapy

Another important approach to optimizing therapy in patients with early CML-CP may be the use of second-generation TKIs as front-line therapy. Several phase II trials are under way studying nilotinib and dasatinib in this setting. The Italian GIMEMA CML Working Party enrolled 73 patients in a phase II study, having the achievement of complete cytogenetic response rate at one year as primary endpoint [77]. All patients and 48/73 (66%) completed three and six months on treatment, respectively. The complete hematologic response rates were 100% and 98%, respectively; the complete cytogenetic response rates were 78% and 96%, respectively. A major molecular response was achieved by 59% after three months and 74% after six months. One patient progressed at six months to accelerated blastic phase with the T315I mutation. A phase II study in patients with newly diagnosed CML-CP at the M. D. Anderson Cancer Center showed that nilotinib (400 mg twice daily) induces a complete cytogenetic response in nearly all patients as early as three months after the start of therapy with a favorable toxicity profile (Table 5.4) [78]. Forty-nine patients

Table 5.4 Cytogenetic and molecular responses by time to dasatinib and nilotinib front line at the M.D. Anderson Cancer Center

M.D. Anderson Cancer Center Experience	Dasatinib N = 50	Nilotinib N = 49
CCyR		
3 mos	78%	93%
6 mos	94%	100%
12 mos	97%	96%
MMR 12 mos	37%	52%

CCyR: complete cytogenetic response; MMR: major molecular response; mos: months.

have been treated for a median of 13 months. Complete cytogenetic responses were achieved, respectively, by 93% and by 100% of patients at three- and six-month evaluations. The rate of complete cytogenetic response at 3, 6, 12, 18 and 24 months compared favorably to those observed in historical controls treated with imatinib (400 mg or 800 mg daily). Major molecular response was observed in 45% at six months and 52% at 12 months. The estimated 24-month event-free survival is 95%. Preliminary data demonstrate that nilotinib was well tolerated with infrequent reports of grade 3/4 hematologic laboratory abnormalities and non-hematologic AEs. Dasatinib has also been evaluated as front-line therapy in a phase II study [79]. Patients with previously untreated CML-CP received dasatinib 50 mg BID (53%) or 100 mg QD (47%). Complete cytogenetic response rates at three and six months were 78% and 94%, respectively. Major molecular response rates of 23% and 36% were observed at three and six months, respectively. Grade 3–4 hematologic toxicity included neutropenia (23%), thrombocytopenia (11%), and anemia (7%) and pleural effusions occurred in 13% (grade 2) and 2% (grade 3) of patients.

Allogenic stem cell transplantation

Allogeneic stem cell transplantation is the only treatment for CML known to be potentially curative. Since the development of modern TKIs, however, allogeneic SCT is more commonly administered after patients have received imatinib and second-generation agents and is an important treatment option following treatment failure. Prior imatinib treatment does not adversely affect OS, progression-free survival (PFS), or non-relapse mortality following allogeneic SCT [80], and indeed the two approaches may be favorably combined. Moreover, second-generation TKIs do not appear to increase transplant-related toxicity [81]. In a study reported recently, 7 out of 10 patients with mutations-dependent imatinib failure CML were alive free of disease after a median follow-up of 19 months post -allogeneic SCT [82]. Current treatment guidelines recommend allogeneic SCT or

inclusion in clinical trials for imatinib-resistant CML patients with the T315I mutation. Allogeneic SCT was attempted in four patients with T315I mutants: two responded, but the other two died following relapse. Therefore, T315I mutations are associated with poor prognoses, particularly in advanced phases, although occasional responses may be achieved through drug therapy or allogeneic SCT.

Decision making

The primary goal of therapy for patients with CML is still achievement of complete cytogenetic response. Those who achieve this goal have a low probability of eventually progressing. Achieving a major molecular response is desirable as it further improves the long-term outcome, but patients who have a complete cytogenetic response are not considered to have failure to imatinib if they do not have a major molecular response. This is because the difference in EFS probability is small, although significant. The timing of this response is also important. Despite initial suggestions from the IRIS trial that a major molecular response at 12 months improved long-term outcome, compared to complete cytogenetic response but no major molecular response, the seven-year follow-up data has shown no difference in outcome using this hallmark. By 18 months, patients who have a complete cytogenetic response and major molecular response have a better probability of EFS than those with complete cytogenetic response but no major molecular response, but the difference is small (95% vs. 86%), and even smaller if considering only transformation to AP or BP or death as an event (99% vs. 96%).

The recommendations by the European LeukemiaNet (http://www.leukemia-net.org/content/home/) have provided a clear framework for decision making and the significance of the definitions of failure and suboptimal response have been demonstrated in two independent series [83, 84]. Patients with suboptimal response to therapy have an inferior outcome, although the significance appears to be heterogeneous, with a more profound adverse prognostic effect for patients with suboptimal response to therapy at earlier time-points (six months) than at later time-points (18 months). It is, however, reasonable to consider treatment modifications for patients who have a suboptimal response to therapy. Treatment guidelines recommend dose escalation of imatinib to 600 or 800 mg/day in cases of suboptimal response [18, 19]. However, it should be acknowledged that there is minimal data available regarding the effectiveness of this approach [24, 25]. For patients with clear failure to imatinib therapy, the current approach is to change therapy to a second-generation TKI, although allogeneic SCT is also an option following treatment failure [18, 19]. Clinical trial data have confirmed the efficacy of dasatinib and nilotinib in patients with imatinib resistance or intolerance, and the superiority of dasatinib versus imatinib dose escalation following imatinib resistance [85, 86]. It is possible that earlier treatment switch to second-line agents, that is, after suboptimal response, could result in more favorable long-term outcomes than with dose-escalated imatinib, but there are currently no clinical data to support this hypothesis.

An important question now is what the response hallmarks are for patients receiving second-generation TKIs. A recent study has hinted at possible treatment goals for second-line treatment. Among patients with CP-CML receiving dasatinib (n = 70) or nilotinib (n = 43) after imatinib failure, those who achieved a major cytogenetic response within 12 months post-imatinib treatment had a significantly higher survival rate than patients with a minor cytogenetic response or complete hematologic response (one-year survival: 97% vs. 84%, respectively; $p = 0.02$) [87]. Moreover, fewer than 10% of patients with no cytogenetic response of any level within three to six months went on to achieve a major cytogenetic response at 12 months, suggesting these patients might require switch to third-line treatment or to allogeneic SCT. However, additional studies are required to confirm these findings.

The selection of second-line TKI therapy should be individualized to each patient, carefully considering drug efficacy and toxicity, as well as patient mutation data. In many cases, a patient's BCR-ABL genotype can serve as a prognostic factor to disease progression. Preliminary analysis from phase II studies suggested that levels of response to new TKIs depend on the type of BCR-ABL kinase domain mutation. The outcome of patients receiving second-generation TKIs depends on the type of mutation, with mutations with predicted intermediate levels of sensitivity (i.e., higher IC50 *in vitro*) having decreased probability of response and event-free survival, particularly in CP [88].

Therapy decision should also take into consideration the potential side effects, in relation to each patient characteristic. Patient compliance is another point to be considered. Finally, allogeneic SCT remains a potential therapeutic modality provided the patient is young, fit, has not achieved a MCyR with second TKI therapy, and a donor match can be quickly identified.

Conclusions

Targeted agents have significantly improved the prognosis in CML. Imatinib represented a significant turning point in the natural history of the disease and in patient survival. However, resistance to imatinib remains a barrier to recovery for some patients. The recent availability of highly potent tyrosine kinase inhibitors has further improved the outcome of many patients. The advent of novel agents, with the possibility of combining drugs with different mechanisms of action will hopefully lead to a further optimization of CML therapy.

References

1 Barnes DJ, Melo JV. (2002) Cytogenetic and molecular genetic aspects of chronic myeloid leukaemia. *Acta Haematol* **108**:180–202.

2 Faderl S, Talpaz M, Estrov Z, Kantarjian HM. (1999) Chronic myelogenous leukemia: biology and therapy. *Ann Intern Med* **131**:207–19.

3 Litzow MR. (2006) Imatinib resistance: obstacles and opportunities. *Arch Pathol Lab Med* **130**:669–79.

4 Rowley JD. (1973) Letter: A new consistent chromosomal abnormality in chronic myelogenous leukaemia identified by quinacrine fluorescence and Giemsa staining. *Nature* **243**:290–93.

5 Koptyra M, Falinski R, Nowicki MO, et al. (2006) BCR/ABL kinase induces self-mutagenesis via reactive oxygen species to encode imatinib resistance. *Blood* **108**:319–27.

6 Hu Y, Liu Y, Pelletier S, et al. (2004) Requirement of Src kinases Lyn, Hck and Fgr for BCR-ABL1-induced B-lymphoblastic leukemia but not chronic myeloid leukemia. *Nat Genet* **36**:453–61.

7 Bhatia R, Holtz M, Niu N, et al. (2003) Persistence of malignant hematopoietic progenitors in chronic myelogenous leukemia patients in complete cytogenetic remission following imatinib mesylate treatment. *Blood* **101**:4701–7.

8 Faderl S, Talpaz M, Estrov Z, et al. (1999) The biology of chronic myeloid leukemia. *N Engl J Med* **341**:164–72.

9 Guilhot F, Chastang C, Michallet M, et al. (1997) Interferon alfa-2b combined with cytarabine versus interferon alone in chronic myelogenous leukemia. *N Engl J Med* **337**:223–9.

10 Kantarjian HM, O'Brien S, Smith TL, et al. (1999) Treatment of Philadelphia chromosome-positive early chronic phase chronic myelogenous leukemia with daily doses of interferon alpha and low-dose cytarabine. *J Clin Oncol* **17**:284–92.

11 Deininger M, Buchdunger E, Druker BJ. (2005) The development of imatinib as a therapeutic agent for chronic myeloid leukemia. *Blood* **105**:2640–53.

12 O'Brien SG, Guilhot F, Goldman JM, et al. (2008) International Randomized Study of Interferon versus STI571 (IRIS) 7-year follow-up: Sustained survival, low rate of transformation and increased rate of major molecular response (MMR) in patients (pts) with newly diagnosed chronic myeloid leukemia in chronic phase (CML-CP) treated with imatinib (IM). *Blood* **112**:186.

13 Druker BJ, Guilhot F, O'Brien SG, et al. (2006) Five-year follow-up of patients receiving imatinib for chronic myeloid leukemia. *N Engl J Med* **355**:2408–17.

14 Kantarjian HM, Talpaz M, O'Brien S, et al. (2006) Survival benefit with imatinib mesylate versus interferon-alpha-based regimens in newly diagnosed chronic-phase chronic myelogenous leukemia. *Blood* **108**:1835–40.

15 Kantarjian H, Talpaz M, O'Brien S, et al. (2004) High-dose imatinib mesylate therapy in newly diagnosed Philadelphia chromosome-positive chronic phase chronic myeloid leukemia. *Blood* **103**:2873–8.

16 Cortes J, Baccarani M, Guilhot F, et al. (2008) A Phase III, randomized, open-label study of 400 mg versus 800 mg of imatinib mesylate (IM) in patients (pts) with newly diagnosed, previously untreated chronic myeloid leukemia in chronic phase (CML-CP) using molecular endpoints: 1-year results of TOPS (Tyrosine Kinase Inhibitor Optimization and Selectivity) Study. *Blood* **112**:335.

17 Baccarani M, Rosti G, Castagnetti F, et al. (2009) Comparison of imatinib 400 mg and 800 mg daily in the front-line treatment of high-risk, Philadelphia-positive chronic myeloid leukemia: a European LeukemiaNet study. *Blood* **113**:4497–504.

18 National Comprehensive Cancer Network (NCCN) clinical practice guidelines in oncology. Chronic Myeloid Leukemia. V.I 2010. At www.NCCN.org/professional/physician-gls/PDF/cml.pdf (last accessed June 2009).

19 Baccarani M, Saglio G, Goldman J, et al. (2006) Evolving concepts in the management of chronic myeloid leukemia: recommendations from an expert panel on behalf of the European LeukemiaNet. *Blood* **108**:1809–20.

20 Apperley JF. (2007) Part I: mechanisms of resistance to imatinib in chronic myeloid leukaemia. *Lancet Oncol* **8**:1018–29.

21 Soverini S, Colarossi S, Gnani A, et al. (2006) Contribution of ABL kinase domain mutations to imatinib resistance in different subsets of Philadelphia-positive patients: By the GIMEMA Working Party on Chronic Myeloid Leukemia. *Clin Cancer Res* **12**:7374–9.

22 Donato NJ, Wu JY, Stapley J, et al. (2004) Imatinib mesylate resistance through BCR-ABL independence in chronic myelogenous leukemia. *Cancer Res* **64**:672–7.

23 Penserga ET, Skorski T. (2007) Fusion tyrosine kinases: a result and cause of genomic instability. *Oncogene* **26**:11–20.

24 Kantarjian HM, Larson RA, Guilhot F, et al. (2009) International Randomized Study of Interferon and STI571 (IRIS) Investigators. Efficacy of imatinib dose escalation in patients with chronic myeloid leukemia in chronic phase. *Cancer* **115**:551–60.

25 Jabbour E, Kantarjian HM, Jones D, et al. (2009) Imatinib mesylate dose escalation is associated with durable responses in patients with chronic myeloid leukemia after cytogenetic failure on standard-dose imatinib therapy. *Blood* **113**:2154–60.

26 Lombardo LJ, Lee FY, Chen P, et al. (2004) Discovery of N-(2-chloro-6-methyl-phenyl)-2-(6-(4-(2-hydroxyethyl)-piperazin-1-yl)-2-methylpyrimidin-4-ylamino)thiazole-5-carboxamide (BMS-354825), a dual

Src/Abl kinase inhibitor with potent antitumor activity in preclinical assays. *J Med Chem* **47**:6658–61.

27 O'Hare T, Walters DK, Stoffregen EP, et al. (2005) In vitro activity of Bcr-Abl inhibitors AMN107 and BMS-354825 against clinically relevant imatinib-resistant Abl kinase domain mutants. *Cancer Res* **65**:4500–5.

28 Bradeen HA, Eide CA, O'Hare T, et al. (2006) Comparison of imatinib mesylate, dasatinib (BMS-354825), and nilotinib (AMN107) in an N-ethyl-N-nitrosourea (ENU)-based mutagenesis screen: high efficacy of drug combinations. *Blood* **108**:2332–8.

29 Guilhot F, Apperley J, Kim DW, et al. (2007) Dasatinib induces significant hematologic and cytogenetic responses in patients with imatinib-resistant or -intolerant chronic myeloid leukemia in accelerated phase. *Blood* **109**:4143–50.

30 Hochhaus A, Baccarani M, Deininger M, et al. (2008) Dasatinib induces durable cytogenetic responses in patients with chronic myelogenous leukemia in chronic phase with resistance or intolerance to imatinib. *Leukemia* **22**:1200–6.

31 Cortes J, Rousselot P, Kim DW, et al. (2007) Dasatinib induces complete hematologic and cytogenetic responses in patients with imatinib-resistant or -intolerant chronic myeloid leukemia in blast crisis. *Blood* **109**:3207–13.

32 Shah NP, Kim D-W, Kantarjian HM, et al. (2008) Dasatinib dose-optimization in chronic phase chronic myeloid leukemia (CML-CP): Two-year data from CA180-034 show equivalent long-term efficacy and improved safety with 100 mg once daily dose. *Blood* **112**:3225.

33 Porkka K, Khoury HJ, Paquette R, et al. (2008) Dasatinib 100 mg once daily (QD) maintains long-term efficacy and minimizes the occurrence of pleural effusion: An analysis of 24-month data in patients with resistance, suboptimal response, or intolerance to imatinib (CA180-034). *Blood* **112**:3242.

34 Mauro MJ, Baccarani M, Cervantes F, et al. (2008) Dasatinib 2-year efficacy in patients with chronic-phase chronic myelogenous leukemia (CML-CP) with resistance or intolerance to imatinib (START-C). *J Clin Oncol* **26**:7009.

35 Hochhaus A, Mueller M, Cortes JE, et al. (2008) Dasatinib efficacy by dosing schedule across individual baseline BCR-ABL mutations in chronic phase chronic myelogenous leukemia (CML-CP) after imatinib failure. *J Clin Oncol* **26**:7014.

36 Soverini S, Colarossi S, Gnani A, et al. (2007) Resistance to dasatinib in Philadelphia-positive leukemia patients and the presence or the selection of mutations at residues 315 and 317 in the BCR-ABL kinase domain. *Haematologica* **92**:401–4.

37 Shah NP, Skaggs BJ, Branford S, et al. (2007) Sequential ABL kinase inhibitor therapy selects for compound drug-resistant BCR-ABL mutations with altered oncogenic potency. *J Clin Invest* **117**:2562–9.

38 Khorashad JS, Milojkovic D, Mehta P, et al. (2008) In vivo kinetics of kinase domain mutations in CML patients treated with dasatinib after failing imatinib. *Blood* **111**:2378–81.

39 Jabbour E, Kantarjian HM, Jones D, et al. (2008) Characteristics and outcome of chronic myeloid leukemia patients with F317L BCR-ABL kinase domain mutation after therapy with tyrosine kinase inhibitors. *Blood* **112**:4839–42.

40 Mueller MC, Erben P, Ernst T, et al. (2007) Molecular response according to type of preexisting BCR-ABL mutations after second line dasatinib therapy in chronic phase CML patients. *Blood* **110**:319.

41 Weisberg E, Manley PW, Breitenstein W, et al. (2005) Characterization of AMN107, a selective inhibitor of native and mutant Bcr-Abl. *Cancer Cell* **7**:129–41.

42 Kantarjian HM, Giles F, Gattermann N, et al. (2007) Nilotinib (formerly AMN107), a highly selective BCR-ABL tyrosine kinase inhibitor, is effective in patients with Philadelphia chromosome-positive chronic myelogenous leukemia in chronic phase following imatinib resistance and intolerance. *Blood* **110**:3540–6.

43 le Coutre P, Ottmann OG, Giles F, et al. (2008) Nilotinib (formerly AMN107), a highly selective BCR-ABL tyrosine kinase inhibitor, is active in patients with imatinib-resistant or -intolerant accelerated-phase chronic myelogenous leukemia. *Blood* **111**:1834–9.

44 Kantarjian HM, Giles F, Bhalla KN, et al. (2008) Nilotinib in chronic myeloid leukemia patients in chronic phase (CMLCP) with imatinib resistance or intolerance: 2-year follow-up results of a phase 2 study. *Blood* **112**:3238.

45 le Coutre PD, Giles F, Hochhaus A, et al. (2008) Nilotinib in chronic myeloid leukemia patients in accelerated phase (CML-AP) with imatinib resistance or intolerance: 2-year follow-up results of a phase 2 study. *Blood* **112**:3229.

46 Giles FJ, Larson RA, Kantarjian HM, et al. (2008) Nilotinib in patients with Philadelphia chromosome-positive chronic myelogenous leukemia in blast crisis (CML-BC) who are resistant or intolerant to imatinib. *J Clin Oncol* **26**:7017.

47 Hochhaus A, Kim D-W, Martinelli G, et al. (2008) Nilotinib efficacy according to baseline BCR-ABL mutations in patients with imatinib-resistant chronic myeloid leukemia in chronic phase (CML-CP). *Blood* **112**:3216.

48 Cortes J, Kantarjian HM, Kim D-W, et al. (2008) Efficacy and safety of bosutinib (SKI-606) in patients with chronic phase (CP) Ph + chronic myelogenous leukemia (CML) with resistance or intolerance to imatinib. *Blood* **112**:1098.

49 Cortes J, Paquette R, Talpaz M, et al. (2008) Preliminary clinical activity in a phase I trial of the BCR-ABL/IGF- 1R/aurora kinase inhibitor XL228 in patients with Ph + + leukemias with either failure to multiple TKI therapies or with T315I mutation. *Blood* **112**:3232.

50 Gontarewicz A, Balabanov S, Keller G, et al. (2007) Simultaneous targeting of aurora kinases and Bcr-Abl by the small molecule inhibitor PHA-739358 is effective in imatinib-resistant mutations including T315I. *Blood* **110**:1042.

51 Gontarewicz A, Balabanov S, Keller G, et al. (2007) PHA-680626 exhibits antiproliferative and pro-apoptotic activity on imatinib-resistant chronic myeloid leukemia cell lines and primary CD34 + cells by inhibition of both Bcr-Abl tyrosine kinase and aurora kinases. *Blood* **110**:4568.

52 Paquette RL, Shah NP, Sawyers CL, et al. (2007) PHA-739358, an aurora kinase inhibitor, induces clinical responses in chronic myeloid leukemia harboring T315I mutations of BCR-ABL. *Blood* **110**:1030.

53 Giles FJ, Cortes J, Jones D, et al. (2007) MK-0457, a novel kinase inhibitor, is active in patients with chronic myeloid leukemia or acute lymphocytic leukemia with the T315I BCR-ABL mutation. *Blood* **109**:500–2.

54 O'Hare T, Eide CA, Adrian LT, et al. (2008) Complete suppression of in vitro resistance by AP24534, a pan-BCR-ABL inhibitor. *Blood* **112**:726.

55 Van Etten RA, Chan WW, Zaleskas VM, et al. (2008) Switch pocket inhibitors of the ABL tyrosine kinase: distinct kinome inhibition profiles and in vivo efficacy in mouse models of CML and B-lymphoblastic leukemia induced by BCR-ABL T315I. *Blood* **112**:576.

56 Spencer A, Prince M, DeAngelo DJ, et al. (2007) Phase IA/II study of oral LBH589, a novel deacetylase inhibitor (DACi), administered on 2 schedules, in patients with advanced hematologic malignancies. *Blood* **110**:907.

57 Dasmahapatra G, Yerram N, Dai Y, Dent P, Grant S. (2007) Synergistic interactions between Vorinostat and Sorafenib in chronic myelogenous leukemia cells involve Mcl-1 and p21CIP1 down-regulation. *Clin Cancer Res* **13**:4280–90.

58 Cortes J, Albitar M, Thomas D, et al. (2003) Efficacy of the farnesyl transferase inhibitor R115777 in chronic myeloid leukemia and other hematologic malignancies. *Blood.* **101**:1692–7.

59 Cortes J, Garcia-Manero G, O'Brien S, et al. (2007) Phase 1 study of tipifarnib in combination with imatinib for patients with chronic myelogenous leukemia in chronic phase after imatinib failure. *Cancer* **110**:2000–6.

60 Borthakur G, Daley G, Talpaz M, et al. (2006) Pilot study of lonafarnib, a farnesyl transferase inhibitor, in patients with chronic myeloid leukemia in the chronic or accelerated phase that is resistant or refractory to imatinib therapy. *Cancer* **106**:346–52.

61 Cortes J, Daley G, 'Brien S, et al. (2007) Phase 1 study of lonafarnib (SCH 66336) and imatinib mesylate in patients with chronic myeloid leukemia who have failed prior single-agent therapy with imatinib. *Cancer* **110**:1295–302.

62 Issa JP, Gharibyan V, Cortes J, et al. (2005) Phase II study of low-dose decitabine in patients with chronic myelogenous leukemia resistant to imatinib mesylate. *J Clin Oncol* **23**:3948–56.

63 Kantarjian HM, O'Brien S, Cortes J, et al. (2003) Results of decitabine (5-aza-2′deoxycytidine) therapy in 130 patients with chronic myelogenous leukemia. *Cancer* **98**:522–8.

64 Kantarjian HM, Talpaz M, Santini V, et al. (2001) Homoharringtonine: history, current research, and future direction. *Cancer* **92**:1591–605.

65 O'Brien S, Kantarjian H, Keating M, et al. (1995) Homoharringtonine therapy induces responses in patients with chronic myelogenous leukemia in late chronic phase. *Blood* **86**:3322–6.

66 Cortes J, Khoury HJ, Corm S, et al. (2008) Safety and efficacy of subcutaneous (SC) omacetaxine mepesuccinate in imatinib(IM)-resistant chronic myeloid leukemia (CML) patients (pts) with the T315I mutation: results of an ongoing multicenter phase II study. *Blood* **112**:3239.

67 Jain N, Reuben JM, Kantarjian H, et al. (2009) Synthetic tumor-specific breakpoint peptide vaccine in patients with chronic myeloid leukemia and minimal residual disease: a phase 2 trial. *Cancer* **115**:3924–34.

68 Maslak PG, Dao T, Gomez M, et al. (2008) A pilot vaccination trial of synthetic analog peptides derived from the BCR-ABL breakpoints in CML patients with minimal disease. *Leukemia* **22**:1613–16.

69 Bocchia M, Gentili S, Abruzzese E, et al. (2005) Effect of a p210 multipeptide vaccine associated with imatinib or interferon in patients with chronic myeloid leukaemia and persistent residual disease: a multicentre observational trial. *Lancet* **365**:657–62.

70 Rojas JM, Knight K, Wang L, Clark RE. (2007) Clinical evaluation of BCR-ABL peptide immunisation in chronic myeloid leukaemia: results of the EPIC study. *Leukemia* **21**:2287–95.

71 Rezvani K, Yong AS, Mielke S, et al. (2008) Leukemia-associated antigen-specific T-cell responses following combined PR1 and WT1 peptide vaccination in patients with myeloid malignancies. *Blood* **111**:236–42.

72 Shah NP, Nicoll JM, Branford S, et al. (2005) Molecular analysis of dasatinib resistance mechanisms in CML patients identifies novel BCR-ABL mutations predicted to retain sensitivity to imatinib: rationale for combination tyrosine kinase inhibitor therapy. *Blood* **106**:1093.

73 Weisberg E, Catley L, Wright RD, et al. (2007) Beneficial effects of combining nilotinib and imatinib in preclinical models of BCR-ABL+ leukemias. *Blood* **109**:2112–20.

74 O'Hare T, Eide CA, Tyner JW, et al. (2007) SGX70393 inhibits Bcr-AblT315I in vitro and in vivo and completely suppresses resistance when combined with nilotinib or dasatinib. *Blood* **110**:535.

75 Fiskus W, Pranpat M, Bali P, et al. (2006) Combined effects of novel tyrosine kinase inhibitor AMN107 and histone deacetylase inhibitor LBH589 against Bcr-Abl-expressing human leukemia cells. *Blood* **108**:645–52.

76 O'Hare T, Eide CA, Tyner JW, et al. (2008) SGX393 inhibits the CML mutant Bcr-AblT315I and preempts in vitro resistance when combined with nilotinib or dasatinib. *Proc Natl Acad Sci U S A* **105**:5507–12.

77 Rosti G, Castagnetti F, Poerio A, et al. (2008) High and early rates of cytogenetic and molecular response with nilotinib 800 mg daily as first-line treatment of Ph-positive chronic myeloid leukemia in chronic phase: results of a phase 2 trial of the GIMEMA CML Working Party. *Blood* **112**:181.

78 Cortes J, O'Brien S, Jones D, et al. (2008) Efficacy of nilotinib (formerly AMN107) in patients (pts) with newly diagnosed, previously untreated Philadelphia chromosome (Ph)-positive chronic myelogenous leukemia in early chronic phase (CML-CP). *Blood* **112**:446.

79 Cortes J, O'Brien S, Borthakur G, et al. (2008) Efficacy of dasatinib in patients (pts) with previously untreated chronic myelogenous leukemia (CML) in early chronic phase (CML-CP). *Blood* **112**:182.

80 Deininger M, Schleuning M, Greinix H, et al. (2006) The effect of prior exposure to imatinib on transplant-related mortality. *Haematologica* **91**:452–9.

81 Jabbour E, Cortes J, Kantarjian H, et al. (2007) Novel tyrosine kinase inhibitor therapy before allogeneic stem cell transplantation in patients with chronic myeloid leukemia: no evidence for increased transplant-related toxicity. *Cancer* **110**:340–4.

82 Jabbour E, Cortes J, Kantarjian HM, et al. (2006) Allogenic stem cell transplantation for patients with chronic myeloid leukemia and acute lymphocytic leukemia after BCR-ABL kinase mutation-related imatinb failure. *Blood* **108**:1421–3.

83 Marin D, Milojkovic D, Olavarria E, et al. (2008) European LeukemiaNet criteria for failure or suboptimal response reliably identify patients with CML in early chronic phase treated with imatinib whose eventual outcome is poor. *Blood* **112**:4437–44.

84 Alvarado Y, Kantarjian H, O'Brien S, et al. (2009) Significance of suboptimal response to imatinib, as defined by the European LeukemiaNet, in the long-term outcome of patients with early chronic myeloid leukemia in chronic phase. *Cancer* **115**:3709–18.

85 Kantarjian H, Pasquini R, Hamerschlak N, et al. (2007) Dasatinib or high-dose imatinib for chronic-phase chronic myeloid leukemia after failure of first-line imatinib: a randomized phase 2 trial. *Blood* **109**:5143–50.

86 Kantarjian H, Pasquini R, Levy V, et al. (2009) Dasatinib or high-dose imatinib for chronic-phase chronic myeloid leukemia resistant to imatinib at a dose of 400 to 600 milligrams daily: two-year follow-up of a randomized phase 2 study (START-R). *Cancer* **115**:4136–47.

87 Tam CS, Kantarjian H, Garcia-Manero G, et al. (2008) Failure to achieve a major cytogenetic response by 12 months defines inadequate response in patients receiving nilotinib or dasatinib as second- or subsequent-line therapy for chronic myeloid leukemia. *Blood* **112**:516–18.

88 Jabbour E, Kantarjian H, Jones D, et al. (2009) Long-term outcome of patients with chronic myeloid leukemia treated with second generation tyrosine kinase inhibitors after imatinib failure is predicted by the in vitro sensitivity of BCR-ABL kinase domain mutations. *Blood* **114**:2037–43.

CHAPTER 6

The Molecular Biology of Acute Myeloid Leukemia

Jerald Radich

Fred Hutchinson Cancer Research Center, Seattle, WA, USA

Introduction

Cancer is a genetic disease, and the study of the molecular biology of leukemia has been the major contributor to our understanding of the genetic basis of malignancy in general. Chronic myeloid leukemia (CML) led the way with the observation that all cases had the Ph chromosome, the reciprocal translocation between chromosomes 9 and 22 [1]. The further elucidation that this translocation led to the chimeric *BCR-ABL* gene was the cornerstone for understanding how aberrant gene regulation could cause fundamental changes in pathways regulating proliferation, differentiation, and apoptosis.

The genetic disturbances in AML are far more heterogeneous than CML. However, the study of the recurrent genetic changes in AML demonstrated how a variety of genetic lesions cause changes in a fairly small number of crucial cellular pathways. The importance of cytogenetic changes to prognosis in AML was clear well before we began to understand the functional consequences of the genetic alterations. Thus, the relatively common translocations of t(15:17) found in AML, and the t(8;21) and inv(16) were long known to be "good" risk cytogenetic changes, compared to patients with normal cytogenetics ("intermediate" risk) or complex genetic changes ("poor" risk) [2]. Our understanding of how these molecular disturbances cause cancer is still incomplete, and our comprehension of the

biological ramifications of other common genetic lesions, such as *FLT3* and *NPM1*, is even less complete [3, 4].

Advances in cytogenetic and molecular techniques have now identified genetic lesions in >70% of AML cases (Table 6.1) [5]. In cases with normal cytogenetics, mutations can be found in over 50% of cases. The mutations generally fall into functional categories that disturb differentiation, proliferation, and apoptosis. When multiple mutations are found, they generally affect different functions, as might be predicted from evolutionary logic [6]. Thus, the *PML-RARA* rearrangement blocks differentiation at the promyelocytic cell stage; these cases often have mutations in the *FLT3* tyrosine kinase gene, which increases proliferative drive. Mutations that affect differentiation are often termed Class I mutations, while those affecting proliferation are Class II lesions. Mutations of tumor suppressor genes, which affect cell cycle and apoptotic controls, are unclassified in this scheme, and this reflects both on our lack of understanding of how these pathways interact, as well as the limitations of a simple model (Figure 6.1).

Further classification of AML has been performed by the use of high-resolution techniques to examine DNA sequence (SNPs, "deep" sequencing), global gene expression, microRNA (miRNA), and methylation studies. Thus, we are developing more and more complicated schemes to classify AML. The

Advances in Malignant Hematology, First Edition. Edited by Hussain I. Saba and Ghulam J. Mufti. © 2011 Blackwell Publishing Ltd. Published 2011 by Blackwell Publishing Ltd.

Table 6.1 Frequent mutations in AML and their function

Mutation	Freq.	Function	"Targeted" drugs?	Prognosis?
Translocation				
t(8;21)	10%	Differentiation		Good
inv.16	10%	Differentiation		Good
t(15;17)	10%	Differentiation	ATRA, arsenic	Good
MLL				
Mutations				
NPM 1	50%	Unknown		Good (if FLTwt)
FLT3 ITD	25%	RTK-Proliferation	FLT3 inhibitors[a]	Bad
FLT3 TKD	5%	RTK-Proliferation	FLT3 inhibitors[a]	Variable
RAS	15%	Proliferation	FTI (tipifarnib)	No
KIT	<5%	RTK-Proliferation	TKI (Imatinib, dasatinib)	Bad if CBF
FMS	<5%	RTK-Proliferation		Unknown
WT1	<5%	Unknown	Immunotherapy[a]	Bad
CEBPA	10%	Differentiation		Good
Expression				
AF1q	25%	Unknown		Bad
BAALC	25%	Unknown		Bad
WT1	25%	Unknown	Immunotherapy[a]	Unknown

[a] Multiple agents/approaches in clinical trials

benefit is obviously that a more complete understanding of the biology of disease may lead to better prognostic schemes, new targeted therapy, and a chance to realize the vaunted goal of "personalized medicine." The downside is that we might find that AML is such a heterogeneous disease that we may change a relatively rare disease into a cluster of exceedingly rare diseases. The latter will not be a very attractive target for drug development.

Recurrent translocations and mutations

Translocations and gene mutations can be identified in the majority of AML cases, and a small subset of genetic lesions are sufficiently common to merit prognostic import. In general, the translocations cause dysregulation of normal transcription pathways, whereas many of the mutations described activate signal transduction pathways, leading to inappropriate proliferation.

RARA translocations

Retinoids are derivatives of vitamin A and are involved in the control of embryonic development, organogenesis, differentiation, cell growth, and apoptosis. The effects of the retinoid ligand are mediated through RAR and RXR receptors. In the absence of ligand, RAR-RXR dimers bind to DNA in complexes that include histone deacetylases (HDAC) [7]. Thus

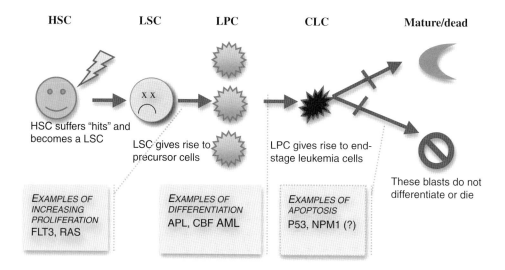

HSC   **LSC**   **LPC**   **CLC**   **Mature/dead**

HSC suffers "hits" and becomes a LSC

LSC gives rise to precursor cells

LPC gives rise to end-stage leukemia cells

These blasts do not differentiate or die

EXAMPLES OF INCREASING PROLIFERATION FLT3, RAS

EXAMPLES OF DIFFERENTIATION APL, CBF AML

EXAMPLES OF APOPTOSIS P53, NPM1 (?)

Figure 6.1 Conceptual (abstract) model of AML. The normal hematopoietic stem cell (HSC) is "hit" by one or more genetic lesions, giving rise to the near mythic leukemia stem cell (LSC). These may proliferate to leukemia progenitor cells (LPC). This gives rise to a committed leukemia cell (CLC). Increases in proliferation, with a block of normal differentiation and apoptosis, cause the accumulation of leukemia cells. Mutations in most/all of these processes may be necessary for leukemia to arise.

in the absence of retinoic acid, RAR-RXR complexes have a transcript repressor function. In the presence of RA, a conformational change occurs in the complex, releasing the co-repressors and allowing recruitment of transcriptional co-activators, including histone acetylases (HATs). Thus, physiologic RA causes a switch from repression to activation of transcription.

In AML, several translocations involving *RARA* on chromosome 17 alter retinoic acid pathways. The most frequent translocation (>95% of this group) involve the zinc finger gene *PML* on chromosome 15, yielding the t(15;17) translocation that defines APL. However, rarely *RARA* partners with the zinc finger protein *PLZF* on chromosome 11, the *NPM1* gene from chromosome 5, or the 5' exons of the nuclear mitotic apparatus protein (NuMa) on chromosome 11 [8–10]. In addition, an interstitial deletion in chromosome 17 can create a fusion of *STAT5B* and *RARA* [11].

The pathogenesis resulting from the creation of a novel fusion gene involving *RARA* is best developed in *PML-RARA*. In this case, it appears that *PML-RARA* is more efficient at recruiting transcriptional repressor complexes, so that normal levels of RA cannot shift the balance from repression to activation. At supra-physiological levels, however, retinoic acid can liberate the co-repressor complexes from *PML-RARA*, allowing recruitment of activators, and transformation of the biology to promoting differentiation and apoptosis. It should be noted that the mechanism of *RARA* function perturbation for the other genetic lesions described above is not known. They are, however, not sensitive to RA.

In APL, both the *PML-RARA* and the reciprocal *RARA-PML* mRNA and protein are expressed. There is increasing evidence that disturbance in normal *PML* function by *PML-RARA* may contribute to the pathogenesis of APL [12]. *PML* is a member of a group of proteins that contain an unusual zinc finger domain (the really interesting gene, or RING, domain). It appears the *PML* is involved with both p53-dependent and independent apoptosis (as *PML* function is essential for both FAS- and TNFA-induced apoptosis). Normal *PML* proteins congregate in subnuclear structures known as *PML* nuclear bodies (PML-NBs), forming a complex with many proteins including the tumor suppressors p53 and pRB, the transcription factor CBP, eiF4E, and DAXX, to name a few. It appears that *PML-RARA* in APL also congregate in NBs, and cause the disruption of the normal *PML* complexes therein. However, *PML* is also produced in several isoforms, many of which function in the cytoplasm. The specific functions of these isoforms, and how they may be affected by *PML-RARA* in APL are unknown.

Core binding factor (CBF) mutations

CBFs are a family of transcription factors comprised of a DNA binding subunit (CBF-alpha) and a non-DNA binding subunit (CBF-beta) [13]. Mutations – either reciprocal translocations or point mutations – affecting either a *RUNX1* (which codes for a CBF-alpha subunit) or *CBFB* (coding for CBF-beta) occur in approximately 20–30% of AML cases [2]. *RUNX1* and *CBFB* are highly evolutionary conserved, and *in vitro* and murine models have demonstrated that both genes are required at an early stage of hematopoetic stem cell development. The most frequent genetic lesion involves the t(8;21) (*RUNX1/-ETO*) or the inv(16)/t(16;16) (*CFBF-MYH11*) translocations; these are considered "favorable risk" AML subtypes, and account for 15–20% of AML cases. The assumption is that these reciprocal translocations disrupt the normal structure and function of CBF, and thus alter the transcription of genes critical in controlling hematopoietic differentiation.

There are several lines of evidence that suggest that CBF mutations are not entirely sufficient to cause leukemia. The first is the coincidence of other mutations in these cases, especially those that activate proliferation pathways (*FLT3*, *RAS*), as well as mutations in other transcription factors (*CEBPA*) [6]. Secondly murine knockout-models with these translocations have quite a long latency, suggesting that the acquisition of additional mutations may be occurring. Lastly, most cases of CBF leukemia can have the translocation detected by sensitive PCR assays years after the achievement of remission [14, 15]. There are a few possible reasons why this might occur (immunologic control of a small leukemia clone; presence of the translocation in lymphoid clones; the persistence of a clone with additional mutations that "freezes" the cells in dormancy), but one distinct possibility is the persistence of a clone bearing the translocation, but not the additional mutations required to achieve full malignant status.

Mixed lineage leukemia gene (*MLL*)

Genetic abnormalities involving the mixed lineage leukemia gene on chromosome 11 q23 are relatively common in AML, particularly in cases arising from previous chemotherapy (especially, but not limited to, treatment with etopoides). *MLL* is quite promiscuous, and over 50 gene partners have been described in the reciprocal translocation [16]. The partner gene of *MLL* largely defines the biology and prognosis [17, 18]. This effect seems most pronounced in pediatric AML. Thus, while the most common t(9;11) translocation is associated with a 50% EFS, extremes of good and poor prognosis are clear [18]. For example, t(1;11) AML involving the AF1q gene (see below) had a 92% EFS(!), while those with t(6;11), involving the AF6 gene, had an EFS of only 11%. In adult AML, it is less clear that different partners (especially the most common t(9;11)) have a clearly distinct prognosis [2, 17]. In addition, duplications of *MLL* can occur in approximately 5% of AML cases, and these are generally associated with adverse risk [19].

"Activating" mutations of kinase-mediated signaling networks

While the CBF mutations primarily affect differentiation, a broad class of "activating" mutations can affect the normal RAS-MAP kinase signaling cascade, affecting both cell proliferation and apoptosis.

Normal signal transduction

Signal transduction pathways translate extracelluar signals (e.g., stimulation to respond to cytokine ligands, interferons) into intracellular action (proliferation, differentiation, survival). In myeloid malignancy signaling through the *RAS* family of GTPases appears to be especially relevant. A highly simplified cartoon of the RAS signal transduction pathway is shown in Figure 6.2. Receptor tyrosine kinases (RTK; e.g., PDGF, Fms, Kit, and *FLT3*) are ligand-binding receptors [20] which signal through H-, K-, and N-ras proteins [21, 22]. These RAS proteins are 21 kd GDP/GTP-binding proteins that serve as a crucial hub of signal transduction The RTK is linked to RAS through the adaptor

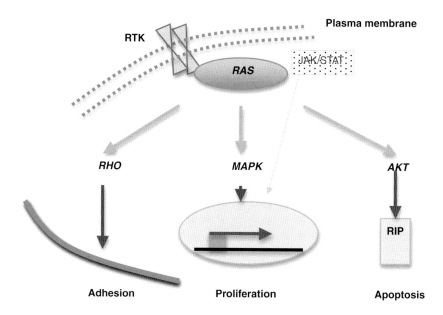

Figure 6.2 Signal transduction. Mutations in the *RTK/ RAS/MAPK* and Jak/STAT signaling pathways are very common in myeloid malignancies. In addition to the mutations common in AML (*FLT3, KIT, RAS*), activation occurs in CML (*BCR-ABL*), CMML (*RAS*) and myeloproliferative syndromes (*JAK2* mutations). Activation of the pathways causes changes in proliferation, apoptosis, adhesion (symbolized by the fuzziness of the plasma membrane) contributing to leukemogenesis. [Not to scale.]

protein Grb2; SOS is a guanine nucleotide exchange protein that promotes RAS-GDP –RAS-GTP phosphate exchange. Conversely, the GTPase activating proteins (GAP) and NF-1 catalyze the conversion of active RAS-GTP back to the inactive RAS-GDP. Thus, an extracellular ligand (e.g., FLT ligand) binds to the RTK, which dimerizes and undergoes autophosphorylation; this in turn phosphylates Grb-2 which when associated with SOS activates RAS. Activated RAS is switched to the inactive RAS-GDP by the GTPase-activating proteins GAP and NF-1.

RAS activation affects several downstream pathways, affecting cell proliferation, differentiation, and apoptosis (reviewed in [22]). The serine/threonine kinase RAF is activated by RAS, activating MAP/ERK kinase (MEK); this in turn activates mitogen-activating protein kinases (MAPK), such as the extracellular signal-regulated kinases ERK 1 and 2. These proteins phosphylate cytoplasmic targets (Rsk, Mnk) that translocate to the nucleus, activating transcription-promoting cell proliferation. RAS activation also influences cytoskeleton organization

through activation of RHO and RAC, and promotes cell cycling through the activation of cyclin-dependent kinases (CDKs). RAS may also inhibit apoptosis by the activation of the c-Akt/PI-3 kinase pathway.

Since the initiation of the signal cascade takes place at the intracellular membrane, RAS undergoes a post-translation modification called prenylation, which adds an isoprenoid moiety to the cytoplasmic RAS [23]. This prenylation is accomplished by the enzymes farnesyl and geranylgeranyl transferases, which add 15- and 17-mer isoprenoids, respectively, to the RAS protein. Prevention of the prenylation RAS is the rationale for the inhibition of farnesyl transferase as a treatment strategy.

Janus kinase-signal transducer and activator of transcription (JAK/STAT) pathways are used by the cytokine receptor superfamily (including erythropoietin, G-CSF, and interferon) [24, 25]. Unlike the RTK receptors, the receptors to these ligands lack their own intrinsic tyrosine kinase activity; binding of ligand to receptor causes autophosphorylation of JAKs, which then phosphorlyate the receptor. These phosphorylated receptors are docking sites for signaling proteins, including STATs, which are in turn activated by phosphorylation. The activated STATs form dimers (either homodimers, or heterodimers with other STATs), translocate into the nucleus, and bind to specific DNA sequences, regulating gene transcription (Figure 6.2). Constitutive activation of STATs has been seen in ~70% of AML cases, and may occur through translocations (e.g., TEL in t (9;11) AML [26]), autocrine (IL-6 [27]), or from RTK activation (FLT3 ITD [28]).

Mutations in the above signaling machinery are relatively common in AML, and represent a common theme of activating mutations.

FLT3 mutations

The internal tandem duplication (ITD) in FLT3 is caused by a duplication of ~5–400 base pairs within exons 14 and 15, placed in a head-to-tail orientation [4, 29, 30]. The majority of ITDs involve codons in the juxtamembrane region of the FLT3 receptor, though ~20–30% occur into the first tyrosine kinase domain (TK-1) [31, 32]. In vitro transduction studies have shown that the FLT3-ITD mutation causes ligand-independent dimerization of FLT3 receptors, leading to auto-phosphorylation and activation of downstream signaling pathways. In addition, missense point mutations of codon D835 within the tyrosine kinase activation loop occurs in 5–10% of AML cases [33, 34]. Deletions, point mutations, and insertions have also been occasionally found within the codons surrounding D835 [35, 36].

The FLT3-ITD mutation is the most common mutation of the RAS signal pathway, with an age-dependent prevalence of 10–35% of AML patients [29, 30, 37–45]. The FLT3-ITD mutation is associated with leukocytosis and high blast counts in patients with normal karyotype, t(15;17) translocations, or t(6;9) translocations. Many studies have found that FLT3-ITD mutations are associated with a poor prognosis (Table 6.1) [40–44, 46, 47]. However, not all FLT3-ITD mutations are created equal. The allelic ratio is the relative amount of mutant to wild-type allele. AML patients harboring high FLT3 allelic ratios (little/no wild-type FLT3) have the worst prognosis [42, 48]. A high allelic ratio may be explained by a simple deletion of the

wild-type gene with loss of heterozygosity (LOH) [48]. However, more commonly homologous recombination of the FLT3-ITD allele occurs, in which the cell, struggling to correct the heterozygous mutation, eliminates the normal allele and duplicates the aberrant allele [42]. In addition, the variation of allelic ratios might occur from several AML subclones within the total AML population; some subpopulations might harbor a FLT3-ITD mutation, while others contain only WT FLT3. This clonal competition could explain why FLT3 mutational status can change between diagnosis and relapse, with some patients developing a new or different FLT3 mutation upon relapse, while others lose their FLT3 mutation altogether [49, 50].

Size may matter in regards to the FLT3-ITD mutation. In some studies, cases with larger ITD have worse prognosis compared to patients with smaller FLT3 ITDs [51, 52]. This may be because the larger ITD cases tend to involve not only the juxtamembrane position of the FLT3 molecule, but also the TK-1 portion of the FLT3 protein. Patients with such mutations have been shown to have an inferior outcome compared to those with mutations that do not involve the TK-1. Presumably this mutation causes further deregulation of normal FLT3 function.

FLT3 tyrosine kinase occurs in 5–10% of AML cases, and these mutations cause ligand-independent activation in vitro (just as FLT3 ITD). However, it is not clear that these mutations have a poor prognosis [34, 42]. Curiously, in one study cases with FLT3-TKD mutations had higher levels of FLT3 mRNA expression than samples with either ITD mutant or WT gene [53].

Ras mutations

Mutations in N-, K-, or H- RAS occur in approximately 10–30% of AML cases [54, 55], myelodysplastic syndrome (MDS) (~5–20%) [56], juvenile CML (20–30%) [57], and CMML (30–50%) [58]. In AML, RAS mutations involve N-ras >K-ras, >H-ras. Point mutations occur in codons 12, 13, and 61 [59], and prevent the hydrolysis of RAS-GTP, keeping RAS in the "on" state. The coincident occurrence of both a FLT3 and RAS mutation in the same cases is very rare, as might be expected since there is no a priori selective advantage to two mutations affecting

Table 6.2 Risk groups based on cytogenetics and mutations

Cytogenetic group	Mutational subsets
Favorable	t(8;21) (*RUNX1-RUNX1T1*)
	inv (16) or t(16;16) (*CBFB-MYH11*)
	NK with *NPM* mutation and wild-type *FLT3*
	NK with *CEBPA* mutation
Intermediate	NK with *NPM* mutation and *FLT3* ITD
	NK with wild-type *NPM* and *FLT3*
	NK with wild-type *NPM* and mutated *FLT3* ITD[a]
Adverse	inv (3) or t(3;3) (*RPN1-EVI1*)
	t(6;9) (*DEK-NUP214*)
	t(v;11) (*MLL* rearrangement)

[a] Note that cases of *FLT3* ITD have their prognostic importance associated with the allelic ration (see text). Thus, cases of *FLT3* ITD with a high allelic ratio (little or no wild-type *FLT3* detected) are at a very high risk of treatment failure.
Cytogenetic classifications: Favorable = CBF, APL; Intermediate = normal karyotype (NK), t(9;11); Adverse = three or more chromosomal abnormalities or involvement of 5q, 7q, or 17q.

the same pathway. However unlike *FLT3-ITD* mutations, *RAS* mutations are not clearly prognostically important [60], suggesting that more than just RTK/RAS signal activation plays an important role in determining disease biology. In both *FLT3* and *RAS* mutations, there may be discordance between diagnosis and relapse. Thus, a patient with either a *RAS* or *FLT3* mutation may relapse without the mutation (or vice versa). This suggests that these mutations are not the primary oncogenic event.

Other tyrosine kinase receptor mutations

Activating point mutations in the kinase domains of *FMS* have been described in 5–10% of selected AML

cases [56, 61]. Deletions, insertions, and point mutations have been found occasionally in the *KIT* receptor, often in cases with a mast cell [62, 63]. Given the relative rarity of these single mutations, their prognostic importance in AML is largely unknown. However, the D816 *KIT* mutation has been found in approximately 10% of CBF leukemia, and this is associated with a poor outcome in these cases otherwise categorized as "favorable" [64].

Other frequent mutations in AML

Nucleophosmin (NPM1) mutations
NPM1 appears to play an important role in the cell cycle and repair pathways involving p53 and ARF. To perform these duties normal *NPM1* shuttles between the cytoplasm and the nucleus. Mutations in *NPM1* are the most common described in AML, occurring in ~30–40% of all cases, and >50% in normal karyotype (NK) AML [3, 65–69]. There are scores of described mutations, but by far the most common is a simple four-base insertion, which inhibits NPM1 migration, causing NPM1 to be stuck in the cytoplasm. There appears to be similar and perhaps complementary biology between *NPM1* and *FLT3*. Both of these: (1) increase in prevalence with age, (2) are found predominately in normal cytogenetic AML, and (3) often co-exist in the same patient. However, while *FLT3* mutations are generally associated with a poor prognosis, *NPM1* mutations appear to be associated with a more favorable prognosis. However, risk appears to be associated with the status of both *NPM1* and *FLT3*. The best prognosis appears to be *NPM1* mutated with wild-type *FLT3*; the worst appears to be *NPM1* wild type, with an *FLT3* mutation. The biology underlying these risk classifications is unknown.

*TET*2 mutations and deletions
Recently mutations in the *TET2* gene (arising in chromosome 4q24) have been discovered in cases of myeloid leukemia. The frequency appears to range from ~20–25% in cases of MDS and "secondary" AML, ~105 in *de novo* AML, and 10–20% in cases of myeloproliferative and CMML [70–72]. In some cases, it appears that mutated *TET2* occurs with a loss

of a 4q24 allele, suggesting that *TET2* is a tumor suppressor gene. Some cases have been found to have a co-existent mutation in *JAK2*, and when subsets of cells were identified, the *TET2* mutation appeared to predate the *JAK2* mutation. The association TET2 mutations and outcome is unclear, as one study found it associated with an inferior prognosis in AML [70], while one study showed it was a favorable prognostic factor in MDS [73].

CEBPA mutations

Mutations in the CAAT/enhancer-binding protein alpha gene occur in ∼5–10% of AML cases [74, 75]. *CEBPA* codes for the C/EBPA leucine zipper class transcription factor, essential to the regulation of proliferation and granulocytic differentiation. Mutations in *CEBPA* occur in the N-terminus, often yielding premature stop codons, or the zipper domain, affecting DNA binding function as well as dimerization potential. In both pediatric and adult AML, CEBPA tend to occur in patients with normal cytogenetics and, in both settings, are associated with an improved outcome compared to patients without a mutation.

Wilms tumor (*WT*1) expression and mutation

WT1 codes for a zinc finger DNA binding protein. Mutations and deletions of *WT1* were first described in the setting of Wilms tumor cases, and the early data suggested that the normal function of *WT1* was that of a tumor suppressor. However, *WT1* is highly expressed in many types of leukemia, especially AML, ALL, and CML. Mutations of WT1 occur in 5–10% of AML cases, more often in those with a normal karyotype [76]. Some studies have suggested that high WT1 expression, or *WT1* mutations, bode for a poor outcome in AML [77–79]. As detailed below, *WT1* expression has been touted as a potentially useful marker of minimal residual disease [80]. In addition, various immune therapies are been addressed to target cells with high *WT1* mRNA levels [80].

Other potentially prognostic genes

AF1q was originally cloned from a t(1;11) AML case, where AF1q was the partner to the MLL gene [81].

AF1q is a mitochondrial membrane protein involved in the control of apoptosis. The role of AF1q is somewhat confusing, as *in vitro* experiments suggest that overexpression facilitates chemotherapy-induced apoptosis, whereas overexpression of AF1q in AML and MDS is associated with a poor prognosis [82–84]. Curiously, in pediatric AML cases with MLL translocations, those with AF1q as the MLL partner have an excellent prognosis [18].

The brain and acute leukemia, cytoplasmic gene (BAALC) has been found to be over-expressed in AML, particularly in normal karyotype AML, where it carries a poor prognosis [85, 86]. The normal function of the *BAALC* gene is not known. The over-expression of the ETS-related gene (*ERG*) has been associated with poor prognosis in NK adult AML [87].

''-Omics" analyses in AML

Most of the work defining different genetic subgroups in AML involves probing for genetic lesions by routine metaphase cytogenetics, fluorescence i*n situ* hybridization (FISH), or molecular tests. More sensitive assays probe form mutations in known genes. However, there are undoubtedly many more lesions in AML that account for its heterogeneity. New molecular techniques can find smaller aberrations in genomic DNA using SNP arrays, or whole genome CGH; and global transcriptional changes can be assessed by mRNA or miRNA expression arrays. Understanding the bridge between DNA structural changes, miRNA expression, mRNA, and protein activity will in all probability link distinct biological pathways to AML behavior. Work in these areas will likely give us a broader understanding of leukemogenesis as well as define new therapeutic targets.

Chromosomal abnormalities

Gross cytogenetic abnormalities involving large swaths of DNA can be detected by metaphase cytogenetics, and the frequency and implication of these changes have been described above and elsewhere in this book. While genomic alterations such as loss of heterozygosity can occur from actual loss of one segment of DNA, other subtle ways of genetic recombination can effectively cause a change in copy number. Uniparental disomy (UPD) is a mechanism of mitotic recombination that tries to correct a new mutation, and in so doing can change a heterozygotic mutation into a homozygotic mutation. Such events have specifically been described in *CEBPA* and *FLT3-ITD* mutations. Acquired UPD is actually relatively common in AML, and has been estimated to occur in 15–20% of cases [88, 89]. Mechanistically, UPD is significant since it can change the gene dosage of a mutation. Looking for finer changes in DNA can be accomplished by SNP or CGH studies, and these have found evidence of abnormalities (compared to matched normal DNA) in >70% of AML cases [90]. Lastly, the ultimate measure of DNA integrity can be accomplished by sequencing the whole genome. Alas, this is prohibitively expensive to do on any significant number of specimens (in fact, for many labs >1 case would "break the bank"). However, in an instructive study, a single case of CN M1 AML was subjected to whole genome sequencing [91, 92]. By sequencing both AML and normal skin from the same patient, they were able to detect 10 mutations in the AML genome: *FLT3* and *NPM1* were mutated, as were eight other genes not previously described in AML cases. Unfortunately, these eight genes were examined in a cohort of 187 other AML cases, and in no case were any of these candidate genes mutated [91]. A second CN M1 AML patient revealed 12 non-synonymous mutations; while two were "old news" (*RAS* and *NPM1*), 10 were novel [92]. One, the IDH1 gene, was subsequently found mutated in 13/80 (16%) CN AML cases. Validation in other pediatric and adult cohorts, as well as the possible prognostic import of IDH1, should prove interesting.

Transcription deregulation

By far the vast majority of "-omics" data in AML uses the application of mRNA expression arrays. Critics dismissed early studies of gene expression profile (GEP) as mere "fishing expeditions." However, GEP studies have done much to understand the genes and pathways involved in specific translocations and mutations, and have huge potential in both identi-

fying new prognostic diagnostics, as well as new targets for therapy (demonstrating, perhaps, that the best way to *catch* fish is *to fish*).

The most straightforward approach has been to associate specific cytogenetic lesions to gene expression and pathways [93–97]. Several studies have performed GEP on various translocations, including the CBF translocations, t(15;17), and *MLL*. GEP discriminates these various genetic lesions with great accuracy, which is comforting given the different clinical biology of these diseases. For the CBF leukemias, GEP suggests different patterns of gene expression, suggesting a different array of secondary "hits" necessary in leukemogenesis [98, 99]. GEP studies examining pathways involved with mutations are a bit more complex in interpretation. For example, while it is easy to assume that all genetic changes involving the RAS/MAPK should yield the same phenotype, we know that this is not true clinically. *FLT3*-ITD mutations tend to have a poor outcome, while *FLT3*-TK mutations have an uneven relationship with outcome, while "downstream" *RAS* mutations have no clear deleterious association with outcome. The GEP studies tend to mirror this disconnect between our simple cartoons of signal cartoon and clinical reality. The studies of *FLT3* mutations are somewhat inconsistent. One study demonstrated that *FLT3*-ITD and TK mutations both cause changes in cell cycle and signal transduction pathways, as well as deregulation of *HOX* genes [100]. The later genes are thought to play a prominent role in hematopoietic stem cell differentiation, and thus deregulation may promote cells to "freeze" in an immature state. However, other studies have suggested that, while *FLT3* mutations have clear expression changes from those of wild-type *FLT3*, subtle differences occur between cases with ITD and TK mutations. For example, *FLT3*-ITD mutations seem to disturb differentiation (*HOXB5*), whereas TK mutations affect transcription factors (*FOXA1*) [101]. There has been no published clear GEP associated with any of the *RAS* mutations. GEP and *NPM1* mutations have also been investigated [102–104]. *NPM1* mutations are involved with genes involved in signaling and apoptosis; curiously, *HOX* transcription factors are also deregulated in *NPM1* mutations.

Patterns of gene expression appear associated with favorable or unfavorable prognosis [98, 99, 105, 106]. Bullinger et al. found several distinct patterns of gene expression; while most mapped to specific cytogenetic lesions, a distinct poor-risk group was found with genes involving the *NOTCH* pathway, with a good outcome group associated with gene expression of monocytic genes, and *VEGF* signaling [98]. These results were subsequently supported in a study of CN AML [106]. Other studies defined good-risk groups by genes associated with *NPM1*, proliferation signaling, and apoptosis, or genes involving *CEBPA* activation [99, 104]. In these studies, poor-risk groups were found to be associated with *MDR* and *EVA1* dysregulation. While these findings are interesting, there are several caveats. The first is that it is unknown if a profile associated with prognosis is strictly linked to a particular treatment, or is transferable to another treatment. This is obviously crucial, for a prognostic fingerprint only relevant to current therapy is not much use in the future (unless therapy never changes). Second, it is not clear yet what components of the profile are essential to prognosis, and what patterns or pathways are "targetable" for new therapeutic strategies.

Despite the marked heterogeneity of AML, it appears that there are some similarities across all AML subtypes. Thus, a recent study of many types of AML examined genes consistently de-regulated in AML, but not in normal CD34 + cells [107]. These 13 genes (including *BIK*, *CCNA1*, *IL3RA*, *WT1* among others) may give insight into new pathways for drug therapy and biological study. Further, genes dramatically upregulated in AML compared to normal bone marrow (e.g., *WT1*, *PRAME*) might prove as worthy targets for minimal residual disease detection [108].

MicroRNA deregulation

MicroRNAs (miRNA) are evolutionarily conversed small non-coding RNAs [109, 110]. Larger 70–100 bp hairpin precursor RNA are processed into 19–25-mer miRNA, which affect gene regulation by either causing mRNA degradation, or blocking protein translation. Thus, structural changes in DNA can cause either an up- or downregulation in miRNA abundance, which can then cause changes in mRNA and protein expression. In addition, up- or downregulation of the expression of large segments of DNA can cause changes in miRNA expression, and with it further changes in mRNA and protein expression.

The patterns of association of miRNA expression and AML subtypes have followed the pattern originally witnessed with the advent of mRNA array studies, though accelerated in pace of discovery. Thus, AML was found to have a different miRNA signature than ALL cells [111]. With that study, there was confidence to proceed to specific classes of AML cases, first concentrating on the frequent cytogenetic lesions. Predictably, different cytogenetic subtypes of AML display different miRNA expression signatures [112, 113]. Thus, cases of t (15;17) were found to have different miRNA profiles from other types of AML cases. However, there is a fair amount of heterogeneity in the miRNA signal found across studies of t(15;17). Surprisingly, common to most studies of t(15;17) are not miRNA associated directly with the breakpoint, but rather, with an area of 14q32 under methylation control [114]. Similarly, CBF leukemia appeared to have a unique signature, with some consistency across studies implicating the involvement of miR-126 and miR-133a [115].

Common oncogene and tumor suppressor mutations also appear to be associated with fairly unique miRNA signatures. For example, miR-155 is upregulated in cases with *FLT3*-ITD mutations [112, 113, 116]. This association probably has biological relevance, as in murine models, miR-155 overexpression causes increased proliferation of hematopoietic cells; in humans, *FLT3*-ITD (and thus, miR-155) is highly associated with elevated blast counts at diagnosis. Mutations in *NPM1* are associated with elevation of miRs that are associated with chromosomal domains housing *HOX* genes [103]. Since *HOX* genes are upregulated in *NPM1* mutations, it is unclear if the concordant miRNA upregulation causes independent functional effects apart from HOX gene deregulation.

Like mRNA, miRNA deregulation has been associated with clinical outcomes. The largest studies are in cases of CN-AML, where a set of 12 miRNAs are associated with outcome [117]. In correlating miRNA expression and mRNA expression, certain miRNA and their gene targets seems significantly associated with outcome. For example, miR-181a and -181b were inversely associated with EFS. Targets of these miRs, *CARD12*, *CASP1*, *IL1B*, and *TLR4*, were found to be associated with outcome in the same AML population. Thus, a network typing of miRNA expression was inversely correlated with mRNA expression.

Epigenetic regulation

Substantial control of gene expression is accomplished by histone modification and DNA methylation [118–120]. The study of epigenetic regulation may be complimentary to gene expression studies, and may be useful in predicting which patients with MDS and AML are potentially sensitive to histone deacetylase inhibition and hypo-methylation therapy [121]. For example, array-based methylation assays have shown that wide-scale aberrant methylation is common in MDS and secondary AML, but far less so in *de novo* AML (indeed, the methylation profile of *de novo* AML was quite similar to normal hematopoietic cells) [122]. This highlights a fundamental biological difference between primary and *de novo* AML, and supports the relative effectiveness of hypomethylating agents in the former condition

compared to the later. In addition, these assays could detect "correction" of the methylation state towards normal within weeks of hypomethlylation therapy.

Patterns of mutations and cytogenetic lesions

Different types of genetic lesions segregate in a non-random fashion, generally revealing the type of biological (dys)functions necessary to create AML (reviewed [123–125]). For example, the *FLT3* mutation is associated with an increase in proliferation, and it is often found (in ~40% of cases) in t(15;17) APL (in ~40% of cases), where the *PML-RARA* acts to block differentiation. Likewise, the proliferative N-*RAS* or *KIT* mutations are often found in the differentiation blocking CBF lesions (~20–40% of cases); but two proliferative mutations (*FLT3* and RAS), are rarely found in the same sample [37, 55, 126]. That being said, *FLT3* and *NPM* may be found together in normal karyotype AML, but in many cases where only *FLT3* or *NPM* mutations are found, the cooperating genetic event is unknown, although in the majority of cases at least two cooperative lesions are apparent [67] (Figure 6.3).

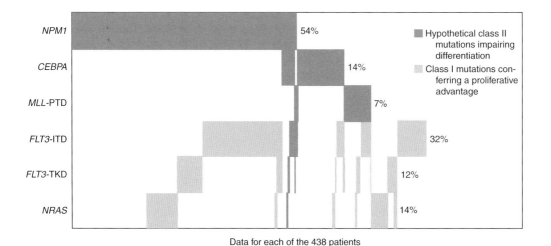

Data for each of the 438 patients

Figure 6.3 Cooperative mutations in normal karyotype (NK) AML. Greater than 80% of NK AML had at least one mutation, with the largest being those with both *NPM1* and *FLT3* mutations. The light gray bars describe "Type 1" mutations, affecting proliferation; the dark gray are "Type 2" mutations, affecting differentiation. (Reproduced from Schlenk [67], with permission from the Massachusetts Medical Society.)

Can AML biology dictate therapy?

With the increasing knowledge of how various mutations contribute to AML comes the obvious insight into new targets for therapy. Indeed, the anticipation is that soon the mutational characterization of each patient's AML will drive the therapeutic decision. The obvious "poster child" for this theme is the treatment of APL with all-trans retinoic acid (ATRA), where supraphysiologic doses of this drug liberates differentiation from the block induced by the *PML-RARA* complex. Given the prevalence of abnormalities of signaling traffic in AML (outlined above), this pathway holds huge potential for targeting. The RTK *FLT3* and *KIT* are obvious targets. Thus far several agents to block *FLT3* mutants have been introduced to the clinic, without huge consequence. This may be because the earlier versions lack potency, or because in AML so many pathways are disturbed, simply shutting down the *FLT3* defect is insufficient. *KIT* mutations in CBF leukemia greatly impairs the relatively favorable prognosis of that mutational class, and several trials are now introducing the TKI inhibitors imatinib or dasatinib, which have considerable inhibitory power against *KIT,* in combination with standard induction therapy.

Conclusion

Our understanding of the genetics of AML has exploded over the last decade. Given the rapid advances in technology, the day when every patient's leukemia will be completely genotyped prior to therapy will soon be upon us. The next challenge will then be to understand how the genetics interact with specific drug combinations in the human patient – where genetic variation in drug metabolism, immunology, and microenvironments influence both the disease and the treatment. This should keep us busy for some time.

References

1 Rowley JD. (1973) A new consistent chromosome abnormality in chronic myelogenous leukemia identified by quinacrine fluorescence and Giemsa staining. *Nature* **243**:209–13.

2 Byrd JC, Mrozek K, Dodge RK, et al. (2002) Pretreatment cytogenetic abnormalities are predictive of induction success, cumulative incidence of relapse, and overall survival in adult patients with de novo acute myeloid leukemia: results from Cancer and Leukemia Group B (CALGB 8461). *Blood* **100**:4325–36.

3 Falini B, Mecucci C, Tiacci E, et al. (2005) Cytoplasmic nucleophosmin in acute myelogenous leukemia with a normal karyotype. *New Engl J Med* **352**:254–66.

4 Stirewalt DL, Radich JP. (2003) The role of *FLT3* in haematopoietic malignancies. *Nature Reviews* **3**:650–65.

5 Haferlach T. (2008) Molecular genetic pathways as therapeutic targets in acute myeloid leukemia. *Hematology* **2008**:400–11.

6 Gilliland DG. (2001) Hematologic malignancies. *Curr Opin Hematol* **8**:189–91.

7 Collins SJ. (1998) Acute promyelocytic leukemia: relieving repression induces remission. *Blood* **91**:2631–3.

8 Chen Z, Guidez F, Rousselot P, et al. (1994) PLZF-RAR alpha fusion proteins generated from the variant t (11;17)(q23;q21) translocation in acute promyelocytic leukemia inhibit ligand-dependent transactivation of wild-type retinoic acid receptors. *Proc Natl Acad Sci U S A* **91**:1178–82.

9 Redner RL, Rush EA, Faas S, Rudert WA, Corey SJ. (1996) The t(5;17) variant of acute promyelocytic leukemia expresses a nucleophosmin-retinoic acid receptor fusion. *Blood* **87**:882–6.

10 Wells RA, Catzavelos C, Kamel-Reid S. (1997) Fusion of retinoic acid receptor alpha to NuMA, the nuclear mitotic apparatus protein, by a variant translocation in acute promyelocytic leukaemia. *Nat Genet* **17**:109–13.

11 Arnould C, Philippe C, Bourdon V, et al. (1999) The signal transducer and activator of transcription STAT5b gene is a new partner of retinoic acid receptor alpha in acute promyelocytic-like leukaemia. *Hum Mol Genet* **8**:1741–9.

12 Salomoni P, Pandolfi P.P. (2002) The role of PML in tumor suppression. *Cell* **108**:165–70.

13 Speck NA, Gilliland DG. (2002) Core-binding factors in haematopoiesis and leukaemia. *Nat Rev Cancer* **2**:502–13.

14 Jurlander J, Caligiuri MA, Ruutu T, et al. (1996) Persistence of the AML1/ETO fusion transcript in patients treated with allogeneic bone marrow transplantation for t(8;21) leukemia. *Blood* **88**:2183–91.

15 Nucifora G, Larson RA, Rowley JD. (1993) Persistence of the 8;21 translocation in patients with acute myeloid leukemia type M2 in long-term remission. *Blood* **82**:712–5.

16 Shih LY, Liang DC, Fu JF, et al. (2006) Characterization of fusion partner genes in 114 patients with de novo acute myeloid leukemia and MLL rearrangement. *Leukemia* **20**:218–23.

17 Schoch C, Schnittger S, Klaus M, et al. (2003) AML with 11q23/MLL abnormalities as defined by the WHO classification: incidence, partner chromosomes, FAB subtype, age distribution, and prognostic impact in an unselected series of 1897 cytogenetically analyzed AML cases. *Blood* **102**:2395–402.

18 Balgobind BV, Raimondi SC, Harbott J, et al. (2009) Novel prognostic subgroups in childhood 11q23/MLL-rearranged acute myeloid leukemia: results of an international retrospective study. *Blood* **114**:2489–96.

19 Dohner K, Tobis K, Ulrich R, et al. (2002) Prognostic significance of partial tandem duplications of the MLL gene in adult patients 16 to 60 years old with acute myeloid leukemia and normal cytogenetics: a study of the Acute Myeloid Leukemia Study Group Ulm. *J Clin Oncol* **20**:3254–61.

20 Lyman SD, Jacobsen SE. (1998) c-kit ligand and *FLT3* ligand: stem/progenitor cell factors with overlapping yet distinct activities. *Blood* **91**:1101–34.

21 Bos JL. (1989) Ras oncogenes in human cancer: a review. *Cancer Res* **49**:4682–9.

22 Stirewalt DL, Meshinchi S, Radich JP. (2003) Molecular targets in acute myelogenous leukemia. *Blood Rev* **17**:15–23.

23 Gelb MH. (1997) Protein prenylation, et cetera: signal transduction in two dimensions. *Science* **275**:1750–1.

24 Ihle JN. (1996) Signaling by the cytokine receptor superfamily in normal and transformed hematopoietic cells. *Adv Can Res* **68**:23–65.

25 Taniguchi T. (1995) Cytokine signaling through non-receptor protein tyrosine kinases. *Science* **268**:251–5.

26 Lacronique V, Boureux A, Valle VD, et al. (1997) A TEL-JAK2 fusion protein with constitutive kinase activity in human leukemia. *Science* **278**:1309–12.

27 Schuringa JJ, Wierenga AT, Kruijer W, Vellenga E. (2000) Constitutive Stat3, Tyr705, and Ser727 phos-

phorylation in acute myeloid leukemia cells caused by the autocrine secretion of interleukin-6. *Blood* **95**:3765–70.

28 Birkenkamp KU, Geugien M, Lemmink HH, Kruijer W, Vellenga E. (2001) Regulation of constitutive STAT5 phosphorylation in acute myeloid leukemia blasts. *Leukemia* **15**:1923–31.

29 Kiyoi H, Towatari M, Yokota S, et al. (1998) Internal tandem duplication of the *FLT3* gene is a novel modality of elongation mutation which causes constitutive activation of the product. *Leukemia* **12**:1333–7.

30 Nakao M, Yokota S, Iwai T, et al. (1996) Internal tandem duplication of the *FLT3* gene found in acute myeloid leukemia. *Leukemia* **10**:1911–8.

31 Breitenbuecher F, Markova B, Kasper S, et al. (2009) A novel molecular mechanism of primary resistance to *FLT3*-kinase inhibitors in AML. *Blood* **113**:4063–73.

32 Kayser S, Schlenk RF, Londono MC, et al. (2009) Insertion of *FLT3* internal tandem duplication in the tyrosine kinase domain-1 is associated with resistance to chemotherapy and inferior outcome. *Blood* **114**:2386–92.

33 Abu-Duhier FM, Goodeve AC, Wilson GA, et al. (2001) Identification of novel FLT-3 Asp835 mutations in adult acute myeloid leukaemia. *Br J Haematol* **113**:983–8.

34 Yamamoto Y, Kiyoi H, Nakano Y, et al. (2001) Activating mutation of D835 within the activation loop of *FLT3* in human hematologic malignancies. *Blood* **97**:2434–9.

35 Frohling S, Scholl C, Levine RL, et al. (2007) Identification of driver and passenger mutations of *FLT3* by high-throughput DNA sequence analysis and functional assessment of candidate alleles. *Cancer Cell* **12**:501–13.

36 Vempati S, Reindl C, Kaza SK, et al. (2007) Arginine 595 is duplicated in patients with acute leukemias carrying internal tandem duplications of *FLT3* and modulates its transforming potential. *Blood* **110**:686–94.

37 Kiyoi H, Naoe T, Yokota S, et al. (1997) Internal tandem duplication of *FLT3* associated with leukocytosis in acute promyelocytic leukemia. Leukemia Study Group of the Ministry of Health and Welfare (Kohseisho). *Leukemia* **11**:1447–52.

38 Xu F, Taki T, Yang HW, et al. (1999) Tandem duplication of the *FLT3* gene is found in acute lymphoblastic leukaemia as well as acute myeloid leukaemia but not in myelodysplastic syndrome or juvenile chronic mye-

logenous leukaemia in children. *Br J Haematol* **105**:155–62.

39 Stirewalt DL, Kopecky KJ, Meshinchi S, et al. (2001) *FLT3*, RAS, and TP53 mutations in elderly patients with acute myeloid leukemia. *Blood* **97**:3589–95.

40 Meshinchi S, Woods WG, Stirewalt DL, et al. (2001) Prevalence and prognostic significance of *FLT3* internal tandem duplication in pediatric acute myeloid leukemia. *Blood* **97**:89–94.

41 Schnittger S, Schoch C, Dugas M, et al. (2002) Analysis of *FLT3* length mutations in 1003 patients with acute myeloid leukemia: correlation to cytogenetics, FAB subtype, and prognosis in the AMLCG study and usefulness as a marker for the detection of minimal residual disease. *Blood* **100**:59–66.

42 Thiede C, Steudel C, Mohr B, et al. (2002) Analysis of *FLT3*-activating mutations in 979 patients with acute myelogenous leukemia: association with FAB subtypes and identification of subgroups with poor prognosis. *Blood* **99**:4326–35.

43 Abu-Duhier FM, Goodeve AC, Wilson GA, et al. (2000) *FLT3* internal tandem duplication mutations in adult acute myeloid leukaemia define a high-risk group. *Br J Haematol* **111**(1):190–5.

44 Kiyoi H, Naoe T, Nakano Y, et al. (1999) Prognostic implication of *FLT3* and N-RAS gene mutations in acute myeloid leukemia. *Blood* **93**:3074–80.

45 Kottaridis PD, Gale RE, Frew ME, et al. (2001) The presence of a *FLT3* internal tandem duplication in patients with acute myeloid leukemia (AML) adds important prognostic information to cytogenetic risk group and response to the first cycle of chemotherapy: analysis of 854 patients from the United Kingdom Medical Research Council AML 10 and 12 trials. *Blood* **98**:1752–9.

46 Iwai T, Yokota S, Nakao M, et al. (1999) Internal tandem duplication of the *FLT3* gene and clinical evaluation in childhood acute myeloid leukemia. The Children's Cancer and Leukemia Study Group, Japan. *Leukemia* **13**:38–43.

47 Kondo M, Horibe K, Takahashi Y, et al. (1999) Prognostic value of internal tandem duplication of the *FLT3* gene in childhood acute myelogenous leukemia. *Med Pediatr Oncol* **33**:525–9.

48 Whitman SP, Archer KJ, Feng L, et al. (2001) Absence of the wild-type allele predicts poor prognosis in adult de novo acute myeloid leukemia with normal cytogenetics and the internal tandem duplication of *FLT3*:

a cancer and leukemia group B study. *Cancer Res* **61**:7233–9.

49 Shih LY, Huang CF, Wu JH, et al. (2002) Internal tandem duplication of *FLT3* in relapsed acute myeloid leukemia: a comparative analysis of bone marrow samples from 108 adult patients at diagnosis and relapse. *Blood* **100**:2387–92.

50 Noguera NI, Breccia M, Divona M, et al. (2002) Alterations of the *FLT3* gene in acute promyelocytic leukemia: association with diagnostic characteristics and analysis of clinical outcome in patients treated with the Italian AIDA protocol. *Leukemia* **16**:2185–9.

51 Schnittger S, Schoch C, Dugas M, et al. (2002) Analysis of *FLT3* length mutations in 1003 patients with acute myeloid leukemia: correlation to cytogenetics, FAB subtype, and prognosis in the AMLCG study and usefulness as a marker for the detection of minimal residual disease. *Blood* **100**:59–66.

52 Stirewalt DL, Kopecky KJ, Meshinchi S, et al. (2006) Size of *FLT3* internal tandem duplication has prognostic significance in patients with acute myeloid leukemia. *Blood* **107**:3724–6.

53 Libura M, Asnafi V, Tu A, et al. (2003) *FLT3* and MLL intragenic abnormalities in AML reflect a common category of genotoxic stress. *Blood* **102**:2198–204.

54 Radich JP, Kopecky KJ, Willman CL, et al. (1990) N-ras mutations in adult de novo acute myelogenous leukemia: prevalence and clinical significance. *Blood* **76**:801–7.

55 Stirewalt DL, Kopecky KJ, Meshinchi S, et al. (2001) *FLT3*, RAS, and TP53 mutations in elderly patients with acute myeloid leukemia. *Blood* **97**:3589–95.

56 Padua RA, Guinn BA, Al-Sabah AI, et al. (1998) RAS, FMS and p53 mutations and poor clinical outcome in myelodysplasias: a 10-year follow-up. *Leukemia* **12**:887–92.

57 Flotho C, Valcamonica S, Mach-Pascual S, et al. (1999) RAS mutations and clonality analysis in children with juvenile myelomonocytic leukemia (JMML). *Leukemia* **13**:32–7.

58 Hirsch-Ginsberg C, LeMaistre AC, Kantarjian H, et al. (1990) RAS mutations are rare events in Philadelphia chromosome-negative/bcr gene rearrangement-negative chronic myelogenous leukemia, but are prevalent in chronic myelomonocytic leukemia. *Blood* **76**:1214–9.

59 Byrne JL, Marshall CJ. (1998) The molecular pathophysiology of myeloid leukaemias: Ras revisited. *Br J Haematol* **100**:256–64.

60 Bacher U, Haferlach T, Schoch C, Kern W, Schnittger S. (2006) Implications of NRAS mutations in AML: a study of 2502 patients. *Blood* **107**:3847–53.

61 Ridge SA, Worwood M, Oscier D, Jacobs A, Padua RA. (1990) FMS mutations in myelodysplastic, leukemic, and normal subjects. *Proc Natl Acad Sci U S A* **87**:1377–80.

62 Gari M, Goodeve A, Wilson G, et al. (1999) c-kit proto-oncogene exon 8 in-frame deletion plus insertion mutations in acute myeloid leukaemia. *Br J Haematol* **105**:894–900.

63 Sperr WR, Walchshofer S, Horny HP, et al. (1998) Systemic mastocytosis associated with acute myeloid leukaemia: report of two cases and detection of the c-kit mutation Asp-816 to Val. *Br J Haematol* **103**:740–9.

64 Schnittger S, Kohl TM, Haferlach T, et al. (2006) KIT-D816 mutations in AML1-ETO-positive AML are associated with impaired event-free and overall survival. *Blood* **107**:1791–9.

65 Dohner K, Schlenk RF, Habdank M, et al. (2005) Mutant nucleophosmin (NPM1) predicts favorable prognosis in younger adults with acute myeloid leukemia and normal cytogenetics: interaction with other gene mutations. *Blood* **106**:3740–6.

66 Gale RE, Green C, Allen C, et al. (2008) The impact of *FLT3* internal tandem duplication mutant level, number, size, and interaction with NPM1 mutations in a large cohort of young adult patients with acute myeloid leukemia. *Blood* **111**:2776–84.

67 Schlenk RF, Dohner K, Krauter J, et al. (2008) Mutations and treatment outcome in cytogenetically normal acute myeloid leukemia. *New Engl J Med* **358**:1909–18.

68 Schnittger S, Schoch C, Kern W, et al. (2005) Nucleophosmin gene mutations are predictors of favorable prognosis in acute myelogenous leukemia with a normal karyotype. *Blood* **106**:3733–9.

69 Thiede C, Koch S, Creutzig E, et al. (2006) Prevalence and prognostic impact of NPM1 mutations in 1485 adult patients with acute myeloid leukemia (AML). *Blood* **107**:4011–20.

70 Abdel-Wahab O, Mullally A, Hedvat C, et al. (2009) Genetic characterization of TET1, TET2, and TET3 alterations in myeloid malignancies. *Blood* **114**:144–7.

71 Tefferi A, Lim KH, Abdel-Wahab O, et al. (2009) Detection of mutant TET2 in myeloid malignancies other than myeloproliferative neoplasms: CMML, MDS, MDS/MPN and AML. *Leukemia* **23**:1343–5.

72 Delhommeau F, Dupont S, Della Valle V, et al. (2009) Mutation in TET2 in myeloid cancers. *New Engl J Med* **360**:2289–301.

73 Kosmider O, Gelsi-Boyer V, Cheok M, et al. (2009) TET2 mutation is an independent favorable prognostic factor in myelodysplastic syndromes (MDSs). *Blood* **114**:3285–91.

74 Frohling S, Schlenk RF, Stolze I, et al. (2004) CEBPA mutations in younger adults with acute myeloid leukemia and normal cytogenetics: prognostic relevance and analysis of cooperating mutations. *J Clin Oncol* **22**:624–33.

75 Preudhomme C, Sagot C, Boissel N, et al. (2002) Favorable prognostic significance of CEBPA mutations in patients with de novo acute myeloid leukemia: a study from the Acute Leukemia French Association (ALFA). *Blood* **100**:2717–23.

76 Yang L, Han Y, Suarez Saiz F, Minden MD. (2007) A tumor suppressor and oncogene: the WT1 story. *Leukemia* **21**:868–76.

77 Bergmann L, Miething C, Maurer U, et al. (1997) High levels of Wilms' tumor gene (wt1) mRNA in acute myeloid leukemias are associated with a worse long-term outcome. *Blood* **90**:1217–25.

78 King-Underwood L, Pritchard-Jones K. (1998) Wilms' tumor (WT1) gene mutations occur mainly in acute myeloid leukemia and may confer drug resistance. *Blood* **91**:2961–8.

79 Summers K, Stevens J, Kakkas I, et al. (2007) Wilms' tumour 1 mutations are associated with *FLT3*-ITD and failure of standard induction chemotherapy in patients with normal karyotype AML. *Leukemia* **21**(3): 550–1; author reply 2.

80 Weisser M, Kern W, Rauhut S, et al. (2005) Prognostic impact of RT-PCR-based quantification of WT1 gene expression during MRD monitoring of acute myeloid leukemia. *Leukemia* **19**:1416–23.

81 Tse W, Zhu W, Chen HS, Cohen A. (1995) A novel gene, AF1q, fused to MLL in t(1;11) (q21;q23), is specifically expressed in leukemic and immature hematopoietic cells. *Blood* **85**:650–6.

82 Strunk CJ, Platzbecker U, Thiede C, et al. (2009) Elevated AF1q expression is a poor prognostic marker for adult acute myeloid leukemia patients with normal cytogenetics. *Am J Haematol* **84**:308–9.

83 Tse W, Joachim Deeg H, Stirewalt D, et al. (2005) Increased AF1q gene expression in high-risk myelodysplastic syndrome. *Br J Haematol* **128**:218–20.

84 Tse W, Meshinchi S, Alonzo TA, et al. (2004) Elevated expression of the AF1q gene, an MLL fusion partner, is an independent adverse prognostic factor in pediatric acute myeloid leukemia. *Blood* **104**:3058–63.

85 Baldus CD, Tanner SM, Ruppert AS, et al. (2003) BAALC expression predicts clinical outcome of de novo acute myeloid leukemia patients with normal cytogenetics: a Cancer and Leukemia Group B study. *Blood* **102**:1613–8.

86 Langer C, Radmacher MD, Ruppert AS, et al. (2008) High BAALC expression associates with other molecular prognostic markers, poor outcome, and a distinct gene-expression signature in cytogenetically normal patients younger than 60 years with acute myeloid leukemia: a Cancer and Leukemia Group B (CALGB) study. *Blood* **111**:5371–9.

87 Marcucci G, Baldus CD, Ruppert AS, et al. (2005) Overexpression of the ETS-related gene, ERG, predicts a worse outcome in acute myeloid leukemia with normal karyotype: a Cancer and Leukemia Group B study. *J Clin Oncol* **23**:9234–42.

88 Gondek LP, Tiu R, O'Keefe CL, et al. (2008) Chromosomal lesions and uniparental disomy detected by SNP arrays in MDS, MDS/MPD, and MDS-derived AML. *Blood* **111**:1534–42.

89 Gupta M, Raghavan M, Gale RE, et al. (2008) Novel regions of acquired uniparental disomy discovered in acute myeloid leukemia. *Genes, Chromosomes Cancer* **47**:729–39.

90 Suela J, Alvarez S, Cifuentes F, et al. (2007) DNA profiling analysis of 100 consecutive de novo acute myeloid leukemia cases reveals patterns of genomic instability that affect all cytogenetic risk groups. *Leukemia* **21**:1224–31.

91 Ley TJ, Mardis ER, Ding L, et al. (2008) DNA sequencing of a cytogenetically normal acute myeloid leukaemia genome. *Nature* **456**:66–72.

92 Mardis ER, Ding L, Dooling DJ, et al. (2009) Recurring mutations found by sequencing an acute myeloid leukemia genome. *New Engl J Med* **361**:1058–66.

93 Armstrong SA, Staunton JE, Silverman LB, et al. (2002) MLL translocations specify a distinct gene expression profile that distinguishes a unique leukemia. *Nat Genet* **30**:41–7.

94 Haferlach T, Kohlmann A, Schnittger S, et al. (2005) AML M3 and AML M3 variant each have a distinct gene expression signature but also share patterns different from other genetically defined AML subtypes. *Genes, Chromosomes Cancer* **43**:113–27.

95 Schoch C, Kohlmann A, Schnittger S, et al. (2002) Acute myeloid leukemias with reciprocal rearrangements can be distinguished by specific gene expression profiles. *Proc Natl Acad Sci U S A* **99**:10008–13.

96 Haferlach T, Kohlmann A, Schnittger S, et al. (2005) Global approach to the diagnosis of leukemia using gene expression profiling. *Blood* **106**:1189–98.

97 Virtaneva K, Wright FA, Tanner SM, et al. (2001) Expression profiling reveals fundamental biological differences in acute myeloid leukemia with isolated trisomy 8 and normal cytogenetics. *Proc Natl Acad Sci U S A* **98**:1124–9.

98 Bullinger L, Dohner K, Bair E, et al. (2004) Use of gene-expression profiling to identify prognostic subclasses in adult acute myeloid leukemia. *New Engl J Med* **350**:1605–16.

99 Valk PJ, Verhaak RG, Beijen MA, et al. (2004) Prognostically useful gene-expression profiles in acute myeloid leukemia. *New Engl J Med* **350**:1617–28.

100 Lacayo NJ, Meshinchi S, Kinnunen P, et al. (2004) Gene expression profiles at diagnosis in de novo childhood AML patients identify *FLT3* mutations with good clinical outcomes. *Blood* **104**:2646–54.

101 Neben K, Schnittger S, Brors B, et al. (2005) Distinct gene expression patterns associated with *FLT3*- and NRAS-activating mutations in acute myeloid leukemia with normal karyotype. *Oncogene* **24**:1580–8.

102 Alcalay M, Tiacci E, Bergomas R, et al. (2005) Acute myeloid leukemia bearing cytoplasmic nucleophosmin (NPMc+ AML) shows a distinct gene expression profile characterized by up-regulation of genes involved in stem-cell maintenance. *Blood* **106**:899–902.

103 Verhaak RG, Goudswaard CS, van Putten W, et al. (2005) Mutations in nucleophosmin (NPM1) in acute myeloid leukemia (AML): association with other gene abnormalities and previously established gene expression signatures and their favorable prognostic significance. *Blood* **106**:3747–54.

104 Wilson CS, Davidson GS, Martin SB, et al. (2006) Gene expression profiling of adult acute myeloid leukemia identifies novel biologic clusters for risk classification and outcome prediction. *Blood* **108**:685–96.

105 Metzeler KH, Hummel M, Bloomfield CD, et al. (2008) An 86-probe-set gene-expression signature predicts survival in cytogenetically normal acute myeloid leukemia. *Blood* **112**:4193–201.

106 Radmacher MD, Marcucci G, Ruppert AS, et al. (2006) Independent confirmation of a prognostic gene-

expression signature in adult acute myeloid leukemia with a normal karyotype: a Cancer and Leukemia Group B study. *Blood* **108**:1677–83.

107 Stirewalt DL, Meshinchi S, Kopecky KJ, et al. (2008) Identification of genes with abnormal expression changes in acute myeloid leukemia. *Genes, Chromosomes and Cancer* **47**:8–20.

108 Steinbach D, Schramm A, Eggert A, et al. (2006) Identification of a set of seven genes for the monitoring of minimal residual disease in pediatric acute myeloid leukemia. *Clin Cancer Res* **12**:2434–41.

109 Bartel DP. (2004) MicroRNAs: genomics, biogenesis, mechanism, and function. *Cell* **116**:281–97.

110 Calin GA, Liu CG, Ferracin M, et al. (2007) Ultraconserved regions encoding ncRNAs are altered in human leukemias and carcinomas. *Cancer Cell* **12**:215–29.

111 Mi S, Lu J, Sun M, et al. (2007) MicroRNA expression signatures accurately discriminate acute lymphoblastic leukemia from acute myeloid leukemia. *Proc Natl Acad Sci U S A* **104**:19971–6.

112 Garzon R, Volinia S, Liu CG, et al. (2008) MicroRNA signatures associated with cytogenetics and prognosis in acute myeloid leukemia. *Blood* **111**:3183–9.

113 Jongen-Lavrencic M, Sun SM, Dijkstra MK, Valk PJ, Lowenberg B. (2008) MicroRNA expression profiling in relation to the genetic heterogeneity of acute myeloid leukemia. *Blood* **111**:5078–85.

114 Dixon-McIver A, East P, Mein CA, et al. (2008) Distinctive patterns of microRNA expression associated with karyotype in acute myeloid leukaemia. *PloS ONE* **3**:e2141.

115 Li Z, Lu J, Sun M, et al. (2008) Distinct microRNA expression profiles in acute myeloid leukemia with common translocations. *Proc Natl Acad Sci U S A* **105**:15535–40.

116 Garzon R, Garofalo M, Martelli MP, et al. (2008) Distinctive microRNA signature of acute myeloid leukemia bearing cytoplasmic mutated nucleophosmin. *Proc Natl Acad Sci U S A* **105**:3945–50.

117 Marcucci G, Radmacher MD, Maharry K, et al. (2008) MicroRNA expression in cytogenetically normal acute myeloid leukemia. *New Engl J Med* **358**:1919–28.

118 Bird A. (2002) DNA methylation patterns and epigenetic memory. *Genes Dev* **16**:6–21.

119 Jenuwein T, Allis CD. (2001) Translating the histone code. *Science* **293**:1074–80.

120 Jones PA, Baylin SB. (2002) The fundamental role of epigenetic events in cancer. *Nat Rev Genet* **3**:415–28.

121 Jiang Y, Dunbar A, Gondek LP, et al. (2009) Aberrant DNA methylation is a dominant mechanism in MDS progression to AML. *Blood* **113**:1315–25.

122 Figueroa ME, Skrabanek L, Li Y, et al. (2009) MDS and secondary AML display unique patterns and abundance of aberrant DNA methylation. *Blood* **114**:3448–58.

123 Haferlach T, Bacher U, Haferlach C, Kern W, Schnittger S. (2007) Insight into the molecular pathogenesis of myeloid malignancies. *Cur Opin Hematol* **14**:90–7.

124 Marcucci G, Mrozek K, Bloomfield CD. (2005) Molecular heterogeneity and prognostic biomarkers in adults with acute myeloid leukemia and normal cytogenetics. *Cur Opin Hematol* **12**:68–75.

125 Mrozek K, Marcucci G, Paschka P, Whitman SP, Bloomfield CD. (2007) Clinical relevance of mutations and gene-expression changes in adult acute myeloid leukemia with normal cytogenetics: are we ready for a prognostically prioritized molecular classification? *Blood* **109**:431–48.

126 Meshinchi S, Stirewalt DL, Alonzo TA, et al. (2003) Activating mutations of RTK/ras signal transduction pathway in pediatric acute myeloid leukemia. *Blood* **102**:1474–9.

CHAPTER 7

Acute Myeloid Leukemia

Martin S. Tallman, Ritesh Parajuli and Jessica K. Altman
Northwestern University Feinberg School of Medicine and Robert H. Lurie Comprehensive Cancer Center, Chicago, IL, USA

Introduction

Overview

Acute myeloid leukemia (AML) is a heterogenous group of disorders that arise from the neoplastic transformation of a hematopoietic stem cell in which the malignant cells appear to either not differentiate, differentiate minimally, or differentiate abnormally. These abnormal cells proliferate and primarily accumulate in the bone marrow and peripheral blood, but may also invade visceral tissues such as the liver, lung, central nervous system (CNS), and skin. The accumulation of immature cells inhibits normal hematopoiesis by unclear mechanisms resulting in neutropenia, anemia, and thrombocytopenia, with the corresponding clinical consequences of infection, fatigue, and bleeding. The disease is usually rapidly fatal if untreated. Intensive investigations during the last two decades have provided insights into the pathogenesis of the disease, and have revealed marked heterogeneity with respect to cytogenetics and molecular genetics of the malignant cells in AML [1]. Such insights have led to new classification systems that categorize patients not only by morphologic features as in the French-American-British (FAB) classification [2–4], but also take into account contemporary information about cytogenetic and molecular genetics and whether the disease arises from an antecedent hematologic disorder or evolves as a result of prior chemotherapy exposure [5].

Treatment of AML includes two main phases, remission induction and post-remission therapy [1]. The latter usually includes multiple cycles of intensive chemotherapy or hematopoietic stem cell transplantation (HSCT). Although allogeneic HSCT appears to be associated with lower relapse rates, transplant-related mortality (TRM) has historically limited the impact of this strategy and studies have yielded conflicting results when the outcome of transplantation is compared to that of intensive post-remission chemotherapy [6].

Despite these strategies, the majority of younger adults and almost all older adults with AML die of their disease. Among patients ≤age 55, large cooperative group studies uniformly show that only approximately 20–30% survive disease-free at five years and, for patients >55, only approximately 10–15% of patients are disease-free at five years [1] (Figure 7.1). Recently, advances in immunophenotyping, karyotype analysis, and molecular biology have led to important developments in tailored and targeted therapy such as all-trans retinoic acid (ATRA) and arsenic trioxide (ATO) for patients with acute promyelocytic leukemia (APL). It is likely that with further insights into the mechanisms of cell cycle control, apoptosis, differentiation, and cellular antigen expression, new targeted therapeutic strategies will be developed and perhaps even the leukemia stem cell will be able to be eradicated [7].

Etiology
Therapy-related AMLs and those evolving from an antecedent hematologic disorder
The etiology of AML is not completely understood in the majority of cases. However, AML evolving from

Advances in Malignant Hematology, First Edition. Edited by Hussain I. Saba and Ghulam J. Mufti. © 2011 Blackwell Publishing Ltd.
Published 2011 by Blackwell Publishing Ltd.

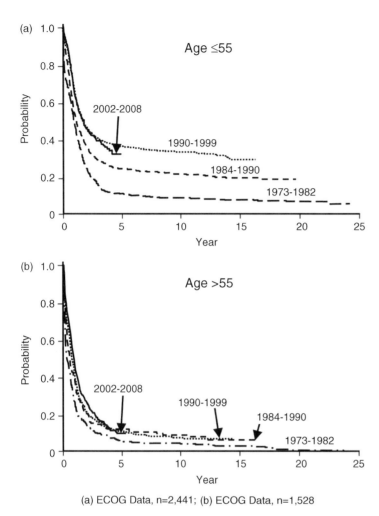

(a) ECOG Data, n=2,441; (b) ECOG Data, n=1,528

Figure 7.1 Overall survival of patients with untreated AML entered on Eastern Cooperative Oncology Group (ECOG) trials between 1973–2008. (A) Patients ≤55 years and (B) Patients >55 years old. This research was originally published in Blood Online. (Reproduced from Tallman et al. [1], with permission from the American Society of Hematology.)

either an antecedent hematologic disorder such as a myelodysplastic syndrome (MDS) or a myeloprolif-erative neoplasm (MPN), or developing after prior exposure to certain chemotherapeutic agents, are increasingly well recognized. Following exposure to cumulating doses of alkylating agents, patients may develop AML with leukemia cells that have chro-mosomal changes including deletions of all or part of chromosomes 5 and/or 7 [8]. Such leukemias tend to have a relatively long latency period and a period of myelodysplasia.

A second, well-recognized, type of therapy-related AML arises after exposure to epipodophylo-toxins or other topoisomerase-II inhibitors. In these cases, the leukemia calls have often translocations involving chromosome 11q23 [9]. These leukemias often have a shorter latency period, do not have a period of myelodysplasia and appear to be derived from a monocytic lineage [8]. The estimated cumu-lative probability of developing therapy-related MDS or AML, in one study, was approximately 8.6% (±2.1%) at six years among 612 patients undergoing high-dose chemotherapy and autolo-gous HSCT for Hodgkin lymphoma and non-Hodgkin lymphoma [10]. The most important risk factor appears to be large cumulative doses of alkylating agents. However, patient age (particularly over age 40 years) and previous radiotherapy, particularly total body irradiation as part of the conditioning regimen, are additional risk factors. Patients

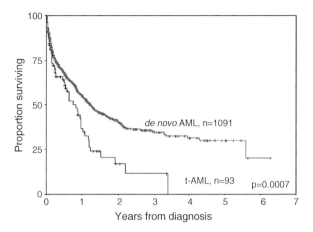

Figure 7.2 Overall survival of 1091 patients with *de novo* AML compared to 93 patients with therapy-related AML. (Reproduced from Schoch et al. [11], with permission from Nature Publishing Group.)

with therapy-related AML have a particularly poor prognosis [11] (Figure 7.2).

Genetic factors
Genetic factors can be implicated in some patients with AML. An increased incidence of AML is present in patients with congenital disorders associated with chromosomal changes including Down syndrome and Klinefelter's syndrome. Other diseases associated with chromosomal instability such as Fanconi's anemia, Bloom's syndrome and ataxia telangiectasia are associated with the development of AML. However, the majority of patients with AML have acquired clonal chromosomal abnormalities, particularly patients with therapy-related AML or whose disease has evolved from a prior MDS [12, 13].

Radiation exposure
Studies from survivors of the atomic bombs in Hiroshima and Nagasaki have confirmed the risk of AML after exposure to radiation. Furthermore, an increased risk is present in patients treated in the past with radiation for ankylosing spondylitis and menorrhagia, radiation workers, and radiologists prior to the era of proper protection.

Viruses and other potential risk factors
The role of viruses in the development of human AML has been implicated, but unclear. An additional important risk factor recently recognized is tobacco exposure, which has been associated with an increased risk of AML in older men [14].

Epidemiology
Acute myeloid leukemia accounts for approximately 15–20% of acute leukemias in children and approximately 80% of the acute leukemias in adults. The incidence is 2.3 per 100 000 population, and increases with age such that there are 12.6 cases per 100 000 over age 65, with a median age of 72 years [15]. Interestingly, APL is one subtype of AML that appears to be associated with a relatively constant incidence regardless of age [16]. In addition, APL may occur more frequently in individuals of Hispanic or Latino origin, suggesting a possible genetic link [17]. Recent data from the Surveillance, Epidemiology, and End Results (SEER) Program of the National Cancer Institute (NCI), however, suggest this may not be the case [18]. In 2007, an estimated 13 400 new cases of AML will occur in the US with a slight predominance in women (5900 estimated new cases in women and 4700 in men). An estimated 9000 patients with AML died of their disease in the US in 2007. Data suggests that African American men may have a worse prognosis with respect to complete remission (CR) rates and overall survival (OS) compared to White and African American women [19].

Cytogenetics and molecular genetics
Cytogenetics
Clonal chromosomal abnormalities identified with high-resolution banding techniques represent the most well-studied independent prognostic factor at diagnosis [20–22]. A number of specific cytogenetic

abnormalities correlate with particular morphologic and clinical features of AML. Together, these define characteristic clinical syndromes of AML, including t (15;17) in APL (M3 in the FAB classification system), inv(16) or t(16;16) in acute myelomonocytic leukemia (M4Eo) with eosinophilia, and t(8;21) in acute myelocytic leukemia (FAB M2) which may be associated with chloromas [23, 24].

Cytogenetic risk groups

The correlation of specific cytogenetic abnormalities with outcome has defined three risk groups which have been validated by many large cooperative group studies (Table 7.1). Patients with AML who have balanced reciprocal translocations between chromosomes 8 and 21, 15 and 17, 16 and 16, or inversion chromosome 16, generally have relatively favorable outcomes in both CR rates and OS when treated with conventional induction chemotherapy and intensive cytarabine consolidation with OS of approximately 55–70% at five years [20, 25]. Patients whose leukemic cells have abnormalities of chromosome 5 or 7 such as 5q-, 7q- or monosomy 5 or 7, complex karyotypes and most 11q23 abnormalities have very unfavorable prognoses with five-year OS of 5–20%. The Cancer and Leukemia Group B (CALGB) suggested that patients with t(9;11)(p22;q23) have a better outcome than patients with other translocations involving band 11q23 [26]. Patients with leukemic cells having a normal karyotype, trisomy 8 or other numeric changes including trisomy 21 or trisomy 22 have an intermediate prognosis with an OS of five years of approximately 30–60%. The most common abnormalities in therapy-related MDS or

Table 7.1 ECOG/SWOG cytogenetic risk groups

Favorable	inv(16); t(15;17) with any abn; t(8;21) lacking del(9q) or complex karyotype
Intermediate	Normal or +8 or +21 or others
Unfavorable	-5/del(5q), -7/del(7q), inv(3q), abn of 11q, 20q, 21q, 17p, del(9q), t(6;9), t(9;22), complex karyotypes with ≥3 abn

Reproduced from Slovak et al. [21], with permission from the American Society of Hematology.

therapy-related AML involve loss of part or all of chromosomes 5 and/or chromosome 7.

Cytogenetic abnormalities associated with characteristic biologic and clinical findings

Several other clonal karyotype abnormalities are associated with characteristic biologic and clinical findings. A balanced reciprocal translocation between chromosomes 6 and 9 has been associated with basophilia and has a particularly poor prognosis [27, 28]. Abnormalities of chromosome 3, including an inversion chromosome 3, or t(3;3), have been associated with thrombocytosis and a very poor prognosis [29, 30].

AML with t(8;21)

One of the best characterized subtypes of AML is FAB M2 with t(8;21). Approximately 20% of adults and 40% of pediatric patients with FAB M2 have leukemic cells with this karyotype. The disease is associated with a younger median age at onset, extramedullary disease, and has a relatively favorable prognosis in the absence of extramedullary disease [25, 31]. Patients with t(8;21) whose cells express CD56 may have a less favorable prognosis [32]. Recent insights in the understanding of the molecular features of leukemogenesis in patients with t(8;21) are discussed below.

Molecular genetics

Many specific chromosomal abnormalities in patients with AML involve rearrangements and often fusion of specific genes that have been implicated in the pathogenesis of AML (Table 7.2) [33]. Studies of the altered function of these genes has provided insights into the pathogenesis of AML as well as the normal function in non-malignant cells [34].

Molecular features of AML with t(8;21)

The balanced reciprocal translocation between chromosomes 8 and 21 is the most common balanced translocation in *de novo* AML, and is associated with a fusion of RUNX1 (formerly known as AML1) and RUNX1T1 (formerly known as ETO for eight;twenty-one) genes (Table 7.3). The AML1 gene (also called CBFA$_2$) codes for the DNA-binding component of

Table 7.2 Recurring structural rearrangements in acute myeloid leukemia

Disease	Chromosome abnormality	Involved genes
AML-M2	t(8;21)(q22;q22)	ETO-AML1
APL-M3, M3v	t(15;17)(q22;q12)	PML-RARA
Atypical APL	t(11;17)(q23;q12)	PLZF-RARA
AMMoL-M4Eo	inv(16;16)(p13q22) or t(16;16)(p13q22	MYH11-CBFB
AMMoL-M4/ AmoL-M5	t(6;11)(q27;q23) t(9;11)(p22;q23)	AF6-MLL[a] AF9-MLL
AMegL-M7	t(1;22)(p13;q13)	
AML	t(3;3)(q21q26)	RPN-EVI1
	or inv(3)(q21q26)	
	t(3;5)(q21;q31)	
	t(3;5)(q25;q34)	MLF1-NPM1
	t(6;9)(p23;q34)	DEK-CAN (NUP214)
	t(7;11)(p15;p15)	HOXA9-NUP98
	t(8;16)(p11;p13)	MOZ-CBP
	t(9;12)(q34;p13)	TEL-ABL
	t(12;22)(p13;q13)	TEL-NM1
	t(16;21)(p11;q22)	TLS(FUS)-ERG
	-5 or del(5q)	
	-7 or del(7q)	
	del(20p)	
	del(12p)	TEL,?p27[KIP1]
Therapy-related AML	-7 or del(7q) and/or -5 or del(5q)	IRF1:
	t(11q23)	MLL
	t(3;21)(q26;q22)	EAP/MDS1/ EVI1-AML1

Reproduced from Rowley JD (1999) *Semin Hematol* 36:59–76, with permission from Elsevier.

Table 7.3 Core binding factor (CBF) leukemias

Translocation	Genes involved
t(8;21)	AML1-ETO
t(3;21)	AML1-EAP, MDS1, EVI1
t(12;21)	TEL (ETV6)
inv(16)/t(16;16)	CBFβ-MYH11

core binding factor β, one subunit of a CBF complex which binds to DNA sequences and activates transcription of a number of genes important in hematopoiesis [35]. The normal function of the ETO gene remains elusive, but the gene is expressed as a nuclear phosphoprotein in brain tissue and in CD34+ hematopoietic progenitor cells. The structure of ETO, as a nuclear zinc-finger-containing protein, implicates its role in a regulator of transcription. ETO can bind nuclear co-repressor N-COR and Sin33A which bind histone deacetylase. These observations suggest that, in healthy cells, ETO functions as an adaptor protein within the nuclear co-repressor complex to stabilize the interaction of these co-repressor proteins. The chimeric fusion protein AML-1/ETO, therefore, appears to repress transcription of genes normally activated by AML-1/CBFβ.

As a result of this translocation, AML fuses to ETO, not normally expressed in hematopoietic cells. Patients with such CBF leukemias with either alterations of the AML-1 or CBF genes such as patients with AML M4EO involving either inv(16) (p13;q22) or t(16;16) (p13;q22) and a fusion between MYH11 and CBFβ genes, appear to have a more favorable prognosis compared to that of patients with either normal or other karyotype abnormalities when given repetitive cycles of intensive consolidation chemotherapy. The activating mutation c-KIT has been reported in the leukemic cells of 13–45% of patients with core binding factor AML [36]. Such patients have a poorer prognosis compared to patients without such a mutation [37] (Figure 7.3). Whether tyrosine kinase inhibitors which can inhibit c-KIT or HSCT will be effective in such patients remains to be determined [38].

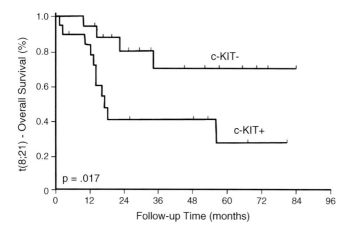

Figure 7.3 Kaplan-Meier plot showing overall survival of patients t(8;21), c-KIT⁻ versus c-KIT⁺ patients. (Reproduced from Cairoli et al. [37], with permission from the American Society of Hematology.)

Molecular features of AML with t(15;17)

Perhaps the best example of how the juxtaposition of two otherwise disparate genes is critical in the pathogenesis of AML is represented by the translocation between chromosomes 15 and 17 in APL. There is a fusion between the retinoic acid receptor α (RARα) gene normally located on chromosome 17 and the PML (promyelocyte) gene normally located in chromosome 15 [39]. The RARα gene is a retinoic acid-dependent transcription factor important in normal myeloid differentiation. Changes in the function of the PML and RARα genes that occur as a result of their fusion result in the recruitment of nuclear corepressors which bind histone deacetylase leading to transcriptional repression. Therefore, the chimeric fusion protein arrests normal differentiation of the promyelocytic stage of myeloid maturation. The administration of pharmacologic doses of the vitamin A derivative, ATRA, results in terminal differentiation of the leukemic promyelocytes into mature granulocytes and hematologic remission.

Molecular features of AML and 11q23

Translocations involving the breakpoint at 11q23 occur frequently in infants with leukemia and in those developing following exposure to chemotherapeutic agents that interact with topoisomerase II (discussed above). Approximately 25 different chromosome bands on 14 different chromosomes have been described in reciprocal translocations or insertions involving 11q23. Approximately 95% of translocations involving 11q23 are associated with the MLL gene. Patients with such translocations may have either AML or ALL [typically t(4;11)]. Several partner genes have been demonstrated in translocation involving 11q23 and the AMLs that result can have different clinical manifestations and outcome [40, 41]. Furthermore, partial tandem duplication of the mixed lineage leukemia (MLL) gene has been discovered in patients with normal karyotypes (approximately 11%).

Molecular genetics in patients with a normal karyotype

Several genes that are expressed in general in the leukemia cells of patients with a normal karyotype have been recently identified. This subtype represents approximately 40% of adult patients with AML [42]. The most studied include fms-like tyrosine kinse-3 (FLT3) [43], nucleophosmin-1 [44, 45], and Wilms tumor-1 (WT1) [46]. The FLT3 internal tandem duplication (ITD) is one of the most frequent molecular mutations in AML. Mutations in the tyrosine kinase domain are also seen, but are much less common and appear to be most common in patients with FAB M4, M5b, and APL [47]. The presence of the FLT3-ITD mutation in a patient with a normal karyotype confers a poor prognosis [48]. However, recent data suggest that FLT3 ITD results in downregulation of equilibrative nucleoside transporter 1 (ENT1) which is responsible for the uptake of ara-C possibly by reduction of its promoter activity by induction of hypoxia inducible factor 1 alpha subunit (HIF-1) [49]. FLT3 inhibitors such as PKC-

Table 7.4 Proposed WHO classification of myeloid neoplasms

Acute Myeloid Leukemias

---

1. AMLs with recurrent cytogenetic translocations

    AML with t(8;21)(q22;q22), AML1 (CBF-alpha)/ETO

    Acute promyelocytic leukemias (AML with t(15;17)(q22; q11) and variants, PML/RAR-alpha)

    AML with abnormal bone marrow eosinophils (inv916) (p13q22) or t(16;16)(p13;q11), CBFβ/MYH11X

    AML with 11q23 (MLL) abnormalities

2. AML with multilineage dysplasia

    With prior myelodysplastic syndrome

    Without prior myelodysplastic syndrome

3. AML and myelodysplastic syndromes, therapy-related

    Alkylating agent-related

    Epipodophylotoxin-related (some may be lymphoid)

    Other types

4. AML not otherwise categorized

    AML minimally differentiated

    AML with maturation

    AML without maturation

    Acute monocytic leukemia

    Acute erythroid leukemia

    Acute panmyelosis with myelofibrosis

5. Acute biphenotypic leukemias

Reproduced from Harris et al. [5], with permission from the American Society of Clinical Oncology.

412 have been shown to reduce the blast percentage in the peripheral blood and bone marrow, but few, if any patients achieve CR with monotherapy [50]. Newer and potentially more potent FLT3 inhibitors such as Sorafenib and AC220 may prove more effective [51–53].

NPM1 gene mutations are frequently associated with FLT3 mutations, but when occurring alone without the FLT3 ITD in patients with a normal karyotype, are associated with a higher CR rate, longer event-free survival and a trend towards OS [44, 45, 54] (Figure 7.4). Such new information that identifies patients with a normal karyotype with a more or less favorable prognosis has prompted a reclassification of the standard cytogenetic risk categories which may influence treatment (Table 7.5).

Mutations in the transcription factor CCAAT/ enhancer-binding protein-alpha (CEBP-alpha) have also been associated with a favorable prognosis in patients with a normal karyotype, but only in those patients with a double mutation [55, 56]. Other gene mutations in patients with normal karyotype AML that confer a poor outcome include ETS-related gene (ERG) [57] and ectopic integration virus-1 (EVI1) [58]. Microarray miRNA expression profiles can identify a specific signature in a group of patients with normal karyotype whose cells express FLT3 ITD, but not NPM1 [59].

Classification systems for AML
French-American-British classification

The French-American-British (FAB) classification was initially described in 1976 and classified AMLs based on morphologic and cytochemical features of the leukemic cell [60]. Cytogenetics and immunophenotyping have emerged as important advances in diagnosis and classification and have supplanted the FAB classification [61]. However, the FAB classification remains useful as a foundation to understand the newer World Health Organization (WHO) classification [5].

World Health Organization (WHO) classification

Recent advances in our understanding of the pathogenesis of AML, as well as insights into karyotype abnormalities and molecular genetics, have led to a new classification generated by the World Health Organization (WHO) that correlates morphology, cytochemistry, immunophenotype, molecular genetics, and clinical features [5, 62] (Table 7.4). Acute myeloid leukemias are classified into the following categories: (1) those with one of the well-characterized cytogenetic or molecular abnormalities; (2) those with multilineage dysplasia; (3) those that are therapy-related (either alkylating agent-induced or epipodophylotoxin-involved);

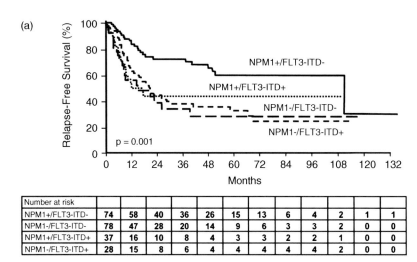

Number at risk												
NPM1+/FLT3-ITD-	74	58	40	36	26	15	13	6	4	2	1	1
NPM1-/FLT3-ITD-	78	47	28	20	14	9	6	3	3	2	0	0
NPM1+/FLT3-ITD+	37	16	10	8	4	3	3	2	2	1	0	0
NPM1-/FLT3-ITD+	28	15	8	6	4	4	4	4	4	2	0	0

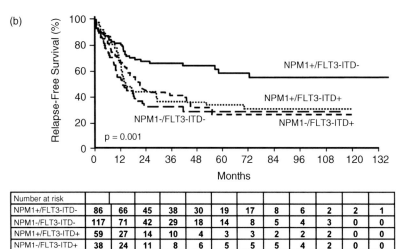

Number at risk												
NPM1+/FLT3-ITD-	86	66	45	38	30	19	17	8	6	2	2	1
NPM1-/FLT3-ITD-	117	71	42	29	18	14	8	5	4	3	0	0
NPM1+/FLT3-ITD+	59	27	14	10	4	3	3	2	2	2	0	0
NPM1-/FLT3-ITD+	38	24	11	8	6	5	5	5	4	2	0	0

Figure 7.4 Treatment results according to the combined NPM1 and FLT3-ITD mutation status. (Reproduced from Dohner et al. [44], with permission from the American Society of Hematology.)

(4) those not otherwise categorized, which includes the FAB morphologic subtypes, acute basophilic leukemia, acute panmyelosis and fibrosis, and acute biphenotypic leukemia. The European Leukemia Net has proposed a classification system for standardized reporting which correlates cytogenetic and molecular genetic data in AML with outcome. (Figure 7.5) [63].

Clinical features

The majority of patients with AML come to medical attention because of the consequences of pancytopenia. Therefore, patients usually present with fatigue or dyspnea, fever or infection, and evidence of bleeding.

Extramedullary disease

Patients with AML may also present with extramedullary disease [64]. Leukemia cutis or infiltration of the gingiva is particularly common in patients whose leukemia cells demonstrate monocytic differentiation, including M5a and M5b. Such patients may also develop CNS disease with either chloromas (also called granulocytic sarcomas) or leukemic meningitis. Some patients with M2 and t(8;21) develop extramedullary disease, particularly orbital chloro-

Table 7.5 Standardized reporting for correlation of cytogenetic and molecular genetic data in AML with clinical data

Genetic group	Subsets
Favorable	t(8;21)(q22;q22); *RUNX1-RUNX1T1* inv(16)(p13.1q22) or t(16;16)(p13.1;q22); *CBFB-MYH11* Mutated *NPM1* without *FLT3*-ITD (normal karyotype) Mutated *CEBPA* (normal karyotype)
Intermediate-I[*]	Mutated *NPM1* and *FLT3*-ITD (normal karyotype) Wild-type *NPM1* and *FLT3*-ITD (normal karyotype) Wild-type *NPM1* without *FLT3*-UD (normal karyotype)
Intermediate-II	t(9;11)(p22;q23); *MLLT3-MLL* Cytogenetic abnormalities not classified as favorable or adverse[†]
Adverse	inv(3)(q21q26.2) or t(3;3)(q21;q26.2); *RPN1-EVI1* t(6;9)(p23;q34); *DEK-NUP214* t(v;11)(v;q23); *MLL* rearranged −5 or del(5q); −7; abnl(17p); complex karyotype[‡]

Reproduced from Dohner H (2010) *Blood* 115:453–74, with permission from American Society of Hematology.

Frequencies, response rates, and outcome measures should be reported by genetic group, and, if sufficient numbers are available, by specific subsets indicated; excluding cases of acute promyelocylic leukemia.

[*] Includes all AMLs with normal karyotype except for those included in the favorable subgroup; most of these cases are associated with poor prognosis, but they should be reported separately because of the potential different response to treatment.

[†] For most abnormalities, adequate numbers have not been studied to draw firm conclusions regarding their prognostic significance.

[‡] Three or more chromosome abnormalities in the absence of one of the WHO designated recurring translocations or inversions, that is, t(15;17), 1(8;21), inv(16) or t(16;16), t(9;11), t(v;11)(v;q23), t(6;9), Inv(3) or t(3;3); indicate how many complex karyotype cases have involvement of chromosome arms 5q, 7q, and 17p.

mas [24]. The leukemic cells from such patients frequently express CD56 or the neural crest adhesion molecule that appears to play a role in the trafficking of leukemic cells. The expression of this antigen appears to confer an unfavorable prognosis [11].

Hyperleukocytosis and leukostasis

Patients may also present with hyperleukocytosis, which has been considered a poor prognostic finding at diagnosis, and is associated with an increased risk of early death and a lower CR rate with induction chemotherapy. The risk of early death is greatest when the white blood cell count (WBC) is greater than 100 000/μL and is approximately 25% [65]. However, although the early death rate may be lower with leukapheresis, it is not clear that such a strategy results in improved OS in such patients. The risk of hyperleukocytosis relates to the potential for leukostasis in which there may be vascular obstruction, hypoxia, and tissue injury attributable to increased blood viscosity leading to microcirculatory obstruction. In addition, leukemia cells may directly invade vessel walls or compete for oxygen in the circulation. This finding is particularly associated with the microgranular variant of APL (M3v) and patients with AML whose leukemic cells show monocytic differentiation. Hyperleukocytosis may also be associated with the 11q23 abnormality and inv(16) (p13;q22), as well as chromosome 6 abnormalities [66].

Coagulopathy

Coagulation abnormalities are not uncommon in patients with newly diagnosed AML. In addition to thrombocytopenia, patients may also present with disseminated intravascular coagulation (DIC). This is particularly common in patients with APL [67, 68], but is also seen in patients with leukemia cells that show monocytic differentiation such as patients with M4 and M5 morphology. Venous thromboembolism in AML may be more common than previously recognized [69].

Metabolic laboratory abnormalities

Metabolic abnormalities are common at presentation and during treatment. Patients may present with tumor lysis syndrome manifested by hyperuricemia, hyperkalemia, hyperphosphatemia, and hypocalcemia with an incidence of approximately

17% [70]. Patients may also rarely present with hypercalcemia, hypokalemia related to renal tubular dysfunction, itself related to production to lysozyme (muramidase).

Clinical evaluation

Evaluation of the bone marrow cells should include routine morphologic review of stained material (such as Wright-Giemsa stain), immunophenotypic analysis usually by flow cytometry, cytogenetics and, in many cases, molecular genetic analysis. The diagnosis of AML is established by the demonstration of at least 20% myeloid blasts in the marrow or peripheral blood (WHO classification criteria) or, in uncommon cases, the biopsy of a chloroma (a myeloid sarcoma by WHO classification discussed above). Patients with balanced reciprocal translocation between t(8;21), inv(16) or t(16;16) and t(15;17) may have the diagnosis of AML established with less than 20% peripheral blood or marrow blasts according to the WHO classification. Because of the life-threatening bleeding diathesis in APL, treatment with ATRA (discussed below) must be started when the diagnosis is first suspected by clinical features and review of the peripheral blood smear and before the diagnosis is confirmed by cytogenetics, molecular genetics, or even by a bone marrow examination [71].

Immunophenotype findings

The myeloid markers CD45, CD13, and CD33 are the most commonly detected by flow cytometry on the surface of AML cells and are expressed on the cells on almost all patients [72–74]. Leukemic cells in AML often express CD11, CD14, and CD15. However, there is no definitive leukemia-specific antigen expression. The leukemia cells may also express CD34, which putatively identifies the hematopoietic stem cell and which confers an unfavorable prognosis. The identification of cell surface phenotype, usually by flow cytometry, is critical in MPO−, esterase− cases of acute leukemia. The diagnosis of AML FAB M0 can only be definitively established by immunophenotyping. The routine immunophenotypic analysis of leukemic cells that are MPO−, esterase− is mandatory to establish a diagnosis of M0 a subtype of AML which cannot otherwise easily be distinguished from ALL.

Aberrant expression of lymphoid markers on the leukemic cells from patients with AML is not uncommon. Terminal deoxynucleotide transferase (Tdt) may be expressed in approximately 25% of patients with AML, and CD7 may be expressed in 16% of patients [72]. Expression of lymphoid markers may be associated with 11q23 abnormalities and immunoglobulin heavy chain (IgH) or T-cell receptor gene rearrangements. This expression is also associated with high WBC at presentation and a poor prognosis.

Correlation of surface antigen expression with morphology, karyotype, and outcome

Immunophenotyping may be useful to detect minimal residual disease (MRD) in patients in apparent CR not identified by karyotype analysis. A study from Spain in patients in CR after induction with aberrant phenotypes at diagnosis used multiparametric flow cytometry to identify the level of MRD. The level of MRD predicted relapse rate and OS.

Treatment of acute myeloid leukemia

Overview

With the exception of APL, which is treated with ATRA commenced emergently at the first suspicion of the diagnosis in combination with chemotherapy, the majority of patients with other subtypes of AML in adults do not usually need to be treated with antileukemic chemotherapy emergently. The treatment of AML consists, in general, of two phases, remission induction followed by multiple cycles of intensive post-remission therapy (in younger adults) as consolidation to eradicate MRD.

The goal of the induction phase is the achievement of CR. The best remission induction chemotherapy includes an anthracycline plus cytarabine. Complete remission is defined as the absence of morphologic evidence of leukemia upon examination of the bone marrow (≤5% blasts identified) with peripheral blood count recovery, and the absence of extramedullary disease. Modifications of conventional induction in an attempt to increase the CR have included more intensive therapy with higher doses of anthracyclines or cytarabine or inclusion of additional active agents. However, with the exception of higher doses of daunorubicin, no regimen has been definitively shown to be more effective than the conventional two-drug induction regimen [75]. Post-remission therapy is administered to prevent or delay relapse of the leukemia and has generally included multiple cycles of intensive chemotherapy, most often HiDAC (high-dose cytarabine).

Induction therapy in younger adults

Complete remission is routinely achieved in more than 50% of patients when an anthracycline and cytarabine are combined. The CALGB established that three days of daunorubicin and seven days of cytarabine were better than two days and five days, respectively, and that 10 days of cytarabine was not better than seven. Daunorubicin at a dose of $30\,mg/m^2$ is inferior to $45\,mg/m^2$ in patients less than age 60 years. Finally, $100\,mg/m^2$ of cytarabine was found to be equally effective as $200\,mg/m^2$ [76].

The Eastern Cooperative Oncology Group (ECOG) has recently reported the results of a randomized trial in which patients less than 61 years of age were treated with cytarabine and daunorubicin at either $45\,mg/m^2$ or $90\,mg/m^2$ [75]. The higher dose of daunorubicin resulted in a higher rate of complete remission (70.6% vs. 57.3%; $P < 0.001$) and improved OS (median, 23.7 vs. 15.7 months; $P = 0.003$) (Figure 7.5). The rates of serious adverse events were similar in the two groups. Therefore, the most widely used induction chemotherapy regimen currently administered is daunorubicin (60–90 mg/m^2/day intravenously (IV) for three days) and cytarabine ($100\,mg/m^2$/day IV for 3 days) and cytarabine ($100\,mg/m^2$ by continuous IV infusion for 7 days). A number of studies with the goal of improving the CR rate have been conducted recently. Some trials have tested new agents such as idarubicin as a substitution for daunorubicin or the addition of etoposide or HiDAC. The EORTC and GIMEMA conducted a prospective trial of daunorubicin, mitoxantrone or idarubicin, combined with cytarabine and etoposide in standard doses for induction in younger patients followed by cytarabine ($500\,mg/m^2$ every 12 hours

for 6 days) plus the same anthracycline as given during induction, as consolidation [77]. Patients in CR then were assigned to either allogeneic or autologous HSCT depending on the availability of a sibling donor. While the CR rates were the same, the DFS and OS were significantly shorted in the daunorubicin arm among patients who did not undergo allogeneic HSCT.

Induction therapy in older adults

The ECOG completed a prospective randomized trial in older adults of daunorubicin versus idarubicin versus mitoxantrone as the anthracycline given together with cytarabine [78]. This trial showed that, among 350 patients, the CR rates achieved with the three different anthracyclines did not differ. There was a trend toward a decreased induction mortality rate on the mitoxantrone arm. In a trial conducted by the Dutch-Belgian Hemato-Oncology Cooperative Group (HOVON), patients 60 years of age and older were randomized to receive either daunorubicin at $45\,mg/m^2$ or $90\,mg/m^2$ with cytarabine in standard doses [79]. The CR rates were 64% in the group that received the escalated dose of daunorubicin and 54% in the group that received the conventional dose ($P = 0.002$); the rates of remission after the first cycle of induction treatment were 52% and 35%, respectively ($P < 0.001$). There was no significant difference between the two groups in the incidence of hematologic toxic effects, 30-day mortality (11% and 12% in the two groups, respectively), or the incidence of moderate, severe, or life-threatening adverse events ($P = 0.08$). Survival end points in the two groups did not differ significantly overall, but patients in the escalated-treatment group who were 60 to 65 years of age, as compared with the patients in the same age group who received the conventional dose, had higher rates of CR (73% vs. 51%), event-free survival (29% vs. 14%), and OS (38% vs. 23%). In a UK Medical Research Council (UK MRC) AML12 trial, 1243 patients, ages 15–59, and 26 patients, ages 60–65, were randomly assigned to receive either daunorubicin or mitoxantrone, each given with cytarabine for one or two courses for induction. All patients achieving CR subsequently received multiple courses of consolidation chemotherapy. There were no significant differences in CR rate, percent

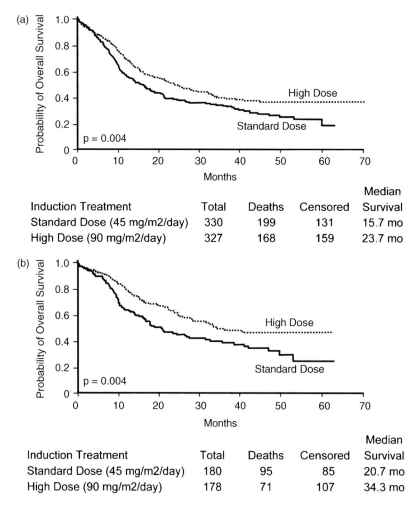

Induction Treatment	Total	Deaths	Censored	Median Survival
Standard Dose (45 mg/m2/day)	330	199	131	15.7 mo
High Dose (90 mg/m2/day)	327	168	159	23.7 mo

Induction Treatment	Total	Deaths	Censored	Median Survival
Standard Dose (45 mg/m2/day)	180	95	85	20.7 mo
High Dose (90 mg/m2/day)	178	71	107	34.3 mo

(a) All Patients; (b) Favorable or Intermediate Cytogenetic Profile.

Figure 7.5 Outcome of younger patients with AML randomized to either daunorubicin 45 mg/m^2/day or 90 mg/m^2/day given with cytarabine 100 mg/m^2/day. (A) All patients. (B) Patients with favorable-risk and intermediate-risk cytogenetics. (Reproduced with permission from Fernandez et al. [75]. Copyright © 2009 Massachusetts Medical Society. All rights reserved.)

of patients dying in CR, rate of resistant disease, relapse rate, DFS or OS between the two induction regimens.

Randomized trials of cytarabine dose during induction

Several prospective randomized trials with relatively large numbers of patients accrued have compared HiDAC with standard induction while employing the same post-remission therapy in both arms [77, 80]. Both studies showed a longer DFS, but not OS, among patients receiving the high-dose regimen.

However, these studies do not provide information as to whether HiDAC must be given in induction or whether it would yield similar outcomes if HiDAC was given as consolidation.

Randomized trials of additional drugs in induction

The Australian Leukemia Study Group (ALSG) compared standard-dose cytarabine plus daunorubicin (7 + 3) to 7 + 3 plus etoposide (75 mg/m^2/day for 7 days, [7 + 3 + 7]) followed by consolidation with the same agents over a shorter time, 5 + 2 versus

$5 + 2 + 5$ [80]. Although there was a significantly longer DFS on the etoposide arm, OS was not improved. The 5- and 10-year OS rates for $7 + 3 + 7$ were 19% and 16%, respectively, compared to 16% and 12%, respectively for $7 + 3$. However, the OS among patients less than age 55 was significantly longer on the $7 + 3 + 7$ arm (P = 0.04) with a 5- and 10-year OS of 25% and 25%, respectively, and 17% and 14% for $7 + 3$. Therefore, in younger patients, intensified induction may improve CR duration and OS without necessarily improving the CR rate. However, caution in interpretation is required given the fact that there was no stratification at randomization based on age.

Long-term follow-up results of the HiDAC + $3 + 7$ versus $7 + 3 + 7$ trial conducted by the ALSG show that the median remission duration was 46 months for HiDAC + $3 + 7$ and 12 months for $7 + 3 + 7$ (P = 0.0007) [80]. The DFS among patients achieving CR at five years was 48% on the HiDAC arm compared to 25% on the $7 + 3 + 7$ arm and there were no relapses on either arm beyond 54 months. The difference in OS between the two arms approached statistical significance (P = 0.053). These data suggest that intensified induction, as administered here, may improve outcome, but such a strategy has not been routinely adopted.

The MRC evaluated the benefits of adding etoposide to an anthracycline-cytarabine-based induction regimen in the AML10 trial [82]. More than 1800 patients age 55 years and younger were randomized to either $7 + 3$ (daunorubicin 50 mg/m^2) + 6-TG for two courses, the first with cytarabine and 6-TG given for 10 days and the second with both agents given for eight days, or $7 + 3$ (daunorubicin 50 mg/m^2) + etoposide (100 mg/m^2/day for five days), for two courses, the first with cytarabine given for 10 days and the second with cytarabine given for eight days. Induction mortality was higher on the etoposide arm (9% vs. 6%, P = 0.06). The CR rates between the two arms did not differ. There were no differences in either DFS (42% at six years for $7 + 3$ and 43% for $7 + 3 + 5$ or OS (40% for both groups)).

Hematopoietic growth factors during induction

Myeloid hematopoietic growth factors
Hematopoietic growth factors have been shown to shorten the period of neutropenia after induction therapy in AML. Many prospective randomized trials have been carried out, but have varied with respect to design, patient age, and induction regimens. In the aggregate experience, these studies suggest that myeloid growth factors shorten the period of neutropenia by two to six days following induction chemotherapy, and in several studies significantly reduce morbidity [83]. However, the CR rate and OS are generally not improved. Therefore, growth factors appear safe with little or no risk of leukemic cell stimulation.

Post-remission therapy

Intensive consolidation chemotherapy
A variety of studies have suggested that increasing the intensity of post-remission therapy prolongs remission duration and improves OS in patients with AML who are younger than 60 years [1]. The CALGB randomly assigned 596 patients in CR to receive four courses of cytarabine at one of three doses: 100 mg/m^2/day by continuous IV infusion for five days; 400 mg/m^2/day by continuous IV infusion for five days, or 3 g/m^2 as a three-hour IV infusion twice daily on days 1, 3, and 5 [84]. High rates of CNS toxicity were observed in patients older than 60 years randomized to the high-dose regimen. DFS was 21% in the 100 mg/m^2 group, 25% in the 400 mg/m^2 group and 39% in the 3 g/m^2 group. The results were most significant in patients with favorable cytogenetics. This trial demonstrated a dose–response relationship for cytarabine in younger patients undergoing post-remission therapy. Although the HiDAC regimen used in this trial has become a popular regimen, after the four courses of HiDAC all patients were to receive four monthly cycles of intensive maintenance therapy and these maintenance cycles are often omitted. Data from the MRC suggest that HiDAC may not be required to achieve similar results [85].

The number of courses of HiDAC required for optimal post-remission therapy is uncertain and remains an important question. The Finnish Leukemia Group randomized patients less than age 65 years in CR after two courses of induction to either four additional consolidation courses after two courses of HiDAC-containing consolidation or observation [86]. No benefit was observed for patients randomized to the longer consolidation regimen, suggesting early intensive consolidation is likely the most important influence on outcome rather than the number of cycles of intensive chemotherapy. In general, two to four cycles of intensive post-remission chemotherapy are given to most patients. However, the optimal doses of agents and schedule have not been determined.

Treatment of CBF AML

The outcome of patients with CBF leukemias may be relatively more favorable when multiple (3–4) cycles of HiDAC ($3g/m^2$ per dose) are administered [87, 88]. The CALGB retrospectively reviewed their experience of patients with M2 AML and t(8;21). The five-year DFS and OS for patients given three to four cycles of HiDAC (71% and 76% respectively) was significantly higher than that for patients given one cycle (37% and 44% respectively (P = 0.03, log-rank test, and P=0.04, long-rank test, respectively). A collaborative report from Southwest Oncology Group (SWOG), ECOG and M.D. Anderson Cancer Center also suggested that patients with CBF AML have a more favorable outcome when consolidated with HiDAC [25] (Figure 7.6).

Hematopoietic stem cell transplantation in AML
Allogeneic hematopoietic stem cell transplantation

HLA-matched sibling transplantation

Hematopoietic SCT is an important, potentially curative, post-remission strategy for many patients with AML. The important benefit attributable to the success of this strategy is referred to as graft-versus-leukemic (GVL) or adoptive immunotherapy, an effect whereby the donor cells recognize the recipient's cells, including leukemia cells, as foreign, with subsequent cytotoxicity, a phenomenon initially described in 1979 [89]. Such an immunologic reaction is also believed to be partly responsible for acute graft-versus-host disease (GVHD) manifested by skin rash, abnormal liver function, abdominal pain, diarrhea, and hematochezia and chronic GVHD manifested by immunosuppression, susceptibility to infections and a collagen vascular disease-like reaction with pigmentary changes and contracture formation [90]. A major focus in current research involves the identification of methods to alter the immunologic environment to exploit GVL effect while minimizing GVHD.

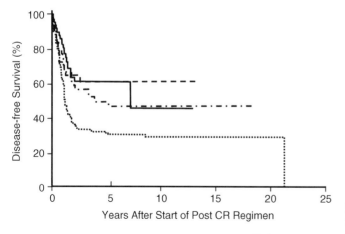

	n	Events	5-year Estimate
—— FA	53	20	61%
- - - HCT	31	12	61%
·-·- HDAC	44	23	50%
········ Other	136	96	31%

Figure 7.6 Kaplan-Meier estimates of disease-free survival of 264 patients with core binding factor acute myeloid leukemia given post-remission therapy with FA, HDAC, HST or other. (Reproduced from Appelbaum et al. [25], with permission from Blackwell Publishing Ltd.)

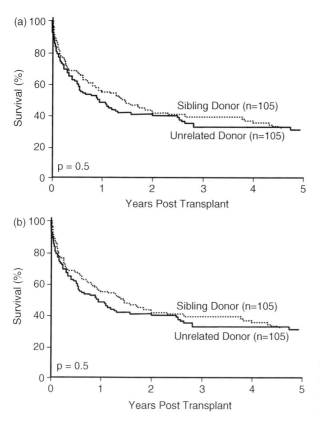

Figure 7.7 Kaplan-Meier curve of DFS (A) and overall survival (B) in URD and MSD allogeneic HSCT for AML. (Reproduced from Moore et al. [92], with permission from Elsevier.)

The role of matched sibling allogeneic HSCT continues to evolve. Several recent studies have contributed important new information. Firstly, matched sibling donor (MSD) allogeneic HSCT appears to improve relapse-free and OS of many patients in first CR who have intermediate- or poor-risk cytogenetics, but not for those with good-risk cytogenetics [91]. Secondly, in the era of high-resolution DNA-based HLA typing, the outcome for patients undergoing MSD and matched unrelated donor (MUD) HSCT appear to be similar [92, 93] (Figure 7.7). This may be also true for older adults [94]. Importantly, many patients who might not otherwise be eligible for an HSCT because of advanced age or comorbid conditions that in the past would preclude transplantation can now undergo non-myeloablative HSCT to promote GVL.

Non-myeloablative transplantation

An additional area of active investigation is the administration of intensive immunosuppressive agents such as fludarabine with less intensive cytotoxic chemotherapy (non-myeloablative) in an effort to permit engraftment of allogeneic hematopoietic stem cells, promote chimerism, and minimize TRM. This strategy may expand the population of patients who may benefit from transplantation (older adults, those with co-morbidities). Preliminary studies suggest such a strategy is feasible, results in engraftment of donor cells with rapid hematologic recovery, and is associated with acceptable risks of GVHD [95–98] (Table 7.6).

Autologous hematopoietic stem cell transplantation

The lack of a suitable HLA-matched donor and TRM limit the application of allogeneic transplantation. Alternatively autologous HSCT is potentially available to all patients and has very low mortality and TRM rates. Despite the lack of potential GVL effect, this approach has been associated with three- to five-year DFS rates of 40–70%. Prospective randomized

Table 7.6 Reduced-intensity conditioning HSCT in high-risk AML and MDS

Study (Ref. No.)	N	Med Age	ED%	DFS %	OS%
Tauro et al. [95]	76	52	9	37	42
Hegenbart et al. [96]	122	58	2	44	48
Oran et al. [97]	112	55	7	NR	44
Valcarel et al. [98]	93	53	8	43	45

HSCT: hematopoietic stem cell transplantation; AML: acute myeloid leukemia; MDS: myelodysplastic syndrome; ED: early death; DFS: disease-free survival; OS: overall survival.

trials have not clearly demonstrated a benefit in outcome compared to intensive consolidation although the relapse rate after autologous HSCT is lower [6]. The role, if any, of purging the stem cells of clonogenic leukemia cells is not established. To decrease the relapse rate following autologous HSCT, investigators have explored post-transplanted immunologic manipulations with interferon or interleukin-2, but any definitive benefits are not established.

Matched unrelated donors

Matched but unrelated donor (MUD) transplant registries have grown and this, coupled with more sensitive tissue-typing techniques, has become an effective approach for more patients [98]. However, there are limitations to this strategy including donor availability, length of time to identify the donor, and significant TRM (historically, approximately 25–30%), and the exact role of MUD transplantation in patients with AML has not been established. Improved OS has been associated with transplantation earlier in the natural history of the disease (e.g., first CR) and in patients with a low tumor burden. The presence of circulating leukemic blasts has been associated with poor outcome. Finally, transplantation of a marrow cell dose above 3.65×10^8/kg has been associated with faster neutrophil and platelet engraftment as well as decreased incidence of severe GVHD. The leukemia-free survival for patients with

AML in remission with poor prognostic features undergoing MUD transplantation with greater than 3.65×10^8 per kilogram of recipient body weight is approximately 45%. Patients undergoing MUD transplantation in CR have a significantly lower risk of relapse than patients transplanted in relapse or after primary induction failure.

Umbilical cord transplants

Hematopoietic stem cells procured from umbilical cords from related and unrelated donors can also restore hematopoiesis with acceptable risks of GVHD [100, 101]. Such stem cells have advantages compared to stem cells procured from adults including the capacity to form more colonies in cultures, a higher cell cycle rate, and autocrine production of growth factors. The immaturity of the lymphocytes from umbilical cords could theoretically reduce the risks of GVHD and allow for more successful HLA-mismatched transplants. This approach has been limited by size of the recipient since it has often been difficult to collect enough stem cells. *Ex vivo* expansion of stem cells is an area of active research that may expand the application of umbilical cell transplantation.

Maintenance therapy

A prospective randomized trial conducted by the ECOG suggested that maintenance therapy with 6-TG plus cytarabine ($60 \, \text{mg/m}^2$ once a week for two years) offered a benefit in remission duration compared to no maintenance treatment (median remission duration of 8.1 vs. 4.1 months (P = 0.003), although no significant survival difference was identified [102]. Buchner and colleagues conducted a randomized trial of 1770 patients who received either induction with one course of standard-dose chemotherapy and one course of HiDAC, or two courses of HiDAC and then either prolonger maintenance or autologous HSCT [103]. The AML9 study conducted by the MRC randomized patients in CR to maintenance treatment for one year with eight courses of cytarabine ($70 \, \text{mg/m}^2$ subcutaneous every 12 hours) and 6-thioguanine ($100 \, \text{mg/m}^2$ orally every 12 hours for five days per month) followed by four courses of COAP (cyclophosphamide, vincristine, cytarabine, and prednisone) or observation. Such therapy delayed, but did not prevent, relapse with no improvement in the OS at five years. Therefore, contemporary studies employing various maintenance regimens consistently show a benefit in DFS, but not OS. Age remains an important predictor of prognosis in AML [104].

Therapy of older adults
Characteristics of AML in older adults
The treatment of older adults (>55 to 60 years of age) deserves separate consideration because of the associations of AML in older adults with unfavorable prognostic factors including the frequent presence of an antecedent hematologic disorder, poor prognosis cytogenetic abnormalities, and the expression of the MDR1 gene, and the lack of tolerance for intensive antileukemic chemotherapy. In a SWOG trial conducted in 211 older patients with AML (median age 68 years), pretreatment leukemic blasts were studied for karyotype and intrinsic drug resistance by quantitating MDR1 expression [105]. Unfavorable cytogenetics were present in 32% of patients and 71% of patients expressed MDR1. Interestingly, patients with *de novo* AML with favorable or intermediate risk cytogenetics and no MDR1 expression had a CR rate of 81%.

Treatment strategies for older adults
Older adults, who are suitable candidates, should be offered either investigational treatments on a clinical trial or conventional-dose induction chemotherapy. Once in CR, the best post-remission approach has not been determined. No benefit in older adults was observed with HiDAC compared to much lower doses of cytarabine in the randomized CALGB trial discussed above [84]. Similarly, no improvement in outcome (OS) was observed in the MRC AML11 trial which tested three induction regimens: DAT (daunorubicin, cytarabine, G-thioguanine) versus ADE (cytarabine, daunorubicin and etoposide) versus MAC (mitoxantrone and cytarabine) each for two cycles [106]. The CR rate was higher for daunorubicin, cytarabine and G-thioguanine than ADE (62% vs. 50%; P = 0.002) or MAC (62% vs. 55%; P = 3.04). In addition, no improvement was observed with G-CSF (vs. placebo) in CR rate. Neither the DFS nor OS differed among patients ran-

domized to either a third cycle of therapy (DAT) or six total courses of additional chemotherapy. Finally, in this trial, 12 months of maintenance interferon was not beneficial. Most investigators would consider some post-remission cytarabine, but the best dose and schedule are unknown. Maintenance chemotherapy has not clearly been demonstrated to improve OS. However, revisiting maintenance therapy with novel agents is an active area of research.

Induction therapy in patients with relapsed or refractory AML

The options for reinduction therapy include: (1) intensive chemotherapy with conventional cytotoxic chemotherapeutic agents; (2) investigational therapies on a clinical trial; (3) immediate HSCT for the individual with a suitable allogeneic donor or cryopreserved autologous stem cells available; (4) palliative intent chemotherapy; or (5) best supportive care. Individuals who received an allogeneic HSCT during remission may be eligible for donor lymphocyte infusions as an immunologic maneuver to generate GVL effect. The determination of the optimal therapy depends, in part, on the duration of the first remission, whether HSCT is planned if a second CR is achieved, and the manner in which the relapse was detected. The likelihood of achieving a second remission is influenced by the duration of the first CR [107]. Individuals with remission less than 6–12 months in duration are best treated with investigational agents on clinical trials or, if feasible, immediate HSCT depending on the marrow blast percentage. Individuals with a remission greater than 18–24 months may be treated with more conventional salvage treatment that commonly includes a HiDAC-containing regimen.

Conventional salvage therapy for the younger adult and healthy older adult
Results of two selected trials for patients with relapsed disease are summarized in Table 7.7. The randomized trial conducted by the SWOG failed to demonstrate a significant benefit to the addition of mitoxantrone to cytarabine (3 g/m^2 every 12 hours for six doses) [108]. The German AML Cooperative

Table 7.7 Results of selected trials of conventional salvage therapy in adults with relapsed or refractory AML

Trial design	SWOG Randomized Phase III [108]		German AML Group Randomized Phase III [103]	
Therapy	HiDAC	HiDAC + Mito	S-HAM cytarabine 3 g	S-HAM cytarabine 1 g
Patients treated	81	81	73	65
CR rate, %	32	44	52	45
DFS (median, m)	9	5	5	3
Mortality, %	10	16	23	11

SWOG: Southwest Oncology Group; HiDAC: high-dose cytarabine; S-HAM: high-dose cytarabine + mitoxantrone; CR: complete remission; DFS: disease-free survival

Group trial compared cytarabine $(3\,g/m^2)$ versus cytarabine $(1\,g/m^2)$ administered twice daily on days 1, 2, 8, and 9 in patients less than 60 years of age. All patients received mitoxantrone. There was no substantial difference is CR rate or median OS. Thus, dose-intense cytarabine should probably be viewed as an essential component of a conventional salvage program, but escalation to $3\,g/m^2$ is probably not justified given the increased toxicity. There appears to be no value to adding standard-dose anthracyclines. However, there are multiple single-arm trials using escalated doses of anthracyclines that may present a reasonable alternative. It is critical to minimize the toxicity and likelihood of persistent complications since many individuals will be offered bone marrow transplantation if another CR is achieved.

New agents for relapsed or refractory AML
Targeted therapy with gemtuzumab ozogamicin

Gemtuzumab ozogamicin (GO) is an immunoconjugate of an engineered human anti-CD33 antibody linked with a potent cytotoxic antibiotic, calicheamicin. This agent warrants discussion because it serves as a paradigm for the development of targeted therapy and was the first drug approved by the FDA for patients with relapsed and/or refractory AML. Calicheamicin is a complex molecule containing four sugar residues, a hexa-substituted aromatic ring containing an odine, a methyl trisulfide, and a novel structural unit called a bicyclic enedieyne. This molecule joins to DNA in a sequence-specific way because the helical carbohydrate groups are complimentary in position to that of DNA. The calicheamicin is activated when the sulfur-bonds are reduced leading to an unstable diradical precursor. Low intracellular pH leads to hydrolases that cleave calicheamicin from the antibody. Calicheamicin binds to DNA and induces double-stranded DNA breaks and subsequent cell death.

In an analysis of 142 patients pooled from three studies of patients in first relapse, remission was achieved in 30% of patients; 16% achieved a CR and 13% a CRp (all criteria for CR except incomplete recovery of platelets). The median time to either CR or CRp was 60 days. The median RFS was 7.2 months for patients achieving CR, 4.4 months for patients achieving CRp, and 6.8 months for both cohorts of patients. Studies evaluating GO in combination with conventional antileukemic chemotherapy in induction therapy have been disappointing [109].

Several new agents currently in clinical trials that appear particularly promising are shown in Table 7.8 and represent the diversity of new agents currently

Table 7.8 Selected new agents for the treatment of AML

Agent	Mechanism	Comments
XIAP antisense oligo	Apoptosis inhibitor of caspases 3/9	Effective w/chemo as early reinduction
CPX-351	Liposomal fixed molar ratio of dauno/ara-C	Phase II rando trial underway
Amonafide	Topo II inhibitor	Phase III trial underway
Sorafenib	Multikinase inhibitor	Can be safely combined with chemo

in clinical trials. These include XIAP, an antisense oligonucleotide [110]; Sorafenib, a multikinase inhibitor [53]; CPX351, a liposome containing a fixed molar ratio of daunorubicin and cytarabine [111], and amonafide, a novel topoisomerase inhibitor which may be particularly effective in patients with therapy-related AML [112].

Supportive care during the treatment of AML

Supportive care during the treatment of patients with AML has improved significantly. During the initial phase of treatment one needs to be vigilant for metabolic complications related to lysis of leukemic cells. The prolonged neutropenia related to the underlying disease and treatment and mucosal injury are major risk factors for infections. Prolonged thrombocytopenia is the major risk factor for hemorrhage, but patients may also have additional coagulation abnormalities such as DIC and fibrinolysis in APL and AML with monocytic differentiation. Finally, patients who receive HiDAC are at risk for unique complications including cerebellar dysfunction, keratitis, and rash.

The cerebellar syndrome typically is characterized by the development of ataxia, dysarthria, dysmetria, or dysdiadochokinesia. The prevalence is greater in older (>60 years) patients, in the presence of hepatic or renal impairment, and with higher doses or shorter infusion times. Patients who receive HiDAC are also at risk for keratitis and should receive corticosteroid eye-drops during and for 24–48 hours after the completion of therapy.

Routine follow-up of patients in CR

Routine follow-up for patients in CR who have completed all therapy generally includes a periodic history, physical examination, and a complete blood count with differential count. One schedule would include the above evaluation every three months for two to three years and, thereafter every six months. Long-term follow-up data suggest that the incidence of relapse after three years in CR is quite small. Bone marrow examinations are generally not recommended unless there has been a change in the peripheral blood counts. Studies have shown little deleterious long-term impact of intensive induction and consolidation chemotherapy on other organs.

References

1 Tallman MS, Gilliland DG, Rowe JM. (2005) Drug therapy for acute myeloid leukemia. *Blood* **106**: 1154–63.

2 Bennett JM, Catovsky D, Daniel MT, et al. (1976) Proposals for the classification of the acute leukaemias. French-American-British (FAB) co-operative group. *Br J Haematol* **33**:451–8.

3 Bennett JM, Catovsky D, Daniel MT, et al. (1985) Criteria for the diagnosis of acute leukemia of megakaryocyte lineage (M7). A report of the French-American-British Cooperative Group. *Ann Intern Med* **103**:460–2.

4 Bennett JM, Catovsky D, Daniel M.T. et al. (1985) Proposed revised criteria for the classification of acute myeloid leukemia. A report of the French-American-British Cooperative Group. *Ann Intern Med* **103**:620–5.

5 Harris NL, Jaffe ES, Diebold J, et al. (1999) World Health Organization classification of neoplastic diseases of the hematopoietic and lymphoid tissues: report of the Clinical Advisory Committee meeting – Airlie House, Virginia, November 1997. *J Clin Oncol* **17**:3835–49.

6 Cassileth PA, Harrington DP, Appelbaum FR, et al. (1998) Chemotherapy compared with autologous or allogeneic bone marrow transplantation in the management of acute myeloid leukemia in first remission. *N Engl J Med* **339**:1649–56.

7 Guzman ML, Rossi RM, Neelakantan S, et al. (2007) An orally bioavailable parthenolide analog selectively eradicates acute myelogenous leukemia stem and progenitor cells. *Blood* **110**:4427–35.

8 Pedersen-Bjergaard J, Rowley JD. (1994) The balanced and the unbalanced chromosome aberrations of acute myeloid leukemia may develop in different ways and may contribute differently to malignant transformation. *Blood* **83**:2780–6.

9 Super HJ, McCabe NR, Thirman MJ, et al. (1993) Rearrangements of the MLL gene in therapy-related acute myeloid leukemia in patients previously treated with agents targeting DNA-topoisomerase II. *Blood* **82**:3705–11.

10 Darrington DL, Vose JM, Anderson JR, et al. (1994) Incidence and characterization of secondary myelodysplastic syndrome and acute myelogenous leukemia following high-dose chemoradiotherapy and autologous stem-cell transplantation for lymphoid malignancies. *J Clin Oncol* **12**:2527–34.

11 Schoch C, Kern W, Schnittger S, Hiddemann W, Haferlach T. (2004) Karyotype is an independent prognostic parameter in therapy-related acute myeloid leukemia (t-AML): an analysis of 93 patients with t-AML in comparison to 1091 patients with de novo AML. *Leukemia* **18**:120–5.

12 Bacher U, Kern W, Schnittger S, et al. (2005) Population-based age-specific incidences of cytogenetic subgroups of acute myeloid leukemia. *Haematologica* **90**:1502–10.

13 Mauritzson N, Albin M, Rylander L, et al. (2002) Pooled analysis of clinical and cytogenetic features in treatment-related and de novo adult acute myeloid leukemia and myelodysplastic syndromes based on a consecutive series of 761 patients analyzed 1976–1993 and on 5098 unselected cases reported in the literature 1974–2001. *Leukemia* **16**:2366–78.

14 Pogoda JM, Preston-Martin S. (2006) Smoking and risk of acute myeloid leukemia in adults. *Cancer Causes Control* **17**:351–2.

15 Juliusson G, Antunovic P, Derolf A, et al. (2009) Age and acute myeloid leukemia: real world data on decision to treat and outcomes from the Swedish Acute Leukemia Registry. *Blood* **113**:4179–87.

16 Vickers M, Jackson G, Taylor P. (2000) The incidence of acute promyelocytic leukemia appears constant over most of a human lifespan, implying only one rate limiting mutation. *Leukemia* **14**:722–6.

17 Douer D. (2003) The epidemiology of acute promyelocytic leukaemia. *Best Pract Res Clin Haematol* **16**:357–67.

18 Matasar MJ, Ritchie EK, Consedine N, Magai C, Neugut AI. (2006) Incidence rates of acute promyelocytic leukemia among Hispanics, blacks, Asians, and non-Hispanic whites in the United States. *Eur J Cancer Prev* **15**:367–70.

19 Sekeres MA, Peterson B, Dodge RK, et al. (2004) Differences in prognostic factors and outcomes in African Americans and whites with acute myeloid leukemia. *Blood* **103**:4036–42.

20 Grimwade D, Walker H, Oliver F, et al. (1998) The importance of diagnostic cytogenetics on outcome in AML: analysis of 1,612 patients entered into the MRC AML 10 trial. The Medical Research Council Adult and Children's Leukaemia Working Parties. *Blood* **92**:2322–33.

21 Slovak ML, Kopecky KJ, Cassileth PA, et al. (2000) Karyotypic analysis predicts outcome of preremission and postremission therapy in adult acute myeloid leukemia: a Southwest Oncology Group/Eastern Cooperative Oncology Group Study. *Blood* **96**: 4075–83.

22 Byrd JC, Mrozek K, Dodge RK, et al. (2002) Pretreatment cytogenetic abnormalities are predictive of induction success, cumulative incidence of relapse, and overall survival in adult patients with de novo acute myeloid leukemia: results from Cancer and Leukemia Group B (CALGB 8461). *Blood* **100**:4325–36.

23 Koeffler HP. (1987) Syndromes of acute nonlymphocytic leukemia. *Ann Intern Med* **107**:748–58.

24 Tallman MS, Hakimian D, Shaw JM, et al. (1993) Granulocytic sarcoma is associated with the 8;21 translocation in acute myeloid leukemia. *J Clin Oncol* **11**:690–7.

25 Appelbaum FR, Kopecky KJ, Tallman MS, et al. (2006) The clinical spectrum of adult acute myeloid leukaemia associated with core binding factor translocations. *Br J Haematol* **135**:165–73.

26 Mrozek K, Heinonen K, Lawrence D, et al. (1997) Adult patients with de novo acute myeloid leukemia and t(9; 11)(p22; q23) have a superior outcome to patients with other translocations involving band

11q23: a cancer and leukemia group B study. *Blood* **90**:4532–8.

27 Slovak ML, Gundacker H, Bloomfield CD, et al. (2006) A retrospective study of 69 patients with t(6;9)(p23; q34) AML emphasizes the need for a prospective, multicenter initiative for rare 'poor prognosis' myeloid malignancies. *Leukemia* **20**:1295–7.

28 Lillington DM, MacCallum PK, Lister TA, Gibbons B. (1993) Translocation t(6;9)(p23;q34) in acute myeloid leukemia without myelodysplasia or basophilia: two cases and a review of the literature. *Leukemia* **7**:527–31.

29 Gascoyne RD, Noble MC, Kalousek DK. (1986) Translocation t(3;3)(q21;q26) and thrombocytosis. *Cancer Genet Cytogenet* **22**:365.

30 Sperr W, Valent P. (2007) Biology and clinical features of myeloid neoplasms with inv(3)(q21q26) or t(3;3) (q21q26). *Leuk Lymphoma* **48**:2096–7.

31 Nguyen S, Leblanc T, Fenaux P, et al. (2002) A white blood cell index as the main prognostic factor in t(8;21) acute myeloid leukemia (AML): a survey of 161 cases from the French AML Intergroup. *Blood* **99**:3517–23.

32 Baer MR, Stewart CC, Lawrence D, et al. (1997) Expression of the neural cell adhesion molecule CD56 is associated with short remission duration and survival in acute myeloid leukemia with t(8;21)(q22; q22). *Blood* **90**:1643–8.

33 Rowley JD. (1999) The role of chromosome translocations in leukemogenesis. *Semin Hematol* **36**:59–72.

34 Haferlach T. (2008) Molecular genetic pathways as therapeutic targets in acute myeloid leukemia. *Hematology (Am Soc Hematol Educ Program)* **2008**:400–11.

35 Nucifora G, Rowley JD. (1995) AML1 and the 8;21 and 3;21 translocations in acute and chronic myeloid leukemia. *Blood* **86**:1–14.

36 Care RS, Valk PJ, Goodeve AC, et al. (2003) Incidence and prognosis of c-KIT and FLT3 mutations in core binding factor (CBF) acute myeloid leukaemias. *Br J Haematol* **121**:775–7.

37 Cairoli R, Beghini A, Grillo G, et al. (2006) Prognostic impact of c-KIT mutations in core binding factor leukemias: an Italian retrospective study. *Blood* **107**:3463–8.

38 Kindler T, Breitenbuecher F, Marx A, et al. (2004) Efficacy and safety of imatinib in adult patients with c-kit-positive acute myeloid leukemia. *Blood* **103**:3644–54.

39 Melnick A, Licht JD. (1999) Deconstructing a disease: RARalpha, its fusion partners, and their roles in the pathogenesis of acute promyelocytic leukemia. *Blood* **93**:3167–215.

40 Schoch C, Schnittger S, Klaus M, et al. (2003) AML with 11q23/MLL abnormalities as defined by the WHO classification: incidence, partner chromosomes, FAB subtype, age distribution, and prognostic impact in an unselected series of 1897 cytogenetically analyzed AML cases. *Blood* **102**:2395–402.

41 Krauter J, Wagner K, Schafer I, et al. (2009) Prognostic factors in adult patients up to 60 years old with acute myeloid leukemia and translocations of chromosome band 11q23: individual patient data-based meta-analysis of the German Acute Myeloid Leukemia Intergroup. *J Clin Oncol* **27**:3000–6.

42 Schlenk RF, Dohner K, Krauter J, F et al. (2008) Mutations and treatment outcome in cytogenetically normal acute myeloid leukemia. *N Engl J Med* **358**:1909–18.

43 Kottaridis PD, Gale RE, Frew ME, et al. (2001) The presence of a FLT3 internal tandem duplication in patients with acute myeloid leukemia (AML) adds important prognostic information to cytogenetic risk group and response to the first cycle of chemotherapy: analysis of 854 patients from the United Kingdom Medical Research Council AML 10 and 12 trials. *Blood* **98**:1752–9.

44 Falini B, Mecucci C, Tiacci E, et al. (2005) Cytoplasmic nucleophosmin in acute myelogenous leukemia with a normal karyotype. *N Engl J Med* **352**:254–66.

45 Dohner K, Schlenk RF, Habdank M, et al. (2005) Mutant nucleophosmin (NPM1) predicts favorable prognosis in younger adults with acute myeloid leukemia and normal cytogenetics: interaction with other gene mutations. *Blood* **106**:3740–6.

46 Gaidzik VI, Schlenk RF, Moschny S, et al. (2009) Prognostic impact of WT1 mutations in cytogenetically normal acute myeloid leukemia: a study of the German-Austrian AML Study Group. *Blood* **113**:4505–11.

47 Bacher U, Haferlach C, Kern W, Haferlach T, Schnittger S. (2008) Prognostic relevance of FLT3-TKD mutations in AML: the combination matters – an analysis of 3082 patients. *Blood* **111**:2527–37.

48 Gale RE, Green C, Allen C, et al. (2008) The impact of FLT3 internal tandem duplication mutant level, number, size, and interaction with NPM1 mutations in a large cohort of young adult patients with acute myeloid leukemia. *Blood* **111**:2776–84.

49 Jin G, Matsushita H, Asai S, et al. (2009) FLT3-ITD induces ara-C resistance in myeloid leukemic cells through the repression of the ENT1 expression. *Biochem Biophys Res Commun* **390**:1001–6 [Epub 2009 Oct 22].

50 Stone RM, DeAngelo DJ, Klimek V, et al. (2005) Patients with acute myeloid leukemia and an activating mutation in FLT3 respond to a small-molecule FLT3 tyrosine kinase inhibitor, PKC412. *Blood* **105**:54–60.

51 Lee SH, Paietta E, Racevskis J, Wiernik PH. (2009) Complete resolution of leukemia cutis with sorafenib in an acute myeloid leukemia patient with FLT3-ITD mutation. *Am J Hematol* **84**:701–2.

52 Zarrinkar PP, Gunawardane RN, Cramer MD, et al. (2009) AC220 is a uniquely potent and selective inhibitor of FLT3 for the treatment of acute myeloid leukemia (AML). *Blood* **114**:2984–92.

53 Metzelder S, Wang Y, Wollmer E, et al. (2009) Compassionate use of sorafenib in FLT3-ITD-positive acute myeloid leukemia: sustained regression before and after allogeneic stem cell transplantation. *Blood* **113**:6567–71.

54 Schnittger S, Schoch C, Kern W, et al. (2005) Nucleophosmin gene mutations are predictors of favorable prognosis in acute myelogenous leukemia with a normal karyotype. *Blood* **106**:3733–9.

55 Preudhomme C, Sagot C, Boissel N, et al. (2002) Favorable prognostic significance of CEBPA mutations in patients with de novo acute myeloid leukemia: a study from the Acute Leukemia French Association (ALFA). *Blood* **100**:2717–23.

56 Wouters BJ, Lowenberg B, Erpelinck-Verschueren CA, et al. (2009) Double CEBPA mutations, but not single CEBPA mutations, define a subgroup of acute myeloid leukemia with a distinctive gene expression profile that is uniquely associated with a favorable outcome. *Blood* **113**:3088–91.

57 Marcucci G, Maharry K, Whitman SP, et al. (2007) High expression levels of the ETS-related gene, ERG, predict adverse outcome and improve molecular risk-based classification of cytogenetically normal acute myeloid leukemia: a Cancer and Leukemia Group B Study. *J Clin Oncol* **25**:3337–43.

58 Lugthart S, van Drunen E, van Norden Y, et al. (2008) High EVI1 levels predict adverse outcome in acute myeloid leukemia: prevalence of EVI1 overexpression and chromosome 3q26 abnormalities underestimated. *Blood* **111**:4329–37.

59 Marcucci G, Radmacher MD, Maharry K, et al. (2008) MicroRNA expression in cytogenetically normal acute myeloid leukemia. *N Engl J Med* **358**:1919–28.

60 Bennett JM, Catovsky D, Daniel MT, et al. (1976) Proposals for the classification of the acute leukemias: French-American-British (FAB) Cooperative Group. *Br J Haematol* **33**:451–8.

61 Tallman MS, Kim HT, Paietta E, et al. (2004) Acute monocytic leukemia (French-American-British classification M5) does not have a worse prognosis than other subtypes of acute myeloid leukemia: a report from the Eastern Cooperative Oncology Group. *J Clin Oncol* **22**:1276–86.

62 Vardiman JW, Thiele J, Arber DA, et al. (2009) The 2008 revision of the World Health Organization (WHO) classification of myeloid neoplasms and acute leukemia: rationale and important changes. *Blood* **114**:937–51.

63 Dohner H, Estey EH, Amaderi S, et al. (2010) Diagnosis and management of acute myeloid leukemia in adults: recommendations from an international expert panel, on behalf of the European Leukemia Net. *Blood* **115**:453–74.

64 Eshghabadi M, Shojania AM, Carr I. (1986) Isolated granulocytic sarcoma: report of a case and review of the literature. *J Clin Oncol* **4**:912–7.

65 Bug G, Anargyrou K, Tonn T, et al. (2007) Impact of leukapheresis on early death rate in adult acute myeloid leukemia presenting with hyperleukocytosis. *Transfusion* **47**:1843–50.

66 Tallman MS. (2004) Extramedullary acute myeloid leukemia infiltrates. *Leuk Res* **28**:1005–6.

67 Watanabe R, Murata M, Takayama N, et al. (1997) Long-term follow-up of hemostatic molecular markers during remission induction therapy with all-trans retinoic acid for acute promyelocytic leukemia. Keio Hematology-Oncology Cooperative Study Group (KHOCS). *Thromb Haemost* **77**:641–5.

68 Tallman MS, Lefebvre P, Baine RM, et al. (2004) Effects of all-trans retinoic acid or chemotherapy on the molecular regulation of systemic blood coagulation and fibrinolysis in patients with acute promyelocytic leukemia. *J Thromb Haemost* **2**:1341–50.

69 Ku GH, White RH, Chew HK, et al. (2009) Venous thromboembolism in patients with acute leukemia: incidence, risk factors, and effect on survival. *Blood* **113**:3911–7.

70 Montesinos P, Lorenzo I, Martin G, et al. (2008) Tumor lysis syndrome in patients with acute myeloid leukemia: identification of risk factors and development of a predictive model. *Haematologica* **93**:67–74.

71 Tallman MS, Altman JK. (2009) How I treat acute promyelocytic leukemia. *Blood* **114**:5126–35.

72 Khalidi HS, Medeiros LJ, Chang KL, Brynes RK, Slovak ML, Arber DA. (1998) The immunophenotype of adult acute myeloid leukemia: high frequency of lymphoid antigen expression and comparison of immunophenotype, French-American-British classification, and karyotypic abnormalities. *Am J Clin Pathol* **109**:211–20.

73 Paietta E. (1995) Proposals for the immunological classification of acute leukemias. *Leukemia* **9**:2147–8.

74 Chang H, Salma F, Yi QL, et al. (2004) Prognostic relevance of immunophenotyping in 379 patients with acute myeloid leukemia. *Leuk Res* **28**:43–8.

75 Fernandez HF, Sun Z, Yao X, et al. (2009) Anthracycline dose intensification in acute myeloid leukemia. *N Engl J Med* **361**:249–59.

76 Rai KR, Holland JF, Glidewell OJ, et al. (1981) Treatment of acute myelocytic leukemia: a study by Cancer and Leukemia Group B. *Blood* **58**:1203–12.

77 Bishop JF, Matthews JP, Young GA, et al. (1996) Randomized study of high-dose cytarabine in induction in acute myeloid leukaemia. *Blood* **87**:1710–7.

78 Rowe JM, Neuberg D, Friedenberg W, et al. (2004) A phase 3 study of three induction regimens and of priming with GM-CSF in older adults with acute myeloid leukemia: a trial by the Eastern Cooperative Oncology Group. *Blood* **103**:479–85.

79 Lowenberg B, Ossenkoppele GJ, van Putten W, et al. (2009) High-dose daunorubicin in older patients with acute myeloid leukemia. *N Engl J Med* **361**:1235–48.

80 Bishop JF, Matthews JP, Young GA, Bradstock K, Lowenthal RM. (1998) Intensified induction chemotherapy with high dose cytarabine and etoposide for acute myeloid leukemia: a review and updated results of the Australian Leukemia Study Group. *Leuk Lymphoma* **28**:315–27.

81 Bishop JF, Lowenthal PM, Joshua D, et al. (1990) Etoposide in acute non-lymphoblastic leukaemia. *Blood* **75**:27–32.

82 Hann I, Stevens R, Goldstone A, et al. (1997) Randomized comparison of DAT versus ADF as induction chemotherapy in children and younger adults with acute myeloid leukemia. Results of the Medical Research Council's 10th AML trial (MRC AML10). Adult and Childhood Leukaemia Working Parties of the Medical Research Council. *Blood* **89**:2311–8.

83 Wadleigh M, Stone RM. (2009) The role of myeloid growth factors in acute leukemia. *J Natl Compr Canc Netw* **7**:84–91.

84 Mayer RJ, Davis RB, Schiffer CA, et al. (1994) Intensive postremission chemotherapy in adults with acute myeloid leukemia. Cancer and Leukemia Group B. *N Engl J Med* **331**:896–903.

85 Burnett AK, Goldstone AH, Stevens RM, et al. (1998) Randomised comparison of addition of autologous bone-marrow transplantation to intensive chemotherapy for acute myeloid leukaemia in first remission: results of MRC AML 10 trial. UK Medical Research Council Adult and Children's Leukaemia Working Parties. *Lancet* **351**:700–8.

86 Elonen E, Almqvist A, Hanninen A, et al. (1998) Comparison between four and eight cycles of intensive chemotherapy in adult acute myeloid leukemia: a randomized trial of the Finnish Leukemia Group. *Leukemia* **12**:1041–8.

87 Byrd JC, Dodge RK, Carroll A, et al. (1999) Patients with t(8;21)(q22;q22) and acute myeloid leukemia have superior failure-free and overall survival when repetitive cycles of high-dose cytarabine are administered. *J Clin Oncol* **17**:3767–75.

88 Byrd JC, Ruppert AS, Mrozek K, et al. (2004) Repetitive cycles of high-dose cytarabine benefit patients with acute myeloid leukemia and inv(16)(p13q22) or t(16;16)(p13;q22): results from CALGB 8461. *J Clin Oncol* **22**:1087–94.

89 Weiden PL, Flournoy N, Thomas ED, et al. (1979) Antileukemic effect of graft-versus-host disease in human recipients of allogeneic-marrow grafts. *N Engl J Med* **300**:1068–73.

90 Sullivan KM, Agura E, Anasetti C, et al. (1991) Chronic graft-versus-host disease and other late complications of bone marrow transplantation. *Semin Hematol* **28**:250–9.

91 Koreth J, Schlenk R, Kopecky KJ, et al. (2009) Allogeneic stem cell transplantation for acute myeloid leukemia in first complete remission: systematic review and meta-analysis of prospective clinical trials. *JAMA* **301**:2349–61.

92 Moore J, Nivison-Smith I, Goh K, et al. (2007) Equivalent survival for sibling and unrelated donor allogeneic stem cell transplantation for acute myelogenous leukemia. *Biol Blood Marrow Transplant* **13**:601–7.

93 Pagel JM, Gooley TA, Petersdorf EW, et al. (2007) Outcome following hematopoietic cell transplantation for patients with AML-CR1: comparison between matched-sibling and unrelated allografts. *Blood* **110**:330a.

94 Schetelig J, Bornhauser M, Schmid C, et al. (2008) Matched unrelated or matched sibling donors result in comparable survival after allogeneic stem-cell transplantation in elderly patients with acute myeloid leukemia: a report from the cooperative German Transplant Study Group. *J Clin Oncol* **26**:5183–91.

95 Tauro S, Craddock C, Peggs K, et al. (2005) Allogeneic stem-cell transplantation using a reduced-intensity conditioning regimen has the capacity to produce durable remissions and long-term disease-free survival in patients with high-risk acute myeloid leukemia and myelodysplasia. *J Clin Oncol* **23**:9387–93.

96 Hegenbart U, Niederwieser D, Sandmaier BM, et al. (2006) Treatment for acute myelogenous leukemia by low-dose, total-body, irradiation-based conditioning and hematopoietic cell transplantation from related and unrelated donors. *J Clin Oncol* **24**:444–53.

97 Oran B, Giralt S, Saliba R, et al. (2007) Allogeneic hematopoietic stem cell transplantation for the treatment of high-risk acute myelogenous leukemia and myelodysplastic syndrome using reduced-intensity conditioning with fludarabine and melphalan. *Biol Blood Marrow Transplant* **13**:454–62.

98 Valcarcel D, Martino R, Caballero D, et al. (2008) Sustained remissions of high-risk acute myeloid leukemia and myelodysplastic syndrome after reduced-intensity conditioning allogeneic hematopoietic transplantation: chronic graft-versus-host disease is the strongest factor improving survival. *J Clin Oncol* **26**:577–84.

99 Sierra J, Martino R, Sanchez B, et al. (2008) Hematopoietic transplantation from adult unrelated donors as treatment for acute myeloid leukemia. *Bone Marrow Transplant* **41**:425–37.

100 Laughlin MJ, Barker J, Bambach B, et al. (2001) Hematopoietic engraftment and survival in adult recipients of umbilical-cord blood from unrelated donors. *N Engl J Med* **344**:1815–22.

101 Laughlin MJ, Eapen M, Rubinstein P, et al. (2004) Outcomes after transplantation of cord blood or bone marrow from unrelated donors in adults with leukemia. *N Engl J Med* **351**:2265–75.

102 Cassileth PA, Lynch E, Hines JD, et al. (1992) Varying intensity of postremission therapy in acute myeloid leukemia. *Blood* **79**:1924–30.

103 Buchner T, Berdel WE, Haferlach C, et al. (2009) Age-related risk profile and chemotherapy dose response in acute myeloid leukemia: a study by the German Acute Myeloid Leukemia Cooperative Group. *J Clin Oncol* **27**:61–9.

104 Appelbaum FR, Gundacker H, Head DR, et al. (2006) Age and acute myeloid leukemia. *Blood* **107**:3481–5.

105 Leith CP, Kopecky KJ, Chen IM, et al. (1999) Frequency and clinical significance of the expression of the multidrug resistance proteins MDR1/P-glycoprotein, MRP1, and LRP in acute myeloid leukemia: a Southwest Oncology Group Study. *Blood* **94**:1086–99.

106 Goldstone AH, Burnett AK, Wheatley K, et al. (2001) Attempts to improve treatment outcomes in acute myeloid leukemia (AML) in older patients: the results of the United Kingdom Medical Research Council AML11 trial. *Blood* **98**:1302–11.

107 Estey EH. (2000) Treatment of relapsed and refractory acute myelogenous leukemia. *Leukemia* **14**:476–9.

108 Karanes C, Kopecky KJ, Head DR, et al. (1999) A phase III comparison of high dose ARA-C (HIDAC) versus HIDAC plus mitoxantrone in the treatment of first relapsed or refractory acute myeloid leukemia. Southwest Oncology Group Study. *Leuk Res* **23**:787–94.

109 Burnett AK, Kell WJ, Goldstone AH, et al. (2006) The addition of gemtuzumab ozogamicin to induction chemotherapy for AML improves disease-free survival without extra toxicity: Preliminary analysis of 1115 patients in the MRC AML15 trial. *Blood* **108**:13a.

110 Schimmer AD, Estey EH, Borthakur G, et al. (2009) Phase I/II trial of AEG35156 X-linked inhibitor of apoptosis protein antisense oligonucleotide combined with idarubicin and cytarabine in patients with relapsed or primary refractory acute myeloid leukemia. *J Clin Oncol* **27**:4741–6.

111 Bayne WF, Mayer LD, Swenson CE. (2009) Pharmacokinetics of CPX-351 (cytarabine/daunorubicin HCl) liposome injection in the mouse. *J Pharm Sci* **98**:2540–8.

112 Burcu M, O'Loughlin KL, Ford LA, Baer MR. (2008) Amonafide L-malate is not a substrate for multidrug resistance proteins in secondary acute myeloid leukemia. *Leukemia* **22**:2110–5.

CHAPTER 8

Acute Promyelocytic Leukemia

Sylvain Thépot, Lionel Ades and Pierre Fenaux

Service d'hématologie clinique, Hôpital Avicenne (Assistance Publique – Hôpitaux de Paris) and Paris 13 University, Bobigny, France

Introduction

First described in 1957 [1], acute promyelocytic leukemia (APL) is a specific type of AML characterized by the morphology of its blast cells, t(15;17) translocation [2] which fuses the *PML* and the *RAR* alpha genes [3]. APL has considerably benefited from therapeutic progress over the last 20 years; a large majority of the patients are now being cured using a combination of all-trans retinoic acid (ATRA) and anthracycline-based chemotherapy. Arsenic derivatives have a growing place in the therapeutic strategy as well, being the reference treatment of relapse, and are starting to play an important role in first-line treatment.

Clinical and biological characteristics of APL

Clinical findings

APL is rare (about 1.5 new cases per million per year), that is, less than 10 % of all AML [4]. Its incidence depends partly on ethnic and environmental factors, and previous exposures are increasingly incriminated (up to 15% of the cases in recent series), especially breast carcinoma treated by topoisomerase-II inhibitors (anthracyclines, mitoxantrone, and less often VP16) [5]. Contrary to other AML, the incidence increases with age until 55 where it reaches a plateau and then decreases [6].

Bleeding or, less often, other signs of bone marrow failure (fever, anemia) and pancytopenia are the most common presenting signs. Bleeding is often severe, due to the combination of thrombocytopenia (secondary to bone marrow failure) and coagulopathy (see below). It can include cutaneous purpura, often suggestive if extensive, and associated with bleeding at injections sites (or, for example, at the site of marrow aspirate). The most severe form of bleeding is central nervous system (CNS) bleeding, which can be a presenting factor. Severe pulmonary bleeding can also develop. Organomegaly is rarely found at diagnosis, except sometimes in hyperleukocytic forms, while involvement of other organs at diagnosis (especially in the CNS and skin) is also rare.

Blood and bone marrow morphology and immunophenotype

The blood count is generally characterized by pancytopenia, leukopenia being found in about 70 % of the cases, while blast cells are not always seen in the blood. Leukocytosis (>10 g/L) is found in only about 25% of the cases, WBC being rarely greater than 100 g/L. On bone marrow examination, blasts are characterized by cell nuclear shape often kidney-shaped or bilobed, and cytoplasm completely occupied by densely packed or even coalescent granules. In some cells, the cytoplasm is filled with fine dust-like granules. At least a proportion of promyelocytic blasts contain several Auer rods, generally in bundles ("faggot cells"). MPO is always strongly positive in

Advances in Malignant Hematology, First Edition. Edited by Hussain I. Saba and Ghulam J. Mufti. © 2011 Blackwell Publishing Ltd. Published 2011 by Blackwell Publishing Ltd.

all blast cells. Flow cytometry has been described as CD34$^{-/+}$ heterogeneous, CD117$^{-/+}$ dim, HLADR$^{-/+}$ dim, CD11b$^-$, low levels of CD15 and frequent coexpression of the T-lineage marker CD2 with myeloid markers CD13+ (heterogeneous) and CD33+ (homogeneous) [7].

An atypical form (called M3 variant or hypogranular form), usually associated with peripheral hyperleukocytosis, is observed in 10–20% and is characterized by paucity or absence of granules, but a prominently bilobed nuclear shape. Careful examination often finds a few cells with several Auer rods.

Cytogenetics and molecular biology

t(15;17)(q22;q12) translocation is observed in more than 95% of the cases, leading to fusion of the retinoic acid receptor alpha (*RARα*) gene on chromosome 17q12 to the promyelocytic leukemia (*PML*) gene on chromosome 15q22, and to a fusion mRNA and chimeric protein PML-RAR, with three different breakpoints at the mRNA level (Bcr1, 2, and 3) (Figure 8.1, showing the typical t(15;17) translocation and different *PML-RARα* breakpoints).

Molecular analysis is mandatory to confirm the presence of the specific PML-RARα fusion and char-

acterize its isoform, especially for subsequent molecular monitoring of minimal residual disease (MRD) during treatment.

Three other different and very rare gene rearrangements can be observed, fusing (very rarely) *RARα* to promyelocytic leukemia zinc finger (*PLZF*, located in 11q23), or (quite exceptionally) *RARα* to nucleophosmin (*NPM*, located in 5q35), or nuclear matrix associated (*NuMA*, located in 11q13) genes.

Confirmation of genetic diagnosis should be performed on leukemia cells from bone marrow (BM). FISH analysis, which can be useful in case of conventional cytogenetic failure, is also preferably performed in BM samples, as is RT-PCR analysis of *PML-RARα* although the fusion transcript is usually readily detectable in peripheral blood (PB).

FLT3 internal tandem duplications are seen in one-third of the cases and are generally associated, in APL, with a higher WBC count, so that they do not add important independent prognostic information to WBC count and currently do not influence management [8, 9].

Molecular pathogenesis

The origin of APL is a balanced reciprocal translocation, t(15;17)(q22;q11-12), leading to a fusion

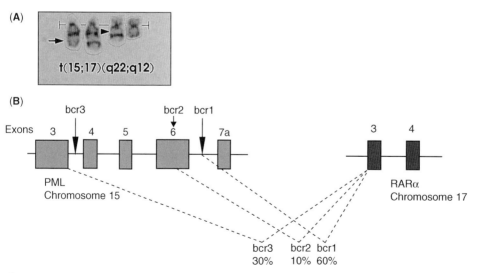

Figure 8.1 Cytogenetics and molecular biology of APL. (A) Conventional cytogenetic with typical t(15;17); (B) different *PML-RARα* breakpoints.

of the promyelocytic leukemia gene (*PML*) on chromosome 15 and the retinoic acid receptor-alpha (*RAR*α) on chromosome 17 [3]. In rare cases, alternative chromosomal translocations generate RARα fusion proteins in which PML is replaced with PLZF, nuclear mitotic apparatus (NUMA), NPM, or signal transducer and activator of transcription 5B (STAT5B) [87].

RARα is a member of the RA nuclear receptor family that acts as ligand-inducible transcription factor by binding to specific response elements (RARE) at the promoter region of target genes. In the absence of ligand, RARα forms heterodimers with the retinoid X receptor (RXR) and recruits a co-repressor complex (CoR) containing Daxx and mSin3A and HDAC activities that induce chromatin condensation and transcriptional repression. Physiological concentrations of RA (1×10^9 M) are able to release the nuclear co-repressors complex from the RAR-RXR and recruit coactivators with HAT activities. This results in hyperacetylation of histones at RARE sites, chromatin remodeling, and transcriptional activation of RARα target genes [88, 89].

PML belongs to a family of proteins containing a distinctive C3HC4 zinc-binding domain referred to as RING finger. PML controls p53-dependent induction of apoptosis, growth suppression, and cellular senescence in response to ionizing radiation and oncogenic transformation. Moreover, PML is required for transcriptional repression mediated by other tumor suppressors such as Rb and Mad [90, 91].

The fusion transcript of PML-RARα is able to form dimers with PML, RXR or another PML-RARα forming a chimeric protein.

The generation of PML–RARα has several effects: firstly, PML-RARα has a higher affinity than wild-type RARα for HDACs, so unphysiologically high doses of ATRA are needed to dissociate the HDAC-containing corepressor complex from PML-RARα (pharmacological doses of ATRA of 10–6 M) [92].

Secondly, as PML-RARα oligomers/dimers bind to retinoid response elements, they act as dominant silencing transcription factors that repress transcription activation mediated by the RAR-RXR hetero-

dimer, which is still produced from the intact *RARα* allele [93, 94].

Thirdly, in order to recruit HDAC activity, PML-RARα is also able to bind the DNA methylating enzymes Dnmt1 and Dnmt3a, leading to the methylation of RA target promoters in APL blasts [95, 96].

Finally, PML function is also disrupted by PML-RARα interactions with the PML expressed from the intact allele, causing nuclear bodies to disintegrate, and leading to the relocalization of nuclear body proteins in aberrant nuclear structures [97, 98].

In patients with the variant t(11;17) leading to the PLZF/RARα fusion, an additional co-repressor complex binding site is present in the PLZF moiety, accounting for stronger transcription repression and resistance to pharmacologic doses of RA. In these cases, HDAC inhibitors have proven effective to restore sensitivity to retinoic acid *in vitro* [99, 100].

Coagulopathy

APL patients can develop fatal hemorrhage during diagnostic evaluation, even before beginning antileukemic therapy or during the first days of induction. It has been published that as many as 3% of APL patients might die of hemorrhage before the onset of therapy [10]. The coagulation/bleeding syndrome at the onset of APL is a complex disorder that combines disseminated intravascular coagulation (DIC), fibrinolysis, and a more general proteolysis. DIC involves the rapid consumption of coagulation factors and platelets and an intravascular clotting activation. Biological clotting tests reveal hypofibrinogenemia, increased fibrinogen-fibrin degradation products (FDP), and prolonged prothrombin and thrombin times. When cytotoxic chemotherapy was the only treatment available, coagulation parameters usually worsened when it was started, resulting in severe hemorrhagic complications. On the contrary, ATRA rapidly improves the hemostatic laboratory parameters and bleeding complications and should, therefore, be started as soon as the diagnosis of APL is suspected upon morphologic examination, without waiting for genetic confirmation of diagnosis.

Prognostic factors in APL

Pretreatment factors associated with a higher risk of relapse include high WBC counts, FAB M3v morphology, presence of the short bcr3 transcript, CD2 and CD34 expression, FLT3 internal tandem duplication and slow and incomplete *in vitro* differentiation of blasts with ATRA [11–16] (Plate 8.1 illustrates a case of APL with rapid and complete differentiation, and one with slow and incomplete differentiation).

Except for slow and incomplete differentiation these parameters are generally correlated to high WBC counts. The Sanz's score is a predictive model that distinguishes three groups for relapse risk based on patient leukocyte and platelet counts at diagnosis: low-risk patients with a WBC count less than 10 g/L and a platelet count greater than 40 g/L; intermediate-risk patients had a WBC count less than 10 g/L and a platelet count less than 40 g/L; and high-risk patients had a WBC count greater than 10 g/L [17]. For therapeutic purposes, low- and intermediate-risk groups are often combined, individualizing the high-risk group characterized by WBC >10g/L that carries a greater risk of early death and relapse. However, some therapeutic improvements in APL have particularly benefited patients with high WBC counts, and, in very recent experiences, their prognosis now appears almost identical to that of patients with lower WBC counts [18].

The major prognostic factor of relapse during or after treatment is the amount of fusion *PML-RARα* mRNA transcript determined by RT-PCR in bone marrow cells, more and more often using a quantitative method [19–23]. However, kinetics of the disappearance of the *PML-RARα* transcript depends upon the sensitivity of the RT-PCR method used. Persistent positivity after consolidation treatment or later on, or a switch to positivity in patients who were negative using low-sensitivity methods (sensitivity of 10^{-3} to 10^{-4}) indicate probable relapse in the following few weeks or months. On the other hand, very sensitive quantitative methods require interpretation based on the detection limit and all for repeated examinations to assess the increase, stability, or decrease of the abnormal signal during follow-up.

First-line treatment of APL

Background: ATRA combined with anthracycline-based chemotherapy in the treatment of newly diagnosed APL

Before the advent of all-trans retinoic acid (ATRA), APL was treated exclusively by conventional chemotherapy using anthracycline +/− cytarabine. With this chemotherapy and intensive platelet support during induction treatment, complete remission (CR) rates of 70–80% were obtained, and about 40% of the patients who achieved CR could be cured of their disease with consolidation chemotherapy, that is, more than any other types of AML [24].

ATRA can differentiate APL blasts both *in vitro* and *in vivo* (Plate 8.1). With ATRA treatment alone, 85–90% of newly diagnosed APL cases can obtain CR, through differentiation of APL blasts into mature granulocytes [24–28]. In addition, ATRA rapidly improves the biological signs of APL coagulopathy. However, in some cases, ATRA also leads to major blood hyperleukocytosis and potentially fatal "ATRA syndrome" (subsequently renamed "leukocyte activation syndrome" (LAS), as it can also be observed with arsenic derivatives). Furthermore, almost all patients relapse unless they receive consolidation chemotherapy. Those findings rapidly lead clinical groups to combine ATRA and classical anthracycline-AraC chemotherapy in the treatment of newly diagnosed APL, in order to reduce the incidence and severity of ATRA syndrome and the incidence of relapse. Many trials, including two randomized trials performed in the 1990s (European APL 91 trial, and a US Intergroup trial), clearly showed that ATRA followed by two to three anthracycline-AraC chemotherapy cycles could reduce the incidence of relapse from 50% with chemotherapy alone to about 25%, while slightly increasing the CR rate from 80% to about 90% [29, 30].

This means, however, that about 10 % of the patients still did not achieve CR, and that about 25 % relapsed with a regimen (combining ATRA and several courses of anthracycline-AraC) that was associated with important myelosuppression, and about 5 % mortality in CR (up to 15–20% in elderly patients). Failure to achieve CR was mainly due to

In vitro differenciation of APL blast cultured with ATRA
0.1 µM during 4-6 days

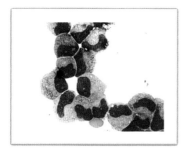

Courtesy of Bruno Cassinat

Low differenciation   High differenciation

Plate 8.1 *In vitro* differentiation of APL blast cultured with ATRA 0.1µM over four to six days. Image courtesy of Bruno Cassinat.

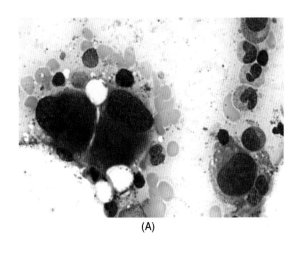

(A)

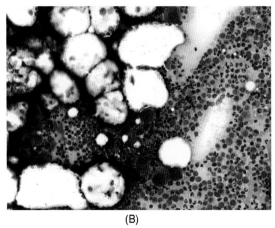

(B)

Plate 10.1 Myelodysplastic syndrome subcategory: 5q minus syndrome. Deletion of a specific portion of the long arm of chromosome 5 results in an important subtype of MDS defined by specific clinico-pathogical findings as well as a defined clinical treatment. Del 5q MDS involves loss of the region within the bands q21 through q32. This subcategory of MDS is characterized clinically by refractory anemia, normal to increased platelets and a relatively prolonged clinical course. Further, pathological characteristics revolve around classical dysplasia in the myeloid and erythroid lineages (A). Additionally, consistent across many Del5q syndromes there is evidence of dysplastic (hypolobulated) megakaryocytes (B) within the bone marrow, and less than 5% myeloblasts. Images courtesy of Lynn Moscinski.

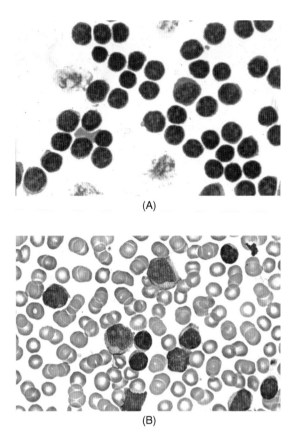

Plate 13.1 (A) A leucapheresis sample from a patient with CLL. Note the monomorphic small lymphocytes with dark condensed chromatin in the nuclei and minimal cytoplasm. Smudge cells are present in this and in (B) which also shows an admixture of prolymphocytes with prominent nucleoli.

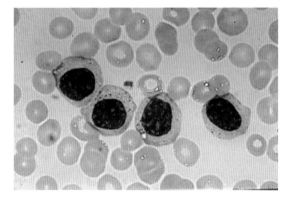

Plate 15.1 Peripheral blood smear in a case of LGL leukemia (Wright-Giemsa, 1000x), displaying circulating large granular lymphocytes characterized by abundant cytoplasm with azurophilic granules.

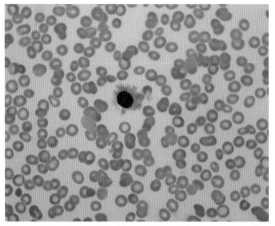

Plate 16.1 Classic hairy cell with a round nucleus, partially condensed chromatin, small nucleolus, and ample rim of blue, agranular cytoplasm with frayed margins (Wright-Giemsa, 1000x).

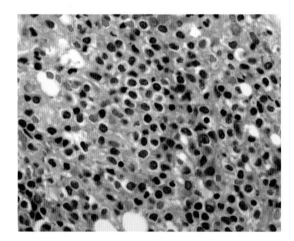

Plate 16.2 Typical histologic appearance of hairy cell leukemia characterized by a monotonous population of lymphoid cells with abundant cytoplasm imparting a well-spaced appearance to the centrally placed nuclei (H&E, 400x).

bleeding (principally in the CNS), infection or LAS rather than leukemic failure, extremely rare (about 1 in 500 cases in confirmed cases of APL.)

Optimization of first-line APL treatment in the late 1990s and early 2000s

The following years were, therefore, used to improve results obtained with this ATRA and anthracycline-based chemotherapy "backbone". Many experiences have reported that early addition of chemotherapy to ATRA, optimal prevention and treatment of LAS, intensive treatment of coagulopathy, and maintenance treatment could further reduce early mortality and the incidence of relapses, while reduction of the intensity of chemotherapy (by the possible avoidance of AraC in most cases) has reduced treatment toxicity. Finally, the most recent years have been characterized by introduction of arsenic derivatives in the first-line treatment of APL by several groups.

With those improvements, reported CR rates are now closer to 95% than 90%, relapse rates have dropped to less than 10% (although they remain a little higher in patients with high WBC counts) and mortality in CR has also diminished, giving the hope that APL may now be cured in the vast majority of cases.

Role of early addition of chemotherapy to ATRA

It has been clearly shown that treatment with ATRA combined with intensive chemotherapy gave better results than intensive chemotherapy alone in newly diagnosed APL, and suspected that ATRA should be started immediately after APL diagnosis. The effectiveness of administration of chemotherapy after or concomitantly with ATRA was uncertain.

Results of a trial randomizing ATRA followed by chemotherapy and ATRA with early addition of chemotherapy (on day 3 of ATRA treatment) in APL with WBC counts below 10g/L showed similar CR rates, but a strong trend for few relapses (21.6% vs. 13.2% at 10 years; p = 0.09) in patients who had early addition of chemotherapy. Early addition of chemotherapy also reduced the incidence of LAS, one of the persisting causes of failure to achieve CR

in APL [31]. In patients with WBC >10g/L, rapid addition of chemotherapy to ATRA appears particularly recommended to avoid the risk of severe LAS [18].

Prophylaxis and treatment of the leukocyte differentiation or activation syndrome (LAS), and other side effects of ATRA

LAS was first described with ATRA [32], but is also seen with arsenic derivatives [101]. Its pathophysiology remains uncertain, but probably includes the release of various cytokines by differentiating leukocytes. Induction of interleukin (IL)-1 alpha and G-CSF secretion by APL cells under ATRA treatment may contribute to hyperleukocytosis *in vivo*, while the secretion of IL-1 alpha, IL-6, tumor necrosis factor (TNF) alpha, and IL-8 – which are involved in leukocyte activation and adherence, and are implicated in the development of adult respiratory distress syndrome (ARDS) – could play a pathogenetic role in LAS [77, 78]. More recently, it has been shown that ATRA induced aggregation of NB4 cells (an APL cell line). This process was mediated by the adhesion molecule lymphocyte function-associated antigen 1 (LFA-1) and intercellular adhesion molecule 2 (ICAM-2) and was reversed by addition of methylprednisolone [79]. These findings suggest that modification of the adhesive properties of APL cells by ATRA could play a role in LAS.

Diagnosis of this syndrome should be clinically suspected in the presence of one of the following symptoms and signs: dyspnea, unexplained fever, weight gain, peripheral edema, unexplained hypotension, acute renal failure, or congestive heart failure, and particularly by a chest radiograph demonstrating interstitial pulmonary infiltrates, or pleuropericardial effusion. Those symptoms are not pathognomonic of the syndrome, as in this context they could be due to bacteremia, sepsis, fungal infection, or congestive heart failure. Incidence of LAS ranges from 10–15% in different series [33, 34]. Symptoms generally occur around 7 and 11 days after drug onset and are generally, but not always, preceded by an increase of WBC. In some cases, LAS occurs very early or, on the contrary, at the time of recovery from aplasia in patients treated with ATRA who received early intensive chemotherapy. LAS is fatal in 5–15 % of the cases. In addition, its occurrence is associated with an increased risk of subsequent relapse [35]. As said above, in our experience (APL 93 trial), early addition of chemotherapy to ATRA in newly diagnosed APL with low WBC counts significantly reduced the incidence of ATRA syndrome [36].

In APL presenting with high WBC counts, very early addition of chemotherapy to ATRA (on day 1 or 2 of ATRA treatment) is recommended by most teams to prevent a risk of severe LAS.

Specific treatment with dexamethasone at a dose of 10 mg twice daily by intravenous injection should be started promptly at the very earliest symptom or sign of LAS [37]. Temporary discontinuation of ATRA or ATO is indicated only in case of severe LAS (i.e., patients developing renal failure or requiring admission to the intensive care unit due to respiratory distress). Otherwise, these differentiating agents can generally be maintained unless progression to overt syndrome or lack of response to dexamethasone is observed. If a favorable response is obtained, dexamethasone should be maintained until complete disappearance of symptoms, and ATRA or ATO then be resumed.

While this preemptive therapy with dexamethasone currently represents a standard approach to treating patients developing LAS, there is no evidence that prophylactic corticosteroids are useful to reduce rates of morbidity and mortality associated with this syndrome. Nevertheless, in uncontrolled studies, very low mortality or morbidity due to LAS was reported following ATRA treatment when corticosteroids were administered prophylactically in patients presenting with WBC count greater than 5 to 10×10^9/L, particularly in our experience [18]. Other side effects of ATRA include dryness of lips and mucosae which is usual but reversible with symptomatic treatment. Increases in transaminases and triglycerides are common, but they have never required treatment discontinuation in our experience. Headache, due to intracranial hypertension, is generally moderate in adults, but may be severe in children and associated with signs of pseudotumor cerebri [38].

Lower ATRA doses (25 mg/m^2 per day) reduce this side effect in children and seem as effective as conventional doses of 45 mg/m^2 per day in inducing CR. Isolated fever frequently develops in the absence of other signs of ATRA syndrome (or infection) and is reversible within 48 hours of ATRA discontinuation.

A few other side effects, including bone marrow necrosis, hypercalcemia, erythema nodosum, marked basophilia, severe myositis, Sweet syndrome, Fournier's gangrene (necrotizing fasciitis of the penis and scrotum), thrombocytosis, and necrotizing vasculitis have rarely been reported with ATRA treatment [39–48].

Optimal treatment of coagulopathy

Intracerebral and pulmonary bleeding are not only the most frequent causes of death early during induction therapy, but they can also occur before the diagnosis of APL has been made and therapy started. To prevent them, supportive measures should be instituted immediately after the diagnosis of APL is suspected. ATRA should be started in order to decrease the risk of severe bleeding and before diagnosis is confirmed [49].

Supportive care consists of massive transfusion of platelets, in order to maintain a platelet count above 50 g/L whenever possible. Fresh frozen plasma and fibrinogen are advocated in case of fibrinogen level below 150 mg/dL. Monitoring is required at least once a day or more. Central venous catheterization, lumbar puncture, and other invasive procedures (e. g., bronchoscopy) should be avoided at this stage of the treatment.

The benefit of heparin, tranexamic acid, or other anticoagulant or antifibrinolytic therapy to attenuate the hemorrhagic syndrome is unclear.

Role of maintenance treatment

Two randomized studies, the APL 93 and US Intergroup trials, showed that maintenance treatment with continuous low-dose chemotherapy (in APL 93 trial), with ATRA (in US and APL 93 trials) or both (in APL 93 trial) significantly decreased the incidence of relapse by comparison to no maintenance, with an additive effect of the two modalities in newly diagnosed APL [31, 37].

Patients with high WBC seemed to particularly benefit from maintenance in APL 93 trial. In patients with WBC>5 g/L, the relapse rate dropped from 64.5% % with no maintenance to 20.5% with combined (ATRA + chemotherapy) maintenance. Interestingly, the effect of the low-dose chemotherapy component of maintenance treatment seemed even more important than that of maintenance ATRA. Long-term results in APL 93 also showed significantly more relapse in patients who discontinued maintenance treatment before one year (for reasons other than relapse) compared to patients who received longer maintenance.

Role of AraC

Classical consolidation chemotherapy cycles combining an anthracycline and AraC are associated with about a 5% mortality in younger adults, which can however reach 15–20% in elderly patients. Further improvement in the outcome of APL would require reduction of this mortality in CR, especially through reduction of the intensity of consolidation chemotherapy. In this perspective, a major attempt has been to avoid AraC during consolidation chemotherapy courses.

Before the ATRA era, a few studies had suggested that chemotherapy with an anthracycline alone, especially idarubicin, provided it was given at relatively high dose, gave similar results as anthracycline-AraC regimens [102, 103].

Since the advent of ATRA, the Spanish PETHEMA group reported the largest experience of ATRA + anthracycline alone chemotherapy in APL patients in two successive trials (LPA 96 and 99 trials) [50, 51]. The induction regimen consisted of ATRA and idarubicin ($12 \, mg/m^2$ x 4) followed by three consolidation courses with idarubicin or mitoxantrone (with ATRA in patients at intermediate or high risk of relapse), and a two-year maintenance combining low-dose 6MP + MTX chemotherapy and ATRA. Those consolidation chemotherapy courses with an anthracycline alone could generally be administered on an outpatient basis and were associated with low morbidity and no mortality. Five-year cumulative incidence of relapse and disease-free were 11% and 84%, respectively. Nevertheless, in patients with WBC>10 g/L and WBC>50 g/L, the five-year cumulative incidence of relapse was 23% and 34% respectively.

In order to confirm those results in a randomized trial, the APL 2000 trial (conducted by the European APL group) randomized, in patients aged ≤60 years with WBC<10 g/L, to either the best treatment group of the APL 93 trial (ATRA with early introduction of anthracycline-AraC chemotherapy – "AraC group"), followed by two consolidation anthracycline-AraC courses and maintenance combining continuous chemotherapy and intermittent ATRA, to the same regimen, but without AraC ("No AraC group"). In the AraC and the no AraC group, respectively, the CR rate was 99% versus 94% (p = 0.066), the two-year cumulative incidence of relapse (CIR) was 4.7% versus 15.9% (p = 0.011), and survival was 97.9% versus 89.6% (p = 0.0066). Those results suggested that, in patients with WBC<10 g/L, that is, at low risk of relapse, using anthracycline alone for chemotherapy instead of the classical anthracycline-AraC combination could lead to an increased risk of relapse. Discrepancies between our results and those of the PETHEMA group studies could be due to the higher cumulative dose of anthracycline administered in the Spanish studies or to a superiority of idarubicin (used in the Spanish trial) over daunorubicin (used in European and US Intergroup trials) in APL. Thus, substituting idarubicin for daunorubicin during induction and consolidation treatment could improve long-term results in APL. Finally, using ATRA during the consolidation course, as in the LPA 99 trial, may have had a positive impact on the risk of relapse.

To better understand those discrepancies, a joint analysis was performed in younger patients included in the Spanish PETHEMA LPA 99 (without AraC) and APL 2000 (with AraC) studies. In low- and intermediate-risk patients, the CR rates, two-year CIR, EFS, and survival were not significantly different in the LPA 99 and APL 2000 trials. In high-risk patients, the CR rate was significantly better in patients included in the APL 2000 trial and the cumulative incidence of relapse was significantly lower than in patient treated in LPA 99 [54].

This analysis suggests than in patients with WBC<10 g/L, the current PETHEMA approach is not associated with more relapses than a classical ATRA + DNR + AraC regimen, while being clearly less myelosuppressive. It also strongly suggests that, if one uses an anthracycline alone, daunorubicin should not be substituted for idarubicin, as it may be less effective in APL. In patients with high WBC counts, APL 2000 results yielded better EFS and survival and a strong trend for fewer relapses than PETHEMA results, suggesting a beneficial role for AraC, possibly at high dose, in this subset of patients [55]. Italian GIMEMA group and German group results, although they were not randomized, also strongly support a role for AraC in reducing the relapse rate in APL with WBC counts greater than 10 g/L [52, 53]. In the ongoing Spanish PETHEMA LPA 2005 trial, which now includes AraC during consolidation in patients with high WBC counts, a great reduction in the risk of relapse has been observed in this subset of patients (Sanz, November 2008, personal communication). As shown below, it is currently being investigated whether arsenic derivatives could be substituted for AraC in this situation.

Role of arsenic derivatives

Arsenic trioxide, the most used arsenic derivative administered in APL, is the treatment of choice for relapsing APL. It is not, in particular, associated with toxicities commonly observed with anthracycline-based chemotherapy, especially myelosuppression (see treatment of relapses). Those results led investigators from China, Iran, India, and from the Western world countries to assess the role of ATO in newly diagnosed APL, either in addition to ATRA and anthracycline-based chemotherapy, particularly in cases with an increased risk of relapse (mainly patients with high WBC counts), or in order to reduce the amount of chemotherapy administered, and even in some cases avoiding any concomitant chemotherapy [56–58].

Using the first approach, a Chinese trial randomized newly diagnosed APL patients for induction between ATRA alone, ATO alone, and the combination of both. Patients who achieved CR then received anthracycline-based consolidation chemotherapy. The CR rate was the same in each of the three treatment arms, but decrease of the fusion transcript was faster and, more importantly, the incidence of relapse significantly lower in patients treated with the ATRA-ATO combination upfront [56]. A US Intergroup trial evaluated the benefit of two additional courses of ATO as first post-remission therapy in a standard treatment based on ATRA and anthracycline-AraC chemotherapy. Three-year EFS was 77% in the ATO arm compared to 59% in the standard arm, and three-year OS was 86% in the ATO arm compared to 77% in the standard arm. The benefit of the addition of two courses of ATO consolidation following remission induction was particularly important in patients presenting with high WBC counts [104].

In the second approach, ATO was used alone or with limited ATRA and chemotherapy. In an Indian trial, patients received ATO as single agent for induction and one consolidation course of 28 days, followed by maintenance courses of 10 days/month for 6 months. The complete remission rate was 86% and the three-year DFS and OS were 87% and 86% respectively [58].

Similar results, but with a higher relapse rate (40% vs. 15%), were observed in an Iranian trial that used the same approach of induction and one consolidation course of ATO alone, but without maintenance treatment. The M.D. Anderson group also reported on 44 patients who received ATO and ATRA for induction (associated with gemtuzumab ozogamycin (GO) in high-risk patients) with 89% CR (all with molecular CR) [59]. In low- and intermediate-risk patients, the CR rate was 96%. Very few relapses (exclusively in high-risk patients) were seen with ATRA-ATO maintenance.

Those reports were impressive, as they constituted the first demonstration that a leukemia could be cured without any chemotherapy. On the other hand, those experiences with ATO as a single agent during induction treatment of APL generally reported relatively high incidences of LAS, sometimes fatal. The risk may even be higher if ATRA is combined to ATO upfront. This complication could probably be avoided by early introduction of chemotherapy or GO, as reported by the M.D. Anderson group [61]. However, given the very high CR rates obtained with ATRA-anthracycline-based chemotherapy, now about 95 % in most trials, we feel that induction protocols without chemotherapy (i.e., with ATO alone or with ATO combined to ATRA) need to be validated in large multicenter trials before they can be recommended outside of specialized centers.

Central nervous system (CNS) prophylaxis

The CNS is the most common site of extramedullary disease in APL [60]. In the European and PETHEMA group experience, 10 of 169 of the relapses observed were extramedullary, mainly in the CNS (n = 9) and, less often, the skin (n = 1). In eight of the cases, the marrow was also involved by the relapse, with the presence of blasts in seven but only marrow relapse in one. Patients with CNS relapse were characterized by younger age, higher WBC count, and treatment without high-dose AraC [61]. Prognosis was poor, with a median survival of 13 months. Because the majority of CNS relapses occurred in patients presenting with hyperleukocytosis, some groups, including ours, include CNS prophylaxis for patients presenting with high WBC counts. This involves using intrathecal MTX + AraC and/or systemic high-dose AraC, although the benefit of this policy has not been established in prospective studies. Intrathecal therapy, in addition, should not be performed during induction treatment due to the bleeding risk, but started only during consolidation treatment.

In patients without hyperleukocytosis, in whom the risk of CNS relapse is extremely low, there is a general consensus to avoid CNS prophylaxis. Finally, preliminary findings suggest that ATO may cross the blood-brain barrier, further supporting its wider use during consolidation first-line treatment of APL [62].

Molecular and cytogenetic evaluation

The molecular status at the end of induction has no predictive value on patient outcome even using low-sensitivity methods (i.e., with the detection threshold between 10^{-3} and 10^{-4}) [63]. After consolidation treatment, molecular evaluation of MRD performed on bone marrow cells using low-sensitivity methods is well correlated to the risk of relapse. Patients with persistent MRD at the end of consolidation using such low-sensitivity methods should be considered for further treatment instead of only mainte-

nance [80]. Of note is that blood analysis is generally less sensitive than marrow analysis, poorly correlated with marrow results and cannot be recommended routinely. Because molecular detection of PML-RAR alpha fusion transcript is well correlated to the risk of relapse, molecular remission as well as molecular relapse have recently been incorporated in response criteria in APL [64]. During maintenance and follow-up in patients with undetectable MRD, conversion to MRD positivity is associated with generally rapid hematologic relapse [81], leading more and more groups to treat those patients without waiting for marrow relapse [82].

Patients at higher risk of relapse (i.e., patients with WBC>10 g/L at diagnosis) should be closely monitored, at least five to six times/year during the first year and every three months during the second and third year. The monitoring of patients at low risk of relapse is nowadays a question of debate. Finally, quantitative RT-PCR techniques (RQ-PCR) are increasingly being used in APL, and efforts are being made to reach consensus on technical approaches [21]. The kinetics of evolution of the fusion transcript may sometimes give more adequate and/or rapid information than the positive versus negative information provided by qualitative PCR. However, the clinical advantage of RQ-PCR over those classical techniques needs to be more firmly determined.

Treatment of relapsing APL

Induction treatment

Arsenic derivatives

Arsenic derivatives, especially ATO, currently constitute the reference induction treatment of APL in first relapse (or subsequent relapses in patients who have not received arsenic derivatives).

ATO induces 80–90 % of second hematological CR, associated with molecular CR after two cycles in most cases (contrary to what is achieved with ATRA alone) [69]. ATO may act on APL cells through several modes of action including induction of differentiation and/or apoptosis, growth inhibition, and angiogenesis inhibition. Like ATRA, ATO triggers the degradation of the PML-RARa fusion protein, but contrary to ATRA, ATO targets the PML part rather than the RARa part of this fusion protein. The safety profile of ATO compares favorably with the safety profile of intensive salvage chemotherapy particularly without profound cytopenia and cardiac failure [65]. Treatment with ATO is associated with electrolyte abnormalities and prolongation of the QT interval which require careful monitoring. Maintenance of the serum potassium above 4.0 mmol/L and serum magnesium above 0.82 mmol/L, well above the lower limit of normal, is mandatory to avoid a risk of cardiac arrythmias, the most severe being *torsades de pointe*. Medications that may cause prolonged QTc interval have to be stopped. If the QTc interval is prolonged longer than 500 milliseconds, ATO should be discontinued. ATO also carries the risk of LAS; however, this is generally less important in relapse than in newly diagnosed patients. If a major increase in WBC counts is seen, preventive and therapeutic measures could be rapidly taken as for first-line treatment.

Other induction treatments of relapse

Even before the ATO era, relatively high rates of second CR could be obtained with intensive anthracycline-based chemotherapy or, in patients who had not received ATRA within a few months of relapse, with ATRA-chemotherapy combinations. This treatment was associated, however, with major toxicity and poorer results of subsequent allogeneic stem cell transplantation (STC) [70].

Preliminary results indicate that GO might be a promising agent in APL patients, particularly in the case of molecular relapse [66]. The M.D. Anderson group also reported interesting results with GO in consolidation with ATO and ATRA after ATO induction in first relapse [59].

Tamibarotène (Am80) is a new synthetic retinoid approximately 10 times more potent than ATRA as an *in vitro* differentiation inducer. This drug is potentially capable of overcoming resistance to ATRA due to its hypermetabolism. In a Japanese trial, it resulted in 58% CR in patient that had relapsed from CR induced by ATRA. However, because all those patients had discontinued ATRA for at least 18 months, it is unclear whether Am80 was superior to

ATRA in this situation, and whether it would be able to overcome resistance to ATRA [67].

It is finally unclear, with the probable exception of GO, if those approaches can be effective in patients who have already received ATO, especially in first relapse.

Consolidation/maintenance treatment

At least two, and sometimes three cycles of ATO (i.e., at least one induction course and one or two consolidation courses, 5 days x 5 weeks) are generally required to achieve molecular remission in relapsing APL. Once this has been obtained, consolidation with autologous or allogeneic STC is strongly recommended to obtain sustained second CR [65]. Because it is associated with few relapses (if stem cells are collected after molecular CR has been achieved) and low toxicity, autologous STC is increasingly advocated at the expense of allogeneic STC. Reaching molecular CR may, however, sometimes require consolidation chemotherapy or GO in addition to ATO before stem cell collection [68]. If molecular CR cannot be obtained, and probably also in younger patients (less than 30 years perhaps), allogeneic SCT should be preferred to autologous SCT. In patients who can be neither allogeneic nor autografted, maintenance treatment should use variable combinations of ATRA, ATO, anthracyclines with or without Ara-C, GO, and maintenance with 6-mercaptopurine and methotrexate, depending in particular on what the patient received before relapse.

The improvement in the treatment of relapsing APL is stressed by results of our group, with a two-year survival of 77% in relapsing APL patients salvaged by ATO (and consolidated by allo, auto or various maintenance regimens), as compared to 51% in a similar population treated before the arsenic era [69].

Treatment in elderly patients and in children

APL in the elderly

As mentioned above, APL is relatively uncommon in older patients, as only 20% of APL patients are aged more than 60. Elderly APL patients are more likely to present with low-risk features than younger patients [71]. In our experience (APL 93 trial) the CR rate was 94% under 60 years compared to 85% after 70 years [72], the difference being exclusively due to a higher incidence of early deaths in older patients, as those patients, like younger ones, had no case of resistant leukemia. The relapse rate was not higher in elderly patients compared to younger adults, but the mortality rate in CR was 19% in patients older than 70 years, mainly due to sepsis secondary to neutropenia [72]. Reducing the intensity of consolidation therapy in elderly patients is, therefore, of utmost importance. The PETHEMA group reported, with their regimen devoid of AraC, a six-year cumulative incidence of relapse of 8.5% in elderly consolidated without AraC, with less than 8.2 % mortality in CR [71].

The intensity of consolidation chemotherapy can probably be even further decreased by using ATO during consolidation courses. On the other hand, as said above for all patients, caution must be exercised during induction treatment if one is to use ATO $+/-$ ATRA without chemotherapy, due to the risk of severe LAS, particularly in this fragile population [59].

APL in children

APL is also rare in children. Compared to the disease in adults, APL in childhood more frequently presents with hyperleukocytosis (approximately 40% in children vs. 20–25% in adults) [73]. The therapeutic strategy in children has generally been similar to that in adults, combining ATRA and chemotherapy [73, 84–86]. Due to the frequent occurrence of headaches, and even clinical features of pseudointracranial hypertension, however, reduced doses of ATRA (i.e., 25 mg/m/d) are often used either systematically or only (and we would favor this latter approach in order to maximize the quantity of ATRA administered) if those symptoms occur [76].

Some attempts have been made to reduce the cumulative dose of anthracyclines in children, because of their potential long-term cardiac toxicity. Preliminary analysis of the US Intergroup study of children treated with ATRA and reduced dose intensity of anthracycline-based chemotherapy have not been encouraging, however [83]. Although ATO

also appears to be effective in pediatric APL [74] there is only very limited experience of this agent in children with newly diagnosed APL, possibly due to the concerns of pediatricians about using a drug with potential long-term side effects [75].

Conclusion

With protocols combining ATRA and idarubicin, intensive supportive care during induction treatment (especially platelet transfusions) and prolonged maintenance, more than 95% of APL patients with WBC counts below 10000/mm^3 reach CR, with less than 10% relapse. Patients with higher WBC counts maintain an early death risk close to 10%, which can be further reduced by rapid introduction of chemotherapy and particularly intensive platelet support. In those patients, AraC or possibly ATO (in addition to maintenance) should be added to idarubicin in order to reduce the relapse rate (to probably no more than 10%). ATO, which remains the gold standard for relapse, can be used during first-line treatment in addition to chemotherapy in order to reduce the relapse risk (in patients with high WBC counts) or, to some extent, be substituted for chemotherapy (in elderly or frail patients) mainly during the consolidation period. On the other hand, we believe that its place during first-line induction treatment has to be further validated in multicenter trials, due in particular to the risk of LAS. Finally, due to the drug armamentarium we have, allogeneic or autologous SCT are now very generally restricted to the consolidation treatment of first relapse.

References

1 Hillestad LK. (1957) Acute promyelocytic leukemia. *Acta Med Scand* **159**:189–94.

2 Rowley JD, Golomb HM, Repp R, et al. (1977) 15/17 translocation, a consistent chromosomal change in acute promyelocytic leukemia. *Lancet* **1**:549–50.

3 De The H, Lavau C, Marchio A. et al. (1991) The PML RAR alpha fusion mRNA generated by the t(15, 17) translocation in acute promyelocytic leukemia encodes a functionally altered RAR. *Cell* **66**:675–84.

4 Ribeiro RC, Rego E. (2006) Management of APL in developing countries: epidemiology, challenges and opportunities for international collaboration. *Hematology (Am Soc Hematol Educ Program)* **2006**:162–8.

5 Beaumont M, Sanz M, Carli PM et al. (2003) Therapy related acute promyelocytic leukemia. A report on 106 cases. *J Clin Oncol* **21**:2123–37.

6 Vickers M, Jackson G, Taylor P. (2000) The incidence of acute promyelocytic leukemia appears constant over most of a human lifespan, implying only one rate limiting mutation. *Leukemia* **14**:722–6.

7 Orfao A, Ortuño F, de Santiago M, Lopez A, San Miguel JF. (2004) Immunophenotyping of acute leukemias and myelodysplastic syndromes. *Cytometry* **58A**:62–71.

8 Callens C, Chevret S, Cayuela JM, et al. (2005) Prognostic implication of FLT3 and Ras gene mutations in patients with acute promyelocytic leukemia (APL): a retrospective study from the European APL Group. *Leukemia* **19**:1153–60.

9 Gale RE, Hills R, Pizzey AR, et al. (2005) Relationship between FLT3 mutation status, biologic characteristics, and response to targeted therapy in acute promyelocytic leukemia. *Blood* **106**:3768–76.

10 De la Serna J, Montesinos P, Vellenga E, et al. (2008) Causes and prognostic factors of remission induction failure in patients with acute promyelocytic leukemia treated with all-trans retinoic acid and idarubicin. *Blood* **111**:3395–402.

11 Asou N, Adachi K, Tamura J, et al. (1998) Analysis of prognostic factors in newly diagnosed acute promyelocytic leukemia treated with all-trans retinoic acid and chemotherapy. *Japan Adult Leukemia Study Group. J Clin Oncol* **16**:78–85.

12 Claxton DF, Reading CL, Nagarajan L, et al. (1992) Correlation of CD2 expression with PML gene breakpoints in patients with acute promyelocytic leukemia. *Blood* **80**:582–6.

13 Paietta E, Andersen J, Gallagher R, et al. (1994) The immunophenotype of acute promyelocytic leukemia (APL): an ECOG study. *Leukemia* **8**:1108–12.

14 Guglielmi C, Martelli MP, Diverio D, et al. (1998) Immunophenotype of adult and childhood acute promyelocytic leukaemia correlation with morphology, type of PML gene breakpoint and clinical outcome. A cooperative Italian study on 196 cases. *Br J Haematol* **102**:1035–41.

15 Murray CK, Estey E, Paietta E, et al. (1999) CD56 expression in acute promyelocytic leukemia: a possible indicator of poor treatment outcome? *J Clin Oncol* **17**:293–7.

16 Cassinat B, Chevret S, Zassadowski F, et al (2001) In vitro all-trans retinoic acid sensitivity of acute promyelocytic leukemia blasts: a novel indicator of poor patient outcome. *Blood* **98**:2862–4.

17 Sanz MA, Lo Coco F, Martin G, et al. (2000) Definition of relapse risk and role of non anthracycline drugs for consolidation in patients with acute promyelocytic leukemia: a joint study of the PETHEMA and GIMEMA cooperative groups. *Blood* **96**:1247–53.

18 Kelaidi C, Chevret S, De Botton S, et al. (2009) Improved outcome of acute promyelocytic leukemia with high WBC counts over the last 15 years: the European APL group experience. *J Clin Oncol* **27**:2668–76.

19 Jurcic JG, Nimer SD, Scheinberg DA, et al. (2001) Prognostic significance of minimal residual disease detection and PML/RAR-α isoform type: long-term follow-up in acute promyelocytic leukemia. *Blood* **98**:2651–6.

20 Diverio D, Rossi V, Avvisati G, et al. (1998) Early detection of relapse by prospective reverse transcriptase-polymerase chain reaction analysis of the PML/RAR alpha fusion gene in patients with acute promyelocytic leukemia enrolled in the GIMEMA-AIEOP multicenter "AIDA" trial. GIMEMA AIEOP Multicenter "AIDA" Trial. *Blood* **92**:784–9.

21 Cassinat B, Zassadowski F, Balitrand N, et al. (2000) Quantitation of minimal residual disease in acute promyelocytic leukemia patients with t(15;17) translocation using real-time RTPCR. *Leukemia* **14**:324–8.

22 Visani G, Buonamici S, Malagola M, et al. (2000) Pulsed ATRA as single therapy restores long term remission PML-RAR alpha-positive acute promyelocytic leukemia patient real time quantification of minimal residual disease. A pilot study. *Leukemia* **15**:1696–700.

23 Gallagher RE, Yeap BY, Bi W, et al (2003) Quantitative real-time RT-PCR analysis of PML-RAR alpha mRNA in acute promyelocytic leukemia: assessment of prognostic significance in adult patients from intergroup protocol 0129. *Blood* **101**:2521–8.

24 Bernard J, Weil M, Boiron M, et al. (1973) Acute promyelocytic leukemia: results of treatment by daunorubicin. *Blood* **41**:489–96.

25 Castaigne S, Chomienne C, Daniel MT, et al. (1990) All-trans retinoic acid as a differentiation therapy for acute promyelocytic leukemias. I. Clinical results. *Blood* **76**:1704–9.

26 Degos L, Chomienne C, Daniel MT, et al. (1990) Treatment of first relapse in acute promyelocytic leukaemia with all-trans retinoic acid. *Lancet* **336**:1440–1.

27 Chen ZX, Xue YQ, Zhang R, et al. (1991) A clinical and experimental study on all-trans retinoic acid-treated acute promyelocytic leukemia patients. *Blood* **78**:1413–19.

28 Warrell R.P. Jr., Frankel SR, Miller W.H. Jr., et al. (1991) Differentiation therapy of acute promyelocytic leukemia with tretinoin (all-trans-retinoic acid). *N Engl J Med* **324**:1385–93.

29 Fenaux P, Le Deley MC, Castaigne S, et al. (1993) Effect of all-trans retinoic acid in newly diagnosed acute promyelocytic leukemia. Results of a multicenter randomized trial. European APL 91 Group. *Blood* **82**:3241–9.

30 Tallman MS, Andersen JW, Schiffer CA, et al. (1997) All-trans retinoic acid in acute promyelocytic leukemia. *N Engl J Med* **337**:1021–8.

31 Fenaux P, Chastang C, Chevret S, et al. (1999) A randomized comparison of all-trans retinoic acid (ATRA) followed by chemotherapy and ATRA plus chemotherapy and the role of maintenance therapy in newly diagnosed acute promyelocytic leukemia. The European APL Group. *Blood* **94**:1192–200.

32 Frankel SR, Eardley A, Lauwers G, et al. (1992) The "retinoic acid syndrome" in acute promyelocytic leukemia. *Ann Intern Med* **117**:292–6.

33 Kanamaru A, Takemoto Y, Tanimoto M, et al (1995) All-trans retinoic acid for the treatment of newly diagnosed acute promyelocytic leukemia. Japan Adult Leukemia Study Group. *Blood* **85**:1202–6.

34 Vahdat L, Maslak P, Miller W.H. Jr., et al. (1994) Early mortality and the retinoic acid syndrome in acute promyelocytic leukemia: impact of leukocytosis, low-dose chemotherapy, PMN/RAR-alpha isoform, and CD13 expression in patients treated with all-trans retinoic acid. *Blood* **84**:3843–9.

35 de Botton S, Dombret H, Sanz M, et al. (1998) Incidence, clinical features, and outcome of all-trans retinoic acid syndrome in 413 cases of newly diagnosed acute promyelocytic leukemia. The European APL Group. *Blood* **92**:2712–8.

36 De Botton S, Coitteux V, Chevret S, et al. (2001) Early onset chemotherapy can reduce the incidence of ATRA syndrome in newly diagnosed acute promyelocytic leukemia (APL). Results of a randomized study. *Blood* **98**:766a.

37 Tallman MS, Andersen JW, Schiffer CA, et al. (1997) All-trans retinoic acid in acute promyelocytic leukemia. *N Engl J Med* **337**:1021–8.

38 Mahmoud HH, Hurwitz CA, Roberts WM, et al. (1993) Tretinoin toxicity in children with acute promyelocytic leukaemia. *Lancet* **342**:1394–5.

39 Hakimian D, Tallman MS, Zugerman C, Caro WA. (1993) Erythema nodosum associated with all-trans retinoic acid in the treatment of acute promyelocytic leukemia. *Leukemia* **7**:758–9.

40 Koike T, Tatewaki W, Aoki A,et al (1992) Brief report: severe symptoms of hyperhistaminemia after the treatment of acute promyelocytic leukemia with tretinoin (all-trans retinoic acid). *N Engl J Med* **327**:385–7.

41 Iwakiri R, Inokuchi K, Dan K, Nomura T. (1994) Marked basophilia in acute promyelocytic leukaemia treated with all-trans retinoic acid: molecular analysis of the cell origin of the basophils. *Br J Haematol* **86**:870–2.

42 Miranda N, Oliveira P, Frade MJ, et al. (1994) Myositis with tretinoin. *Lancet* **344**:1096.

43 Tomas JF, Escudero A, Fernandez-Ranada JM. (1994) All-trans retinoic acid treatment and Sweet syndrome. *Leukemia* **8**:1596.

44 Arun B, Berberian B, Azumi N, et al. (1998) Sweet's syndrome during treatment with all-trans retinoic acid in a patient with acute promyelocytic leukemia. *Leuk Lymphoma* **31**:613–615.

45 Levy V, Jaffarbey J, Aouad K, Zittoun R. (1998) Fournier's gangrene during induction treatment of acute promyelocytic leukemia, a case report. *Ann Hematol* **76**:91–2.

46 Mori A, Tamura S, Katsuno T, et al. (1999) Scrotal ulcer occurring in patients with acute promyelocytic leukemia during treatment with all-trans retinoic acid. *Oncol Rep* **6**:55–8.

47 Kentos A, LeMoine F, Crenier L, et al. (1997) All-trans retinoic acid induced thrombocytosis in a patient with acute promyelocytic leukaemia. *Br J Haematol* **97**:685.

48 Paydas S, Sahin B, Zorludemir S, Hazar B. (1998) All-trans retinoic acid as the possible cause of necrotizing vasculitis. *Leuk Res* **22**:655–7.

49 Tapiovaara H, Matikainen S, Hurme M, Vaheri A. (1994) Induction of differentiation of promyelocytic NB4 cells by retinoic acid is associated with rapid increase in urokinase activity subsequently downregulated by production of inhibitors. *Blood* **83**:1883–91.

50 Sanz MA, Lo-Coco F. (2000) Definition of relapse risk and role of nonanthracycline drugs for consolidation in patients with acute promyelocytic leukemia: a joint study of the PETHEMA and GIMEMA cooperative groups. *Blood* **96**:1247–53.

51 Sanz A, Martin G, Gonzalez M, et al. (2004) Risk-adapted treatment of acute promyelocytic leukemia with all-trans retinoic acid and anthracycline mono-chemotherapy: a multicenter study by the PETHEMA group. *Blood* **103**:1237.

52 Lo-Coco F, Vignetti M, Avvisatti G, et al. (2004) Front-line treatment of acute promyelocytic leukemia with AIDA induction followed by risk-adapted consolidation: results of the AIDA 2000 trial of the Italian GIMEMA group. *Blood* **104**:392.

53 Lengfelder E, Reichert A, Schoch C, et al. (2000) Double induction strategy including high dose cytarabine in combination with all-trans retinoic acid: effects in patients with newly diagnosed acute promyelocytic leukemia. German AML Cooperative Group. *Leukemia* **14**:1362–70.

54 Adès L, Sanz MA, Chevret S, et al. (2008) Treatment of newly diagnosed acute promyelocytic leukemia (APL): a comparison of French-Belgian-Swiss and PETHEMA results. *Blood* **111**:1078–84.

55 Adès L, Chevret S, Raffoux E, et al. (2006) Is cytarabine useful in the treatment of acute promyelocytic leukemia? Results of a randomized trial from the European Acute Promyelocytic Leukemia Group. *J Clin Oncol* **24**:5703–10.

56 Shen ZX, Shi ZZ, Fang J, et al. (2004) All-trans retinoic acid/As2O3 combination yields a high quality remission and survival in newly diagnosed acute promyelocytic leukemia. *Proc Natl Acad Sci U S A* **101**:5328–35.

57 Ghavamzadeh A, Alimoghaddam K, Ghaffari SH, et al. (2006) Treatment of acute promyelocytic leukemia without ATRA and/or chemotherapy. *Ann Oncol* **17**:131–4.

58 Mathews V, George B, Lakshmi KM, et al. (2006) Single-agent arsenic trioxide in the treatment of newly diagnosed acute promyelocytic leukemia: durable remissions with minimal toxicity. *Blood* **107**:2627–32.

59 Estey E, Garcia-Manero G, Ferrajoli A, et al. (2006) Use of all-trans retinoic acid plus arsenic trioxide as an alternative to chemotherapy in untreated acute promyelocytic leukemia. *Blood* **107**:3469–73.

60 Evans GD, Grimwade DJ. (1999) Extramedullary disease in acute promyelocytic leukemia. *Leuk Lymphoma* **33**:219–29.

61 de Botton S, Sanz MA, Chevret S, et al. (2005) Extramedullary relapse in acute promyelocytic leukemia treated with all-trans retinoic acid and chemotherapy. *Leukemia* **20**:35–41.

62 Au WY, Tam S, Fong BM, et al. (2008) Determinants of cerebrospinal fluid arsenic concentration in patients with acute promyelocytic leukemia on oral arsenic trioxide therapy *Blood* **112**:3587–90.

63 Santamaria C, Chillon MC, Fernandez C, et al. (2007) Relapse-risk stratification in acute promyelocytic leukemia patients by PML-RAR transcript quantification. *Haematologica* **92**:316–23.

64 Cheson BD, Bennett JM, Kopecky KJ, et al. (2003) Revised recommendations of the International Working Group for Diagnosis, Standardization of Response Criteria, Treatment Outcomes, and Reporting Standards for Therapeutic Trials in Acute Myeloid Leukemia. *J Clin Oncol* **21**:4642–9.

65 Sanz MA, Fenaux P, Lo-Coco F. (2005) Arsenic trioxide in the treatment of acute promyelocytic leukemia. A review of current evidence. *Haematologica* **90**:1231–5.

66 Lo-Coco F, Cimino G, Breccia M, et al. (2004) Gemtuzumab ozogamicin (Mylotarg) as a single agent for molecularly relapsed acute promyelocytic leukemia *Blood* **104**:1995–9.

67 Tobita T, Takeshita A, Kitamura K, et al. (1997) Treatment with a new synthetic retinoid, Am80, of acute promyelocytic leukemia relapsed from complete remission induced by all-trans retinoic acid. *Blood* **90**:967–73.

68 Douer D, Hu W, Giralt S, et al. (2003) Arsenic trioxide (trisenox) therapy for acute promyelocytic leukemia in the setting of hematopoietic stem cell transplantation. *Oncologist* **8**:132–140.

69 Thomas X, Pigneux A, Raffoux E, et al. (2006) Superiority of an arsenic trioxide-based regimen over a historic control combining all-trans retinoic acid plus intensive chemotherapy in the treatment of relapsed acute promyelocytic leukemia. *Haematologica* **91**:996–7.

70 de Botton S, Fawaz A, Chevret S, et al. (2005) Autologous and allogeneic stem cell transplantation as salvage treatment of acute promyelocytic leukemia initially treated with all-trans retinoic acid: a retrospective analysis of the European Acute Promyelocytic Leukemia Group. *J Clin Oncol* **23**:120–6.

71 Sanz MA, Vellenga E, Rayón C, et al. (2004) All-trans retinoic acid and anthracycline monochemotherapy

for the treatment of elderly patients with acute promyelocytic leukemia. *Blood* **104**:3490–3.

72 Adès L, Chevret S, De Botton S, et al. (2005) Outcome of acute promyelocytic leukemia treated with all-trans retinoic acid and chemotherapy in elderly patients: the European group experience. *Leukemia* **19**:230–3.

73 de Botton S, Coiteux V, Chevret S, et al. (2004) Outcome of childhood acute promyelocytic leukemia with all-trans retinoic acid and chemotherapy. *J Clin Oncol* **22**:1404–12.

74 Fox E, Razzouk BI, Widemann BC, et al. (2008) Phase 1 trial and pharmacokinetic study of arsenic trioxide in children and adolescents with refractory or relapsed acute leukemia, including acute promyelocytic leukemia or lymphoma. *Blood* **111**:566–73.

75 George B, Mathews V, Poonkuzhali B, et al. (2004) Treatment of children with newly diagnosed acute promyelocytic leukemia with arsenic trioxide: a single center experience. *Leukemia* **18**:1587–90.

76 Castaigne S, Lefebvre P, Chomienne C, et al. (1993) Effectiveness and pharmacokinetics of low-dose all-trans retinoic acid (25 mg/m^2) in acute promyelocytic leukemia. *Blood* **82**:3560–63.

77 Dubois C, Schlageter MH, de Gentile A, et al. (1994) Modulation of IL-8, IL-1 beta, and G-CSF secretion by all-trans retinoic acid in acute promyelocytic leukemia. *Leukemia* **8**:1750–7.

78 Dubois C, Schlageter MH, de Gentile A, et al. (1994) Hematopoietic growth factor expression and ATRA sensitivity in acute promyelocytic blast cells. *Blood* **83**:3264–70.

79 Larson RS, Brown DC, Sklar LA. (1997) Retinoic acid induces aggregation of the acute promyelocytic leukemia cell line NB-4 by utilization of LFA-1 and ICAM-2. *Blood* **90**:2747–56.

80 Grimwade D, Lo Coco F. (2002) Acute promyelocytic leukemia: a model for the role of molecular diagnosis and residual disease monitoring in directing treatment approach in acute myeloid leukemia. *Leukemia* **16**:1959–73.

81 Diverio D, Rossi V, Avvisati G, et al. (1998) Early detection of relapse by prospective reverse transcriptase-polymerase chain reaction analysis of the PML/RARa fusion gene in patients with acute promyelocytic leukemia enrolled in the GIMEMA-AIEOP multicenter "AIDA" trial. *Blood* **92**:784–9.

82 Gallagher RE, Yeap BY, Bi W, et al. (2003) Quantitative real-time RT-PCR analysis of PML-RAR alpha mRNA in acute promyelocytic leukemia: assessment of prognostic significance in adult patients from intergroup protocol 0129. *Blood* **101**:2521–8.

83 Powell BL, Moser B, Stock W, et al. (2007) Larson effect of consolidation with arsenic trioxide (As2O3) on event-free survival (EFS) and overall survival (OS) among patients with newly diagnosed acute promyelocytic leukemia (APL): North American Intergroup Protocol C9710. *J Clin Oncol* **25**:2.

84 Testi AM, Biondi A, Lo Coco F, et al. (2005) GIMEMA-AIEOPAIDA protocol for the treatment of newly diagnosed acute promyelocytic leukemia (APL) in children *Blood* **106**:447–53.

85 Ortega JJ, Madero L, Martín G, et al. (2005) Treatment with all-trans retinoic acid and anthracycline monochemotherapy for children with acute promyelocytic leukemia: a multicenter study by the PETHEMA Group. *J Clin Oncol* **23**:7632–40.

86 Mann G, Reinhardt D, Ritter J, et al. (2001) Treatment with all-trans retinoic acid in acute promyelocytic leukemia reduces early deaths in children. *Ann Hematol* **80**:417–22.

87 Redner RL. (2002) Variations on a theme: the alternate translocations in APL. *Leukemia* **16**:1927–32.

88 Dilworth FJ, Chambon P. (2000) Nuclear receptors coordinate the activities of chromatin remodeling complexes and coactivators to facilitate initiation of transcription. *Oncogene* **20**:3047–54.

89 Glass CK, Rosenfeld MG. (2000) The co-regulator exchange in transcriptional function of nuclear receptors. *Genes Dev* **14**:121–41.

90 Zhong S, Salomoni P, Pandolfi P.P. (2000) The transcriptional role of PML and the nuclear body. *Nat Cell Biol* **2**:E85–90.

91 Gurrieri C, Capodieci P, Bernardi R, et al. (2004) Loss of the tumor suppressor PML in human cancers of multiple histologic origins. *J Natl Cancer Inst* **96**:269–79.

92 Pandolfi P.P. (2001) In vivo analysis of molecular genetics of acute promyelocytic leukemia. *Oncogene* **20**:5726–35.

93 Minucci S, Maccarana M, Cioce M, et al. (2000) Oligomerization of RAR and AML1 transcription factors as a novel mechanism of oncogenic activation. *Mol Cell* **5**:811–20.

94 Lin RJ, Evans RM. (2000) Acquisition of oncogenic potential by RAR chimeras in acute promyelocytic leukemia through formation of heterodimers. *Mol Cell* **5**:821–30.

95 Di Croce L. Raker VA, Corsaro M, et al. (2002) Methyl-transferase recruitment and DNA hypermethylation of target promoters by an oncogenic transcription factor. *Science* **295**:1079–82.

96 Villa R, Morey L, Raker VA, et al. (2006) The methyl-CpG binding protein MBD1 is required for PML-RAR alpha function. *Proc Natl Acad Sci U S A* **103**:1400–5.

97 Pearson M, Carbone R, Sebastiani C, et al. (2000) PML regulates p53 acetylation and premature senescence induced by oncogenic RAS. *Nature* **406**:207–10.

98 Zhong S, Muller S, Ronchetti S, et al. (2000) Role of SUMO-1-modified PML in nuclear body formation. *Blood* **95**:2748–52.

99 He LZ, Tolentino T, Grayson P, et al. (2001) Histone deacetylase inhibitors induce remission in transgenic models of therapy resistant acute promyelocytic leukemia. *J Clin Invest* **108**:1321–30.

100 Lo-Coco F, Ammatuna E. (2006) The biology of acute promyelocytic leukemia and its impact on diagnosis and treatment. *Hematology* **2006**:156–61.

101 Camacho LH, Soignet SL, Chanel S et al. (2000) Leukocytosis and the retinoic acid syndrome in patients with acute promyelocytic leukemia treated with arsenic trioxide. *J Clin Oncol* **18**:2620–5.

102 Head D, Kopecky KJ, Weick J, et al. (1995) Effect of aggressive daunomycin therapy on survival in acute promyelocytic leukemia. *Blood* **86**:1717–28.

103 Avvisati G, Petti MC, Lo Coco F, et al. (2002) Induction therapy with idarubicin alone significantly influences event-free survival duration in patients with newly diagnosed hypergranular acute promyelocytic leukemia: Final results of the GIMEMA randomized study LAP 0389 with 7 years of minimal follow-up. *Blood* **100**:3141–6.

104 Powell BL, Moser B, Stock W, et al. (2007) Effect of consolidation with arsenic trioxide (As2O3) on event-free survival (EFS) and overall survival (OS) among patients with newly diagnosed acute promyelocytic leukemia (APL): North American Intergroup Protocol C9710. *J Clin Oncol* **25**(Suppl): Abstract 2.

CHAPTER 9

A Pluralistic Approach to the Study of Myelodysplastic Syndromes: Evolving Pathology of the Seed via the Soil

Naomi Galili, Raymond Cruz, Jamie Stratton, Jessica Clima, Ghulam Sajjad Khan and Azra Raza

Columbia University Medical Center, New York, NY, USA

Introduction

Despite the great heterogeneity in the clinical presentation and pathology of the marrow cells in patients with MDS, the unifying concepts of clonal expansion of an abnormal stem cell accompanied by excessive proliferation in the presence of excessive apoptosis have been the underlying hypothesis that has driven mechanistic and translation research in the past two decades. The mutation(s) responsible for the acquired growth advantage of a specific stem cell has not been identified but is assumed to be similar to those that are associated with other cancers, that is, activation of an oncogene or elimination of a tumor suppressor gene (or both) via deletion, mutation, or changes in chromatin structure. Thus the initiating event has been assigned to the precursor hematopoietic cell. The role of the tumor microenvironment, however, is now emerging as a significant player in the establishment of a "permissive milieu" for clonal expansion to occur. The cellularity of stromal cells, which compose the marrow microenvironment, is known to decrease with age. MDS, a disease that predominates in the elderly, may thus be the result of a combination of aberrant stromal cell-derived growth and differentiation signals to a

"primed" stem cell ultimately leading to a monoclonal disease. It is thus possible that the mutations in the stem cell itself are secondary to the changes in the microenvironment. It should be noted that approximately 40% of women over the age of 65 have been found to have monoclonal hematopoiesis without any evidence of having MDS. In other words, oligo- or monoclonality appears to be a consequence of aging and, possibly, an altered microenvironment. These observations have led to the idea of involvement of both the *seed and soil* in MDS evolution but, until recently, there has only been indirect experimental data to support the theory.

If we assume that MDS is a disease of the hematopoietic stem cell and its microenvironment, then it is important to examine the biologic studies that have been done to characterize each of these compartments. Kinetic studies conducted as early as the 1980s demonstrated that MDS marrow is generally hyperproliferative [1–3]. The clonal cells appeared to be cycling well, but later were shown to be predisposed to a premature programmed cell death [4–6]. This apoptotic death appeared to be cytokine-induced and thus led to one of the first clues regarding the possible involvement of the bone

---

Advances in Malignant Hematology, First Edition. Edited by Hussain I. Saba and Ghulam J. Mufti. © 2011 Blackwell Publishing Ltd. Published 2011 by Blackwell Publishing Ltd.

marrow microenvironment. After reviewing the proliferation and apoptosis studies in more detail below, we will present published data on the emerging new pathology of ribosomal dysregulation in MDS followed by a summary of what specific abnormalities of the seed and the soil could be engineered in animal models to mimic the human disease.

Excessive proliferation-apoptosis mediated through cytokines

The paradox of MDS has been that despite a hyper- or normocellular marrow, the patients present with varying peripheral cytopenias. In the early 1980s, the thymidine analogs bromo- and iododeoxyuridine were administered *in vivo* for investigation of detailed cell cycle kinetics in patients with MDS and AML [1, 2]. Contrary to the expectation that peripheral cytopenias would turn out to be the result of a failing marrow, it was shown that these cells were rapidly proliferating. In fact, the MDS marrows had more cells synthesizing DNA (S-phase cells) than a normal marrow or even AML marrow cells. The conundrum now was what caused the paucity of cells in the blood in the presence of such a rapidly multiplying bone marrow compartment. While it was hypothesized that the hematopoietic cells could be dying before reaching the peripheral blood, it was not until the discovery of cell death via programmed suicidal self-destruction that a high death rate was actually demonstrated in MDS marrow cells. It was shown that the maturing hematopoietic cells are eliminated prematurely through apoptotic death in the marrow, resulting in peripheral cytopenias [4, 5]. Furthermore, this programmed cell death was shown to be mediated by abnormal pro-inflammatory cytokine signaling with tumor necrosis factor alpha (TNFα) initiating an apoptotic cascade through autocrine and paracrine interactions [6–9]. This finding presents yet a second paradox; how can clonal expansion occur in cells that are primed to die? The propensity to undergo apoptosis is not shared equally by the daughter cells of a specific MDS clone. The sensitivity to apoptotic signals varies from the highly sensitive to highly resistant as shown by the finding that peripheral blood granu-

locytes from MDS patients could be even more resistant to apoptosis than normal granulocytes. Additionally, it is possible that the signaling outcome of TNFα is to stimulate proliferation in early progenitor cells while inducing apoptosis in the differentiated cells [6]. In either case, all the peripheral blood myeloid cells in the MDS patient are resistant to programmed cell death, have been able to differentiate and leave the marrow, and are derived from the single abnormal clone. Surprisingly, these abnormalities of excessive proliferation and excessive apoptosis were present across all MDS subtypes and until recently, represented the only biologic characteristic unifying the heterogeneous syndromes presenting with myelodysplasia. More importantly, these biologic insights were translated into the development of novel anticytokine and anti-apoptotic treatment strategies leading to the successful use of thalidomide [10] and its derivative, lenalidomide in MDS [11, 12].

Ribosomal biogenesis is deregulated in the *seed* of MDS

While approximately 50% of MDS patients present with cytogenetic abnormalities of chromosomes 5, 7, 8, and 20, the genetic mutations that accompany them are not well understood. Focus has been directed to genes that are involved in proliferation and apoptosis but, while specific gene mutations have been found in a percentage of patients, none has been shown to be specifically characteristic of MDS and the multiple subtypes. Recent studies suggest, however, that a totally unexpected biologic pathway may be the unifying genetic abnormality that is responsible for the marrow phenotype seen in MDS.

Initial clues came with the study of patients that carry a deletion in one allele of the long arm of chromosome 5 (del(5q)). The deletion, which occurs in 10–15% of patients, is found in two regions, the more telomeric (the commonly deleted region or CDR) being associated with a specific subtype of MDS; the 5q- syndrome [13]. Patients with 5q- syndrome are typically female with macrocytic anemia and often thrombocytosis, refractory anemia, megakaryocytic hyperplasia with nuclear hypolobation, and an isolated interstitial deletion of chromosome 5. These patients rarely transform to AML and have long survival. The CDR, a 1.5MB interval, contains 40 genes, including two ribosomal genes, RBM22 and RPS14 [13]. Extensive study did not find mutations in any of these genes in the undeleted allele that would account for disease evolution, but Boultwood et al. hypothesized that downregulated expression of several genes including the ribosomal genes and the deregulation of their pathway could be associated with 5q- syndrome (haplo-insufficiency) [14]. Support for this hypothesis came from previous studies of genetic mutations in congenital anemias including dyskeratosis congenital [15], cartilage-hair hypoplasia [16], Diamond-Blackfan anemia [17], and Shwachman-Diamond syndrome [18, 19]. In all these diseases, mutations have been found in genes that are part of the ribosome biogenesis pathway. The causative role of RPS14 in 5q- syndrome was subsequently demonstrated by Ebert et al. [20]. Using RNAi to selectively inhibit each of the 40 genes in the CDR by approximately 50% to represent haploinsufficiency, they found that RPS14 suppression in normal human CD34 + marrow cells resulted in a phenotype similar to 5q- syndrome. Most importantly, when RPS14 was overexpressed in CD34 + marrow cells from 5q- syndrome patients, the aberrant phenotype was rescued. In addition, these studies demonstrated that impaired expression of the RPS14 protein produced a block in 18S ribosomal RNA processing resulting in deficient formation of the 40S ribosomal subunit. How could disrupted ribosome biogenesis account for the phenotype of 5q-syndrome? Normal erythropoiesis requires rapid proliferation of erythroid precursors, which, in turn, demands continuous protein synthesis. Thus, disruption in the generation of ribosomes would decrease protein synthesis and could account for the severe anemia associated with 5q- syndrome. Megakaryocytes, however, are produced at slower rates, and could accumulate the ribosomal proteins despite the reduction in gene dosage. In fact, many patients with 5q- syndrome present with thrombocytosis in addition to anemia. Subsequent studies have now shown that multiple genes associated with the ribogenesis pathway may also be deregulated in del(5q) patients [21], as well as in other subtypes of MDS [22] and thus may represent an additional unifying component of the disease together with proliferation and apoptosis.

Is there a molecular connection between the biologic characteristics of excessive proliferation, premature excessive apoptosis, and defective ribogenesis in the hematopoietic cells of MDS patients?

The answer is yes; there is one gene that serves as the nodal point for multiple cellular functions that is emerging as the key player. The p53 tumor suppressor protein family plays an integral part in stringent control of the cell cycle becoming activated in response to a variety of cellular stress signals. A number of studies have shown that deregulated ribosome biogenesis results in increased levels of p53 expression (the ribosome stress response) and can trigger apoptosis in a lineage specific manner [23–25]. Additionally, p53 has been shown to exert control on protein translational events directly. P53 signaling is mediated via interaction with the MDM2 protein (murine double minute 2). MDM2, a ubiquitin ligase, binds to p53 and signals p53 for degradation. However, MDM2 can also bind to several ribosomal proteins, sequestering MDM2 and allowing increase in p53 protein. If free ribosomal protein accumulates in the cell due to impaired ribosomal biogenesis, p53 level will increase and activate the apoptotic pathway. When this occurs in the MDS erythroid precursor cells, the patient becomes anemic. Alternatively, synthesis of proteins essential for erythrocyte differentiation, especially hemoglobin, may be perturbed by ribosomal imbalance and again the patient will develop anemia. It is likely that both mechanisms play a role in MDS evolution. However, RPS14 haploinsufficiency cannot explain the growth advantage acquired by the mutated cell, resulting in clonal expansion [20]. Reduced RPS14 expression does not appear to be a transforming event and thus additional genes are most likely associated with disease.

Recent studies have demonstrated the importance of miRNA genes miR-145 and miR-146a found in or near the CDR in producing the phenotype of 5q-syndrome [26]. It should be noted, however, that the MDS cell is proliferating and expanding in an increasingly abnormal microenvironment and thus it is not clear what contributes to the growth advantage of the cell. In other words, is it the seed or the soil, or some combination of both.

Are abnormalities of the seed sufficient to explain the entire syndrome of myelodysplasia?

A reductionist approach is particularly attractive to experimentalists because it would allow them to manipulate a single gene product to generate *in vitro* and *in vivo* models for study and which may also serve as a potential therapeutic target. Unfortunately, such exclusive focus on a single target essentially oversimplifies an otherwise highly complex biologic system. For example, investigating the seed to the exclusion of the soil might ignore one half of the equation. One way to address the contribution of the seed versus the soil in the pathogenesis of MDS is to examine the mouse models that have been generated using specific abnormalities from either component.

Mouse models of MDS

Traditionally, basic studies of biology and pathogenesis of cancer have been carried out either *in vitro* in cells isolated from the human tumor or in a murine model that replicates many of the human environmental characteristics of the disease. While neither approach is perfect, much of the mutational and causal events resulting in disease have been discovered first in these models and later confirmed in humans. Importantly, therapeutic agents can undergo preclinical efficacy testing in the mouse using large numbers of animals with various drug modalities.

One of the major perplexities in MDS is that, while the MDS cells proliferate rapidly to overwhelm the bone marrow, it has not been possible

to grow the MDS cells *in vitro* or to cause disease *in vivo* in an immunodeficient mouse model. The lack of the necessary growth factors and survivor signals from the tumor microenvironment and/or suppressive immune factors of the host have been attributed to these failures. Attributing the low engraftment to NK cells, B- and T-cells of the host, the NOD-SCID mouse that lacks these activities has been used by several groups [27–31].

Using 5q- precursor stem cells, only 12% of the mice showed any engraftment and no disease developed in those recipients [27]. No engraftment was found in this model when trisomy 8 MDS cells were used, although the authors attribute this to the possibility that the trisomy 8 was an event characteristic of a more mature cell and not a true stem cell [28]. Other studies have tried to express human cytokines in the mice receiving MDS stem cells to increase engraftment [29–31] but with little success. Even when low levels of engraftment were detected, the mice did not develop a disease phenotype, possibly due to the low numbers of human abnormal cells.

An alternative approach to generate a murine model of MDS is to genetically engineer the mouse to express (transgenic or knockin models) or not to express (knockout) the gene of interest. Chimeric mice that carry a single allele or homozygous mice that carry the desired mutation on both alleles can then be generated to study the effects of gene dosage. It is also possible to generate mice with promoters that allow the gene mutation(s) to be restricted to specific cell lineages and in designated stages of differentiation. Multiple studies of this sort have been performed in attempt to recapitulate the phenotype of MDS in general and the various subtypes. Thus, a successful mouse model would need to show that the animal develops a clonal stem cell disorder of ineffective hematopoiesis resulting in peripheral cytopenia(s) with morphologic dysplasia and a tendency for evolution to AML.

Targeting the *seed* of MDS by single gene disruption

The "two-hit model of leukemogenesis" was first proposed in 2002 [32]; in this hypothesis two classes of mutations are required for the development of AML. Class 1 mutations provide growth or survival advantage to the cell while class 2 mutations block hematopoietic differentiation. This theory has been supported by numerous studies although rare exceptions to the two-hit model of myeloid leukemia have been described. In an extension of this hypothesis, mutations of a single class 1 gene such as Jak 2 would be expected to produce a myeloid proliferative disease with excessive proliferation and decreased apoptosis. However, for MDS where apoptosis is increased, mutations of class 2 would be expected. Thus many of the mouse models for MDS have looked at the perturbation of class 2 type genes.

EVI1

EVI1 is a transcription factor gene located on the human chromosome 3, a region that is karyotypically abnormal in a small proportion of patients with MDS. Studies using both mouse and human cell lines have shown that EVI1 blocks differentiation of hematopoietic progenitor cells to granulocytes and erythroid cells while promoting differentiation along the megakaryocte lineage [33]. Overexpression of EVI1 in a mouse transplant model [34] resulted in pancytopenia at 7–8 months after marrow transplant eventually leading to death at 10–12 months. Examinations of the spleens showed increased size, increased numbers of immature erythrocytes, iron deposition, and increased numbers of apoptotic cells. As in the human disease, the marrow showed ineffective hematopoiesis characterized by megakaryocytic and erythroid hyperplasia and dyserythropoiesis. Unlike patients with MDS, however, there was no evolution of the disease to AML in these mice. Further study showed that the binding of EVI1 to Gata1 inhibited the expression of the EpoR gene resulting in defective erythropoiesis while binding to Pu.1 inhibited myelopoiesis. [35]

Npm1

NPM1 is a nucleolar protein gene located on chromosome 5q35, a region frequently deleted in patients with MDS. The gene plays a role in regulation of p53, and centrosome duplication (implicating genetic instability) as well as in ribosome biogenesis. It was thus a likely candidate for mutational modeling for

MDS [36, 37]. Deletion of the gene on both alleles results in embryonic lethality approximately by day 12. However, chimeric mice developed erythroid morphologic abnormalities similar to MDS at 6–18 months, although peripheral counts remained normal. The marrow morphology was one of erythroid and megakaryocytic dysplasia. With a two-year follow-up, 22% of the animals had transformed to leukemia of which 17% were myeloid, 4% B-cell, and 2% T-cell. Thus, while this model seems to recapitulate many of the features of human MDS, the fact that the mice did not develop anemia, the cytopenias that affects the majority of patients with MDS is a confounding factor.

NUP98

The nucleporin 98 gene NUP98 on 11p15 is frequently found as a partner of chromosomal translocations in hematopoietic malignancies. In MDS, a translocation with the homeobox-containing gene HOXD13 created a fusion gene [38] that was then used to create a mouse model [39]. In mice receiving retrovirus transduced bone marrow cells expressing the fusion protein, subsets of lymphocytes were decreased and myeloid cells were increased. Erythroid precursors were decreased in colony-forming spleen assays, and the mice developed myeloproliferative disease. Transformation to AML did not occur, however. In contrast to this model, transgenic mice created with the hematopoietic promoter Vav1 developed anemia, neutropenia, and lymphopenia with hypercellular or normocellular marrows by four to seven months [40]. The marrow exhibited dysplasia similar to the human form of MDS and approximately 50% of the animals progressed to leukemia by 10–14 months. While the majority of the leukemias were AML, some B- and T-cell leukemias also developed. The differences seen between the retrovirus model and the transgenic model have not as yet been fully explained, but the transgenic mice recapitulate many features of the human disease.

AML1 (RUNX1)

Two different mutations of the AML1 (RUNX1) gene (essential for normal hematopoiesis) have been identified in patients with MDS or MDS/AML [41].

Using retroviral models [42], the first mutation results in truncation of the C-terminus of the protein and the mice showed pancytopenia with erythroid dysplasia but little myeloid dysplasia. The second mutation in the runt domain of the protein also resulted in pancytopenia, hepatosplenomegaly, leukocytosis and marked dysplasia. A proportion (60%) of these mice progressed to AML by 14 months and some were shown to have integration sites at the Evi1 locus. When BM cells were transfected with both the runt domain mutation of AML1 and Evi1, the transformation to AML was shortened to three to five months suggesting that the two genes interact during transformation of MDS to AML.

Miscellaneous

Other models, including the knockdown of Pten/Ship (second messenger regulating genes) [43], Dido1 (gene upregulated in apoptosis) deletion [44], SALL4G (transcription facto gene) overexpression [45], inducible BCL2 and NRAS [46], Arid4a (chromatin modification gene) deletion [47], Polg mutation (polymerase gene for mitochondrial DNA) [48] and TGF-β (inflammatory cytokine gene) transgene [49, 50], have all recapitulated some of the aspects of MDS and could be useful for testing specific biologic or therapeutic actions.

Large-scale chromosome engineering

The 5q- syndrome subtype of MDS is characterized by deletion of the CDR on chromosome 5. The region of synteny is divided into two different chromosomes in the mouse; chromosome 11 and 18. Using nested random deletions in embryonic stem cells, mice deficient in one allele (haploinsufficiency) of overlapping segments of syntenic CDR were generated [51]. The only mice to display changes in their hematopoiesis were the mice that had a deletion of an 8-gene interval including RPS14 on chromosome 18. These mice developed macrocytic anemia, together with a mild thrombocytopenia. Additional study showed that p53 expression

was elevated as was apoptosis in the marrow cells. The marrows were depleted of common myeloid and granulocyte-monocyte progenitor cells. Crossing these mice with p53 knockout mice resulted in complete rescue of the hematopoietic stem cell population, providing support for the link of ribosomal stress due to decreased expression of RPS14 with p53 activation. In contrast to 5q- syndrome MDS, however, the engineered mice exhibit thrombocytopenia although the reason for this remains under study.

Targeting the *soil* can generate a MDS-like phenotype

The presence of an increasingly abnormal stromal microenvironment and a mutationally primed stem cell are now considered to be pivotal events contributing to the evolution of MDS. The animal models described above have all been based on abnormalities in the parenchymal cells which lead to an MDS-like phenotype. What about changes in the mesenchymal or stromal cells? Mouse models have shown that specific mesenchymal cells of the bone marrow are integral players in the regulation of the stem cell niche [52, 53]. These cells express the Sp7 transcription factor essential for osteoblast differentiation and niche formation. Using the promoter of the Sp7 gene, a mouse model was created in which Dicer1, a gene that controls miRNA biogenesis, was deleted specifically in osteoprogenitor cells, without altering hematopoietic stem cells [54]. By weeks 4–6, osteoblast and osteoclast differentiation was impaired and by week 8, 30% of the animals died. The peripheral blood counts revealed pancytopenia with varying degrees of anemia due to extramedullary hematopoiesis in the spleen. The marrow was found to be normo- to hypercellular and thus the animals displayed all the clinical signs in ineffective hematopoiesis. Morphologic findings of striking dysplasia in neutrophils, platelets, and megakaryocytes together with increased apoptosis and proliferation confirmed the MDS diagnosis. Most importantly, when hematopoietic cells from mDicer1 mutant mice were transplanted to a different strain of wild-type mice, no disease phenotype developed despite successful engraftment. Thus, this model demonstrates that the MDS phenotype of the mutant mice is dependent solely on the abnormal microenvironment. These findings further suggest that the microenvironment can be the initiating site of signals that cause eventual genetic alterations in the hematopoietic stem cells, leading to clonal expansion and disease evolution. Further expression profiling studies of the mutated osteoprogenitor cells revealed that Sbds, a gene mutated in the congenital disease Shwachman-Diamond syndrome, is underexpressed. Sbds abnormalities have been shown to affect ribosome biogenesis. Patients with this disease have both marrow failure and a propensity for developing leukemia. In fact, MDS developed in mice when the Sbds gene was deleted. These results suggest that the MDS-like phenotype resulting from mutation of Dicer1 in osteoprogenitor cells may be through the perturbation of pathways controlled by Sbds. For the first time there is direct experimental proof for the hypothesis suggested more than 15 years ago, that it is only in the context of an abnormal micro-environment (as evidenced by the production of pro-inflammatory cytokines) that a "primed" stem cell can gain growth advantage and evolve into MDS [4].

Are mouse models sufficiently faithful to the human disease?

Mouse models are extremely valuable for understanding the biologic mechanisms of disease evolution as well as for developing novel therapeutic strategies. In order to serve these two purposes, the models need to mimic the human disease as faithfully as possible. Unfortunately, there are inadequacies in each of the models described above:

• EVI1 mouse model: Over-expression of EVI1 in human MDS is associated with a higher incidence of transformation to acute leukemia. These mice do not evolve to AML.
• Npm1: Haploinsufficiency results in dysplasia but not in cytopenia, and thus anemia, the main feature of human MDS is not seen. The mice will, however, eventually transform to acute leukemia.

• Nup98: A transgenic model of the NUP98-HOXD13 under control of the Vav promoter resulted in many of the features of MDS with fairly rapid progression to AML and ALL. However this translocation is extremely rare in MDS and, thus, is not a common feature of the human disease.
• Aml1(Runx1): Retroviral transduction of mutated gene in two different domains showed that only the mutation in the runt domain results in an MDS-like phenotype, while both types of mutations are found in the human disease.
• RPS14 deleted region: Haploinsufficiency of the 8-gene region that includes RPS14 recapitulated many of the features of 5q- syndrome and demonstrates the pivotal role of p53 in disease evolution. However, the mice develop thrombocytopenia, which is not characteristic of the human disease. On the contrary, patients with 5q- syndrome often show slightly elevated platelet counts.
• Dicer1 deletion specifically in osteoprogenitor cells: The phenotype of these mice results in hematopoietic insufficiency, with many of the features of MDS which may be due to interaction with the gene shown to be mutated in congenital Shwachman-Bodian-Diamond syndrome (SBDs). The SBDs gene has not been shown to be mutated in MDS, although common pathways such as ribosome biogenesis may be perturbed in both. This model does, however, show the pivotal role played by cells of the micro-enviroment in disease evolution.

As shown by the summary above, no single mouse model accurately recapitulates all facets of the human syndromes. The most plausible explanation for the failure to do so obviously relates to the complexity and heterogeneity of MDS which cannot be neatly packaged into a seed or soil compartment but is a consequence of highly intricate interactions between the two.

A new paradigm for MDS: seed *via* soil

Everything should be made as simple as possible, but
no simpler . . . *Albert Einstein*
Trying to understand a highly interactive system like the bone marrow with its seeds and soil acting

together to produce billions of cells every hour by concentrating on the study of single genes is like the three blind men trying to describe the elephant. Taking a pluralistic rather than a reductionist view of the problem at hand, our contention is that even if the initiating event occurs in one compartment, its clonal expansion cannot progress without the cooperation of the other. The question is not whether the etiology resides within the seed and/or the soil but rather how the clinical syndromes result from the pathology of the seed *via* the soil. Systems biology, which combines the expertise of multiple disciplines including computer science and engineering, offers one way to tackle this complexity by developing disease models that can predict the *emergent* properties of individual characteristics in combination. In the final analysis, however, *Man must remain the measure of all things*, and so even the outcomes predicted by systems biology must be confirmed through observations of the human disease itself. Which brings us to the most important final conclusion: there is little that can substitute for the study of freshly obtained human bone marrow.

References

1 Raza A, Preisler HD, Mayers GL, Bankert R. (1984) Rapid enumeration of S-phase cells by means of monoclonal antibodies. *N Engl J Med* **310**:991.

2 Raza A, Spiridonidis C, Ucar K, et al. (1985) Double labeling of S-phase murine cells with bromodeoxyuridine and a second DNA-specific probe. *Cancer Res* **45**:2283–7.

3 Raza A, Maheshwari Y, Preisler HD. (1987) Differences in cell cycle characteristics among patients with acute nonlymphocytic leukemia. *Blood* **69**:1647–53.

4 Raza A, Gezer S, Mundle S, et al. (1995) Apoptosis in bone marrow biopsy samples involving stromal and hematopoietic cells in 50 patients with myelodysplastic syndromes. *Blood* **86**:268–276. [First study to show that apoptosis of the marrow cells could account for the peripheral cytopenias of MDS despite the hypercellular marrow.].

5 Raza A, Mundle S, Shetty V, et al. (1996) Novel insights into the biology of myelodysplastic syndromes: Excessive apoptosis and the role of cytokines. *Int J Hematol* **63**:265–78.

6 Raza A, Gregory SA, Preisler HD. (1996) The myelodysplastic syndromes in 1996: complex stem cell disorders confounded by dual actions of cytokines. *Leuk Res* **20**:881–90.

7 Mundle SD, Ali A, Cartlidge J, Reza S, et al. (1999) Evidence for involvement of tumor necrosis factor-α in apoptotic death of bone marrow cells in myelodysplastic syndromes. *Am J Hematol* **60**:36–47.

8 Claessens YE, Bouscary D, Dupont JM, et al. (2002) In vitro proliferation and differentiation of erythroid progenitors from patients with myelodysplastic syndromes: evidence for Fas-dependent apoptosis. *Blood* **99**:1594–601.

9 Campioni D, Secchiero P, Corallini F, et al. (2005) Evidence for a role of TNF-related apoptosis-inducing ligand (TRAIL) in the anemia of myelodysplastic syndromes. *Am J Pathol* **166**:557–63.

10 Raza A, Meyer P, Dutt D, et al. (2001) Thalidomide produces transfusion independence in long-standing refractory anemias of patients with myelodysplastic syndromes. *Blood* **98**:958–65.

11 List A, Dewald G, Bennett J, et al. (2006) Lenalidomide in the myelodysplastic syndrome with chromosome 5q deletion. *Myelodysplastic Syndrome-003 Study Investigators. N Engl J Med* **355**:1456–65.

12 Raza A, Reeves JA, Feldman EJ, et al. (2008) Phase 2 study of lenalidomide in transfusion-dependent, low-risk, and intermediate-1 risk myelodysplastic syndromes with karyotypes other than deletion 5q. *Blood* **111**:86–93.

13 Boultwood J, Fidler C, Strickson AJ, et al. (2002) Narrowing and genomic annotation of the commonly deleted region of the 5q- syndrome. *Blood* **99**:4638–41.

14 Boultwood J, Pellagatti A, Cattan H, et al. (2007) Gene expression profiling of CD34 + cells in patients with the 5q- syndrome. *Br J Haematol* **139**:578–89.

15 Heiss NS, Knight SW, Vulliamy TJ, et al. (1998) X-linked dyskeratosis congenita is caused by mutations in a highly conserved gene with putative nucleolar functions. *Nat Genet* **19**:32–8.

16 Ridanpää M, van Eenennaam H, Pelin K, et al. (2001) Mutations in the RNA component of RNase MRP cause a pleiotropic human disease, cartilage-hair hypoplasia. *Cell* **104**:195–203.

17 Draptchinskaia N, Gustavsson P, Andersson B, et al. (1999) The gene encoding ribosomal protein S19 is mutated in Diamond-Blackfan anaemia. *Nat Genet* **21**:169–75.

18 Boocock GR, Morrison JA, Popovic M, et al. (2003) Mutations in SBDS are associated with Shwachman-Diamond syndrome. *Nat Genet* **33**:97–101.

19 Austin KM, Leary RJ, Shimamura A. (2005) The Shwachman-Diamond SBDS protein localizes to the nucleolus. *Blood* **106**:1253–8.

20 Ebert BL, Pretz J, Bosco J, et al. (2008) Identification of RPS14 as a 5q- syndrome gene by RNA interference screen. *Nature* **451**:335–9.

21 Pellagatti A, Hellström-Lindberg E, Giagounidis A, et al. (2008) Haploinsufficiency of RPS14 in 5q- syndrome is associated with deregulation of ribosomal- and translation-related genes. *Br J Haematol* **142**:57–64.

22 Sohal D, Pellagatti A, Zhou L, et al. (2008) Down-regulation of ribosomal proteins is seen in non 5q-MDS. *Blood* **112**:854.

23 McGowan KA, Li JZ, Park CY, et al. (2008) Ribosomal mutations cause p53-mediated dark skin and pleiotropic effects. *Nat Genet* **40**:963–70.

24 Vousden KH, Prives C. (2009) Blinded by the light: the growing complexity of p53. *Cell* **137**:413–31.

25 Starczynowski DT, Kuchenbauer F, Argiropoulos B, et al. (2010) Identification of miR-145 and miR-146a as mediators of the 5q- syndrome phenotype. *Nat Med* **16**:49–58.

26 Pellagatti A, Marafioti T, Paterson JC, et al. (2010) Induction of p53 and up-regulation of the p53 pathway in the human 5q- syndrome. *Blood* **115**:2721–3.

27 Nilsson L, Astrand-Grundström I, Arvidsson I, et al. (2000) Isolation and characterization of hematopoietic progenitor/stem cells in 5q-deleted myelodysplastic syndromes: evidence for involvement at the hematopoietic stem cell level. *Blood* **96**:2012–21.

28 Nilsson L, Astrand-Grundström I, Anderson K, et al. (2002) Involvement and functional impairment of the CD34(+)CD38(–)Thy-1(+) hematopoietic stem cell pool in myelodysplastic syndromes with trisomy 8. *Blood* **100**:259–67.

29 Benito AI, Bryant E, Loken MR, et al. (2003) NOD/SCID mice transplanted with marrow from patients with myelodysplastic syndrome (MDS) show long-term propagation of normal but not clonal human precursors. *Leuk Res* **27**:425–36.

30 Thanopoulou E, Cashman J, Kakagianne T, et al. (2004) Engraftment of NOD/SCID-beta2 microglobulin null mice with multilineage neoplastic cells from patients with myelodysplastic syndrome. *Blood* **103**:4285–93.

31 Kerbauy DM, Lesnikov V, Torok-Storb B, Bryant E, Deeg HJ. (2004) Engraftment of distinct clonal MDS-derived hematopoietic precursors in NOD/SCID-beta2-microglobulin-deficient mice after intramedullary transplantation of hematopoietic and stromal cells. *Blood* **104**:2202–3.

32 Kelly LM, Kutok JL, Williams IR, et al. (2002) PML/RARalpha and FLT3-ITD induce an APL-like disease in a mouse model. *Proc Natl Acad Sci U S A* **99**:8283–8.

33 Buonamici S, Chakraborty S, Senyuk V, Nucifora G. (2003) The role of EVI1 in normal and leukemic cells. *Blood Cells Mol Dis* **31**:206–12.

34 Buonamici S, Li D, Chi Y, et al. (2004) EVI1 induces myelodysplastic syndrome in mice. *J Clin Invest* **114**:713–9.

35 Laricchia-Robbio L, Fazzina R, Li D, et al. (2006) Nucifora G. Point mutations in two EVI1 Zn fingers abolish EVI1-GATA1 interaction and allow erythroid differentiation of murine bone marrow cells. *Mol Cell Biol* **26**:7658–66.

36 Grisendi S, Bernardi R, Rossi M, et al. (2005) Role of nucleophosmin in embryonic development and tumorigenesis. *Nature* **437**:147–53.

37 Sportoletti P, Grisendi S, Majid SM, et al. (2008) Npm1 is a haploinsufficient suppressor of myeloid and lymphoid malignancies in the mouse. *Blood* **111**:3859–62.

38 Raza-Egilmez SZ, Jani-Sait SN, Grossi M, et al. (1998) NUP98-HOXD13 gene fusion in therapy-related acute myelogenous leukemia. *Cancer Res* **58**:4269–73.

39 Pineault N, Buske C, Feuring-Buske M, et al. (2003) Induction of acute myeloid leukemia in mice by the human leukemia-specific fusion gene NUP98-HOXD13 in concert with Meis1. *Blood* **101**:4529–38.

40 Lin YW, Slape C, Zhang Z, Aplan PD. (2005) NUP98-HOXD13 transgenic mice develop a highly penetrant, severe myelodysplastic syndrome that progresses to acute leukemia. *Blood* **106**:287–95.

41 Osato M. (2004) Point mutations in the RUNX1/AML1 gene: another actor in RUNX leukemia. *Oncogene* **23**:4284–96.

42 Watanabe-Okochi N, Kitaura J, Ono R, et al. (2008) AML1 mutations induced MDS and MDS/AML in a mouse BMT model. *Blood* **111**:4297–308.

43 Moody JL, Xu L, Helgason CD, Jirik FR. (2004) Anemia, thrombocytopenia, leukocytosis, extramedullary hematopoiesis, and impaired progenitor function in Pten+/-SHIP-/- mice: a novel model of myelodysplasia. *Blood* **103**:4503–10.

44 Fütterer A, Campanero MR, Leonardo E, et al. (2005) Dido gene expression alterations are implicated in the induction of hematological myeloid neoplasms. *J Clin Invest* **115**:2351–62.

45 Ma Y, Cui W, Yang J, et al. (2006) SALL4, a novel oncogene, is constitutively expressed in human acute myeloid leukemia (AML) and induces AML in transgenic mice. *Blood* **108**:2726–35.

46 Omidvar N, Kogan S, Beurlet S, et al. (2007) BCL-2 and mutant NRAS interact physically and functionally in a mouse model of progressive myelodysplasia. *Cancer Res* **67**:11657–67.

47 Wu MY, Eldin KW, Beaudet AL. (2008) Identification of chromatin remodeling genes Arid4a and Arid4b as leukemia suppressor genes. *J Natl Cancer Inst* **100**:1247–59.

48 Chen ML, Logan TD, Hochberg ML, et al. (2009) Erythroid dysplasia, megaloblastic anemia, and impaired lymphopoiesis arising from mitochondrial dysfunction. *Blood* **114**:4045–53.

49 Sanderson N, Factor V, Nagy P, et al. (1995) Hepatic expression of mature transforming growth factor beta 1 in transgenic mice results in multiple tissue lesions. *Proc Natl Acad Sci U S A* **92**:2572–6.

50 Zhou L, Nguyen AN, Sohal D, et al. (2008) Inhibition of the TGF-beta receptor I kinase promotes hematopoiesis in MDS. *Blood* **112**:3434–43.

51 Barlow JL, Drynan LF, Hewett DR, et al. (2010) A p53-dependent mechanism underlies macrocytic anemia in a mouse model of human 5q- syndrome. *Nat Med* **16**:59–66.

52 Calvi LM, Adams GB, Weibrecht KW, et al. (2003) Osteoblastic cells regulate the haematopoietic stem cell niche. *Nature* **425**:841–6.

53 Zhang J, Niu C, Ye L, et al. (2003) Identification of the haematopoietic stem cell niche and control of the niche size. *Nature* **425**:836–41.

54 Raaijmakers MH, Mukherjee S, Guo S, et al. (2010) Bone progenitor dysfunction induces myelodysplasia and secondary leukaemia. *Nature* **464**:852–7.

CHAPTER 10

Myelodysplastic Syndrome: A Review of Current Care

Kenneth H. Shain, Alan F. List and Rami S. Komrokji
Department of Malignant Hematology, H. Lee Moffitt Cancer Center and Research Institute, Tampa, FL, USA

Introduction

Myelodysplastic syndrome (MDS) represents a collection of bone marrow malignancies affecting hematopoietic stem cells with a highly variable morbidity and mortality. The inherent heterogeneity of MDS is highlighted by the broad range of clinical disease courses; MDS can present as a "near chronic disease" with an *unaltered* lifespan or as a disease with unfettered progression with less than a six-month median survival [1]. As our understanding of MDS continues to expand, so does our ability to appropriately diagnose and treat.

MDS is an age-dependent hematopoietic malignancy characterized by: (1) peripheral blood cytopenias secondary to ineffective hematopoiesis, (2) dysplastic hematopoietic cells, (3) increased proliferative fraction of bone marrow myeloblasts in higher risk disease, and (4) frequently associated with clonal cytogenetic abnormalities. These features likely reflect the establishment of clonal bone marrow progenitors with increased proliferative potential, impaired differentiation capacity with accelerated apoptotic cellular attrition culminating in bone marrow failure and ineffective hematopoiesis. Aberrant hematopoiesis presents as peripheral blood cytopenias (anemia, thrombocytopenia, and neutropenia) with associated signs and symptoms. Fatigue, weakness, and dyspnea are the most common clinical signs of anemia – the most frequent

cytopenia affecting MDS patients throughout the course of their disease [2, 3]. Chronic or recurrent infections related to neutropenia or neutrophil dysfunction afflict 50% of newly diagnosed patients and remain the leading cause of death [2]. Progressive bruising or bleeding associated with thrombocytopenia is observed in approximately 66% of patients throughout the course of the disease. Appropriate diagnosis of MDS is paramount as the disorder is associated with significant morbidity, mortality, and risk of transformation to AML. In the sections below we will discuss the epidemiology, clinico-pathology, and disease characteristics that are considered in the design of appropriate treatment algorithms.

Epidemiology/etiology

A number of recent epidemiological studies have helped characterize the populations at risk for MDS [3–6]. MDS is primarily a disease of older adults with a median age of >70 years old with approximately 80% of affected individuals older than 60 years of age. Approximately 10 000 new MDS cases are diagnosed on an annual basis. One recent epidemiological study examined the US Surveillance, Epidemiology and End Result (SEER) program from 2001–2003 demonstrating an incidence of MDS (excluding CMML) of 3.4/100 000 with a median age at diagnosis of 76 [2]. The age-adjusted incidence

Advances in Malignant Hematology, First Edition. Edited by Hussain I. Saba and Ghulam J. Mufti. © 2011 Blackwell Publishing Ltd.
Published 2011 by Blackwell Publishing Ltd.

in this study ranged from 0.1/100 000 in patients less than 30 years of age to as high as 36.3/100 000 in persons over the age of 80 years, illustrating the close correlation between age and risk of MDS (a trend consistent across multiple studies) [5–7]. Male gender also appears to portend an increased risk and a worse prognosis [2]. Race is also associated with differing risk (white [3.5] >black [3.0] >Asian [2.6] >Native American [1.3] per 100 000). Together, these data suggest that increasing age, gender (male), and race contribute to the incidence of MDS.

This myeloid neoplasm evolves as a *de novo* (or primary) hematologic malignancy of the bone marrow in the majority of cases (~80%). However, in the context of *successful* chemotherapy treatment of non-Hodgkin lymphoma, Hodgkin lymphoma, multiple myeloma, breast cancer or other cancers, a growing percentage of cases are considered secondary or arising from prior radiation or chemotherapy. Treatment-related MDS (t-MDS) is a distinct entity (relative to *de novo* MDS) generally characterized by a younger age of onset, more severe cytopenias, high rate of poor-risk cytogenetics, and poor outcome. Alkylating agents and topoisomerase-II inhibitors appear to be the highest risk antecedent agents, each with characteristic presentations [2]. Alkylating agent-related MDS is associated with a relatively delayed onset of cytopenias, approximately five to seven years, and frequently presents with chromosome 5 and 7 anomalies. In contrast, topoisomerase-II inhibitor-related MDS presents more rapidly, in the order of six months to two years and with balanced translocations involving chromosome 11q23. It is important to note that the latency period in t-MDS can vary between 1–25 years irrespective of the eliciting drug [2, 6]. Primary or *de novo* MDS has been linked to multiple etiologic agents including exposure to benzene, tobacco smoke (containing benzene among other compounds), agricultural pesticides, herbicides, and fertilizers, as well as radiation. Further, known familial syndromes like Fanconi anemia, Shwachman-Diamond syndrome, and Diamond-Blackfan syndrome are associated with an increased risk for MDS [2]. Although rare, specific kindreds have been identified with an increased risk of MDS arising from germ-line mutations involving the genes RUNX1, TERT/TERC, and TET2 [8].

Pathophysiology

As stated above, multiple potential environmental stressors and specific chemotherapeutic agents may increase the risk of developing MDS. To this end, it is believed that MDS arises, in most cases, from a genetic event or alteration within senescent hematopoietic stem cells. Reports have suggested that an initial genetic "hit" may occur in a very early hematopoietic progenitor capable of multiple lines of differentiation [9, 10]. However, subsequent/additional genetic or epigenetic events are necessary for proliferation of the malignant progenitor. Allelic haploinsufficiency contributes to the hematologic phenotype, the best example of which involves the RPS14 gene which alone recapitulates the hematologic features of the 5q- syndrome [11].

Accelerated apoptosis is the hallmark of early disease. Stromal defects and altered T-cell homeostasis are other factors that contribute to the premature apoptosis. Diagnosis is dependent upon identification of dysplasia in greater than 10% of cells of any lineage. Erythroid dysplasia is characterized by nuclear budding, megaloblastic changes, and ringed sideroblasts. Myeloid dysplasia may manifest as dysgranulopoiesis characterized by nuclear hypolobation (pseudo-Pelger-Huet or *pelgeroid* appearance), irregular segmentation, hypogranulation, an increased percentage of marrow myeloblasts, and Auer rods. Dysmegakaryopoiesis is characterized by micromegakaryocytes, nuclear hypolobation or multinucleation with nuclear dispersion (Plate 10.1). Although these findings are required for the diagnosis, it is not difficult to imagine that, with the heterogeneity of MDS, diagnosis remains unclear at times.

Two MDS variants occur with sufficient frequency to warrant discussion; hypoplastic MDS and MDS with myelofibrosis [12, 13]. Neither of these entities is incorporated in the classification or prognostic scoring systems, but they have important clinical distinctions. A relatively hypoplastic bone marrow adjusted for age may be identified in approximately

10% of MDS cases. In hypoplastic MDS, the decreased cellularity is frequently associated with controversy upon diagnosis secondary to a high degree of similarity to aplastic anemia [14]. Hypoplastic MDS has yet to be shown to alter disease course/prognosis, but studies suggest significant benefit from immunosuppressive therapeutics [12]. In contrast to hypoplastic MDS, MDS associated with marrow fibrosis (hyperfibrotic MDS) has a more aggressive clinical course with increased bone marrow myeloblasts, multilineage dysplasia, and high AML transformation rate [13]. This subgroup is observed in 10–17% of cases. This is an important subtype to recognize, given that even in the absence of increased blasts it portends an unfavorable prognosis.

Classification

MDS represents a heterogeneous group of disorders. As we have learned more about the disease(s) and the range of clinical outcomes, our need to appropriately stage and classify these diseases has grown. Further, a concise and reproducible staging/classification system is paramount for communication of clinical research/studies to practice. This has led to a continuing evolution of the morphologic classification of MDS from the FAB (French-American-British) classification of the 1980s and 1990s to the WHO (World Health Organization) system initially published in 2001 and, now, to the recently amended WHO classification in 2008 [15, 16].

Three decades ago the first widely accepted classification system for MDS was constructed based on an appreciation of the clinical and pathological characteristics of MDS. In the early 1980s, Bennett et al. expanded the FAB classification system of MDS to include five major subtypes (Table 10.1) [17]. These included Refractory Anemia (RA), RA with Ringed Sideroblasts (RARS), Refractory Anemia with Excess Blasts (RAEB), Refractory Anemia with Excess Blasts in Transformation (RAEB-T), and Chronic Myelomonocytic Leukemia (CMML). Bennett and colleagues based this schema on three primary characteristics: (1) the presence and percentage of peripheral blood and bone marrow myeloblasts, (2) the pres-

ence of ringed sideroblasts, and (3) increased circulating monocytes. The FAB classification system also corresponded with disease overall survival and frequency of AML transformation. However, significant prognostic heterogeneity within the subcategories was evident. Although this schema was an important initial step, it had inherent limitations as a prognostic tool. In 2001, the WHO classification system was adopted based on the foundation of the FAB and incorporated new aspects of MDS morphology and biology [18]. Within the lower risk group(s) of MDS, a number of alterations were established. The association between increased morbidity and mortality in patients with dysplasia beyond the erythroid lineage observed in RA and RARS was incorporated in the category(s) refractory cytopenia with multilineage dysplasia (RCMD) with or without ringed sideroblasts (RCMD with RS; ≥15% RS) [19–21]. A new category was delineated based on the favorable prognosis of MDS patients with isolated deletion of a specific region on the long arm of chromosome 5 (5q-) involving bands q21 through q32. This subcategory of MDS is characterized clinically by refractory anemia, normal to increased platelets with dysplastic (hypolobulated) megakaryocytes within the bone marrow (Plate 10.1), and less than 5% myeloblasts [18, 22]. The absolute bone marrow and peripheral blood myeloblast criteria for AML was reduced to ≥20%, thereby eliminating the RAEB-T category. RAEB was further divided into two groups; RAEB-1 with <5% peripheral blood myeloblasts and/or 5–9% bone marrow myeloblasts, and RAEB-2 with 5–19% peripheral blood and 10–19% bone marrow myeloblasts. Lastly, CMML, atypical chronic myelogenous leukemia (aCML) and juvenile myelomonocytic leukemia (JMML) were annexed to a distinct WHO category denoted myelodysplastic/myeloproliferative disorders (MDS/MPD). This version of the WHO classification system served to integrate MDS nomenclature internationally; however, with expanding information and experience further enhancements have led to the recently published contemporary WHO classification guidelines for the *next* decade.

The most recent WHO classification guidelines recognize seven MDS categories (Table 10.2). These include Refractory Anemia with Unilineage Dyspla-

Table 10.1 Myelodysplastic syndrome classification: FAB

FAB Subtype	Peripheral Blood Blast (%)	Bone Marrow Blast (%)
Refractory Anemia (RA)	<5	<5
RA with Ringed Sideroblasts (RARS)	<5	<5
Refractory Anemia with Excess Blasts (RAEB)	<5	5–20
Refractory Anemia with Excess Blasts in Transformation (RAEB-T)	>5	21–30
CMML	<5	5–20

(Adapted from Bennett J M et al. (1982) *Brit J Haemotol* 51:189–99.)

sia (RCUD); Refractory Anemia (RA); Refractory Neutropenia (RN); Refractory Thrombocytopenia (RT); RCMD, RARS, RAEB-1, RAEB-2, MDS associated with isolated del(5q), and MDS unclassified. CMML remains within the myelodysplastic/myeloproliferative neoplasms category with JMML, atypical CML – also known now as BCR-ABL-1 negative CML, and MDS/MPN unclassified [16]. In contrast to "lower risk" MDS subcategories, the classification schema for higher risk RAEB-1 and RAEB-2 have changed little in the most recent WHO update.

RCUD is intended to encompass lower risk MDS presenting with unilineage dysplasia, including RA, RN, and RT. This subcategory of MDS is a characterized by refractory single lineage cytopenias, unilineage dysplasia, <5% blasts, and with <15% ring sideroblasts in the bone marrow. The term ringed has been changed to "ring" to describe sideroblasts in the

Table 10.2 Myelodysplastic syndrome classification: WHO, 2008

WHO Subtype	Peripheral blood	Bone marrow
Refractory Anemia with Unileage Dysplasia(RCUD); Refractory Anemia (RA); Refractory Neutropenia (RN); Refractory Thrombocytopenia (RT)	Unicytopenia or bicytopenia; no or rare blasts (<1%) *(Bicytopenia can be observed; however, pancytopenia should be classified as MDS-U)*	Unilineage dyslplasia in ≥10% of cells; <5% blasts; <15% ringed sideroblasts
Refractory Cytopenia with Multilineage Dysplasia (RCMD)	Cytopenia(s) (Bicytopenia or Pancytopenia); no or rare blasts (<1%); no Auer rods (AR); <1 monocytes	Dysplasia in 2 or 3 myeloid cell lineages (≥10%); <5% blasts; no AR; +/-15% RS
RA with Ringed Sideroblasts (RARS)	Anemia	RA; >15% ringed sideroblasts
Refractory Anemia with Excess Blasts (RAEB)-1	Cytopenia(s); <5% blasts; no Auer rods; <1 monocytes	Unilineage or Multilineage Dysplasia; 5–9% blasts; no AR
Refractory Anemia with Excess Blasts (RAEB)-2	Cytopenia(s); 5–19% blasts; +/-Auer rods; <1 monocytes	Unilineage or Multilineage Dysplasia; 10–19% blasts; +/- AR
MDS Associated with Isolated del (5q)	Anemia; <5% blasts; normal or increased platelets; no or rare blasts (<1%)	Increased megakaryocytes with hypolobulated nuclei; <5% blasts; no AR
Presumptive MDS with minimal cytogenetic criteria	Cytopenia; no or rare blasts(<1%)	Unequivocal dysplasia in <10% of cells of ≥1 myeloid cell lineages when accompanied by cytogenetic abnormality considered a presumptive evidence for a diagnosis of MDS; <5% blasts

2008 guidelines; the identification of ≥15% ring sideroblasts with alternate lineage of dysplasia constitutes RARS, representing approximately 3–11% of MDS and a favorable prognosis (median overall survival 69–108 months) [20]. Classically, RARS has only anemia but, in some cases, neutropenia or thrombocytopenia may be present in the face of erythroid unilineage dysplasia.

RCMD represents approximately 30% of MDS with a highly heterogeneous disease course likely secondary to the frequency of associated chromosomal anomalies. RCMD is characterized by cytopenia(s), no or rare myeloblasts in the peripheral blood, absence of Auer rods (AR) and without an absolute monocytosis within the peripheral blood. Analysis of the bone marrow should demonstrate dysplasia in two or three myeloid cell lineages (≥10%), <5% blasts, and no AR. However, unlike RA, ≥15% ringed sideroblasts can be seen.

MDS associated with isolated del(5q) and presumptive MDS with minimal cytogenetic criteria are the only categories characterized by *specific* cytogenetic anomalies. Criteria for MDS associated with isolated del(5q) remains the same as the previously named 5q- syndrome [18, 22]. Presumptive MDS with minimal cytogenetic criteria is characterized by cytopenias in the absence of myeloblasts in the peripheral blood and less than 5% myeloblasts within the bone marrow without convincing dysplasia in 10% or more of any myeloid lineage. However, a cytogenetic abnormality consistent with a diagnosis of MDS must be present. The anomaly (ies) consist of both balanced and unbalanced cytogenetic alterations (Table 10.3) [16]. Together, the above described WHO classification grouping begin to highlight the key characteristics in determining the fate of individual MDS patients.

Clinical assessment and prognosis

To further delineate prognosis of MDS patients, Greenberg et al. developed the International Prognostic Scoring System (IPSS) using an international data set of over 800 patients managed solely with supportive care. The IPSS was designed to assess risk for transformation to AML and survival in treatment

Table 10.3 Chromosomal abnormalities in MDS

Abnormality	Abnormality	Percentage
Unbalanced and Presumptive MDS	-7 or del(7)	10
	-5 or del(5)	10
	i(17p) or t(17p)	3–5
	-13 or del(13)	3
	Del(11q)	3
	del(12p) or t(12p)	3
	del(9p)	1–2
	idic(X)(q13)	1–2
Unbalanced and Not Presumptive MDS	+8	10
	del(20)	5–8
	-Y	5
Balanced	t(11:16)(q23;p13.3)	–
	t(3;21)(q26.2;q22.1)	–
	t(1;3)(p36.3;q21.2)	1
	t(2;11)(p21;q23)	1
	inv(3)(q21q26.2)	1
	t(6;9)(p23;q34)	1

naïve *de novo*/primary MDS at initial diagnosis (Table 10.4) [1]. The IPSS creates four risk strata based on cumulative scores termed Low-Risk, Intermediate-1, Intermediate-2, and High-Risk (LR, INT-1, INT-2, and HR). It is important to note that, although the initial IPSS dictated specific risk rates, the system was created in an era without treatment options and has not been reaffirmed in the era of lenalidomide and hypomethylating agents. To this end, the IPSS is generally utilized as a tool to dictate treatment goals more than as an absolute prognosticator. The score is derived from a weighted tabulation based on the following characteristics: cytopenias, percentage of myeloblasts within the bone marrow, and karyotype, therefore capturing hematologic, morphological, and genetic features. The

Table 10.4 International Prognostic Scoring System (IPSS)

	Score Value				
Prognostic indicator	0	0.5	1	1.5	2
Bone marrow blasts (%)	<5	5–10	–	11–20	21–30
Karyotype[a]	Good	Inter-mediate	Poor	–	–
Cytopenias[b]	0–1	2–3	–	–	–

	IPSS			
	Low	Int-1	Int-2	High
Score	0	0.5–1	1.5–2	>2.5
Percent MDS	33	38	22	7
Median survival (months)[c]	5.7	3.5	1.1	0.4
Progression to AML (25%)[c]	9.4	3.3	1.1	0.2

[a] Karyotype: Good → Normal (46XX or XY); -Y; del(5q); del(20) [*alone*] Intermediate → *All* that is not Poor or Good [*other*]
Poor → Complex (>3); Chromosome 7 anomalies
[b] Cytopenia: ANC <1800; Hemoglobin <10; Platelets <100
[c] Without therapy
(Adapted from Greenberg et al. (1997) [1]; Sanz GF et al. (1998) *Haematologica* **83**:358–68.)

IPSS remains the current standard in delineating treatment options in MDS. Retrospective analysis suggests that it is valid at points of restaging; however, it was developed for initial evaluation of *de novo* MDS. Further, the IPSS is limited by our changing understanding of MDS and to the *weight* that myeloblast percentage and karyotypic anomalies contribute to overall prognosis. To this end, a number of alternative prognostic scoring systems have been developed. Although these studies have not yet defined a new standard, they highlight the continuing need to improve on current guidelines.

One such study by Malcovati et al. explored predictive determinants for survival and leukemia evolution in MDS along a temporal continuum, that is, a time-dependent prognostic scoring system [23], thus addressing a concern that the IPSS could not address, namely, changing prognostic features

through the course of the disease. The authors showed that WHO category, karyotype (based on IPSS criteria), and additionally transfusion dependence (defined as requiring at least one RBC transfusion every eight weeks over a period of four months) were the most significant prognostic indicators by multivariate analysis. This WHO classification-based prognostic scoring system (WPSS) identified five prognostic risk groups with median survivals ranging from 12 to 103 months. More recently, a collaborative effort delineated a new proposal for a novel risk stratification model in MDS [15]. This risk model was intended to encompass a larger percentage of patients including secondary MDS, previously treated MDS, and CMML with leukocytosis (>12 000) in addition to *de novo* treatment naïve patients as in the previous prognostic model. This analysis examined 1915 patients randomly divided into two groups (958 in the study group and 957 in the test group). Multivariant analysis identified poor performance status, older age, thrombocytopenia, anemia, percentage of bone marrow myeloblasts, leukocytosis, karyotypic anomalies (chromosome 7 and complex cytogenetics) as well as prior transfusions and negative risk factors. This prognostic system allotted points for poor performance status, age, platelets, anemia, bone marrow blasts, WB, karyotype, and transfusions (Table 10.5). Four groups were identified; a low-risk group (0–4 points), intermediate -1 (5–6), intermediate-2 (7–8), and high risk (≥9) characterized by 54-, 25-, 14-, and 6-month median survival and 63%, 34%, 16%, and 4% 3-year overall survival respectively. Importantly, these prognostic

Table 10.5 Myelodysplastic syndrome risk score[a]

Prognostic factor	Abnormality	Points
Performance status	≥2	2
Age (years)	60–64	1
	≥ 65	2
Platelets	< 30	3
	30–49	2
	50–199	1
Hemaglobin	< 12	2
WBCs	>20 000	2
Bone marrow blasts (%)	5–10	1
	11–29	2
Karyotype	Chromosome 7 abnormality or complex (≥3)	3
Prior transfusion	Yes	1

[a] Four groups were identified (0–15); a *low-risk* group (0–4 points), *intermediate-1* (5–6), *intermediate-2* (7 8), and *high risk* (≥9). These groups are characterized ay 54-, 25-, 14-, and 6-month median survival and 63%, 34%, 16%, and 4% 3-year overall survival respectively.
(Adapted from Kantarjian et al. (2008) *Cancer* 113:1351–61.)

parameters held true in secondary MDS, previously treated MDS, and CMML with leukocytosis. Significantly, this study demonstrated that a relatively simple prognostic system can be developed to aid in prognosticating across the spectrum of MDS, and it facilitates a dynamic model for risk modeling, accounting for evolution of MDS with or without treatment.

Management

Management of patients with MDS parallels the heterogeneous nature of the disease itself. Management can span from anticipatory monitoring to supportive care with growth factors, transfusions, and antibiotics; to active treatment with hypomethylating agents, lenalidomide, and finally hematopoietic stem cell transplant (Tables 10.6 and 10.7). Management decisions are guided by risk stratification, the dynamics and severity of an individual's cytopenias, comorbidities, as well as the patient's preference. Below we will discuss treatment strategies as well as the management algorithms as outlined by the National Comprehensive Cancer Network (NCCN) and practiced at our institution [24].

Supportive care
Patients are frequently diagnosed as a consequence of the symptoms related to cytopenias (anemia>neutropenia>thrombocytopenia). To this end, assessment of an individual's symptoms and their impact on quality of life is paramount. With the goal of improving quality of life, frequently supportive measures involve more than the obvious utilization of clinical monitoring, erythroid stimulating agents (ESA), myeloid growth factors (MGFs), transfusion of blood products, and antibiotics, but also psychosocial support and frequent assessment of quality of life with appropriate timing of iron chelation. Appropriate utilization of these measures is of vital importance for the interests of the patient as well as the burden of the healthcare system.

Erythroid stimulating agents (ESAs)
The development of ESAs (epoetin alpha and darbepoetin) has facilitated a significant improvement in

Table 10.6 Seminal trials utilizing hypomethylating agents

Trial	Overall response rate	Overall survival	Ref.
CALGB 9221	Azacitidine vs. BSC	21 vs. 12 months	Silverman et al. [42]
CALGB 8421, 8921, & 9221	Azacitidine vs. BSC	19.3 vs. 12.9 months[a]	Silverman et al. [43]
AZA-001	Azacitidine vs. conventional care (induction, oral cytarabine, BSC)	24.5 vs. 15 months	Fenaux et al. [44]
Lyons et al.	Azacitidine 5 vs. $5+2+2$ vs. $5+2+5$[b]	NA	Lyons et al. [45]
Kantarjian et al.	Decitabine vs. BSC	*de novo* MDS: 12.6 vs. 9.4 & HR MDS: 9.3 vs. 2.8 months[c]	Kantarjian et al. [49]
Kantarjian et al.	Decitabine 20 mg/m2 IV ×5 vs. 20 mg/m2 SC×5 vs. 10 mg/m2 SC× 10[d]	NA	Kantarjian et al. [50]

[a] MDS-t patients redefined by WHO 2002 criteria
[b] Patients were randomly assigned to one of three arms (1) a five-day regimen (5) of azacitidine (75 mg/m2) on days 1–5 of a 28-day cycle (5); (2) a 7-day regimen $(5+2+2)$ of azacitidine, on (75 mg/m2) 1–5 and 8–9 of a 28-day cycle with no drug on days 6 and 7 to account for the weekend; and (3) a 10-day regimen $(5+2+5)$ with a reduced dose of azacitidine (50 mg/m2) on days 1–5 and 8–12 of a 28-day cycle skipping days 6 and 7
[c] Post-hoc retrospective analysis demonstrated specific survival benefit in *de novo* MDS (12.6 vs. 9.4 months; p = 0.04) and high-risk MDS (9.3 vs. 2.8 months; p = 0.01)
[d] The differing regimens were standard (at the time) vs .20 mg/m2 IV × 5days, 20 mg/m2 subcutaneously for 5 days, or 10 mg/m2 IV for 10 days.

Table 10.7 Seminal trials utilizing lenalidomide

Trial	Conditions	Hematologic response	Ref.
MDS-001	Lenalidomide vs. BSC (all)	46%[a]	List et al. [80]
MDS-003	Lenalidomide vs. BSC (del (5q))	67%[b]	List et al. [56]
MDS-002	Lenalidomide vs. BSC (non-del (5q))	26%	Raza et al. [57]
Adès et al.	Lenalidomide (higher risk; del (5q))[c]	27% (67%)[d]	Adès et al. [59]

[a] 5q- received the greatest benefit with 83% HR, normal cytogenetics 57%, and complex cytogenetics with 12%
[b] With transfusion independence (TI) as the primary end point the trial, intent to treat analysis demonstrated that transfusion requirements were obviated in 67% (CI 59-74%; 72% with isolated 5q-; 48% + 1; and 67% in >2) of patients by 4.6 weeks (1-49 weeks).
[c] This phase II study examined the effects of lenalidomide in higher risk MDS (60% HR & 40% INT-2 by IPSS
[d] Hematologic response in higher risk MDS with isolated del 5q (6/9 with isolated del 5q; 1/11 with one additional mutation, and 0/27 with complex cytogenetics including del 5q.

the quality of life for scores of individuals with MDS. These agents are heavily utilized in the MDS and case control studies suggest that they confer a survival advantage in addition to improved quality of life [25–28]. Responses to ESAs ranges from 15–55% depending on the study examined [28–30]. Importantly, optimal response to these agents can be predicted based on IPSS (LR and INT-1), EPO levels <500 and a transfusion burden of less than two units of packed red blood cells (pRBCs) per month [25, 26]. This response score assigns points for specific serum EPO concentrations and transfusion burden, dividing patients into three response categories: poor, intermediate, and good with response rates of 7%, 23%, and 74%, respectively. This study highlights the need for judicious antecedent response stratification for the use of these agents for maximal response in those that may benefit. To this end, NCCN suggests that ESAs be utilized in patients with LR or INT-1 risk MDS, with EPO levels <500 and/or with a transfusion burden of less than two units pRBCs per month. Response to these agents should occur by 4–6 weeks with reassessment of dosing at that time [24]. Initial dose escalation and ESA utilization should be discontinued if no response is observed by 12 weeks [26]. It is also important to remember that ESAs are not without risk and, therefore, patients need careful monitoring.

Myeloid growth factors

Although the myeloid growth factors G-CSF and GM-CSF have yet to demonstrate disease-modifying activity alone, they significantly enhance erythropoiesis when utilized in combination with ESAs [31–33]. The biological rationale stems from reports documenting G-CSF-mediated development of early precursors into EPO-responsive progenitor cells [31]. Initial reports demonstrated that treatment of anemia in MDS patients with G-CSF and EPO resulted in an erythroid response in 42% of patients [31]. Moreover, lower levels of pretreatment endogenous erythropoietin correlated with response. More recently, Balleari et al. demonstrated that response rates in low-risk MDS patients increased from 40% with ESA alone to 73.3% in combination with myeloid growth factors [33]. Further, 44.4% of patients unresponsive to ESA subsequently responded to combined therapy. Casadevall and colleagues found that increased response to combination therapy equated to increased medical cost, suggesting that although the combination is effective, the use of these agents should be individualized [32]. Lastly, although MDS-associated neutropenia remains relatively growth factor resistant, myeloid growth factors are not infrequently used in MDS patients with febrile neutropenia or active infection(s).

Platelet growth factors

Thrombocytopenia is observed in approximately two-thirds of MDS patients through the course of their disease and can be associated with significant morbidity. With the identification of the c-mpl agonists, romiplostim and eltrombopag, a significant amount of interest has developed in investigating the possible role for these agents in supportive care [34]. Currently, neither of the thrombopoietin receptor agonists is approved for use in MDS, although both have received FDA approval in chronic immune thrombocytopenic purpura (ITP). In MDS, an interim analysis of a placebo-controlled phase II study examining romiplostim support in low- or intermediate-risk patients receiving azacitidine revealed a decrease in thrombocytopenic events and platelet transfusions in the romiplostim arms relative to placebo [35]. Two adverse events were observed in the romiplostim arms, including a rash and an arthralgia. Of note, although no reported deaths occurred in the romiplostim arm, the only transforming event in the study to date occurred in the romiplostim arm. In a phase I/II single agent dose-escalating study, platelet responses were reported in 41% of patients treated with romiplostim. The clinical trial raised safety concerns owing to elevations in bone marrow or peripheral blood blast percentage in more than 20% of patients. Eltrombopag, is an orally bioavailable thrombopoietin receptor agonist that binds at a site distinct from that of other receptor ligands. Preclinical studies suggest that eltrombopag may have intrinsic anti-leukemic effect and blocks the stimulatory effects of native thrombopoietin in AML cells, making it an attractive agent for investigation in MDS. Although thrombopoietic agents have significant potential in supportive care in this disease, to date, these agents do not have an indication in MDS.

Iron overload

In MDS, anemia is one of the most important and likely causes of morbidity. Secondary to ineffective erythropoiesis and clinical sequelae of anemia, red blood cell transfusions are an important supportive modality for MDS. Transfusions are fraught with potential acute transfusion-associated side effects, as well as long term sequelae [3]. One important factor to consider with chronic transfusions is iron overload. Excess iron can contribute to significant comorbidities secondary to parenchymal iron deposition leading to cardiac, hepatic, thyroid, hypothalamic, and endocrine pancreatic dysfunction. Transfusion-dependent patients have a decreased overall survival [15, 23, 36]. Iron overload occurs due to the inability of the human body to excrete excess iron. Chelating agents such as deferoxamine and deferasirox reduce serum ferritin in MDS patients [36–38]. Two studies suggested that iron chelation therapy is associated with better overall survival in lower-risk MDS. No prospective randomized clinical trials have addressed this issue yet [39, 40].

Current guidelines suggest initiation of iron chelation therapy following reaching a cumulative transfusion threshold of 20–30 units of red blood cells and/or once serum ferritin is greater than 1000–2000 mg/L in patients with lower-risk MDS or potential transplant candidates [36]. Importantly, secondary to potential side effects, hepatic, renal function, as well as auditory and ophthalmic testing is indicated with the use of deferasirox [41]. Significantly, in addition to BSC, disease-specific modalities have recently been adopted that have revolutionized clinical practice.

Hypomethylating agents

The hypomethylating agents azacitidine and decitabine are important additions to therapy for MDS. Collectively, these agents are referred to as hypomethylating compounds, based on the ability of these drugs to reverse epigenetic tumor suppressor gene silencing. Azacitidine (5-azacitidine) is a cytosine nucleoside analog with potential for both RNA and DNA incorporation. Decitabine (5-aza-2'-deoxycytidine) is a cytosine analog that is DNA selective. Covalent bonds formed between deoxycytidine nucleotides and DNA methyltransferase depletes the enzyme and, as a consequence, reverses methylation of tumor suppressor genes (hypomethylation) facilitating the activity of azacitadine and decitabine in MDS. Although this is the presumed mechanism of action, it does not exclude other means by which these agents function such as direct cytotoxicity. Currently, the hypomethylating agents are used in individuals with higher risk MDS or preparation for hematopoietic stem cell transplant (Table 10.6) [24]. Moreover, hypomethylating agents are also recommended for use in individuals with lower risk MDS associated with anemia or thrombocytopenia refractory to ESAs or lenalidomide. Within this section we will discuss important studies facilitating their collective utilization in the treatment of MDS.

Azacitidine

Azacitidine was the first FDA-approved drug for use in MDS. Azacitidine is currently FDA approved for the treatment of all FAB disease categories of MDS, RA, RARS (if accompanied with neutropenia, thrombocytopenia, or requiring transfusions), RAEB, RAEB in transition (RAEB-t), and CMML. Approval of azacitidine followed a number of studies, including the CALGB 9221study that demonstrated hematologic benefit and decreased rate of progression to AML [42–44]. The CALGB 9221 study was a randomized phase III study of 191 patients with MDS comparing 5-azacitidine given as 75 mg/m^2 subcutaneously for seven days in 28-day cycles and best supportive care (BSC). If, after four months of BSC, there was evidence for disease progression or increasing transfusion support, those individuals could cross-over to azacitidine treatment [42]. Silverman and colleagues demonstrated significant superiority for azacitidine in several important parameters. Overall response rates (CR + PR (partial remission)) were 23% (CR 7%, PR 16%) and 0% in the azacitidine and BSC arms, respectively. Further, of the 49 patients that crossed over, an ORR of 14% was observed (CR 10%, PR 4%). Median time to transformation to AML was increased from 12 months to 21 months (p<0.007), with an associated decrease in rate of transformation to AML from 24% to 3% in the first six months. Utilization of azacitidine conferred independence from transfusion in 45% of patients initially dependent on blood products. The quality of life (QOL) measures of fatigue, physical function, dyspnea, positive affect, and psychological distress were improved in the azacitidine arm over BSC. A follow-up, retrospective analysis of three CALGB studies (CALGB 8421, 8921, and 9221) utilizing the WHO diagnostic criteria as well as the International Working Group (IWG) criteria for hematologic response had similar findings. More recently, a larger international multicenter phase III trial involving 358 MDS patients compared treatment with azacitidine to three conventional care strategies: BSC, low-dose cytarabine, or intensive AML CT [44]. Eligibility in the AZA-001 was restricted to patients with higher risk MDS stratified by FAB system (primarily RAEB, RAEB-t, and CMML) and IPSS (INT-2 and HR) with overall survival as the primary end point [44]. In this intention to treat (ITT) analysis, Fenaux et al. demonstrated that median OS was significantly extended in the azacitidine group as compared to conventional therapy, 24.5 months versus 15 months respectively. Furthermore, at two years of follow-up, 50.8% of the azacitidine group were alive compared to 26% of the conventional therapy group. Important secondary end points, including response (OR, CR, and PR), time to AML transformation, and transfusion independence, also favored the azacitidine arm. The CR/PR rate was 29% for azacitidine and 12% for conventional therapy (CR 17%/PR 12% vs. CR 8%/PR 4%). Transformation to AML was delayed by 4–5 months (azacitidine: 13 months vs. conventional therapy: 7.6 months). Hematologic response rates also favored the azacitidine arm with 45% of azacitidine group and only 11% of individuals in the conventional care arm becoming transfusion independent. This report was the first, and to date, the only study demonstrating a survival benefit in higher risk MDS.

The success of azacitidine in MDS has stimulated questions on the most appropriate or efficient dosing regimen. Currently, azacitidine is given as consecutive day treatment for seven days of a 28-day cycle at 75 mg/m^2 either subcutaneously or intravenously. However, the growing utilization of azacitidine in the community in lower risk disease in order to obtain hematologic improvement has facilitated discussion regarding the cumbersome dosing regimen. As with most early studies, the seven-day schedule was designed in academic settings and was primarily limited to higher risk MDS. Many community oncologists are more limited in terms of weekend capabilities and support staff. Moreover, in lower risk disease where hematologic response is all that *may* be necessary, alternate dosing schedules with reduced toxicity and greater compliance may be warranted. These details have facilitated an intriguing study comparing three schedules of azacitidine [45]. This study encompasses a different subset of MDS patients with the majority of patients with RA or RARS. The major end points in this study were hematologic improvement (IWG criteria), transfusion independence, and safety. Patients were randomly assigned to one of three arms: (1) a five-day regimen of azacitidine (75 mg/m^2) on days 1–5 of a 28-day cycle (5); (2) a seven-day regimen (5 + 2 + 2) of azacitidine (75 mg/m^2) on days 1–5 and 8–9 of a 28-day cycle with no drug on days 6 and 7 (the weekend); and (3) a 10-day regimen (5 + 2 + 5) with a reduced dose of azacitidine (50 mg/m^2) on days 1–5 and 8–12 of a 28-day cycle omitting the weekend. Each arm was scheduled for six cycles, at which time responding patients could continue to receive maintenance azacitidine using the 5-day schedule at 4 week or 6week cycles. To date, only the response rate between induction arms has been evaluated. Hematologic response was noted in 44%, 45%, and 56% in the 5, 5 + 2 + 2, and 5 + 2 + 5 arms respectively. Transfusion independence was observed in 50% (5), 55% (5 + 2 + 2), and 64% (5 + 2 + 5) of patients who were previously dependent on red blood cell products. Adverse events were also reported with >1 grade 3–4 adverse event in 58%, 77% and 84% in the 5, 5 + 2 + 2, and 5 + 2 + 5 arms respectively (neutropenia (+/-febrile), anemia, and thrombocytopenia). These results demonstrate that, although equivalent responses were observed, the 5-day regimen had significantly fewer adverse events relative to the 7-

or 10-day regimens. It should be emphasized survival was not an end point of the study and these regimens should not be consider congruous to the 7-day dosing regimens impact on survival in higher risk patients. This trial provides an interesting avenue to further optimize the efficiency of azacitidine therapy in both lower and higher risk MDS and suggests that differing regimens may fit specific risk categories.

In addition to the specific regimen utilized, it is also important to comment on the temporal action of azacitidine. Unlike primary induction chemotherapy with rapid response to therapy, treatment with azacitidine had a median time to response of 64 days and median best response of 93 days in the CALGB studies. This translated into a median interval to PR of 7 cycles with a range between 2 and 19 cycles and a median time to CR of 8 cycles ranging from 8–15 cycles. Extending this work, Silverman et al. more recently examined the effects of continued azacitidine treatment in higher risk MDS [46]. Examination of 179 higher risk MDS patients (RAEB, RAEB-T, and CMML) with IPSS of INT-2 or HR following azacitidine subcutaneous injection ($75 \, mg/m^2$ 7/28-day cycles) demonstrated a CR, PR, or hematologic improvement in 51% (91 patients). Of these, the median number of cycles needed to achieve a first response was three, with 81% of patients achieving first response by six cycles and 90% by nine cycles. In 57% of individuals, the first response was the optimal response; however, in the remainder of patients (43%) a median of four additional cycles of treatment were necessary to achieve optimal response. These patterns of response are important to consider in treatment decisions. The data outlined above suggests that, although responses may be documented early in treatment courses, continued therapy will net gains in response in a significant proportion of patients and would be warranted in the absence of unacceptable toxicity or disease progression. Moreover, the delays in response may be indicative of the unique mechanism of action of azacitidine in hypomethylation of formerly dormant tumor suppressor genes. This pattern is also observed, to some extent, with decitabine suggesting a class effect (as discussed below). To this end, knowledge and experience in the use of azacitidine are important for optimal patient care.

Decitabine

Decitabine is the second hypomethylating agent the FDA approved for treatment of MDS. Although decitabine has a similar presumed mechanism of action, its exclusive incorporation into DNA may manifest as slightly different clinical outcomes. It is important to note that the most widely adopted dosing regimen differs from that utilized in the seminal studies defining its role in MDS therapy. Decitabine was initially examined in two phase II studies in higher risk MDS patients in Europe [47, 48]. The positive results of these studies led to a phase III trial in the US comparing $15 \, mg/m^2$ IV over three hours every eight hours for three consecutive days and best supportive care in INT-1, INT-2, and HR MDS [49]. In this study, a 30% response rate was noted with 9% CR, 8% PR, and 13% hematologic improvement. Despite the response rate, median time to death and transformation to AML was not significantly altered. Further analysis demonstrated that specific benefit was seen in *de novo* MDS (12.6 vs. 9.4 months; $p = 0.04$) and high-risk MDS (9.3 vs. 2.8 months; $p = 0.01$). A subsequent retrospective study comparing decitabine to intensive chemotherapy in higher risk MDS did yield a two-year survival rate of 47% and 21% respectively in patients matched with similar baseline characteristics [49]. However, the dosing regimen was rather intensive with prolonged myelosuppression, which fostered exploration of alternate effective regimens specifically appropriate for outpatient administration with a lower toxicity profile. Kantarjian et al. compared three schedules using reduced cumulative decitabine dosing regimens [50]. This report examined 95 patients with INT-1, INT-2, and HR MDS with 32% with secondary MDS. The differing regimens were $20 \, mg/m^2$ IV for 5 days, $20 \, mg/m^2$ subcutaneously for 5 days, and $10 \, mg/m^2$ IV for 10 days. Complete response and marrow CR rates were highest for the five-day intravenous schedule, that is, 39%, versus 21%, and 24%.

The EORTC Leukemia and German MDS Study Groups examined the effects of the approved-dose decitabine regimen ($15 \, mg/m^2$ IV x 3 days of a 6-

week cycle) in elderly patients (>70 years old) with INT-2 (55%) and HR (38%) disease who were not eligible for intensive chemotherapy versus supportive care [51]. This phase III study yielded an overall response rate (CR, PR, and hematological improvement) of 35% in the decitabine arm as compared to supportive care. Further, PFS was improved from 0.25 to 0.55 years in the decitabine arm (p = 0.004; 95% CI, 0.52–0.88). In contrast, overall survival or the median time to transformation to AML or death was not significantly altered between decitabine and supportive care (0.73 vs. 0.51 years; p = 0.24; CI 95%, 0.64–1.12). The authors speculated that, although the PFS is statistically improved in the decitabine arm (versus supportive care), the inability to demonstrate an improved overall survival may stem from the limited dosing schedule. These studies highlight the lack of a disease-modifying effect that impacts survival with the original decitabine schedule and, perhaps, suggest the existence of distinct biological differences between the FDA-approved hypomethylating agents.

Immune modulatory and immunosuppressive therapy

Lenalidomide

Lenalidomide is the third FDA-approved agent and another important therapeutic tool in the MDS armamentarium (Table 10.7). This immune modulatory derivative of thalidomide has proven particularly successful in the treatment of a specific subset of red blood cell transfusion-dependent patients with deletion of the long arm of chromosome 5 (del(5q)) with LR and INT-1 MDS. The precise mechanism of action of lenalidomide in del(5q) MDS has been a topic of focused investigation. Lenalidomide selectively inhibits the *in vitro* growth of del(5q) MDS progenitors [52], whereas in MDS with alternate karyotypes and normal bone marrow CD34 cells, lenalidomide and its analog, pomalidomide, promote erythroid lineage competence and colony-forming capacity [53, 54]. Analysis of *in vitro* drug-induced changes in gene expression has shown that lenalidomide upregulates expression of several genes in del(5q) erythroblasts, including the haplodeficient secretion protein acidic cysteine-rich

(*SPARC*) gene encoded within the common deleted region interstitial chromosome 5 deletion [52]. Although the *SPARC* gene product has antiproliferative and antiangiogenic effects, its precise role, if any, in mediating the apoptotic response to lenalidomide in del(5q) MDS is not clear. Recent investigations have implicated inhibition of two cell cycle regulatory phosphatases (i.e., *Cdc25C* and *PP2 A*-Cα) that are haplodeficient in del(5q) MDS, as key targets underlying the karyotype-dependent cytotoxicity of lenalidomide [55]. Indeed, selective suppression of gene expression by short hairpin RNA (shRNA) promotes selective sensitivity to lenalidomide-induced apoptosis in both a cell-line model and primary MDS bone marrow cells with a normal karyotype. These findings suggest that haploinsufficiency for critical druggable gene products underlies therapeutic specificity of lenalidomide in del(5q) MDS. Three important studies have served to define the niche for lenalidomide in therapy for lower risk MDS: MDS-001, MDS-003, and MDS-002.

MDS associated with isolated del(5q) portends a relatively good prognosis. However, patients are frequently resistant to supportive care with ESA, requiring significant transfusion support. Deletions in 5q represent 15% lower risk MDS (whether alone or in combination with one or more (complex) cytogenetic changes). The utility of lenalidomide in MDS was promoted via a single center phase I/II study, MDS-001 [56]. This clinical trial examined the safety and efficacy of lenalidomide in 43 patients who failed conventional therapy. Seventy-four percent of patients were transfusion dependent, 46% with abnormal cytogenetics and 28% with deletion 5q. All patients had failed treatment with ESAs or had a poor ESA response profile. The study tested three dosing regimens of oral lenalidomide [56]. A major hematologic response as measured by transfusion independence or a greater than a 2 g/dl rise in hemoglobin for at least eight weeks was reported in 49% of patients. Further, major hematologic responses were durable in del(5q) MDS and this was associated with cytogenetic response. Individuals with del(5q) MDS received the greatest benefit with 83% experiencing a major erythroid response, compared to 57% in patients with normal, and 12% in patients with a complex karyotype. Response rate differed by IPSS category with an erythroid response in 68% of LR MDS patients, 50% of INT-1, and 20% of INT-2. Specific treatment-related toxicities included grade 3–4 neutropenia and thrombocytopenia in 65% and 74% of patients, respectively. These parameters were thought to be important hallmarks of drug activity and were assessed carefully in subsequent clinical trials [56].

The multicenter phase II MDS-003 study represents the pivotal study that secured FDA approval of lenalidomide for the treatment of lower risk del (5q) MDS. In this study, 148 primarily transfusion-dependent (84%) lower risk patients with del(5q) were treated with 10 mg lenalidamide 21 days of a 28-day cycle (amended to 10 mg daily based on the analysis of MDS-001) [56]. Overall, 74% of participants had an isolated del(5q), whereas 17% had an additional chromosomal abnormality and two or more anomalies were present in 8% of patients. With transfusion independence (TI) as the primary end point of the trial, ITT analysis demonstrated that transfusion requirements were obviated in 67% (CI 59–74%; 72% with isolated 5q-; 48% +1; and 67% in >2) of patients by a median interval of 4.6 weeks of study treatment (1–49 weeks). Further, a cytogenetic response (>50% reduction in expression of 5q- clones) was observed in 73% of the evaluable patients (77% with isolated 5q-; 67% +1; and 50% in >2). Again, grade 3–4 neutropenia (55%) and thrombocytopenia (44%) were commonly observed, largely in the initial eight weeks of lenalidomide treatment. As hypothesized, the presence of a greater than 50% decrease in platelets from baseline and/or a greater than 75% reduction ANC (absolute neutophil count) portended a greater likelihood of TI. It is important to note that, although neutropenia and thrombocytopenia apparently predict response, they remain significant dose-limiting toxicities with necessity for close monitoring and appropriate dose reductions or interruptions in therapy. Together, these studies have established an important role for lenalidomide in the management of MDS associated with isolated del(5q).

Evidence from MDS-001 suggested that lenalidomide may also have a role in non-5q- MDS. Therefore, the question remained, is there a role for lenalidomide in non-5q deletion MDS? A third study, MDS-002 was designed similarly to MDS-003 in transfusion-dependent lower risk MDS patients. In this study, however, the population was restricted to lower risk MDS patients without chromosome 5 anomalies [57]. MDS-002 yielded TI with lenalidomide in 26% of participants. Although this represents a significantly lower percentage than the response rate observed in MDS-003 (67%), the response is similar to that observed with ESA in unselected patients [58]. These results suggest that lenalidomide may have an important role in therapy for ESA unresponsive non-5q- MDS. It is also important to note that, although observed, neutropenia and thrombocytopenia did not correlate with TI as observed in MDS-003. The differences in activity and toxicity between del(5q) and non-del(5q) MDS patients suggests a dual mechanism of action. In del (5q), suppression or eradication of the clone seems to be the dominant mechanism of action, while promoting erythroid differentiation is noted in non-del(5q) patients.

Based on the above outlined studies, the NCCN recommends lenalidomide in anemic lower risk del (5q) MDS patients with or without additional chromosomal anomalies in the absence of clinically significant thrombocytopenia or neutropenia. Lenalidomide may also be considered in lower risk non-del (5q) MDS refractory to ESA (+/− MGFs). However, a recent phase II study demonstrated the successful treatment (27% HR) of INT-2 and HR MDS patients with del(5q) with lenalidomide [59]. Although these are preliminary results, they indicate that lenalidomide may also play a role in higher risk MDS patients who harbor the del(5q) chromosomal abnormality.

Myelosuppression is mostly anticipated during the first few months of treatment; weekly complete blood counts should be monitored for the first eight weeks. Dose interruption may be required (more in patients with del(5q)) usually within three to four weeks of starting therapy. Patients with impaired renal function were originally excluded from the above-mentioned clinical trials. Recommendations for dose adjustment in patients with renal impairment have been published [60].

Antithymocyte globulin and cyclosporine

Specific subsets of MDS harbor characteristics of autoimmune diseases – specifically hypoplastic MDS, paroxysmal nocturnal hemaglobinuria (PNH), and aplastic anemia (AA). This population of individuals can be identified by a younger age (<60), brief duration of transfusion requirements, HLA-DR phenotype, and hypocellular marrow [61, 62]. A significant number of these patients are noted to have a concomitant clonal expansion of hematopoietic inhibitory T-lymphocytes. Further, reversal of peripheral blood cytopenias and bone marrow suppression has been associated with immune suppressive therapy-mediated attenuation of clonal T-lymphocytes [63]. As such, the use of immune suppressive agents such as ATG and cyclosporine (CsA) has grown into favor as treatment for this group of MDS patients [64–66]. The use of ATG/CsA appears to benefit only a small subset of MDS patients [67]; however, identification of the appropriate population may facilitate lasting responses in this younger cache of individuals [62]. To this end, the National Comprehensive Cancer Network (NCCN) recommends the utilization of ATG/CsA in lower risk MDS patients (LR and INT-1 younger age (<60), positive HLA-DR phenotype, evidence of a PNH clone and a hypocellular marrow). Hematologic improvement is seen in approximately one-third of MDS patients treated with ATG $+/-$ cyclosporine. Most responses are seen in the erythroid lineage; however, response is not lineage-specific and hematologic responses are often durable. Age has emerged as the strongest predictive factor for response as demonstrated by long-term follow-up studies by the National Institutes of Health. Lower CD4: CD8 ratio, arising from CD4+ depletion from homeostatic proliferation, is suggested as an immune signature that may identify potential responders to immunosuppressive therapy [68, 69].

Hematopoietic stem cells transplant (HSCT)

Allogeneic HSCT remains the only potentially curative treatment modality in MDS. However, the decision of when and who to refer for HSCT remains difficult. Patients with higher risk MDS who are at greatest risk for death or AML transformation within months are generally recommended for early allogeneic HSCT. But, as is frequently the case, a large percentage of these patients are not appropriate candidates. Individuals with lower risk disease may benefit from HSCT, however the balance between morbidity and mortality of transplant and quality of life gained with current therapies makes this procedure a difficult decision. Based on results of a decision analysis model, the NCCN recommends that MDS patients less than 60 years of age with IPSS of INT-2 and HR should proceed to HLA-matched sibling HSCT as long as they: (1) have a compatible donor, and (2) have limited co-morbidities that would increase the risks of the procedure. For patients with lower risk disease (LR and INT-1) a trial of therapy should be attempted with close monitoring, reserving HSCT until the time of disease progression or exhaustion of standard therapy [24, 70]. Oliansky et al. recently published a systematic evidence-based review analyzing timing of the HSCT decision [71].

Therapies on the horizon

Although significant strides have been made in therapy for MDS, disease management remains a challenge. As such, continued investigation and development of new modalities of therapy is paramount. These endeavors involve exploration of both novel biological targets and new combinations of currently utilized modalities. Strategies include attempts to improve current response rates by combination therapies and novel agents, or to develop tools to better select responders for a certain type of therapy.

The success of the hypomethylating agents in MDS opened the door to clinical trials examining the activity of other agents with putative roles in chromatin remodulating [72, 73]. One such agent is the histone deacetylase valproic acid. Supported by robust preclinical data demonstrating increased activity of DMTI and HDACs *in vitro* [74], two phase II studies have been carried out examining the dual epigenetic modification in MDS and AML [75, 76]. Issa et al. examined the efficacy of dual epigenetic modification in MDS and AML [75]. In this study, decitabine alone or decitabine and valproate were compared. No significant difference was noted in either overall survival (14.9 vs. 14.9 months) or median time to first response (64 vs. 57 days). The combination was also associated with significantly increased rates of neurotoxicity. The authors concluded that the combination may increase time to first response but had no effect on overall survival, and suggested that alternate and more specific HDAC inhibitors may offer greater activity. Garcia-Manero et al. reported a 37% response rate in a phase I/II study examining the combination of azacitidine and a novel oral isotype selective HDAC inhibitor, MGCD0103 [76]. A third HDAC inhibitor, vironostat, is also under active investigation in MDS both alone and in combination with azacitidine [77, 78]. With a large number of HDAC inhibitors and previous success of epigenetic modifiers, continued investigation may reveal important advances for MDS therapy. Further, the success of current therapeutic modalities suggests that multi-agent regimens may provide additional benefit. A phase I study is examining the feasibility of combining lenalidomide and azacitidine in higher risk MDS [79]. Together, these studies illustrate the momentum created by the identification of biologically active hypomethylating agents and lenalidomide; ideally, leading to the next generation of MDS therapeutics.

Conclusion

MDS is an age-dependent hematopoietic malignancy with inherent morbidity, increased mortality, and increased risk of transformation to AML. Management of this disorder ranges from observation, to supportive care with growth factors, transfusions and antibiotics, to active therapy and hematopoietic stem cell transplant. Azacitidine, decitabine, and lenalidomide have contributed greatly to improving the outcome and quality of life for patients with this disorder. Continued investigation is paramount to identify the next generation of successful treatments.

References

1 Greenberg P, Cox C, LeBeau MM, et al. (1997) International scoring system for evaluating prognosis in myelodysplastic syndromes. *Blood* **89**:2079–88.

2 Ma X, Does M, Raza A, Mayne ST. (2007) Myelodysplastic syndromes: incidence and survival in the United States. *Cancer* **109**:1536–42.

3 Komrokji RS, Matacia-Murphy GM, Ali NH, et al. (2010) Outcome of patients with myelodysplastic syndromes in the Veterans Administration population. *Leuk Res* **34**:59–62.

4 Rollison DE, Howlader N, Smith MT, et al. (2008) Epidemiology of myelodysplastic syndromes and chronic myeloproliferative disorders in the United States, 2001-2004, using data from the NAACCR and SEER programs. *Blood* **112**:45–52.

5 Germing U, Strupp C, Kuendgen A, et al. (2006) Prospective validation of the WHO proposals for the classification of myelodysplastic syndromes. *Haematologica* **91**:1596–604.

6 Strom SS, Velez-Bravo V, Estey EH. (2008) Epidemiology of myelodysplastic syndromes. *Semin Hematol* **45**:8–13.

7 Aul C, Gattermann N, Schneider W. (1992) Age-related incidence and other epidemiological aspects of myelodysplastic syndromes. *Br J Haematol* **82**:358–67.

8 Delhommeau F, Dupont S, Della Valle V, James C, et al. (2009) Mutation in TET2 in myeloid cancers. *N Engl J Med* **360**:2289–301.

9 Tiu R, Gondek L, O'Keefe C, Maciejewski JP. (2007) Clonality of the stem cell compartment during evolution of myelodysplastic syndromes and other bone marrow failure syndromes. *Leukemia* **21**:1648–57.

10 Nilsson L, Astrand-Grundstrom I, Arvidsson I, et al. (2000) Isolation and characterization of hematopoietic progenitor/stem cells in 5q-deleted myelodysplastic syndromes: evidence for involvement at the hematopoietic stem cell level. *Blood* **96**:2012–21.

11 Ebert L, Prentz J, Bosco J. (2007) Identification of RPS14 as the 5q-syndrome gene by RNA interference screen. *Blood* **110**:8a.

12 Lim ZY, Killick S, Germing U, et al. (2007) Low IPSS score and bone marrow hypocellularity in MDS patients predict hematological responses to antithymocyte globulin. *Leukemia* **21**:1436–41.

13 Della Porta MG, Malcovati L, Boveri E, et al. (2009) Clinical relevance of bone marrow fibrosis and CD34-positive cell clusters in primary myelodysplastic syndromes. *J Clin Oncol* **27**:754–62.

14 Young NS, Calado RT, Scheinberg P. (2006) Current concepts in the pathophysiology and treatment of aplastic anemia. *Blood* **108**:2509–19.

15 Kantarjian H, O'Brien S, Ravandi F, et al. (2008) Proposal for a new risk model in myelodysplastic syndrome that accounts for events not considered in the original International Prognostic Scoring System. *Cancer* **113**:1351–61.

16 Swerdlow SH, Campo E, Harris NL,et al. (eds.) (2008) *WHO Classification of Tumours of Haematopoietic and Lymphoid Tissues* (4th ed.). Lyon: IARC.

17 Varela BL, Chuang C, Woll JE, Bennett JM. (1985) Modifications in the classification of primary myelodysplastic syndromes: the addition of a scoring system. *Hematol Oncol* **3**:55–63.

18 Vardiman JW, Harris NL, Brunning RD. (2002) The World Health Organization (WHO) classification of the myeloid neoplasms. *Blood* **100**:2292–302.

19 Gattermann N, Aul C, Schneider W. (1990) Two types of acquired idiopathic sideroblastic anaemia (AISA). *Br J Haematol* **74**:45–52.

20 Germing U, Gattermann N, Strupp C, et al. (2000) Validation of the WHO proposals for a new classification of primary myelodysplastic syndromes: a retrospective analysis of 1600 patients. *Leuk Res* **24**:983–92.

21 Balduini CL, Guarnone R, Pecci A, et al. (1998) Multilineage dysplasia without increased blasts identifies a poor prognosis subset of myelodysplastic syndromes. *Leukemia* **12**:1655–6.

22 Van den Berghe H, Cassiman JJ, David G, et al. (1974) Distinct haematological disorder with deletion of long arm of no. 5 chromosome. *Nature* **251**:437–8.

23 Malcovati L, Germing U, Kuendgen A, et al. (2007) Time-dependent prognostic scoring system for predicting survival and leukemic evolution in myelodysplastic syndromes. *J Clin Oncol* **25**:3503–10.

24 V.1.2009. National Comprehensive Cancer Network, at www.nccn.org (last accessed October 12, 2010).

25 Hellstrom-Lindberg E, Gulbrandsen N, Lindberg G, et al. (2003) A validated decision model for treating the anaemia of myelodysplastic syndromes with erythropoietin + granulocyte colony-stimulating factor: significant effects on quality of life. *Br J Haematol* **120**:1037–46.

26 Steensma DP, Tefferi A. (2007) Risk-based management of myelodysplastic syndrome. *Oncology (Williston Park)* **21**:43–54; discussion 57–8, 62.

27 Park S, Grabar S, Kelaidi C, et al. (2008) Predictive factors of response and survival in myelodysplastic syndrome treated with erythropoietin and G-CSF: the GFM experience. *Blood* **111**:574–82.

28 Jadersten M, Malcovati L, Dybedal I, et al. (2008) Erythropoietin and granulocyte-colony stimulating factor treatment associated with improved survival in myelodysplastic syndrome. *J Clin Oncol* **26**: 3607–13.

29 Stasi R, Abruzzese E, Lanzetta G, et al. (2005) Darbepoetin alfa for the treatment of anemic patients with low- and intermediate-1-risk myelodysplastic syndromes. *Ann Oncol* **16**:1921–7.

30 Giraldo P, Nomdedeu B, Loscertales J, et al. (2006) Darbepoetin alpha for the treatment of anemia in patients with myelodysplastic syndromes. *Cancer* **107**:2807–16.

31 Negrin RS, Stein R, Vardiman J, et al. (1993) Treatment of the anemia of myelodysplastic syndromes using recombinant human granulocyte colony-stimulating factor in combination with erythropoietin. *Blood* **82**:737–43.

32 Casadevall N, Durieux P, Dubois S, et al. (2004) Health, economic, and quality-of-life effects of erythropoietin and granulocyte colony-stimulating factor for the treatment of myelodysplastic syndromes: a randomized, controlled trial. *Blood* **104**:321–7.

33 Balleari E, Rossi E, Clavio M, et al. (2006) Erythropoietin plus granulocyte colony-stimulating factor is better than erythropoietin alone to treat anemia in low-risk myelodysplastic syndromes: results from a randomized single-centre study. *Ann Hematol* **85**:174–80.

34 Tiu RV, Sekeres MA. (2008) The role of AMG-531 in the treatment of thrombocytopenia in idiopathic thrombocytopenic purpura and myelodysplastic syndromes. *Expert Opin Biol Ther* **8**:1021–30.

35 Kantarjian H, Giles, F., Greenberg, P, et al. (2008) Effect of romiplostim in patients with low or intermediate risk MDS receiving azacitidine. *Blood* **112**:224.

36 Dreyfus F. (2008) The deleterious effects of iron overload in patients with myelodysplastic syndromes. *Blood Rev* **22**:S29–34.

37 Gattermann N, Schmid M, Porta MD, et al. (2008) Efficacy and safety of deferasirox (exjade(r)) during 1 year of treatment in transfusion-dependent patients with myelodysplastic syndromes: results from EPIC trial. *Blood* **112**:633.

38 List AF, Baer MR, Steensma D, et al. (2008) Iron chelation with deferasirox (Exjade(R)) improves iron burden in patients with myelodysplastic syndromes (MDS). *Blood* **112**:634.

39 Leitch HA. (2007) Improving clinical outcome in patients with myelodysplastic syndrome and iron overload using iron chelation therapy. *Leuk Res* **31**:S7–9.

40 Rose C, Brechignac S, Vassilief D, et al. (2007) Positive impact of iron chelation therapy (ct) on survival in regularly transfused MDS patients. A prospective analysis by the GFM. *Blood* **110**:249.

41 Jabbour E, Garcia-Manero G, Taher A, Kantarjian HM. (2009) Managing iron overload in patients with myelodysplastic syndromes with oral deferasirox therapy. *Oncologist* **14**:489–96.

42 Silverman LR, Demakos EP, Peterson BL, et al. (2002) Randomized controlled trial of azacitidine in patients with the myelodysplastic syndrome: a study of the Cancer and Leukemia Group B. *J Clin Oncol* **20**:2429–40.

43 Silverman LR, McKenzie DR, Peterson BL, et al. (2006) Further analysis of trials with azacitidine in patients with myelodysplastic syndrome: studies 8421, 8921, and 9221 by the Cancer and Leukemia Group B. *J Clin Oncol* **24**:3895–903.

44 Fenaux P, Mufti GJ, Hellstrom-Lindberg E, et al. (2009) Efficacy of azacitidine compared with that of conventional care regimens in the treatment of higher risk myelodysplastic syndromes: a randomized, open-label, phase III study. *Lancet Oncol* **10**:223–32.

45 Lyons RM, Cosgriff TM, Modi SS, et al. (2009) Hematologic response to three alternative dosing schedules of azacitidine in patients with myelodysplastic syndromes. *J Clin Oncol* **27**:1850–6.

46 Silverman LR, Fenaux P, Mufti GJ, et al. (2008) The effects of continued azacitidine (AZA) treatment cycles on response in higher risk patients (pts) with myelodysplastic syndromes (MDS). *Blood* **112**:227.

47 Wijermans PW, Krulder JW, Huijgens PC, Neve P. (1997) Continuous infusion of low-dose 5-Aza-2′-deoxycytidine in elderly patients with high-risk myelodysplastic syndrome. *Leukemia* **11**:S19–23.

48 Wijermans P, Lubbert M, Verhoef G, et al. (2000) Low-dose 5-aza-2′-deoxycytidine, a DNA hypomethylating agent, for the treatment of high-risk myelodysplastic syndrome: a multicenter phase II study in elderly patients. *J Clin Oncol* **18**:956–62.

49 Kantarjian HM, O'Brien S, Shan J, et al. (2007) Update of the decitabine experience in higher risk myelodysplastic syndrome and analysis of prognostic factors associated with outcome. *Cancer* **109**:265–73.

50 Kantarjian H, Oki Y, Garcia-Manero G, et al. (2007) Results of a randomized study of 3 schedules of low-dose decitabine in higher-risk myelodysplastic syndrome and chronic myelomonocytic leukemia. *Blood* **109**:52–7.

51 WijerMans P, Suciu, S., Baila, L, et al. (2008) Low-dose decitabine versus best supportive case in elderly patients with intermediate or high-risk MDS not eligible for intensive chemotherapy: final results of the randomized phase III study (06011) of the EORTC Leukemia and German MDS Study Groups. *Blood* **112**:226.

52 Pellagatti A, Jadersten M, Forsblom AM, et al. (2007) Lenalidomide inhibits the malignant clone and up-regulates the SPARC gene mapping to the commonly deleted region in 5q- syndrome patients. *Proc Natl Acad Sci U S A* **104**:11406–11.

53 Ebert BL, Galili N, Tamayo P, et al. (2008) An erythroid differentiation signature predicts response to lenalidomide in myelodysplastic syndrome. *PLoS Med* **5**:e35.

54 Moutouh-de Parseval LA, Verhelle D, Glezer E, et al. (2008) Pomalidomide and lenalidomide regulate erythropoiesis and fetal hemoglobin production in human CD34+ cells. *J Clin Invest* **118**:248–58.

55 Wei S, Chen X, Rocha K, et al. (2009) A critical role for phosphatase haplodeficiency in the selective suppression of deletion 5q MDS by lenalidomide. *Proc Natl Acad Sci U S A* **106**:12974–9.

56 List A, Dewald G, Bennett J, et al. (2006) Lenalidomide in the myelodysplastic syndrome with chromosome 5q deletion. *N Engl J Med* **355**:1456–65.

57 Raza A, Reeves JA, Feldman EJ, et al. (2008) Phase 2 study of lenalidomide in transfusion-dependent, low-risk, and intermediate-1 risk myelodysplastic syndromes with karyotypes other than deletion 5q. *Blood* **111**:86–93.

58 Golshayan AR, Jin T, Maciejewski J, et al. (2007) Efficacy of growth factors compared to other therapies for low-risk myelodysplastic syndromes. *Br J Haematol* **137**:125–32.

59 Adès L, Boehrer S, Prebet T, et al. (2009) Efficacy and safety of lenalidomide in intermediate-2 or high-risk myelodysplastic syndromes with 5q deletion: results of a phase II study. *Blood* **113**:3947–52.

60 Chen N, Lau H, Kong L, et al. (2007) Pharmacokinetics of lenalidomide in subjects with various degrees of renal impairment and in subjects on hemodialysis. *J Clin Pharmacol* **47**:1466–75.

61 Saunthararajah Y, Nakamura R, Nam JM, et al. (2002) HLA-DR15 (DR2) is overrepresented in myelodysplastic syndrome and aplastic anemia and predicts a response to immunosuppression in myelodysplastic syndrome. *Blood* **100**:1570–4.

62 Kasner MT, Luger SM. (2009) Update on the therapy for myelodysplastic syndrome. *Am J Hematol* **84**: 177–86.

63 Kochenderfer JN, Kobayashi S, Wieder ED, et al. (2002) Loss of T-lymphocyte clonal dominance in patients with myelodysplastic syndrome responsive to immunosuppression. *Blood* **100**:3639–45.

64 Yazji S, Giles FJ, Tsimberidou AM, et al. (2003) Antithymocyte globulin (ATG)-based therapy in patients with myelodysplastic syndromes. *Leukemia* **17**:2101–6.

65 Stadler M, Germing U, Kliche KO, et al. (2004) A prospective, randomised, phase II study of horse antithymocyte globulin vs. rabbit antithymocyte globulin as immune-modulating therapy in patients with low-risk myelodysplastic syndromes. *Leukemia* **18**:460–5.

66 Melchert M, List A. (2008) Targeted therapies in myelodysplastic syndrome. *Semin Hematol* **45**:31–8.

67 Steensma DP, Dispenzieri A, Moore SB, et al. (2003) Antithymocyte globulin has limited efficacy and substantial toxicity in unselected anemic patients with myelodysplastic syndrome. *Blood* **101**:2156–8.

68 Sloand EM, Wu CO, Greenberg P, et al. (2008) Factors affecting response and survival in patients with myelodysplasia treated with immunosuppressive therapy. *J Clin Oncol* **26**:2505–11.

69 Zou JX, Rollison DE, Boulware D, et al. (2009) Altered naive and memory CD4+ T-cell homeostasis and immunosenescence characterize younger patients with myelodysplastic syndrome. *Leukemia* **23**:1288–96.

70 Cutler CS, Lee SJ, Greenberg P, et al. (2004) A decision analysis of allogeneic bone marrow transplantation for the myelodysplastic syndromes: delayed transplantation for low-risk myelodysplasia is associated with improved outcome. *Blood* **104**:579–85.

71 Oliansky DM, Antin JH, Bennett JM, et al. (2009) The role of cytotoxic therapy with hematopoietic stem cell transplantation in the therapy of myelodysplastic syndromes: an evidence-based review. *Biol Blood Marrow Transplant* **15**:137–72.

72 Garcia-Manero G, Yang H, Bueso-Ramos C, et al. (2008) Phase I study of the histone deacetylase inhibitor vorinostat (suberoylanilide hydroxamic acid [SAHA]) in patients with advanced leukemias and myelodysplastic syndromes. *Blood* **111**:1060–6.

73 Klimek VM, Fircanis S, Maslak P, et al. (2008) Tolerability, pharmacodynamics, and pharmacokinetics studies of depsipeptide (romidepsin) in patients with acute myelogenous leukemia or advanced myelodysplastic syndromes. *Clin Cancer Res* **14**:826–32.

74 Fabre C, Grosjean J, Tailler M, et al. (2008) A novel effect of DNA methyltransferase and histone deacetylase inhibitors: NFkappaB inhibition in malignant myeloblasts. *Cell Cycle* **7**:2139–45.

75 Issa JP, Castoro, R, Ravandi-Kashani F, et al. (2008) Randomized phase II study of combined epigenetic therapy: decitabine vs. decitabine and valproic acid in MDS and AML. *Blood* **112**:228.

76 Garcia-Manero G, Assouline S, Cortes J, et al. (2008) Phase I study of the oral isotype specific histone deacetylase inhibitor MGCD0103 in leukemia. *Blood* **112**:981–9.

77 Silverman LR, Verma A, Odchimar-Reissig, et al. (2008) A phase I trial of the epigenetic modulators vorinostat, in combination with azacitidine in patients with MDS and AML: A study of the New York Cancer Consortium. *Blood* **112**:3656.

78 Garcia-Manero G, Silverman LB, Gojo I, et al. (2008) A randomized Phase IIa study of vorinostat in patients with low or intermediate-1 risk MDS: preliminary results. *Blood* **112**:5084.

79 Sekeres MA, List, AF, Cuthbertson, D, et al. (2008) Final results from a phase I combination study of lenalidomide and azacitidine in patients with higher risk MDS. *Blood* **112**:221.

80 List A, Kurtin S, Roe DJ, et al. (2005) Efficacy of lenalidomide in myelodysplastic syndromes. *N Engl J Med* **352**:549–57.

CHAPTER 11

Supportive Care in Myelodysplastic Syndrome

Hussain I. Saba, Arshia A. Dangol and Donald C. Doll
James A. Haley Veterans' Hospital, and H. Lee Moffitt Cancer Center and Research Institute, University of South Florida College of Medicine, Tampa, FL, USA

Supportive care in MDS

Myelodysplastic syndromes (MDS) are a group of heterogeneous hematopoietic stem cell diseases associated with dysplasia and ineffective hematopoiesis. This leads to peripheral cytopenias and bone marrow failure with, in many instances, clonal cytogenetic abnormalities [1]. Myelodysplastic syndrome is a disease of the elderly, since more than 80% of patients are diagnosed over the age of 60 years. Indeed, according to the SEER data from 2001 through 2003, approximately 86% of MDS were diagnosed in individuals aged ≥60 years (median age at diagnosis 76 years) [2]. Men had a significantly higher incidence than women (4.5 vs. 2.7 per 100 000 per year), which translates to about 10 000 new cases of MDS annually in the US. The incidence rate increased with age and was highest among whites and in non-Hispanics [3]. The overall relative three-year survival rate for MDS was 45%, with males experiencing poorer survival than females [3]. Recent cross-sectional surveys among US hematology and medical oncology specialists, as reported by Sekeres et al. [4], are in accord with the aforementioned findings. The authors noted that, among recently diagnosed MDS patients, 55% were male, the median age at diagnosis was 71 years, and 10% had MDS secondary to chemotherapy, radiation therapy, or environmental exposure. More than 50% of all newly diagnosed and established patients used erythropoiesis-stimulating agents [4]. Transformation to acute myeloid leukemia may also occur with varying risk in patients with myelodysplasia.

Several classification systems have evolved for the classification of myelodysplastic syndromes [5]. MDS was originally classified by the French-American-British (FAB) classification system according to clinical and pathological features [6]. In the year 2000, the World Health Organization revised the FAB classification system in an attempt to provide more uniform and accurate prognostic information [7, 8]. This classification system, termed the WHO classification of MDS, was followed by the International Prognostic Scoring System (IPSS), which remains the most comprehensive prognostic scoring system as of this time for MDS. This scoring system is based upon a score generated from evaluation of the number of bone marrow blasts, karyotype, and the number of cytopenias, and stratifies patients into four risk groups according to survival and risk of AML transformation [9].

The bone marrow failure and peripheral cytopenias observed in MDS can lead to anemia, thrombocytopenia and neutropenia, with increased risk of fatigue, bleeding, and infection (Table 11.1). It has been reported that more than 85% of MDS patients are anemic, with associated weakness, fatigue, and decreased pulmonary function and cardiac compli-

Advances in Malignant Hematology, First Edition. Edited by Hussain I. Saba and Ghulam J. Mufti. © 2011 Blackwell Publishing Ltd. Published 2011 by Blackwell Publishing Ltd.

Table 11.1 Problems associated with cytopenias and dysfunctional blood cells

Anemia

- Fatigue

- Exacerbation of heart failure, angina

- Shortness of breath, decreased pulmonary function

Thrombocytopenia

- Platelet dysfunction

- Active bleeding

- Potential risk of bleeding

Neutropenia

- Active infection

- Risk of infections

  — Immune suppression

  — Gram negative sepsis

  — Aspergillosis

cations [10]. Leukopenia/neutropenia remains another dominant cytopenia, leading to an increased risk and active infection in MDS patients. Thrombocytopenia and its potential for bleeding can also occur in MDS patients. The Sekeres et al. report indicated that the median platelet count was 100 000/mm^3 in their study [4]. Data by Kantarjian et al. support these findings, as 67% of patients referred to their center with MDS at M.D. Anderson had thrombocytopenia [11]. Leukopenia and neutropenia may predispose to infections, further compromising the MDS patient [12, 13]. The risk of infection in patients with MDS has long been known. Pomeroy et al. reported that infections occurred at a rate of approximately one per patient year of observation and that infection was the most common cause of death in MDS [14]. Of note is that miliary tuberculosis without pulmonary involvement may occur in MDS patients and may be a cause of fever of unknown origin [15]. If the diagnosis is not recognized and left untreated, the results may be fatal. Recently, a clinical syndrome characterized by monocytopenia with susceptibility to dis-

seminated non-tubercular mycobacterial infections, papilloma viruses, fungal infections, and myelodysplasia has been reported by Vinh et al. [16]. Of the 18 patients with this clinical phenotype, 9 developed myelodysplasia/leukemia.

Cytopenias occur more frequently in more advanced disease. Kao et al. analyzed 815 patients from the International MDS Risk Analysis Workshop database, and reported that the hemoglobin level was directly related to IPSS risk. Patients with a hemoglobin less than or equal to 8 g/dL or platelet counts less than 20 000/µl were noted to have higher clinical risk, lower overall survival and increased progression to AML [17].

Currently, there is no cure for MDS except for stem cell transplant, which is available for only a minority of patients. Other treatment options include chemotherapy akin to acute myeloid leukemia (AML), hypomethylating agents (azacytidine and decitabine), and immune modulating drugs (antithymocyte globulin, cyclosporine, thalidomide and its derivatives) and others [18]. Chemotherapy may increase the degree of cytopenias observed in MDS patients, and supportive care addresses the treatment of these cytopenias and their complications documented as a result of the underlying myelodysplasia or its treatment with chemotherapy or other cytotoxic modalities. As a result of either the disease itself or treatment, the majority of MDS patients acknowledge the need for and/or require supportive care of some type to help alleviate morbidity and mortality, and improve their QOL [19, 20].

The importance of supportive care has been illustrated in a study by Passweg et al. [21]. In this report, 88 transfusion-dependent MDS patients were randomized to best supportive care (BSC, transfusions + iron chelation) or antithymocyte globulin + cyclosporine (ATG + CSA). Although hematologic response was better in the ATG + CSA group (31%) versus 13% in the BSC group and transfusion-free survival probability was similar in both groups, the overall survival probability estimates at two years was actually improved for supportive care (49% ATG + CSA vs. 61% BSC). Supportive care for MDS patients remains an essential component of management, even in patients receiving intensive

Table 11.2 Modes of supportive care delivery in MDS patients

Supportive care	Underlying requirement	Method of delivery
Ongoing observation	Monitor for progression or complications	Clinic visits, blood work
Psychosocial support	Depression, anger issues	Consult to psychologist or social worker
Hematological	Anemia	Transfusions of red cells
		Growth factor use
	Iron overload	Iron chelation therapy
	Neutropenia	Growth factors (G-CSF, GM-CSF)
	Infection	Antibiotics
	Thrombocytopenia	Transfusions, antifibrinolytics, IL-6, IL-11, recombinant megakaryocyte growth factor and development factor (rHuTPO) and its pegylated form (PEG-rHu-MGDF, romiplostim (AMG531), eltrombopag

therapy, with the goal to reduce morbidity and mortality from cytopenia(s), while providing an acceptable QOL.

Several aspects of supportive care delivery are depicted in Table 11.2.

Anemia in MDS and role of supportive care in management

Scoring systems to predict overall survival in MDS incorporate the number of peripheral cytopenias in the score [7–9, 22]. Anemia is the most common complication observed in MDS patients. It has been reported that 80% of MDS patients are anemic at the time of diagnosis, with more than 40% requiring red blood cell transfusions regularly at some time during the course of their disease [23]. The impact of anemia on QOL can have multiple adverse outcomes [24]. For example, negative effects related to the patient's level of fatigue may lead to depression, anxiety, and anger that may affect both the patient and family [19, 25]. Anemia has also been shown to have a negative impact on survival in older individuals and in MDS patients [5, 8, 9, 26–28]. In 2008, Kao et al. examined 815 MDS patients in the

International MDS Risk Analysis Workshop database, and reported that the overall survival of patients was inversely related to hemoglobin level [17]. Median overall survival was 4.9 years in patients with hemoglobin levels greater than 10 g/dL, while patients with a hemoglobin less than or equal to 8 had an overall survival of only 1.5 years.

The incidence of red cell transfusion dependency was reported to increase as the IPSS category progressed to the higher risk groups. In one study transfusion dependency was reported in 39% of low-risk patients. This increased to 79% in the high-risk IPSS group [29]. Transfusion dependence has been shown to have a negative impact on survival [30–32]. In a study by Cermak et al., the authors concluded that the administration of only 1 unit of RBC every 4–8 weeks had a significant negative impact on survival [33].

Anemia caused by bone marrow abnormalities related to MDS can be further amplified in patients undergoing chemotherapy. Groopman and Itri, in a comprehensive review of chemotherapy trials, reported a relatively high incidence of mild to moderate anemia [34]. This report included studies that utilized a variety of chemotherapeutic combinations for a second neoplastic disorder (e.g., breast cancer, lung cancer, lymphomas, colorectal cancer, and others). Other investigators have also noted the problem of anemia in chemotherapy patients [35–38]. As a result, supportive care for the treatment of anemia remains a high priority in both untreated and treated MDS patients.

Management for anemia in MDS patients includes red cell transfusions and the use of hematopoietic growth factors, such as erythropoietin and its long acting analog darbepoetin. Myeloid growth factors (i.e., G-CSF and GM-CSF) may also have a role in the treatment of anemia in MDS patients. Red cell transfusions may be the only mode of therapy for anemia in MDS and about 40% of patients receive transfusions for their disease [26]. An International MDS Foundation survey of 30 centers disclosed that 39–79% of MDS patients, depending upon their IPSS score, are transfusion dependent. Although red cell transfusions are an accepted supportive intervention for anemic patients, this therapeutic intervention is not without complications. Such complications include transfusion reactions, antibody production, and the risk of infection from blood-borne pathogens, such as HIV and hepatitis. A now commonly recognized and important side effect of red cell transfusions in MDS patients has been the problem of iron overload [39, 40]. It has been estimated that each unit of transfused blood contains approximately 200–250 mg of iron [41] and that a major cause of iron overload in MDS is regular red blood cell transfusions [42]. In fact, 20 units of red cells may result in iron overload in some patients [43].

For anemic MDS patients, erythroid stimulating agents (ESAs) (e.g., erythropoietin, darbepoetin) may be a more viable support option. Erythropoietin is a natural glycoprotein secreted via the kidney which stimulates erythropoiesis and has been shown to be effective in the treatment of anemia in hematologic malignancies [44]. Recently, recombinant erythropoietin (rhEPO) has been produced and marketed for the treatment of anemia. Typically, rhEPO is administered subcutaneously (SQ) either daily or three times/week (150 U/kg or 10 000 U fixed dose) [45, 46]. Hellstrom-Lindberg, in a 1995 meta-analysis of 17 studies of 205 MDS patients, concluded that, while the overall response was low (16%), it appeared that

there was a subpopulation of MDS patients who responded to treatment [47]. Subsequent studies helped to clarify the possible differences, and it has been observed that low- to intermediate-risk MDS patients appear to have a better response to treatment with erythropoietin alone than other subtypes [48]. Mundle et al. performed a meta-analysis on the effectiveness of EPO in achieving transfusion independence (TI) in MDS patients. The highlights of this analysis are shown on Table 11.3.

The studies reviewed included the time period of 1990–2006, and comprised both IWG response criteria and those that did not. As depicted in Table 11.3, the analysis showed that EPO monotherapy resulted in an average post-therapy reduction of 25.8% in RBC units (IWG: 34.3%, non-IWG: 17.3%) used per month. An average of 23.4% (IWG: 28.8, non-IWG: 17.9) of the patients became transfusion independent post-therapy [49]. Kwon et al. reported that 47.5% (19/40) of the patients responded to therapy with standard dose erythropoietin, and 18% (3/16) of the non-responsive patients improved with double-dose EPO [50]. The authors noted, however, that this was an unexpectedly high response rate. Erythroid response to EPO has been shown to increase in patients receiving prolonged administration (minimum 26 weeks), although this effect has been debated [45, 51]. In addition, several studies have shown the efficacy of once weekly dosing of rhEPO in MDS [52–54]. As with any therapeutic intervention, the risk of adverse events must be considered in relation to the anticipated benefit. Potential risks associated with erythropoietin include hypertension, cardiovascular events, seizures, and thrombosis [55, 56]. Furthermore, possible association of compromised survival of MDS patients with transfusions has also been considered [30–33].

Darbepoetin is a recombinant erythropoietin with increased activity and a longer half-life compared to rhEPO. This longer half-life makes it an attractive alternative for many patients and their physicians. Studies have shown that darbepoetin is equally or more effective than rhEPO in the treatment of anemia in MDS patients [53, 57–59]. Patton et al. reported the results of a retrospective cohort study involving 263 MDS patients who had received either 200 μg of darbepoetin alfa every two weeks or 40 000 units epoetin alfa weekly [57]. A major

Table 11.3 MDS-related transfusion-dependent anemia treatment with epoetin alfa

Study group	Non-IWG studies EPO	IWG studies EPO	IWG studies EPO + G/GM-CSF
No. of studies (evaluable patients)	12 (268)	7 (195)	6 (115)
Baseline EPO (mean ± SD)	687.2 ± 684.7	374.3 ± 72.2	288 ± 172.1
Baseline Hb (mean ± SD)	8.5 ± 0.6	7.9 ± 0.4	8.1 ± 0.4
Mean monthly pre-therapy RBC units	2.71	2.37	2.33
Post-EPO tx-independent pts, % (95% CI)	17.9 (10.9–24.9)	28.8 (12.6–45.1)	24.8 (11.8–37.8)
Mean post-EPO reduction in RBC units/month, %	17.3	34.3	10.4

response was observed in 46% of the previously untreated patients receiving darbepoetin alfa compared to 35% in those receiving epoetin alfa. There was no difference in mean hemoglobin or changes in hemoglobin levels between the two treatment groups. Giraldo et al. [10] performed a retrospective Spanish study on 81 MDS patients treated with darbepoetin (75–300 mg SQ once per week) for 16 weeks (Table 11.4). They reported that 55% of the patients had a response, with 30.4% major responses and 24.6% minor responses. Sixty-five percent of the EPO-naïve patients responded in this study. Most responses (65.8%) occurred in less than

Table 11.4 Darbepoetin in MDS

- Retrospective Spanish study of 81 MDS patients
- Once-weekly darbepoetin (75–300 µg SQ) for 16 weeks
- Results:
  - — 55% responded
    - ○ 30.4% major responses
    - ○ 24.6% minor responses
  - — 64% of EPO-naïve patients and 45.7% of EPO-treated patients responded
  - — Most responses (65.8%) occurred ≤ Week 8
  - — No darbepoetin-related adverse events occurred

or equal to week 8, and no darbepoetin-related adverse events occurred.

In a phase II QOL study by Olivia et al., 33 of the patients were treated for a minimum of 8 weeks (150 µg s.c. weekly, doubled in non-responders) [60]. Of these 33, 17 patients responded at 8 weeks (30% minor responses, 21% major) at the initial dose. Seven of the patients (53%) were considered transfusion dependent prior to therapy. The number of responders after dose doubling was 56% at 24 weeks. In this clinical trial, three of six (50%) patients previously unresponsive to epoetin responded to darbepoetin therapy. Darbepoetin has also been reported to improve QOL, with specific improvements in level of fatigue, physical ability, functional ability, social aspects, and overall total scores [60–62].

Although therapeutic intervention with darbepoetin may be more advantageous than rhEPO due to dosing schedule, the cost of darbepoetin appears higher. In a Canadian/US retrospective analysis study on 193 patients receiving erythropoietic growth factors (146 EPO, 47 darbepoetin) from January 2004 to March 2006, Laliberte et al. determined that the cumulative drug cost in his study population was lower in the EPO group compared to the darbepoetin group by US$2022 (29%; EPO US$4882 vs. darbepoetin US$6904; p = 0.01) [63]. It is hoped that this cost difference will be reduced as time progresses.

Musto et al. [64] have also shown that a change in the schedule and dose of darbepoetin, from the usual 150–300 µg once per week to higher doses at longer intervals (500 µg s.c. every 3 weeks), may result in a response in previously non-responsive MDS patients. Additional studies are warranted to confirm this result.

Granulocyte colony-stimulating factor (G-CSF) is a glycoprotein that stimulates the production of granulocytes and stem cells. Studies have shown that combining G-CSF with EPO in patients who have failed therapy with EPO alone may stimulate erythropoiesis in MDS patients (Table 11.5) [65–70].

Although the addition of G-CSF may increase the ability of some patients to respond to erythropoietin, the effect of this response on long-term survival in

Table 11.5 Response to EPO + G-CSF in MDS

Study	Evaluable patient no.	Number of responders	Response rate/ subtype	
Negrin et al., 1996 [65]	44	48%	RA	38%
			RARS	48%
			RAEB	10%
			RAEB-T	4%
Hellstrom-Lindberg et al., 1998 [66]			RA	20%
	47	38%	RARS	46%
			RAEB	37%
Jadersten et al., 2005 [67]	123	39%	RA	23%
			RARS	42%
			RAEB	35%
Nair et al., 2006 [68]	55	65%	N.R.	
Park et al., 2006 [69]	104	58%	N.R.	
Balleari et al., 2006 [70]	15	73.3%	N.A.	

MDS and its subtypes is unclear. Nair et al. did not report a survival benefit in their study, and noted that the progression to AML in their Indian patient population was slightly higher than that documented in other reports [68]. In 2005, Jadersten et al. reported that RA and RARS patients treated with EPO + G-CSF had a longer median survival than RAEB patients receiving EPO + G-CSF, low IPSS risk patients had a longer survival than IPSS INT-1 patients undergoing similar therapy, and that there was a significant difference between patients in the good and intermediate predictive groups for erythroid response [67]. The authors also reported that 29% of the transfusion-dependent patients became transfusion independent. Although differences were observed within treatment groups, there was no significant difference between survival and AML progression when treated and non-treated (supportive care) groups were compared. In a subsequent trial, the authors reported a survival benefit in patients with low transfusion requirement (<2 units/month) but less benefit was observed in those patients with a higher transfusion requirement [71]. These results support the data of Hellstrom-Lindberg et al., who showed that the response rate in patients requiring two or more transfusions/month was 21.7% versus 50% in those requiring less than two transfusions per month [66]. Thus, patients who require fewer transfusions may have better responses and survival than those who require many transfusions [72].

Iron overload in MDS and its management

Although iron overload is a well-known complication of MDS, the role of iron chelation therapy in MDS has recently generated considerable mistrust and controversy. In 2008, Cazzola et al. reported the results of an Italian study on the impact of iron overload in 840 MDS patients. The authors concluded that secondary iron overload significantly affected patient's risk of non-leukemic death and overall survival [39]. Complications associated with secondary iron overload include hepatomegaly, hepatic fibrosis, and an increased risk of cardiac complications [73–75]. Other problems of iron over-load have included diabetes, failure of sexual development, and osteoporosis [76].

Considering the multifaceted complications and long-term health risks associated with iron overload, it is reasonable to assume that iron chelation therapy may have a positive impact on lower risk MDS patients. Iron chelation therapy may decrease the body's stored iron and may reduce the complications associated with the disease. In a 2007 study, Leitch et al. [77] investigated the impact of iron chelation on 178 MDS patients. The study concluded that iron chelation therapy improved the leukemia-free survival and the overall survival of MDS patients. The four-year overall survival was 64% in patients treated with iron chelation therapy as compared to 49% in the control group (p = 0.01). The medial survival in the chelation group was not reached at the time of publication (226 weeks), while it was 40.5 months in the control group [77]. A prospective study of Rose et al. [78] has also indicated a positive impact of iron chelation on survival in regularly transfused, mainly low- and intermediate-1 risk MDS patients. The medial overall survival from diagnosis was 115 months in chelation patients versus 51 months in non-chelation patients (p < 0.0001). Higher risk MDS patients may not benefit from chelation therapy due to the severity of underlying disease (MDS) and shortened life span associated with it [79]. Further prospective clinical trials are warranted to help elucidate the affect of iron overload in MDS and other disease states where patients are dependent upon red cell transfusions.

The NCCN recommends iron chelation for MDS patients who have received more than 20 to 30 red cell transfusions, particularly for those MDS patients considered to be in the lower IPSS risk categories (low, INT-1) [80]. The members of the MDS platform of the Austrian Society of Haematology and Oncology have published recommendations for the treatment of iron overload [81]. They recommend that chelation therapy be considered for MDS patients if (1) the serum ferritin is >2000 ng/ml without active inflammation or liver disease, (2) patients have transfusion-dependent anemia, (3) life expectancy is more than two years, (4) planned chemotherapy or transplant, and (5) if organopathy is present as a result of iron overload. A caveat to these recommendations is that, in cases with the presence of organopathy, iron chelation should be considered even if life expectancy is less than the recommended two years.

Iron overload has historically been treated with slow subcutaneous or intravenous deferoxamine infusions. Deferoxamine is normally administered as a continuous infusion pump for three to five days each week. Compliance has been a major problem with this mode of administration, Thuret reported on a prospective, epidemiological cross-sectional study in France of 278 patients with thalassemia, sickle cell disease, or myelodysplastic syndromes, although good compliance was reported with deferoxamine administration in 67% to 87% of the patients [82]. In a survey of thalassemia major patients with iron overload and deferoxamine infusion by Caro et al. [83], 65% of patients reported unhappiness with the use of the drug. In the same study, more than half of the patients stated that deferoxamine infusions had some type of negative impact on their lives. Despite these limitations, a Canadian study in 2007 on 178 MDS patients reported the advantage of iron chelation, as the four-year overall survival in patients with deferoxamine was 64%, compared to 49% in controls [84]. Aspects of deferoxamine infusions that may affect compliance and QOL include length of infusion period, need for long-term pump use, and/or side effects, such as rashes, bruises, headaches, decreases in blood counts due to hematological toxicity and shortness of breath [85]. Cases of auditory and visual neurotoxicity have also been reported with infusions of high-dose deferoxamine [86, 87].

Oral iron chelating agents and iron overload in MDS

Oral iron chelating agents have been under investigation and are now available in an attempt to circumvent the problems associated with deferoxamine while still allowing patients to benefit from iron chelation therapy.

Deferiprone is an oral iron chelator taken three times daily, with a half-life of three hours. While the drug has been approved in Europe as secondary therapy for iron overload in patients for whom deferoxamine therapy is unacceptable, this drug is not FDA approved for use in the US. Results of studies have suggested that the use of deferiprone may be associated with adverse events including liver fibrosis and agranulocytosis [88, 89]. The toxicity of this drug is still debatable [90, 91].

Deferasirox (ICL670, Exjade) is another orally administered iron chelator, administered once a day due to its longer half-life of 12–16 hours, with minimal adverse events [92]. It has been shown to be an effective therapeutic intervention in thalassemia, MDS, and other transfusions-dependent diseases [93]. Side effects of oral deferasirox therapy as reported in phase I, II, and III trials have been acceptable [94–96]. A retrospective analysis by Faris et al. of 294 patients using deferasirox concluded that MDS patients treated with deferasirox were treatment compliant, an important consideration in the choice of iron chelation therapy [97].

Treatment of patients with oral deferasirox, rather than subcutaneous deferoxamine, may also prove to be more cost effective, as suggested by Mody-Patel et al. [98]. These authors showed that an actual saving of US$389.48 occurred per MDS patient with deferasirox.

Exjade (deferasirox) was approved in the US by the FDA in November 2005 for the treatment of iron overload. The FDA reported adverse events in patients receiving deferasirox (Exjade) therapy, including hepatic, renal, and hematological events considered to be life threatening or disabling. Of note, 19 deaths were observed [99]. Subsequently, an FDA Medwatch Alert update announced that the prescribing information for Exjade had been amended to include a warning regarding information about the post-marketing reports of hepatic failure and a recommendation that serum creatinine and blood counts should be carefully monitored in patients undergoing iron chelation with Exjade [100]. Nonetheless, it appears that iron chelation is advantageous in some MDS populations, with the benefits outweighing the risks. Of note, it has also been suggested that iron chelation therapy may also lower infection risk, improve the outcome of stem cell transplantation, and delay leukemic transformation [101]. It has been suggested that erythropoietin administration may help mobilize stored iron in patients receiving concomitant iron chelation therapy [102].

Myeloid growth factors (G-CSF and GM-CSF): their support for MDS

Leukopenia and neutropenia remain a major complication in myelodysplasia that can lead to infection and not uncommonly sepsis or death. Myeloid growth factors have been utilized in an attempt to improve neutropenia and combat infectious complications. The following role of myeloid growth factors has been postulated for their efficacy in MDS:

1 Effect on residual but normal hematopoietic clones in the marrow of MDS patients. Stimulation of these clones could improve the cytopenias.

2 Their action on MDS clones could induce maturation and proliferation and may lead to extinction of the MDS clones.

3 Myeloid growth factors could sensitize the MDS clones and lead to their cytotoxic extinction.

4 Myeloid growth factors could accelerate hematopoietic recovery following injury or cytotoxic insults of bone marrow by chemotherapeutic agents in the treatment of MDS.

Earlier studies on myeloid growth factors have revealed that these agents have the ability to improve white cell counts. As of 1991, 232 MDS patients with leukopenia were studied, and the results revealed a dose-dependent increase in the white blood cells. In some cases, ANCs increased to mean normal levels. With GM-CSF, increased blood counts were observed in monocytes, eosinophils, lymphocytes, and reticulocytes as well as in neutrophils in 20% of the patients. A platelet count increase above baseline was also observed in 6% of MDS patients treated with GM-CSF. During that time, G-CSF was used in 73 patients and 90% had increases in their ANC levels above normal and no change was observed in the eosinophils, monocytes, or lymphocytes. Five of 15 patients on long-term maintenance for 6–16 months developed AML, 1 with RAEB and 4 with RAEB-t.

There has been concern that the use of myeloid growth factors in MDS patients could enhance and increase the risk of evolution to AML and could be detrimental for their outcome. However, in a study in 1993 [103] using G-CSF versus placebo which included 102 high-risk MDS patients who were stratified for RAEB and RAEB-t, results negated this contention, as AML transformation did not increase in MDS groups treated with myeloid growth factor (G-CSF). This was supported by a subsequent study by Jaderstan et al., indicating that the use myeloid growth factors in the management of MDS is not a risk of conversion to AML [104].

The role of myeloid growth factor in sensitizing MDS to the cytotoxic action of chemotherapy has also been examined. We undertook a phase III trial sponsored by ECOG of a combination of GM-CSF with intermediate dose cytarabine and mitoxantrone chemotherapy to assess the efficacy of GM-CSF-mediated sensitization of MDS clones [105]. This trial was sponsored by ECOG and included RAEB, RAEB-t, and CMML patients. The trial, however, was associated with significant toxicity to the level that the study was terminated. Subsequent clinical investigations, however, have shown that combining myeloid growth factors with chemotherapy for high-risk MDS and/or AML may not be deleterious and could be beneficial in response efficacy and improving overall survival [104, 106, 107].

Thrombocytopenia and its management in MDS

Thrombocytopenia in patients with myelodysplastic syndrome has been reported with a range of 40–65%, with a median frequency of 65% before therapeutic intervention [11]. Also, platelet function may be abnormal in MDS patients [108] making the presence of moderate to severe thrombocytopenia of greater concern. A minority of patients diagnosed with MDS may present with solitary thrombocytopenia. In a retrospective chart review by Sashida et al. of 146 sequential MDS patients, it was reported that 13 patients (8.9%) presented with isolated thrombocytopenia and two of these patients had initially been diagnosed with ITP [109].

Therapeutic interventions for the management of MDS may increase the percentage of patients with thrombocytopenia, or exacerbate the underlying thrombocytopenia. In this regard, thrombocytopenia has been related to MDS treatment with Revlimid, Vidaza, Zarnestra, Dacogen, and others [11]. The severity of thrombocytopenia may vary, as illustrated by Kao and Greenberg [110]. In this study, 815 MDS patients were examined for the degree of thrombocytopenia and overall survival. Univariate analysis showed that the majority of thrombocytopenic MDS patients (63%) had mildly decreased platelet counts (100–150 K). Twenty percent of the patients had platelet counts ranging from 50–99 K, 12% from 20–49 K, and 5% less than 20 K. A survival of 3.9 years was observed for patients with a platelet count from 100–150 K, whereas overall survival decreased as the platelet count level diminished. Patients with <20 K platelets had an overall survival of 0.9 years.

Mild thrombocytopenia does not require any intervention unless the bleeding risk increases (e.g., surgical procedure) or the patient becomes symptomatic. Therapeutic modalities for the treatment of MDS-related thrombocytopenia include splenectomy, Interleukin-6 (IL-6), recombinant megakaryocyte growth factor and development factor, and its pegylated form (PEG-rHu-MGDF), and Interleukin-11. More recently, drugs such as romiplostim (AMG531) and eltrombopag have been evaluated in MDS-associated thrombocytopenia.

Splenectomy is a common therapeutic intervention for patients with ITP [111]. In 2001, Bourgeois et al. reported the results of splenectomy in six MDS patients with platelet counts ranging from 5–30K who failed to respond to other treatments [112]. Platelets in these patients increased to 55–160 K three months post-surgery. Of the six patients, two had normal platelet counts 10 and 52 months post-surgery, three relapsed with disease progression, and one died of sepsis. Abdul-Wahab reported a case of two siblings with familial MDS, one of whom had massive splenomegaly and underwent splenectomy with amelioration of the cytopenia [113].

Interleukin-6 is a cytokine with the ability to induce the maturation of megakaryocyte precursors, although it does not have a direct effect on the proliferation of megakaryocytic progenitors [114, 115]. In a phase I study of IL-6 in 22 thrombocytopenic MDS patients, Gordon et al. reported that eight patients (36%) had improvement of their platelet count, although toxicities including fatigue, fever, elevated alkaline phosphatase, severely limited its usability [116].

Recombinant human thrombopoietin (rHuTPO) and its pegylated form (pegylated recombinant megakaryocyte growth and development factor, PEG-rHuMGDF) have also been utilized in thrombocytopenic patients with MDS with variable results [117]. In a study by Komatsu et al., increased platelet counts were demonstrated in one-third of MDS and aplastic anemia patients treated with daily IV dosage of PEG-rHuMGDF for 14 days [118]. However, antibody production has been associated with its use in some patients receiving intensive chemotherapy [119, 120].

Interleukin-11 (IL-11, Neumega) is a thrombopoietic cytokine that stimulates the production and maturation of megakaryocytic progenitors, leading to increased platelet production [121]. A pilot study of low dose IL-11 (50 mcg/kg/d SQ) in patients with bone marrow failure, 5 of 11 MDS patients achieved a response. The median platelet count increase was 95 K greater than baseline and the response durations ranged from 12–30+ weeks [122]. Tsimberidou et al. [123] reported platelet responses in 6 of 14 MDS patients (43%). Patients received at least two courses of daily recombinant IL-11 (Neumega, 10 mcg/kg SQ) followed by a two-week rest period. Platelet counts increased to a mean maximum of 147 K from a mean baseline of 42K, with a mean increase of 105 K. Of the MDS patients in this report, there were three major platelet responses, two minor responses and one patient with a multilineage response. The duration of response was 1.4–7.1 months, with a mean duration of 3.4 months [123].

Romiplostim (AMG531) is a recombinant protein that mimics endogenous thrombopoietin (TPO), directly binding to and activating the platelet thrombopoietin receptor, leading to the proliferation and differentiation of megakaryocytes [124]. Kantarjian et al. presented data on the use of romiplostim at doses ranging from 300–1500 mcg/week SQ in thrombocytopenic, low-risk MDS patients [125]. Nineteen of 44 patients (46%) had a durable platelet response with a median duration of response of 37 weeks (range 13–56 weeks). Temporary blast count increases occurred in four patients who were treated with higher dose romiplostim (2: 1500 mcg, 1: 1000 mcg, and 1: 700 mcg). Two cases (5%) of AML occurred during the study. Based on the findings and comparisons of absolute platelet counts in each cohort, the 700 mcg dose was selected for future studies.

Recently, a new platelet growth factor has been under investigation. Eltrombopag (Promacta) is an oral platelet growth factor that has the ability to increase platelet counts in patients with chronic ITP and Hepatitis C-associated thrombocytopenia [126–129]. A total of 73% (43/61) patients with a baseline platelet count of <30 K achieved a platelet count of greater than or equal to 50 K. In general, eltrombopag was well tolerated, with the majority of adverse events being mild. The most common side effect was headache. *In vivo* effects of eltrombopag on platelet function suggest that it increases the platelet count via the release of new platelets into the circulation, but these platelets are not activated or stimulated by the study drug [130–132]. Long-term safety and efficacy has led to the FDA granting priority review for eltrombopag (Promacta) for the short-term treatment of patients with chronic ITP [133], although this drug has not yet been investigated in MDS patients but studies are in process. *In vitro* data of eltrombopag on bone marrow cells from patients with AML and MDS have been reported [134]. Results showed that eltrombopag is capable of stimulating megakaryopoiesis in bone marrow cells of patients with AML and MDS.

Danazol is a synthetic hormone used to treat endometriosis, and has been reported to increase platelet counts in patients with ITP [135–137]. Clinical trials of danazol have been reported. Buzaid et al. treated 18 evaluable MDS patients with 800 mg danazol daily, but only three patients (17%) had a non-clinically significant increase in platelet count [138]. Chabannon et al. reviewed 76 MDS patients treated with danazol, and concluded that it is not a beneficial therapeutic intervention [139]. In contrast, Marini and associates treated 16 MDS patients with danazol (600 mg/day, p.o., 12 weeks). Eight patients were thrombocytopenic at baseline, and the thrombocytopenia resolved in 5/8 (62%). Interestingly, anemia improved in 4/14 patients (29%), and the reticulocyte counts increased in 6/13 (46%) patients, as well [140]. A double-blind, placebo-controlled study by Aviles on 50 evaluable patients with MDS treated with danazol versus placebo also noted increases in hemoglobin, granulocytes, platelets, and survival in the danazol group [141]. Chan et al. evaluated 33 MDS patients treated with danazol for six or more weeks. They showed that 76% of the patients (25/33) had an increase in platelet count after six weeks of treatment. After 12 weeks, the number of responders was 72% (21/29 patients) [142]. Side effects of danazol from these studies have been reported to be minor, but masculinization in females could be of concern. Overall, danazol may be a viable treatment option for some thrombocytopenic MDS patients.

Therapeutic agents in MDS and supportive care

One of the hallmarks of myelodysplastic syndrome is ineffective hematopoiesis involving one or more cell lines leading to anemia, thrombocytopenia and/or neutropenia and, in many patients, requiring supportive care as described in this chapter. Patients receiving therapeutic intervention may require supportive care involving transfusions and/or antibiotics. For example, Jain et al. studied the potential benefit of anti-infective prophylaxis in patients with AML or high-risk MDS who were receiving targeted therapy. Results demonstrated that mortality was significantly higher in patients who did not receive any anti-infective prophylaxis [143].

Active therapeutic intervention, although not curative, may benefit MDS patients via improving their cytopenias. Pilatrino et al. studied the role of the HDAC inhibitors valproic acid and all-trans retinoic acid on 11 evaluable older patients with AML or MDS. Hematologic improvement was observed in 6/11 (55%) patients, including 5 with a major platelet response and platelet transfusion independence (TI)

for ≥2 months and 3 with a minor erythroid response and approximately a 50% reduction in transfusion requirements [144]. Immunosuppressive agents (e.g., cyclosporin A and others) may also be beneficial in cytopenias associated with MDS. Chen et al., in a multicenter prospective study of 32 MDS patients, reported that treatment with 3--6 mg/kg/day of cyclosporine A improved hematologic parameters in 20 of the 32 patients (62.5%). Survival for responders was improved compared to non-responders. After 36 months of follow-up in this study, there was only one death in 20 responders in the cyclosporine group compared to seven deaths in 12 responders. The responders of cyclosporine showed a significantly longer survival time with a p-value of 0.01 [145]. The potential benefit of cyclosporine A efficacy in low-risk MDS patients was also suggested by a Japanese study [146]. Twenty low-risk MDS patients were treated with cyclosporine A for 24 weeks, resulting in hematologic improvement in 10 of 19 patients. Results included eight erythroid, six platelet, and one neutrophil response, respectively. Further studies are needed to help elucidate and confirm these findings.

Thalidomide has been used to treat MDS patients and has immunosuppressive and anti-angiogenic properties. In 2002, Strupp et al. published the results of a pilot study of thalidomide for the treatment of MDS [147]. Thirty-four MDS patients received thalidomide at a median dose of 400 mg/day, with 19 of 29 evaluable patients showing hematologic improvement (9 partial hematologic remissions). Responders became TI within two months of thalidomide therapy, and two responders no longer required iron-chelating therapy for prevention of hemosiderosis. All responders reported improved QOL. Musto et al. have also reported that treatment of 25 transfusion-dependent MDS patients with thalidomide led to TI in six patients [148]. Lenalidomide, an immunomodulatory thalidomide deritivative, has produced dramatic results in MDS patients with 5q syndrome. List et al. [149] reported 67% TI in MDS patients with the 5q abnormality undergoing treatment with lenalidomide. In addition, results of a trial in 214 patients with non-5q-MDS treated with lenalidomide noted TI in 26% of patients [150].

Hypomethylating agents and their supportive role in MDS

DNA methylation is a common epigenetic modification playing an important role in gene expression in mammalian cells. As a part of normal development, certain genes may be silenced through methylation of the cytosine residue in their promoter region (CPG islands). However, in some hematopoietic neoplasms, including MDS, hypermethylation can inactivate genes essential for control of normal cell growth, differentiation or apoptosis. A group of enzymes called DNA methyl-transferases (DNMTs) catalyze the methylation of cytosine residues in the newly synthesized DNA, thus replicating the methylating signal. In recent years, there has been interest in pharmacologic therapy targeting this mechanism by inhibiting DNMT, resulting in hypomethylation of the DNA and re-expression of the tumor suppressor gene.

Cytosine analogs such as 5-azacytidine and decitabine have been shown to inhibit DNMT and are being used against MDS as well as AML and other cancers. Multiple genes appear to be hypermethylated in MDS, including P15^{INK4B} which encodes a cell cycle inhibitor. Evidence suggests that P15^{INK4B} may allow leukemia cells to escape the inhibitory signal in the bone marrow. Decitabine treatment has been shown to reverse hypermethylation of P15^{INK4B}, allowing the re-establishment of normal P15^{INK4B} protein expression. In addition, hypomethylation of P15^{INK4B} has been associated with hematological response, supporting pharmacologic hypomethylation and demethylation as a possible mechanism for clinical response. Decitabine appears to have dual mechanisms of action depending upon the dose used. At both lower and high dose, decitabine incorporates into DNA; however, at high dose, decitabine inhibits cell proliferation through non-reversible covalent linking with DNA synthesis. Lower doses of decitabine induce hypomethylation, thereby promoting cell proliferation and re-expression of tumor suppression gene, stimulating immune mechanisms and suppression of tumor growth.

Treatment of MDS patients with azacytidine (Vidaza) have also been shown to improve TI in MDS. Silverman et al. [151] reported the results of CALGB studies involving the treatment of MDS patients with azacytidine. The authors concluded that treatment of MDS patients with either IV or subcutaneous azacitidine resulted in platelet and/or red cell TI in some patients. Likewise, Rossetti et al. [152] documented that azacitidine treatment yielded overall hematological improvement in 51% of patients. Of note, the addition of G-CSF to azacitidine, either with or without erythropoietin, increased the overall hematological response rate to 84%. Another hypomethylating agent, 5-aza-deoxycytidine (decitabine, Dacogen) has also shown improvement of thrombocytopenia and anemia in MDS patients who responded to this agent [153–155].

Dacogen was approved in the year 2004, based upon the multicenter randomized trial conducted on 170 MDS patients (156). In this pivotal North American multicenter trial, 89 patients received the drug decitabine plus supportive care and 81 patients were randomized to receive standard supportive care alone. The dose of decitabine in this trial was 45 mg daily in a 3-hour IV infusion, the dose used in a previous European trial on MDS. The overall response in this trial was 17% with 8% CR and 9% PR. An additional 13% of the patients treated with decitabine in this trial had hematological improvement. The response in the supportive care arm was 0%. The median time to progression to AML or death in the patients receiving decitabine was delayed and was 17.5 months versus 7.8 months in non-responders (p = 0.01). One hundred percent of the responders as well as the patients with hematological improvement became red-cell and platelet-transfusion independent. Furthermore, all responders to decitabine evaluable for cytogenetic abnormalities had a complete cytogenetic response. Based upon the results of this trial, decitabine achieved approval by the FDA for use in all categories of MDS patients. Although decitabine was approved at a 45 mg daily dose as per this trial, it was considered by the group that the response could be improved by reducing the dose of this hypomethylating agent. Therefore, in the next randomized trial, 5-day regimens with 10 mg IV, 20 mg IV, and 20 mg subcutaneous injection were compared (157). It was discovered that the low-dose intensity schedule of decitabine was more efficacious, as the dose of 20 mg

IV daily for five days led to 34% CR as compared to 8% in the previous study, and 73% of the MDS patients in this study exhibited an objective response.

Summary

Supportive care plays a major role in the management of myelodysplastic syndrome patients and can increase the overall QOL. Supportive care includes antimicrobial, antiviral, and antifungal agents, red cell and platelet transfusions, use of growth factors (ESA, G-CSF, GM-CSF, and platelet stimulating agents) and treatment of transfusion-related iron overload, which may compromise survival. Therefore, treatment of iron overload with oral chelating agents is recommended in patients with a heavy transfusion burden. Myeloid growth factor use enhancing the MDS progression to AML has been a concern, but recent data appears to negate this concern and their use in high-risk patients has been beneficial. New platelet growth factors that could be beneficial in preventing bleeding complications in MDS patients are in trials at this stage. Supportive care should be actively employed in both low- and high-risk MDS patient care, particularly as there is no therapeutic cure except for stem cell transplant for MDS patients at this time. Supportive care as discussed in this chapter remains an integral component of an MDS management program.

References

1 Saba HI. (1996) Myelodysplastic syndromes in the elderly: the role of growth factors in management. *Leuk Res* **20**:203–19.

2 Ma X, Does M, Raza A, et al. (2007) Myelodysplastic syndromes. Incidence and survival in the U. S. *Cancer* **109**:1536–42.

3 Rollison DE, Howlader N, Smith MT, et al. (2008) Epidemiology of myelodysplastic syndromes and chronic myeloproliferative disorders in the U.S., 2001–2009, using data from ASSCCR and SEER programs. *Blood* **112**:45–52.

4 Sekeres MA, Schooner M, Kantarjian H, et al. (2008) Characteristics of U.S. patients with myelodysplastic syndromes: Results of six cross-sectional physician surveys. *J Natl Cancer Inst* **100**:1542–51.

5 Saba H.I. (2001) Myelodysplastic syndromes in the elderly. *Cancer Control* **8**:79–102.

6 Bennett JM, Catovsky D, Daniel MT, et al. (1982) Proposals for the classification of the myelodysplastic syndromes. *Br J Haematol* **51**:189–99.

7 Harris NL, Jaffe ES, Diebold J, et al. (1999) The World Health Organization classification of neoplastic disease of the hematopoietic and lymphoid tissues. Report of the Clinical Advisory Committee meeting, Airlie House, Virginia. November, 1997. *J Clin Oncol* **17**:3835–49.

8 Steesma DP, Tefferi A. (2003) The myelodysplastic syndrome(s): a perspective and review highlighting current controversies. *Leuk Res* **27**:95–120.

9 Greenberg P, Cox C, LeBeau M.M. et al. (1997) International scoring system for evaluating prognosis in myelodysplastic syndromes. *Blood* **89**:2079–88.

10 Giraldo P, Nomdedeu B, Loscertales J, et al. (2006) Aranesp in Myelodysplastic Syndromes (ARM) Study Group. Darbepoetin alpha for the treatment of anemia in patients with myelodysplastic syndrome. *Cancer* **107**:2807–16.

11 Kantarjian HM, Giles F, List AF, et al. (2007) The incidence and impact of thrombocytopenia in myelodysplastic syndrome. *Cancer* **15**:1705–14.

12 Catenacci DV, Schiller GJ. (2005) Myelodysplasic syndromes: a comprehensive review. *Blood Rev* **19**:301–19.

13 Kuendgen A, Strupp C, Aivado M. (2006) Myelodysplastic syndromes in patients younger than age 50. *J Clin Oncol* **24**:5358–65.

14 Pomeroy C, Oken MM, Rydell RE, Filice GA. (1991) Infection in the myelodysplastic syndromes. *Am J Med* **90**:338–44.

15 Neonakis IK, Alexandrakis MG, Gitti Z, et al. (2008) Miliary tuberculosis with no pulmonary involvement in myelodysplastic syndromes: a curable, yet rarely diagnosed, disease: case report and review of the literature. *Ann Clin Microbiol Antimicrob* **7**:8.

16 Vinh DC, Patel SY, Uzel G, (2010) Autosomal dominant and sporadic monocytopenia with susceptibility to mycobacteria, fungi, papillomaviruses, and myelodysplasia. *Blood* **115**:1519–29.

17 Kao JM, McMillan A, Greenberg PL. (2008) International MDS Risk Analysis Workshop (IMRAW)/IPSS re-analyzed: Impact of depth of cytopenias on clinical outcomes in MDS. *Am J Haematol* **83**:765–70.

18 NCCN *Clinical Practice Guidelines in Oncology: Myelodysplastic Syndromes*, V2.2010. National Comprehensive

Cancer Network, at www.nccn.org (last accessed October 13, 2010).

19 Thomas ML. (1998) Quality of life and psychosocial adjustment in patients with myelodysplastic syndromes. *Leuk Res* **1001**:S41–S47.

20 Hellstrom-Lindberg E. (2005) Update on supportive care and new therapies: Immunomodulatory drugs, growth factors and epigenetic-acting agents. *Hematology (Am Soc Hematol Educ Program)* **2005**:161–6.

21 Passweg JR, Giagounidis A, Simcock M, et al. (2007) Immunosuppression for patients with low and intermediate-risk myelodysplastic syndrome: A prospective randomized multicenter trial comparing antithymocyte globulin + cyclosporine with best supportive care: SAKK 33/39. *Blood* **110**:461.

22 Lau LG, Chng WJ, Liu TC, et al. (2004) Clinico-pathological analysis of myelodysplastic syndromes according to the French-American-British classification and International Prognostic Scoring System. *Ann Acad Med Singapore* **33**:589–95.

23 Brechignax S, Hellstrom-Lindberg E, Bowen D.T. et al. (2004) Quality of life and economic impact of red blood cell (RBC) transfusions on patients with myelodysplastic syndromes (MDS). *Blood* **104**:4716.

24 Szende A, Schaefer C, Goss T.F. et al. (2009) Valuation of transfusion-free living in MDS: results of health utility interviews with patients. *Health and Quality of Life Outcomes* **7**:81–8.

25 Steesma DP, Heptinstall KV, Johnson VM, et al. (2007) Common troublesome symptoms and their impact on quality of life in patients with myelodysplastic syndromes (MDS): results of a large internet-based survey. *Leuk Res* **5**:691–8.

26 Landi F, Russo A, Danese P, et al. (2007) Anemia status, hemoglobin concentration, and mortality in nursing home older residents. *J Am Med Dir Assoc* **8**:322–7.

27 Zakai MA, Katz R, Hirsh C, et al. (2005) A prospective study of anemia status, hemoglobin concentration, and mortality in an elderly cohort: the Cardiovascular Health Study. *Ann Intern Med* **165**:2214–20.

28 Lorand-Metze I, Pinheiro MP, Ribeiro E, de Paula EV, Metz K. (2004) Factors influencing survival in myelodysplastic syndromes in a Brazilian population: comparison of FAB and WHO classifications. *Leuk Res* **28**:587–94.

29 Kurtin SE. (2007) Myelodysplastic syndromes: diagnosis, treatment planning, and clinical management. *Oncology* **21**:41–8.

30 Alessandrino EP, Della Porta MG. Bacigalupo A, et al. (2010) Prognostic impact of pre-transplantation transfusion history and secondary iron overload in patients with myelodysplastic syndrome undergoing allogeneic stem cell transplantation: a GITMO study. *Haematologica* **95**:476–84.

31 Cazzola M, Malcovatti L. (2005) Myelodysplastic syndromes – coping with ineffective hematopoiesis. *New Engl J Med* **352**:536–8.

32 Malcovati L. (2007) Impact of transfusion dependency and secondary iron overload on the survival of patients with myelodysplastic syndromes. *Leuk Res* **31**:S2–6.

33 Cermak J, Kacirkova R, Mikulenkova D, Michalova K. (2009) Impact of transfusion dependency on survival in patients with early myelodysplastic syndrome without excess of blasts. *Leuk Res* **11**:1469–74.

34 Groopman JE, Itri LM. (1999) Chemotherapy-induced anemia in adults: incidence and treatment. *J Natl Cancer Ins* **91**:1616–34.

35 Ludwig H, Van Belle S, Barrett-Lee P, et al. (2004) The European Cancer Anaemia Survey (ECAS): a large, multinational, prospective survey defining the prevalence, incidence, and treatment of anaemia in cancer patients. *Eur J Cancer* **40**:2293–306.

36 Goldrick A, Olivotto IA, Alexander CS, et al. (2007) Anemia is a common but neglected complication of adjuvant chemotherapy for early breast cancer. *Curr Oncol* **14**:227–33.

37 Kitano T, Tada H, Nishimura T, et al. (2007) Prevalence and incidence of anemia in Japanese cancer patients receiving outpatient chemotherapy. *Int J Hematol* **86**:37–41.

38 Laurie SA, Jeyabalan N, Nicholas G, MacRae R, Dahrouge S. (2006) Association between anemia arising during therapy and outcomes of chemoradiation for limited small-cell lung cancer. *J Thorac Oncol* **1**:146–51.

39 Cazzola M, Della Porta MG, Malcovati L. (2008) Clinical relevance of anemia and transfusion iron overload in myelodysplastic syndromes. *Hematology (Am Soc Hematol Educ Program)* **2008**:166–75.

40 Malcovati L. (2009) Red blood cell transfusion therapy and iron chelation in patients with myelodysplastic syndromes. *Clin Lymphoma Myeloma* **9**:S305–11.

41 Cappellini MD. www.touchbriefings.com/pdf/2460/cappellini.pdf (accessed February 22, 2008).

42 Gattermann N. (2007) Guidelines on iron chelation therapy in patients with myelodysplastic syndromes and transfusional iron overload. *Leuk Res* **31**: S10–15.

43 Porter JB. (2001) Practical management of iron over-load. *Br J Haematol* **115**:239–52.

44 Straus DJ. (2002) Epoetin alfa as a supportive measure in hematologic malignancies. *Semin Hematol* **39**:25–31.

45 Stasi R, Brunetti M, Terzoli E, Abruzzese E, Amadori S. (2004) Once-weekly dosing of recombinant human erythropoietin alpha in patients with myelodysplastic syndromes unresponsive to conventional dosing. *Annals Onc* **15**:1684–90.

46 Rizzo JD, Lichtin AE, Woolf SH, et al. (2002) Use of epoetin in patients with cancer: evidence-based clinical practice guidelines of the American Society of Clinical Oncology and the American Society of Hematology. *Blood* **100**:2303–20.

47 Hellstrom-Lindberg E. (1995) Efficacy of erythropoietin in the myelodysplastic syndromes: a meta-analysis of 205 patients from 17 studies. *Br J Haematol* **89**:67–71.

48 Italian Cooperative Study Group for rHuEpo in Myelodysplastic Syndromes (1998) A randomized double-blind placebo-controlled study with subcutaneous recombinant human erythropoietin in patients with low-risk myelodysplastic syndromes. *Br J Haematol* **103**:1070–4.

49 Mundle S, Lefebvre P, Duh MS, et al. (2007) Treatment of MDS-related transfusion-dependent anemia with epoetin alfa: a meta-analysis perspective. *Blood* **110**:1471.

50 Kwon M, Ballesteros M, Perez I, et al. (2007) Unexpected response to erythropoietin therapy in intermediate-low IPSS myelodysplastic syndromes. *Blood* **110**:4867.

51 Rizzo JD, Somerfield MR, Hagerty KL, et al. (2008) American Society of Hematology/American Society of Clinical Oncology 2007 clinical practice guideline update on the use of epoetin and darbepoetin. *J Clin Oncol* **26**:132–49.

52 Terpos E, Mougiou A, Kouraklis A, et al. (2002) Prolonged administration of erythropoietin increases erythroid response rate in myelodysplastic syndromes: a phase II trial in 261 patients. *Br J Haematol* **118**:174–80.

53 Ross SD, Allen IE, Probst CA, et al. (2007) Efficacy and safety of erythopoiesis-stimulating proteins in myelodysplastic syndrome: A systematic review and meta-analysis. *Oncologist* **12**:1264–73.

54 Musto P, Falcone A, Sanpaolo G, et al. (2003) Efficacy of a single, weekly dose of recombinant erythropoietin in myelodysplastic syndromes. *Br J Haematol* **122**:269–71.

55 Food and Drug Administration (FDA). Erythropoiesis-stimulating agents (ESA) safety alert. Press release. November 22, 2006.

56 Procrit [package insert] (2010). Thousand Oaks, CA: Amgen Inc.

57 Patton JR, Mun Y, Wallace JF. (2005) Darbepoetin alfa maintains hemoglobin levels in patients with myelodysplastic syndrome: Results of a retrospective cohort study after therapeutic substitution from epoetin alfa. *J Support Onc* **3**:28–9.

58 Gabrilove J, Paquette R, Lyons RM, et al. (2006) The efficacy and safety of darbepoetin alfa for treating anemia in low-risk myelodysplastic syndrome patients: results after 53/55 weeks. *Br J Haematol* **133**:513–19.

59 Moyo V, Lefebvre P, Duh MS, Yektashenas B, Mundle S. (2008) Erythropoiesis-stimulating agents in the treatment of anemia in myelodysplastic syndromes: a meta-analysis. *Ann Hematol* **87**:527–36.

60 Olivia EN, Latagliata R, Danova M, et al. (2006) Darbepoetin for the treatment of myelodysplastic syndromes: Efficacy and improvements in quality of life. *Blood* **108**:2667.

61 Littlewood T, Kallich J, San Miguel J, Hendricks L, Hedenus M. (2006) Efficacy of darbepoetin alfa in alleviating fatigue and the effect of fatigue on quality of life in anemic patients with lymphoproliferative malignancies *J Pain Symptom Management* **31**:317–25.

62 Stasi R, Abruzzese E, Lanzetta G, Terzoli E, Amadori S. (2005) Darbepoetin alfa for the treatment of anemic patients with low- and intermediate-1-risk myelodysplastic syndromes. *Ann Oncol* **16**:1921–7.

63 Laliberte F, McKenzie SR, Bookhart BK, Duh MS, Lefebvre P. (2007) Drug utilization and cost considerations of erythropoiesis-stimulating agents in patients with myelodysplastic syndromes. *Blood* **110**:4611.

64 Musto P, Campioni L, Guariglia R, et al. (2007) High dose Darbepoetin Q3W, alone or in combination with peg-filgrastim, for myelodysplastic syndromes unresponsive to recombinant erythropoietin. *Leuk Res* **31**: S117.

65 Negrin RS, Stein R, Doherty K, et al. (1996) Maintenance treatment of the anemia of myelodysplastic syndromes with recombinant human granulocyte colony-stimulating factor and erythropoietin: Evidence for in vivo synergy. *Blood* **87**:4076–81.

66 Hellstrom-Lindberg E, Ahlgren T, Beguin Y, et al. (1998) Treatment of anemia in myelodysplastic syndromes with granulocyte colony-stimulating factor plus erythropoietin: Results from a randomized phase II study and long-term follow-up of 71 patients. *Blood* **92**:68–75.

67 Jadersten M, Montgomery SM, Dybedal I, et al. (2005) Long-term outcome of treatment of anemia in MDS with erythropoietin and G-CSF. *Blood* **106**:803–11.

68 Nair V, Mishra DK, Das SN, et al. (2006) Eythropoietin (EPO) and granulocyte colony stimulating factor (G-CSF) based therapy in patients with low-risk MDS: a single centre experience from India. *Blood* **108**:4869.

69 Park S, Grabar S, Kelaidi C, et al. (2008) Predictive factors of response and survival in myelodysplastic syndrome treated with erythropoietin and G-CSF: the GFM experience. *Blood* **111**:574–82.

70 Balleari E, Rossi E, Clavio M, et al. (2006) Erythropoietin plus granulocyte colony-stimulating factor is better than erythropoietin alone to treat anemia in low-risk myelodysplastic syndromes: results from a randomized single-centre study. *Ann Hematol* **85**:174–80.

71 Jadersten M, Malcovati L, Dybedal I, et al. (2008) Erythropoietin and granulocyte colony-stimulating factor treatment associated with improved survival in myelodysplastic syndrome. *J Clin Oncol* **26**:3607–13.

72 Sekeres M, Schoonen M, Kantarjian H, et al. (2008) Characteristics of US patients with myelodysplastic syndromes: results of six cross-sectional physician surveys. *J Natl Cancer Inst* **100**:1542–51.

73 Pullarkat V. (2009) Objectives of iron chelation therapy in myelodysplastic syndromes: more than meets the eye? *Blood* **114**:5251–5.

74 Greenberg PL. (2006) Myelodysplastic syndromes: Iron overload consequences and current chelation therapies. *JNCCN* **4**:91–6.

75 Gattermann N. (2009) The treatment of secondary hemochromatosis. *Dtsch Arztebl Int* **106**:499–504.

76 Abetz L, Baladi JF, Jones P, Rafail D. (2006) The impact of iron overload and its treatment on quality of life: results from a literature review. *Health and Quality of Life Outcomes* **4**:73–8.

77 Leitch HA, Wong DHC, Leger CS, et al. (2007) Improved leukemia-free and overall survival in patients with myelodysplastic syndrome receiving iron chelation therapy: a subgroup analysis. *Blood* **110**:1469.

78 Rose C, Brechignac S, Vassilief D, et al. (2007) Positive impact of iron chelation therapy (CT) on survival in regularly transfused MDS patients. A prospective analysis by the GFM. *Blood* **110**:249.

79 Chee CE, Steensma DP, Wu W, Hanson CA, Tefferi A. (2008) Neither ferritin nor number of red blood cell transfusions affect survival in refractory anemia with ringed sideroblasts. *Am J Hematol* **83**:611–3.

80 National Comprehensive Cancer Network Practice Guidelines in Oncology: Myelodysplastic Syndromes, v2.2008. http://www.nccn.org/professionals/physician_gls/PDF/mds.pdf (accessed February 25, 2008).

81 Valent R, Krieger O, Stauder R, et al. (2008) Iron overload in myelodysplastic syndromes (MDS) – diagnosis, management, and response criteria: a proposal of the Austrian MDS platform. *Euro J Clin Invest* **38**:143–9.

82 Thuret I, Brun-Strang C, Bachir D, et al. (2006) Patient characteristics, quality-of-life and compliance with deferoxamine in patients with transfusional iron overload: results of ISOSFER study. *Blood* **108**:5513.

83 Caro JJ, Ward A, Green TC, et al. (2002) Impact of thalassemia major on patients and their families. *Acta Haematologica* **107**:150–7.

84 Leitch H, Goodman T, Wong K, et al. (2007) Improved survival in patients with myelodysplastic syndrome (MDS) receiving iron chelation therapy. *Blood* **108**:78a.

85 Alymara V, Bourantas D, Chaidos A, et al. (2004) Effectiveness and safety of combined iron-chelation therapy with deferoxamine and deferiprone. *Hematology J* **5**:475–9.

86 Olivieri NF, Buncic JR, Chew E, et al. (1986) Visual and auditory neurotoxicity in patients receiving subcutaneous deferoxamine infusions. *N Engl J Med* **314**:869–73.

87 Desferal® [product insert T2006-3], Novartis, Revised February 2006.

88 Olivieri NF, Brittenham GM, Matsui D, et al. (1995) Iron-chelation therapy with oral deferiprone in patients with thalassemia major. *N Engl J Med* **332**:918–22.

89 Franchini M, Veneri D. (2004) Iron-chelation therapy: an update. *Hematol J* **5**:287–92.

90 Kontoghiorghes GJ. (2001) Clinical use, therapeutic aspects and future potential of deferiprone in thalassemia and other conditions of iron and other metal toxicity. *Drugs Today* **37**:23–35.

91 Cohen AR. (2006) New advances in iron chelation therapy. *Hematology (Am Soc Hematol Educ Program)* **2006**:42–7.

92 Cappellini MD. (2005) Iron-chelating therapy with the new oral agent ICL670. *Best Pract Res Clin Haematol* **1**:289–98.

93 Porter J, Galanello R, Saglio G, et al. (2007) Relative response of patients with myelodysplastic syndromes and other transfusion-dependent anaemias to defer-asirox (ICL670): a 1-yr prospective study. *Euro J Hae-matol* **80**:168–76.

94 Nisbet-Brown E, Olivieri NF, Giardina PJ, et al. (2003) Effectiveness and safety of ICL670 in iron-loaded patients with thalassemia: a randomized, double-blind, placebo-controlled, dose-escalation trial. *Lancet* **362**:495–6.

95 Galanello R, Piga A, Forni GL, et al. (2006) Phase II clinical evaluation of deferasirox, a once-daily oral chelating agent, in pediatric patients with beta-thalassemia major. *Haematologica* **91**:1343–51.

96 Cappellini MD, Cohen A, Piga A, et al. (2006) A phase III study of deferasirox (ICL670), a once-daily oral iron chelator, in patients with beta-thalassemia. *Blood* **107**:3455–62.

97 Faris RJ, McCrone D, Mody-Patel N, Barghout V, Dutta S. (2007) Compliance and persistency with a new iron chelator in patients with myelodysplastic syndromes. *J Clin Oncol* **25**:17510.

98 Mody-Patel N, Goldberg SL, Barghout V. (2007) Defer-asirox for myelodysplastic syndrome patients with transfusional iron overload: a budget impact analysis. *J Clin Oncol* **25**:17019.

99 FDA Drug Safety Newsletter, Volume 1, Fall 2007. http://www.fda.gov/Drugs/DrugSafety/DrugSafety-Newsletter/ucm118813.htm (accessed February 25, 2008).

100 FDA Medwatch Alert December 13, 2007, at: http://www.drugs.com/fda/exjade-defasirox-12361.html (accessed February 26, 2008).

101 Pullarkat V. (2009) Objectives of iron chelation therapy in myelodysplastic syndromes: more than meets the eye? *Blood* **114**:5251–5.

102 Cermak J. (2006) Erythropoietin administration may potentiate mobilization of storage iron in patients on oral iron chelation therapy. *Hemoglobin* **30**:105–12.

103 Greenberg P, Taylor K, Larson R, et al. (1993) Phase III randomized multicenter trial of G-CSF vs. observation for myelodysplastic syndromes (MDS). *Blood* **82**:196a.

104 Ossenkoppele GJ, Vanderbhoit B, Verhoef G.E. et al. (1999) A randomized study of granulocyte colony-stimulating factor applied during and after chemo-therapy in patients with poor risk myelodysplastic syndromes: A report from the HOVON Cooperative Group [Dutch-Belgium Hemato-Oncology Coopera-tive Group]. *Leukemia* **13**:1207–13.

105 Bennett JM, Young MS, Paietta E, et al. (1998) Phase II trial of high dose cytosine arabinoside, mitoxantrone (S-HAM) and granulocyte-macrophage colony stim-ulating factor (GM-CSF) in patients with high risk myelodysplastic syndromes (MDS). A study of the Eastern Cooperative Oncology Group (ECOG), E3996. *Blood* **92**:630a.

106 Estey EH, Thail PF, Pierce S, et al. (1999) Randomized phase II study of fludarabine + cytosine arabinoside + idarubicin ± all-trans retinoic acid ± granulocyte colony-stimulating factor in poor prognosis newly diagnosed acute myeloid leukemia and myelodysplas-tic syndrome. *Blood* **93**:2478–84.

107 Witz F, Sadoun A, Perrin MC, et al. (1998) A placebo-controlled study of recombinant human granulocyte-macrophage colony-stimulating factor administered during and after induction treatment for de novo acute myelogenous leukemia in elderly patients. *Blood* **91**:2722–30.

108 Lintula R, Rasi V, Ikkala E, Borgström GH, Vuopio P. (1981) Platelet function in preleukaemia. *Scand J Haematol* **26**:65–71.

109 Sashida G, Takau TI, Nishimaki N, et al. (2003) Clin-ico-hematologic features of myelodysplastic syn-drome presenting as isolated thrombocytopenia: an entity with a relatively favorable prognosis. *Leuk Lym-phoma* **44**:653–8.

110 Kao JM, McMillan A, Greenberg PL. (2007) Interna-tional MDS Risk Analysis Workshop (IMRAW)/IPSS re-analyzed: Impact of depth of cytopenias on clinical outcomes in MDS. *Blood* **110**:2457.

111 Schwartz SI. (1985) Splenectomy for thrombocytope-nia. *World J Surg* **9**:416–21.

112 Bourgeois E, Caulier MT, Rose C, Dupretal. (2001) Role of splenectomy in the treatment of myelodys-plastic syndromes with peripheral thrombocytopenia: a report on six cases. *Leukemia* **15**:950–3.

113 Abdul-Wahab J, Naznin M, Suhaimi A, Amir-Hamzah AR. (2007) Favorable response to splenectomy in famil-ial myelodysplastic syndrome. *Singapore Med J* **48**:e206.

114 Ishibashi T, Kimura H, Uchida T, et al. (1989) Human interleukin-6 is a direct promoter of maturation of

megakaryocytes in vitro. *Proc Natl Acad Sci U S A* **86**:5953–7.

115 Kimura H, Ishibashi T, Uchida T, et al. (1990) Interleukin-6 is a differentiation factor for human megakaryocytes in vitro. *Eur J Immunol* **20**:1927–31.

116 Gordon MD, Nemunaitis J, Hoffman R, et al. (1995) A Phase I trial of recombinant human interleukin-6 in patients with myelodysplastic syndromes and thrombocytopenia. *Blood* **85**:3066–76.

117 Will B, Kawahara M, Luciano JP, et al. (2009) Effect of the nonpeptide thrombopoietin receptor agonist Eltrombopag on bone marrow cells from patients with acute myeloid leukemia and myelodysplastic syndrome. *Blood* **114**:3899–908.

118 Komatsu N, Okamoto T, Yoshida T, et al. (2000) Pegylated recombinant human megakaryoctye growth and development factor (PEG-rHuMGDF) increased platelet counts (plt) in patients with aplastic anemia (AA) and myelodysplastic syndrome (MDS). *Blood* **96**:296a.

119 Basser RL, O'Flaherty E, Green M, et al. (2002) Development of pancytopenia with neutralizing antibodies to thrombopoietin after multicycle chemotherapy supported by megakaryocyte growth and development factor. *Blood* **99**:2599–602.

120 Li J, Yang C, Xia Y, et al. (2001) Thrombocytopenia caused by the development of antibodies to thrombopoietin. *Blood* **98**:3241–8.

121 Du X, Williams DA. (1997) Interleukin-11: review of molecular, cell biology, and clinical use. *Blood* **89**:3897–908.

122 Kurzrock R, Cortes J, Thomas DA, et al. (2001) Pilot study of low-dose interleukin-11 in patients with bone marrow failure. *J Clin Oncol* **19**:4165–72.

123 Tsimberidou AM, Giles FJ, Khouri I, et al. (2005) Low-dose interleukin-11 in patients with bone marrow failure: update of the M.D. Anderson Cancer Center experience. *Ann Onc* **16**:139–45.

124 Kantarjian H, Fenaux P, Sekeres MA, et al. (2010) Safety and efficacy of romiplostim in patients with lower-risk myelodysplastic syndrome and thrombocytopenia. *J Clin Oncol* **28**:437–44.

125 Kantarjian H, Fenaux P, Sekeres MA, et al. (2007) Phase 1/2 study of AMG-531 in thrombocytopenic patients (pts) with low-risk myelodysplastic syndrome (MDS): Update including extended treatment. *Blood* **110**:250.

126 Bussel JB, McHutchison J, Provan D, et al. (2007) Safety of eltrombopag, an oral non-peptide platelet growth factor, in the treatment of thrombocytopenia: Results of four randomized, placebo-controlled studies. *Blood* **110**:1299.

127 Bussel JB, Cheng G, Saleh MN, et al. (2007) Eltrombopag for the treatment of chronic idiopathic thrombocytopenic purpura. *New Engl J Med* **357**:2237–47.

128 Bussel JB, Cheng G, Kovaleva L, et al. (2007) Long-term safety and efficacy of oral eltrombopag for the treatment of subjects with idiopathic thrombocytopenic purpura (ITP): Preliminary data from the EXTEND study. *Blood* **110**:566.

129 Bussel JB, Provan D, Shamsi T, et al. (2009) Effect of eltrombopag on platelet counts and bleeding during treatment of chronic idiopathic thrombocytopenic purpura: A randomized, double-blind, placebo-controlled trial. *Lancet* **373**:641–8.

130 Psaila B, Bussel JB, Cheng G, et al. (2007) In vivo effects of eltrombopag on human platelet function. *Blood* **110**:1301.

131 Kantarjian H, Giles F, Greenberg P, et al. (2008) Effect of romiplostim in patients (pts) with low or intermediate risk myelodysplastic syndrome (MDS) receiving azacytidine. *Blood* **112**:224.

132 Erhardt JA, Erickson-Miller CL, Aivado M, et al. (2009) Comparative analyses of the small molecule thrombopoietin receptor agonist eltrombopag and thrombopoietin on in vitro platelet function. *Exp Hematol* **37**:1030–7.

133 http://www.drugs.com/nda/promacta_080303.html (accessed March 25, 2010).

134 Will B, Kawahara M, Luciano JP, et al. (2009) Effect of the nonpeptide thrombopoietin receptor agonist Eltrombopag on bone marrow cells from patients with acute myeloid leukemia and myelodysplastic syndrome. *Blood* **114**:3899–908.

135 Ronnberg L, Ylostalo P, Jarvinen PA. (1979) Effects of danazol in the treatment of severe endometriosis. *Postgrad Med J* **55**:21–6.

136 Ahn YS, Harrington WJ, Simon SR, et al. (1983) Danazol for the treatment of idiopathic thrombocytopenic purpura. *N Engl J Med* **308**:1396–9.

137 Buelli M, Cortelazzo S, Viero P, et al. (1985) Danazol for the treatment of idiopathic thrombocytopenic purpura. *Acta Haematol* **74**:97–8.

138 Buzaid AC, Garewal HS, Lippman SM, et al. (1987) Danazol in the treatment of myelodysplastic syndromes. *Eur J Haematol* **39**:346–8.

139 Chabannon C, Molina L, Pegourie-Bandelier B, et al. (1994) A review of 76 patients with myelodysplastic syndromes treated with danazol. *Cancer* **73**:3073–80.

140 Marini B, Bassan R, Barbui T. (1988) Therapeutic efficacy of danazol in myelodysplastic syndromes. *Eur J Cancer Clin Oncol* **24**:1481–9.

141 Aviles A, Rubio ME, Gomez J, Medina ML, Gonzalez-Llaven J. (1989) Randomized study of danazol vs. placebo in myelodysplastic syndromes. *Arch Invest Med* **20**:183–8.

142 Chan G, DiVenuti G, Miller K. (2002) Danazol for the treatment of thrombocytopenia in patients with myelodysplastic syndrome. *Am J Hematol* **71**:166–71.

143 Jain N, Mattiuzzi GN, Cortes J, et al. (2007) Benefit of anti-infective prophylaxis in patients with acute myeloid leukemia or high-risk myelodysplastic syndrome receiving frontline "targeted therapy". *Blood* **110**:2858.

144 Pilatrino C, Cilloni D, Messa E, et al. (2005) Increase in platelet count in older, poor-risk patients with acute myeloid leukemia or myelodysplastic syndrome treated with valproic acid and all-trans retinoic acid. *Cancer* **104**:101–9.

145 Chen S, Jiang B, Da W, Gong M, Guan M. (2007) Treatment of myelodysplastic syndrome with cyclosporin A. *Int J Hematol* **85**:11–17.

146 Ishikawa T, Tohyama K, Nakao S, et al. (2007) A prospective study of cyclosporine A treatment of patients with low-risk myelodysplastic syndrome: presence of CD55(-) CD59(-) blood cells predicts platelet response. *Int J Hematol* **86**:150–7.

147 Strupp C, Germing U, Aivado M, et al. (2002) Thalidomide for the treatment of patients with myelodysplastic syndromes. *Leukemia* **16**:1–6.

148 Musto P, Falcone A, Sanpaolo G, et al. (2002) Thalidomide abolishes transfusion-dependence in selected patients with myelodysplastic syndromes. *Haematologica* **87**:884–6.

149 List A, Dewald G, Bennett J, et al. (2006) Hematologic and cytogenetic response to lenalidomide in myelodysplastic syndrome with chromosome 5q deletion. *N Engl J Med* **355**:1456–65.

150 Raza A, Reeves JA, Feldman EJ, et al. (2008) Phase 2 study of lenalidomide in transfusion-dependent, low-risk, and intermediate-1 risk myelodysplastic syndromes with karyotypes other than deletion 5q. *Blood* **111**:86–93.

151 Silverman LR, Peterson BL, Holland JF, et al., (2006) and the Cancer and Leukemia Group B (CALGB) Transfusion independence in patients with myelodysplastic syndromes treated with azacitidine. *J Clin Oncol* **24**:6576.

152 Rossetti JM, Falke E, Shadduck RK, Latsko JM, Kramer W. (2006) G-CSF increases hematological response among patients with myelodysplasia treated with azacitidine. *Blood* **108**:4868.

153 Saba HI, Wijermans PW. (2005) Decitabine in myelodysplastic syndromes. *Semin Hematol* **42**:S23–31.

154 Saba H. (2007) Decitabine in the treatment of myelodysplastic syndromes. *Ther Clin Risk Manag* **3**:807–17.

155 Kantarjian H, Issa JPJ, Rosenfeld CS, et al. (2006) Decitabine improves patient outcomes in myelodysplastic syndromes: results of a phase III randomized study. *Cancer* **106**:1794–80.

156 Saba H, Rosenfeld C, Issa JP, et al. (2004) First report of the phase III North American trial of decitabine in advanced myelodysplastic syndrome (MDS). *Blood* **104**:23a.

157 Kantarjian H, Oki Y, Garcia-Manero G, et al. (2007) Results of a randomized study of three schedules of low-dose decitabine in higher risk myelodysplastic syndrome and chronic myelomonocytic leukemia. *Blood* **109**:52–7.

PART 3

Lymphoid Malignancies

CHAPTER 12

Molecular Biology of Chronic Lymphoproliferative Disorders

Monique A. Hartley-Brown and Lubomir Sokol
Department of Medical Hematology and Oncology, University of South Florida and Department of Malignant Hematology, H. Lee Moffitt Cancer Center and Research Institute, Tampa, FL, USA

Chronic lymphocytic leukemia

Definition

Chronic lymphocytic leukemia (CLL) is a disease of the elderly population, and the most common adult leukemia in the Western world, with an incidence of 2–6 cases per 100 000 person-years [1]. The pathophysiology of the disease involves an accumulation of an excessive number of clonal B-cells, overexpressing the antiapoptotic B-cell lymphoma-2 (Bcl-2) protein [2]. Over 90% of CLL cells are considered to be arrested in the G0/G1 phase. It has been postulated that CLL consists of two clinical subsets distinguished by the presence of somatic mutations in the immunoglobulin (Ig) variable region (V) genes [3]. Unmutated CLL is probably derived from a naïve B-cell that has interacted with antigen but the stimulus was insufficient to create a germinal center. This subtype is frequently characterized by IgHV1-69 usage and ZAP-70 expression. Patients with this condition have a worse prognosis compared to the mutated subtype. On the other hand, mutated CLL subtype presumably originates from the memory B-cell that underwent somatic mutation after interaction with antigen and antigen selection at germinal center. The malignant T-cells of this subtype preferentially use IgHV4-34 genes and have an absence of ZAP-70 expression.

Etiology

It was hypothesized that the B-cell receptor (BCR)-mediated stimulation with putative antigen plays an important role in the natural history of CLL [4]. This hypothesis was supported by studies that revealed highly restricted immunoglobulin heavy chain variable region (IgHV) gene repertoire of CLL cells compared to normal adult B-cell repertoire [5, 6].

Patients with CLL expressing IgHV1-69 gene were found to share closely homologous complementarity determining region 3 (CDR3) sequences on IgH and light (L) chains [7]. Overexpression of IgHV1-69 was associated with unmutated CLL and IgHV4-34 in mutated CLL subtypes, respectively [8]. Although physiological aging was associated with increased B-cell populations expressing IgHV4-34, this was not confirmed for IgHV1-69 expression which seems to be CLL-specific [4, 9]. It was reported that more than 20% of unrelated CLL cases carried stereotyped receptors [10]. This data supports a role of putative environmental antigen or autoantigen in etiopathogenesis of this disease.

Immunophenotype

Common CLL immunophenotypic markers include CD5, CD23, CD20low, CD79a, CD43, CD22low, CD11clow, sIgMlow. Typical CLL cells are negative for FMC7 [1, 11]. Atypical variants of CLL include

---

Advances in Malignant Hematology, First Edition. Edited by Hussain I. Saba and Ghulam J. Mufti. © 2011 Blackwell Publishing Ltd. Published 2011 by Blackwell Publishing Ltd.

CD5 or CD23 negativity, positivity for FMC7, CD11c or CD79b and strongly expressed sIg [1].

Cytogenetics/FISH

Cytogenetic and FISH testing is important in this disease. FISH methodology has the proficiency of recognizing over 80% of the clonal cytogenetic abnormalities present in CLL cells [1]. Solo deletion 13q and normal karyotypes are favorable prognostic profiles in CLL, whereas deletion 11q and deletion 17p fare a poor prognosis [12]. Of these clonal aberrations, the most common is deletion 13q14.3, occurring in approximately 50% of patients, and trisomy 12 in about 20% [13]. The other frequent cytogenetic abnormalities (such as deletion 11q22-23, deletion 17p13 and deletion 6q21), constitute the majority of the cytogenetic abnormalities exhibited in the remaining 30% of CLL patients.

MicroRNAs (miRNAs)

Despite the extensive research in the field of molecular pathogenesis of CLL, those causative mutations responsible for this disease have not yet been described. A recent discovery of a novel abundant class of small non-coding RNAs (microRNAs) that regulate the expression of their target mRNAs at the post-transcriptional level was rapidly applied to cancer research [14]. Dysregulation in miRNA expression has emerged as significant in determining mechanisms underlying the development of many solid cancers and leukemias, since these small molecules can act either as oncogenes or tumor suppressors [14].

miRNAs are initially apart of a much longer primary miRNA transcript. The primary miRNA undergoes digestion by two different ribonucleases specific to miRNA; nuclear-restricted Drosha and cytoplasmic Dicer [15]. The product of this digestion process is a hairpin precursor miRNA of approximately 70 nt. In the cytoplasm, the precursor miRNA is digested by Dicer and undergoes maturation with other silencing proteins [16]. The final mature miRNA varies from 19–24 nt in length. Mature miRNAs base pair within the 3′-UTR regions (three prime untranslated region) of the target messenger RNAs, thus regulating gene expression.

Calin et al. reported that miR15 and miR16 are located at chromosome 13q14 region, which is deleted in more than 50% of patients with CLL. They showed that both genes are deleted or down-regulated in approximately 68% patients with CLL [17, 18] (Figure 12.1).

The same group described a unique miRNA expression signature composed of 13 genes that differentiated cases of CLL with low versus high expression of ZAP-70, and cases with unmutated IgVH– region gene from those with mutated IgVH. This signature also correlated with disease progression.

They detected a germ-line C-T homozygous substitution in the miR-16-1 precursor in two patients. This mutation resulted in decreased expression of miR-16-1 *in vitro* and *in vivo*. Germ-line or somatic mutations were found in 5 of 42 miRNAs (miR-16-1, miR-27b, miR-29b-2, miR-187, miR-206) in 11 of 75 patients with CLL, but not in 160 control subjects without cancer. Using fluorescence in situ hybridization, they also found monoallelic deletion at 13q14.3 in most CLL cells from these patients harboring miRNA mutations [19].

MiR15 and miR16 genes that are localized within a 30kb region of each other have a high content of AU-rich elements (AREs) [18]. High content of AREs suggest a genetic area readily susceptible to mutation. The close association of these two miRNAs has made it difficult to elucidate the role of pathogenesis for each miRNA separately. Interestingly, patients with poor prognosis have increased levels of miR15a/16-1, suggestive of an inhibitory effect on tumor suppressor genes and the development of the more aggressive disease [20].

A proposed mechanism by which both genes could result in the evolution of CLL is via bcl-2 upregulation and, therefore, inhibition of apoptosis [2]. However, some studies have shown no correlation between low expression of miR15a/ miR16-1 and upregulation of bcl-2. Therefore, more studies are necessary to correctly discern a plausible mechanistic pathway in which these two miRNAs play an important pathogenic role.

Another miRNA of significance in CLL is miR-NA106b. Induction of this gene has been shown to downregulate a specific E3-ubiquitin lipase, causing

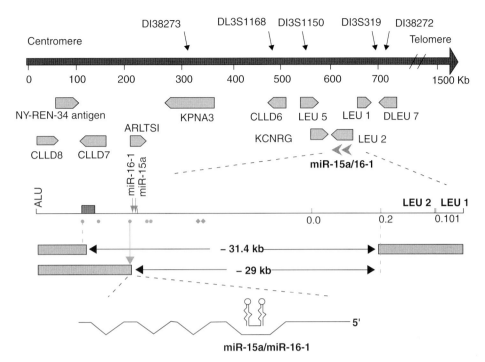

Figure 12.1 miR-15a/miR-16-1 cluster found within the 13q14.3 deletion region in CLL cells. *DLEU7*-deleted in lymphocytic leukemia, 7; *DLEU1*-deleted in lymphocytic leukemia, 1; *DLEU2*- deleted in lymphocytic leukemia, 2; miR-15a-microRNA gene 15a; miR-16-1-microRNA gene 16-1; *KCNRG*-potassium channel regulator; *LEU5*(*RFP2*, ret finger protein 2); *CLLD6* (C13orf1, chromosome 13 open reading frame 1); *KPNA3*-karyopherin alpha 3, importin alpha 4); *ARLTS1* (*ARL11*, ADP-ribosylation factor-like 11); *CLLD7* (*RCBTB1*, regulator of chromosome condensation [RCC1] and BTB [POZ] domain containing protein 1); *NY-REN-34* antigen (PHF11, PHD finger protein 11), *CLLD8* (SETDB2, SET domain, bifurcated 2). (Reproduced from Calin GA et al. [17], with permission from Elsevier.)

accumulation of TAp73, a proapoptotic intracellular substrate of p53, resulting in apoptosis [21].

Marton et al. reported reduced expression of miR-181a, let7a, and miR-30d, with associated overexpression of miR-155 in patients with CLL [22].

Fulci et al. detected overexpression of miR-21 and miR-155 in patients with CLL compared to normal controls with no evidence of gene amplification in corresponding genomic loci [23]. Increased expression of miR-155 has been detected in human B-cell lymphomas, and upregulation of this miRNA resulted in development of B-cell malignancy in mice [23–25].

Zenz et al. studied miR-34a and miR-34b/c expression in 60 patients with CLL. They demonstrated that downregulation of miR-34a is associated with p53 inactivation, chemotherapy-refractory disease, impaired response to DNA damage, and resistance to apoptosis, independently of 17p deletion/TP53 mutation [26].

Stomatopoulos et al. reported that expression levels of miR-29c and miR-223 decreased significantly with progression of disease from Binet Stage A to C. They developed a quantitative real-time PCR score of poor prognostic markers combining miR-29c, miR-223, ZAP70, and lipoprotein lipase (LPL). Using this score, they were able to predict treatment-free survival (TFS) and overall survival (OS) in patients with both the good and poor prognosis subgroups of CLL [27].

Ghosh et al. found constitutive expression of HIF-1alpha under normoxia in CLL cells. Low levels of von Hippel-Lindau protein, which is responsible for HIF-1 alpha degradation, were also detected in CLL cells compared to normal B-cells. miRNA-92-1, which downregulates VHL transcript, was found to be overexpressed in CLL cells, suggesting that miRNA-92-1 regulation is responsible for autocrine VEGF secretion in this disease [28].

Mraz et al. found that a downregulation of miRNA-29c, miRNA-34a, and miRNA-17-5 was associated with an aggressive subtype of CLL with aberrant TP53 gene. These miRNAs target important factors, including BCL-2, TCL-1, and MCL-1, implicated in apoptotic pathways important for survival of malignant CLL cells [29].

A gene signature cluster of 60 genes specific to CLL, including well-known oncogenes such as *MCL1, JUN, SCAP2, TRA1, PDCD61P, RAD51C,* and *HSPA1A/1B,* has been discovered. *MCL1* is known to be a member of the bcl-2 class of proteins, essential in B-cell survival and resistance to chemotherapy [20]. The relevance of these oncogenes in CLL pathogenesis is, as yet, still unclear. Altogether, this data suggests that the dysregulation of expression of miRNAS is implicated in the pathology of sporadic and familial CLL.

Biological markers/intracellular pathways replicated

Several biological markers have been shown to have a prognostic significance in CLL. Notably, three of these markers have evolved as important in this disease, specifically (1) mutation of IgVH region gene, (2) zeta-associated protein-70 (ZAP70) expression, and (3) CD38+ expression [30].

IgVH (immunoglobulin heavy chain variable region)

The IgVH gene is encoded for on chromosome 14, and consists of a variable (V), diversity (D), and joining (J) segments [31]. The Ig molecule consists of heavy and light chains, of which all three VD and J gene segments encode for Ig heavy chains, while only V and J gene segments encode for the Ig light chain. Multiple copies of the VD and J genes exist and allow for the generation of many different combinations that represent different antigen-binding sites for many different antigens [32]. This VDJ recombination is a normal process in B-cells, allowing for the capability to identify and bind to many different antigenic stimuli. In CLL, a somatic IgVH mutation is present in over 50% of cases, and these patients tend to have a better prognosis than those with unmutated IgVH gene [33–35]. One theory suggests that this difference in IgVH mutational status is secondary to the B-cell maturation stage during transformation to the malignant cell type [8, 34–36]. This theory suggests that the pre-germinal center B-cells, likely driven by T-cell independent antigens, are the precursor cells for the unmutated CLL phenotype; while the post-germinal center B-cells, T-cell dependently driven, are the precursor cells for the mutated CLL phenotype [8, 34, 35]. Furthermore, mere usage of the VH3.21 gene is a self-sufficient poor prognostic marker [12].

ZAP70 (zeta-associated protein 70)

ZAP70 is a 70 kd tyrosine kinase encoded by the ZAP70 gene normally expressed in T-cells. This protein is important in T-cell signaling and not normally found in B-cells. In normal T-cells there is T-cell receptor (TCR) ligation followed by activation of immunoreceptor tyrosine-based activation motifs (ITAMs), to which the ZAP70 is recruited activated [37]. Activation of ZAP70 results in cytoplasmic signaling through various pathways including the mitogen-activated protein kinase (MAPK) pathway [38]. In CLL cells, a phosphorylation of ZAP70 appears to result in similar cytoplasmic signal transduction via the B-cell receptor (BCR) complex [39–41]. The outcome of activation of MAPK and similar pathways is unregulated cell growth and apoptotic inhibition. Studies have shown that patients with ZAP70 positive CLL express a more aggressive phenotype compared to the indolent ZAP70 negative patients [30]. A pivotal study by Weistner et al. illustrated a direct correlation of ZAP70 overexpression, via quantitative mRNA analysis in CLL, with unmutated IgVH illustrating a 71% positive predictive value and 100% negative predictive value [42].

CD38

Another possible surrogate marker for IgVH mutational status is the overexpression of CD38.

Expression of both ZAP70 mutation and high CD38 positivity has been illustrated to correlate with expression of unmutated IgVH [43, 44]. CD38 is a cell surface receptor protein with enzymatic activity important in the regulation of cytoplasmic calcium and intracellular interactions [45, 46]. It has been shown to be important in T-cell signaling pathways such as ERK and SYK pathways [45]. The activation of these pathways allows for increased CLL cell survival and proliferation [47]. The CD38 ligand, CD31, is found on stromal cells. The interaction of CD38 and its ligand results in upregulation of cytoplasmic proteins that sustain CLL cell growth [45, 48, 49]. Greater than 30% positivity in CD38 expression in CLL has been associated with a poor prognostic outcome [35, 46]. Additionally, there is an overlap between the CXCL12 chemokine pathway and that controlled by CD38 and ZAP70, allowing for superior cell survival [46].

Familial CLL

Available literature shows more than 10% of CLL patients have a first-degree relative with the disease based on history [50]. Such patients have a 2–7 fold overall risk increase for developing CLL in their lifetime. This is especially important for relatives at an age less than 40 years old [1]. The mutated IgVH gene has been reported to be more prevalent amongst familial CLL patients, compared to acquired cases (68% vs. 47%) [51]. Calin et al. reported that up to 15% of patients with a family history of CLL or other malignancy expressed a germ-line mutation involving miRNA mutations, of which miR16-1 was included [20]. Supportive studies, in NZB mice that naturally develop CLL, allowed for isolation of an aberrant miR16-1 locus giving further credence to the importance of these miRNA genes in familial CLL [20].

More recently, Langren et al. evaluated 9717 CLL patients and matched controls. Over 1500 single nucleotide polymorphisms (SNPs) were analyzed for apoptotic, DNA repair, immune, and other oncogenic pathways. They found an increased relative risk of 8.5 for CLL in the familial cohort (95% CI = 6.1–11.7), compared to controls. SNP analysis elucidated many genes including *IL-10*, *BCL-2*, *TRAIL*, and *TRAILR1*, which were statistically significantly associated with familial CLL [52].

Conversely, data from other studies have compared biological markers including IgVH mutational status, gene usage, CD38, and ZAP70 expression, between familial and acquired CLL patients. One particular study evaluated tissue samples from 3328 CLL patients, 468 familial and 995 acquired cases. They found no statistically significant difference between the groups in any of the parameters studied, suggesting that CLL, regardless of hereditary status, may have derived from a common group of biological pathogenic pathways [52].

The conflicting data indicates the need for further study in this area, but the inheritance pattern strongly supports the theory that the presence of CLL in a first-degree relative predisposes the individual to an increased risk of disease development. The determination of whether familial CLL behaves differently/more aggressively than acquired CLL is as of yet unclear. To date, eight genes have been identified and evaluated for alterations at the DNA and RNA level in patients with sporadic and familial CLL, these include: *Leu-1*(BCMS or EST70/*Leu-1*), *Leu-2* (ALT-1 or 1B4/*Leu-2*), *Leu-5*(CAR), *CLLD7*, *LOC51131 (putative zinc finger protein NY-REN-34 antigen)* and *CLLD8* [18].

Sellick et al. used a high-density SNP genome-wide linkage analysis in 206 families and identified susceptibility loci for CLL in 2q21.2, 6p22.1, and 18q21.1 [53]. Future discovery of causative mutations in suspected genes in familial CLL should undoubtedly help us in understanding the pathobiology of more frequent sporadic CLL.

Therapeutic targets

Fludarabine, cyclophosphamide, and rituximab (FCR) is a standard therapeutic regimen with the highest response rate in untreated patients with CLL. The T-cell leukemia/lymphoma-1 (TCL1) gene, is an oncogene commonly targeted in cells with the chromosomal 14q31.2 mutation [54]. Murine studies have identified that this oncogene plays a role in the development of CLL [55]. TCL1 imparts its effects via the antiapoptotic AKT pathway [56, 57]. Additionally, elevated expression of TCL1 has been correlated with unmutated IgVH, deletion 11q, and ZAP70 positivity [58, 59]. This alludes to the fact that over-expression of TCL1 leads to a more aggressive, treatment-resistant CLL phenotype [60]. Reports suggest that CLL with strong TCL1 expression on immunohistochemistry may respond poorly to the potent chemoimmunotherapy regimen FCR [61].

More promising is the evidence to support use of alemtuzumab in CLL positive for deletion 17p [62]. Reversely, patients with 17p deletion frequently demonstrate resistance to alkylators and purine analog chemotherapy [63].

In the age of targeted therapy one agent of interest in CLL treatment is denileukin diftitox, an anti-CD25 targeted toxin. Frankel et al. treated 22 patients with CLL with denileukin diftitox, with 1/22 (4%) complete remission, and 5/22 (23%) partial remission, with minimal toxicities observed [64]. Currently, standard CLL treatment involves use of alkylators, fludarabine, and monoclonal antibodies, all of which remain non-curative [65]. It is hoped that identification of molecular biomarkers, culprit signature gene cluster regions, and miRNAs specific to CLL will ultimately help in future development of novel therapeutics in CLL [20].

Hairy cell leukemia

Definition

Hairy cell leukemia (HCL) is a rare indolent chronic B-cell malignancy encompassing only 2% of the lymphoid leukemias [1]. HCL affects approximately 0.33 cases per 100 000 person-years in the US, with the mean age of affected adults being around 50 years [66]. Clinically, HCL is often characterized by pancytopenia and splenomegaly. Additionally, there is bone marrow and liver infiltration of the HCL cells, with few to no HCL cells in the peripheral blood [67]. Unique to HCL is the development of bone marrow fibrosis [68].

HCL cells, like CLL cells, contain rearranged Ig variable genes expressed as switched immunoglobulin isotypes, suggesting germinal center (GC) transition with isotype switch recombination and somatic hypermutation [69]. Coexpression of multiple Ig isotypes occur in around 40% of patients [67]. Deletion of the DNA sequence between upstream (IgM and IgD) and downstream (IgA and IgG) Ig isotypes prevents repeat expression of the upstream isotypes, and thus arrests development of HCL cells during Ig isotype switching before deletion recombination and GC exit. These discoveries indicate a connection between the GC cells and HCL cells, historically. Additionally, given the apparently close relationship between these cells, inferences have been proposed suggesting derivation of HCL cells from splenic marginal zone memory B-cells [67].

Etiology

The etiology for the development of hairy cell leukemia is not fully understood. Radiation exposure and exposure to specific organic compounds have been implicated. Epstein-Barr virus has also been considered causative, however adequate biologic evidence remains insufficient [70, 71]. Cytogenetic aberrations specific to chromosome 5, such as trisomy 5 or deletion 5q13, is noted in a large number of patients with hairy cell leukemia. In one study the chromosome 5 aberrations were as high as 40% [72].

The normal precursor B-cell clone from which hairy cell arises is yet unknown. However, somatic mutations in HCL have been identified in 85% of cases [1]. Studies suggest that hairy cells are derived from mature activated B-cell clonal population. The most popular candidate for this theory is the marginal zone B-cell, given the extensive immunophenotypic and morphologic similarities between hairy cells and marginal zone B-cells. Additionally, PCA-1 antigenic expression is present for both cell types [73]. Hairy cells differ, however, by TRAP positivity. Yamaguchi and colleagues have described a polyclonal B-cell population with lymphocytic profile similar to hairy cells – Japanese variant [74, 75].

Immunophenotype

The majority of HCL cases (~92%) can be identified through immunohistochemistry and cytogenetics [76]. Immunophenotypically HCL cells typically express mature B-cell markers such as CD20, CD22, the integrin receptors CD11c and CD103, as well as CD25 [1]. Cyclin D1 is usually weakly expressed. T-bet, Annexin A1 (ANXA1), DBA.44, and FMC-7 expression are also commonly seen, whereas CD10 and CD5 are usually negative. ANXA1 is highly specific for HCL [1]. HC2 and 9C5 are also two specific markers for HCL [76, 77]. CD52 expression has been observed in some cases, resulting in the use of alemtuzumab in certain patients [76].

Cytogenetics/FISH

Many clonal cytogenetic aberrations may be seen in HCL, but to date none have been identified as predominantly HCL specific [1].

Microarray

Microarray analysis in HCL is as yet a poorly explored domain. To date the only information of importance obtained from microarray in HCL is as a possible screening tool to quickly identify HCL from other B-cell lymphoproliferative disorders [78].

Biologic markers/intracellular pathways

HCL cells are slow growing, with a high expression of bcl-2 [67]. This growth latency is consistent with HCL cells being derived from memory B-cells – which are usually quiescent [79]. In addition to bcl-2, there is upregulation of cyclin D1 encoded by the CCND1 gene. This gene is essential in cell cycle progression from G1 to S phase. Additionally, CCND1 is only expressed in malignant cells, not normals [80]. The G1 to S phase transition requires activation of the phosphatidylinositol-3 kinase (PI3k)-AKT pathway, which explains the increased expression of cyclin D1, and conversely the decreased expression of p27, a tumor suppressor gene [67, 81] (Figure 12.2).

FLT3 and interleukin-3 (IL-3) also activate the PI3k-AKT pathway and HCL cells are known to overexpress IL-3 receptor-α (IL-3R-α), as well as FLT3 [82]. The IL-3 activates the PI3k-AKT pathway by phosphorylating BAD (bcl-2-antagonist of cell death), deactivating this pro-apoptotic protein [83]. In concert, the MAPK pathway in HCL cells is also upregulated. Protein kinase C (PKC) is often highly expressed, resulting in the inactivation of the p38-MAPK-JNK pathway. There is also SRC-dependent activation of the extracellular signal-regulated kinase (MEK-ERK) pathway [84]. The effects of both pathways, not only protects the HCL cells from apoptosis but also protects the cells and allow for constitutive proliferation [84].

Ap1/JUND, a transcription factor complex found downstream in the MEK-ERK cascade, is important for the expression of CD11c [85]. Therefore, high expression of CD11c suggests constitutive activation of the MEK-ERK pathway which results in improved cell survival, proliferation, and cyto-protection. Additionally, ERK activation results in upregulation of transcription of cyclin D1 [81].

Fibroblast growth factor 2 (FGF2) also appears to play an essential role in HCL cell growth [86]. FGF2 has both cyto-proliferative and cyto-protective properties, and is produced by HCL cells. Additively, HCL cells overexpress the FGF2 receptor (FGFR1) [79]. Activation of FGFR1 in mouse models results in ERK2 activation, which in turn causes increased mitosis. The PI3k-AKT pathway has also been shown to be activated by FGF2 [87]. Other cell surface receptors such as CD44v3 and syndecan 3 aberrantly expressed by HCL cells have been shown to facilitate the binding of FGF2 with FGFR1 [88]. Furthermore, HCL cells overexpress both cytoplasmic and nuclear FGF2, utilizing both its intracellular/gene regulatory and extracellular signaling effects to improve cell proliferation and survival [79].

HCL cells thrive in the bone marrow, suggesting the microenvironment is contributing to cell survival. The HCL cells express integrin receptors by which they adhere to the bone marrow stroma via vibronectin or fibronectin. This interaction has been shown to confer resistance of HCL cells to interferon α-induced apoptosis [68]. HCL cells also bind via α4β1/VCAM-1 interaction to endothelial cells, which are found abundantly expressed in areas such as the spleen, liver, and bone marrow stroma [76].

Familial variant

Currently, there is no literary evidence identifying a familial form of HCL.

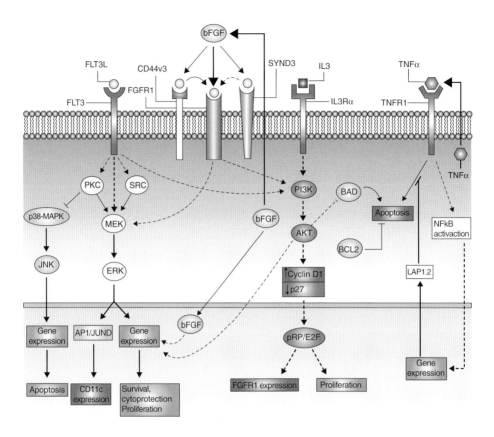

Figure 12.2 Hairy cell leukemia signaling pathways. Apoptosis is inhibited via BCL2, which is activated using mitogen-activated protein kinase (MAPK) pathways. Nuclear factor (NF)-κB is also activated by TNF (tumor necrosis factor)-α, contributing to escape from apoptosis and HCL proliferation. (Reproduced from Tiacci E et al. [67], with permission from Nature Publishing Group.)

Therapeutic targets

Purine analogs (such as pentostatin and cladribine) and interferon-α (INF-α) are known therapeutic agents to which HCL responds favorably [67]. The purine analogs are the first line of therapy because INF-α treatment is less effective, with an inferior ORR of 64% and rare CR rates of 10% [72]. Of note, switching therapy from cladribine to pentostatin and vice versa is reasonable as patients refractory to one drug often respond to the other [76, 89, 90].

Novel targeted therapies include the use of rituximab, a monoclonal anti-cd20 antibody. As monotherapy, rituximab use in HCL results in variable CR

of 13–55%, and ORR from 26–75% [91, 92]. The proposed mechanism of action of rituximab is through neutralization or polymorphism of the IgG FCγ receptor [93].

Epratuzemab, a complementarity-determining region-grafted humanized IgG-1k version of the murine monoclonal antibody is currently being evaluated in phase I/II trials for other indolent NHLs, and HCL is a promising target [93, 94]. Other novel therapeutics includes BL22 and HA22; both are monoclonal anti-CD22 antibodies linked to pseudomonas exotoxin A. HA22 has more affinity for CD22 [95]. Use of BL22 in a study by Kreitman and colleagues achieved CR in 11/16 patients and PR in 2/16 patients, with the major adverse effect being reversible HUS syndrome in two patients [96].

Lmb-2 is an immunotoxin that targets CD25, currently being evaluated for use in refractory patients in early phase clinical trials [97, 98]. Alemtuzumab, an anti-CD52 antibody, has been tried anecdotally showing favorable response in patients with CD52 positive HCL [76, 95].

The lack of prognostically significant and HCL-specific clonal cytogenetic abnormalities has led to some difficulty in finding effective therapeutic targets in this disease [1]. Additionally, to date, microarray analysis has yet to be helpful in identifying any gene signatures specific to HCL that may be of therapeutic importance.

Large granular lymphocytic leukemia

Definition

Large granular lymphocytic leukemia (LGLL) is a malignancy of clonal large granular lymphocytes. It is a rare disease, representing only 2–3% of mature lymphocytic leukemias [1]. Median age of patients manifesting this disease is approximately 60 years [79]. The disease has indolent clinical course in a majority of patients [99–103]. LGLL is often associated with autoimmune diseases such as rheumatoid arthritis, Sjogren syndrome, lupus erythematodes [99]. There are two main types of LGLL, the T-cell variant (85%) and NK-cell variant (15%) [99]. Clinically, patients present with recurrent infections due to neutropenia, anemia, thrombocytopenia and/or splenomegaly [102, 104–107]. The LGLL cells are known to cause direct normal tissue destruction leading to cytopenias and autoimmune disorders [104, 106–109].

Etiology

The etiology of LGLL is not well understood. Chronic activation of T-cells with autoantigen or viral antigens has been suggested as a possible initial event. Wlodarski et al. hypothesized that clonal CTL (cyto-toxic T-lymphocytes) proliferation can occur randomly in the context of autoimmune process. They studied immunodominant clonotypes in a cohort of 56 patients with LGL leukemia and 4 subjects with unspecified neutropenia and compared sequences of their antigen-specific portion of the T-cell receptor (TCR), the variable beta-chain (VB) complementarity-determining region 3 (CDR3) against a clonotypic database containing CDR3 regions of 26 healthy controls. The results suggested a non-random clonal selection in T-LGLL. Two patients had identical immunodominant CDR3 sequence suggesting a possibility of common antigen-triggering expansion of leukemic LGLs [110].

A role of retroviruses such as HTLV-1 and 2 in pathogenesis of LGLL was also investigated. Human T-cell leukemia virus II(HTLV-II) sequences have been detected only in two patients with T-LGLL [111]. Seroindeterminate reactivity against HTLV-I envelope epitope BA21 has been described in about 50% of patients with T-LGLL. However, most patients with LGLL were not infected with prototypical members of the HTLV family [112, 113].

Immunophenotype

The malignant T-LGLL cells arises from antigen-primed cytotoxic T-cells most commonly coexpressing CD3, CD8, and CD57, and TCR-alpha/beta markers.

An antigen-primed effect results in downregulation of homing receptors such as CCR7 and CD62 ligand, with upregulation of effector proteins such as perforin, granzymes, and NKγ2D receptor [114–118]. The LGLL cells also characteristically express CD16 in as much as 80% of cases [1]. Normally, these cells would die after antigen stimulation. However, malignant LGLs are thought to lose their homeostatic drive towards apoptosis; hence, a clonal population of persistently activated T-LGLL cells evolve [119].

KIR/KIR-L

Killer-immunoglobulin-like receptors (KIRs) are heterogeneously expressed on NK cells and small subsets of memory cytotoxic T-cells. These receptors bind human-leucocyte antigen (HLA)-I in an allele-specific manner and promote self-tolerance [120]. Inhibitory KIRs suppress cytotoxicity after binding to its corresponding HLA-I ligand in contrast to stimulatory KIRs, which promote cytotoxicity.

Nowakowski et al. performed HLA-I genotyping in seven T-LGLL cases in which malignant LGLs expressed a single KIR isoform. Five cases demonstrated absence of HLA-I antigen for the expressed KIR isoform, resulting in KIR/HLA-I mismatch. Cytopenias were detected in all five patients with KIR/HLA-I mismatch, suggesting that this phenomenon might play a role in inhibition of hematopoiesis [121].

Nearman et al. reported significantly increased frequency of mismatches between KIR/KIR-L and their specific HLA ligands in T-LGLL. A mismatch between inhibitory KIR3DL2 and HLA-A3/11 was more frequent, possibly leading to self-intolerance. Interestingly, a mismatch between stimulatory KIR 2DS1 and HLA-C2 allele was decreased resulting in reduced silencing of cytotoxic activity. Both mismatches could be responsible *in vivo* for cytopenias frequently detected in some patients with T-LGLL [122].

Cytogenetics/FISH

The vast majority of patients with T-LGLL have normal karyotype. Any chromosomal abnormality detected should be interpreted cautiously in the context of bone marrow morphology due to increased association of LGLL with MDS.

Microarray profiling

Shah et al. compared microarray gene expression profile of naïve normal and activated normal peripheral blood mononuclear cells (PBMNC) with LGLs from 30 patients with LGLL. A significant dysregulation of expression of apoptotic genes was found, suggesting a possible role in failure of activation-induced cell death in leukemic LGLs. Microarray pathway-based analysis revealed a dysregulation of proapoptotic and antiapoptotic sphingolipid-mediated signaling in LGLs. Sphingosine 1-phosphate (S1P) receptor-5 was the predominant S1P receptor detected on LGLs. Functional antagonist (FTY720) of S1P signaling pathway induced apoptosis in leukemic LGLs suggesting a role of sphingolipid-mediated signaling in survival of LGLs [123].

Yu et al. recently reported that a promoter of putative tumor suppressor gene TSC-22 was hypermethylated in primary murine T- and NK cell LGLL. This epigenetic silencing led to downregulation of TSC-22 expression. Treatment of mice bearing T- or NK cell LGL with 5-aza-2′deoxycytidine resulted in increased mice survival [124]. This report suggested that epigenetic silencing could play a role in the pathogenesis of human LGLL and that administration of hypomethylating agents could be used therapeutically in patients with this disease.

Wlodarski and colleagues have shown increased expression of CD31/PECAM-1, MCL-1, CD137/TNFRS9, and CXL-2 in the majority of T-LGLL. In addition, there was overexpression of CCR-2, CD40, CD86, CD302, and HAVCR-2 in many LGLL patients [125]. These genes are a potential signature for LGLL, which may lead to identifying a biomechanism of pathogenesis that could be therapeutically advantageous. Of importance, was the discovery that upregulation of genes encoding cytokines, like IFN-γ, and chemokines, namely CXCL-10 and CXCL-8, via the PI3K/AKT anti-apoptotic pathway, was a part of this miRNA gene signature [125]. Incidentally, viral transformations can result in the same outcome wherein there is upregulation of the PI3K/AKT pathway, inhibiting apoptosis [126].

Additionally, Rodriguez-Caballero and colleagues have shown, through microarray analysis, chronic antigenic stimulation of T-cells by CMV can result in monoclonal expansion *in vitro*. This was specifically shown in patients with a known HLA-DR B10701 genotype. This data strongly suggests an association between the development of T-LGLL and environmental antigens [127].

Biomolecular markers/intracellular pathways

In vitro studies have illustrated the bone marrow cytotoxicity in LGLL is mainly mediated in two ways:

namely, direct inhibition of hematopoiesis via recognition of hematopoietic progenitors or cytokine/chemokine secretion resulting in suppression of hematopoiesis [128]. Of note, the LGLL cells have been shown to exhibit similar intracellular signal pathway dysregulation as cells affected by viruses [129]. One such virus that is closely being evaluated in relation to the evolution of LGLL is the HTLV-1 virus, a related lymphotrophic retrovirus [129]. LGLL cells exhibit high levels of Fas, but the cells are resistant to apoptosis via the Fas ligand pathway. This resistance can be overcome *in vitro* by HTLV-1 activation of the Fas pathway, suggesting a putative role for HTLV-1 in the pathogenesis of LGLL via the Fas ligand pathway [109]. CD137 was identified via isolation from an HTLV-1-activated lymphocyte population, and is known to be associated with clonal expansion and development of LGLL after antigenic stimulation [130]. CD137 also plays a significant role in autoimmune diseases [131].

The HHV-8, herpes viruses have similarly been implicated in the evolution of LGLL [132]. HHV-8 is known to upregulate the CXCL-8 chemokine, which is seen overexpressed in LGLL. In addition, in one study, CD38 expression in T-cell LGLL was 7.06-fold higher compared with normal T-cells [133]. Persistent Parvovirus infection is associated with overexpression of CD38, perforin, and CD57 [134], which is analogous to T-LGLL phenotype. Another surface protein, CD32a, was found overexpressed in LGLL and its ligation results in T-cell stimulation and cytokine secretion [135].

PECAM, also known as CD31, is the CD38 ligand and it stimulates integrin-dependent adhesion and transmigration of leukocytes through vascular cells. It tends to also be overexpressed in TCR-stimulated T-cells [136–138]. Both elevated CD137 and CD31 overexpression are found in LGLL, suggesting the malignant clones are derivatives of autoantigen-primed lymphocytes [121].

Most recently, two proteins, DAP10 and DAP12, have been identified as directly linked to the process of tissue destruction often seen in T-LGLL. NKγ2D receptor ligand-binding directly activates DAP10 and DAP12, which then activate downstream cytoplasmic signals in the SYK, ERK/MAPK, and PI3K-AKT pathways, causing cytokine production, granule mobilization, and cell lysis [107, 139]. This was shown independently of TCR involvement or antigen presentation [128].

Familial LGL leukemia

T-LGLL appears to be an acquired disease in the vast majority of reported patients. Only rare familial cases have been described. Loughran et al. reported LGLL in a mother and her son. Viral studies suggested that, in this family, LGL leukemia was not associated with prototypical HTLV-I or HTLV-II infection [140].

Dysregulation of apoptosis in T-cell LGLs

Under physiological conditions, FasL/Fas receptor-mediated apoptosis limits survival of antigen-stimulated T-lymphocytes and maintains T-cell homeostasis. A constitutive expression of FasL by leukemic LGLs was reported in contrast to normal healthy controls [141]. Lamy et al. demonstrated that LGL leukemic cells are resistant to Fas-mediated apoptosis despite expression of Fas (CD95). Causative mutations were not detected either in Fas or FasL in LGLL patients [142].

FasL/Fas receptor triggers apoptosis via the induction of a death-inducing signaling complex (DISC). Fas-resistance was described in cells with overexpression of the DISC inhibitory protein c-FLIP. Recently, Yang et al. demonstrated that the LGLL patients express increased levels of c-FLIP and reduced capacity for Fas-mediated DISC formation [142, 143].

Schade et al. studied a role of proapoptotic phosphatidylinositol-3 kinase/AKT pathway in T-LGLL cells and compared it to resting CTLs from healthy donors. Patients with LGLL showed increased levels of phosphorylated AKT compare to normal CTL. Inhibition of this pathway with LY294002 (PI3K inhibitor) resulted in induction of apoptosis in T-LGLL cells, suggesting that this pathway might play a key role in a resistance to homeostatic apoptosis described in leukemic LGLs [144].

Zhang et al. constructed a T-LGLL survival signaling network by integrating the signaling path-

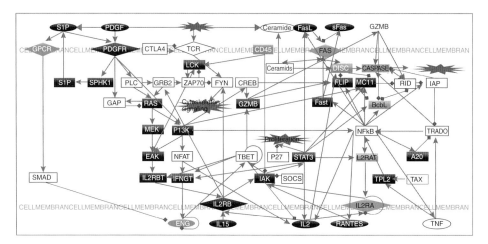

Figure 12.3 T-cell LGL signaling pathways. NODES: Black line: upregulated or constitutively active pathways; broken line: downregulated or inhibited pathways; dotted line: deregulated pathways (either positively or negatively); gray line: unknown/unchanged. LINES: Black: inhibition; dotted line: activation. SHAPE OF NODES: Rectangular: intracellular; ellipse: extracellular; diamond: receptors. (Reproduced from Zhang R et al. [145], with permission from the National Academy of Sciences.)

ways implicated in normal CTL activation and the known dysregulation of survival signaling in leukemic T-LGLs. They validated data in laboratory experiments and showed that IL-15 and PDGF were able to reproduce all of the other signaling abnormalities [145] (Figure 12.3).

New therapeutic targets

Multiple therapies are being evaluated in this disease, mostly based on affecting the immunomodulatory T-cells. Tipifarnib is one such agent. This drug inhibits farnesyl protein transferase, thus inhibiting activation of Ras, resulting in apoptosis, anti-angiogenesis, and cell growth inhibition.

Another drug of interest is a humanized monoclonal antibody to MiK-β-1, which is thought to interact via IL-2R/IL-15Rβ receptor binding. This is a therapeutic target of interest in autoimmune diseases as well as in LGLL [146].

Alemtuzumab, methotrexate, cyclosporine, and cyclophosphamide are all being used in clinical trials to determine how best to treat the cytopenias in patients with LGLL. Of these four, methotrexate has shown significant promise, with over 50% of patients treated obtaining a complete response;

however, ongoing therapy is often necessary to maintain response [147]. To date, no phase III clinical trials have been done and no standard regimen is available for treating this disease.

Conclusions

In summary, research in the molecular biology of chronic lymphoproliferative disorders such as CLL, HCL, and T-LGLL may have a significant impact on understanding of the pathobiology and identifying curative therapeutics for these disorders. High-throughput mRNA and miRNA profiling assays have become useful tools for predicting diagnosis, prognosis, and response to treatment in various hematologic malignancies including chronic lymphoproliferative disorders. The most extensive research in this group of diseases has been done in CLL. Discovery and functional characterization of several miRNAs implicated in pathobiology of CLL could be utilized in the future as therapeutic molecular targets for tailoring individual treatment in a growing era of personalized medicine.

References

1 Swerdlow SH, Campo E, Harris NL,et al. (eds.) (2008) *WHO Classification of Tumours of Haematopoietic and Lymphoid Tissues*, pp. 312-6. IARC: Lyon.

2 McConkey DJ, Chandra J, Wright S, et al. (1996) Apoptosis sensitivity in chronic lymphocytic leukemia is determined by endogenous endonuclease content and relative expression of BCL-2 and BAX. *J Immunol* **156**:2624-30.

3 Stevenson FK, Caligaris-Cappio F. (2004) Chronic lymphocytic leukemia: revelations from the B-cell receptor. *Blood* **103**:4389-95.

4 Johnson TA, Rassenti LZ, Kipps TJ. (1997) Ig VH1 genes expressed in B cell chronic lymphocytic leukemia exhibit distinctive molecular features. *J Immunol* **158**:235-46.

5 Kipps TJ, Tomhave E, Pratt LF, et al. (1989) Developmentally restricted immunoglobulin heavy chain variable region gene expressed at high frequency in chronic lymphocytic leukemia. *Proc Natl Acad Sci U S A* **86**:5913-7.

6 Damle RN, Ghiotto F, Valetto A, et al. (2002) B-cell chronic lymphocytic leukemia cells express a surface membrane phenotype of activated, antigen-experienced B lymphocytes. *Blood* **99**:4087-93.

7 Thorselius M, Krober A, Murray F, et al. (2006) Strikingly homologous immunoglobulin gene rearrangements and poor outcome in VH3-21-using chronic lymphocytic leukemia patients independent of geographic origin and mutational status. *Blood* **107**:2889-94.

8 Fais F, Ghiotto F, Hashimoto S, et al. (1998) Chronic lymphocytic leukemia B cells express restricted sets of mutated and unmutated antigen receptors. *J Clin Invest* **102**:1515-25.

9 Potter KN, Orchard J, Critchley E, et al. (2003) Features of the overexpressed V1-69 genes in the unmutated subset of chronic lymphocytic leukemia are distinct from those in the healthy elderly repertoire. *Blood* **101**:3082-4.

10 Stamatopoulos K, Belessi C, Moreno C, et al. (2007) Over 20% of patients with chronic lymphocytic leukemia carry stereotyped receptors: pathogenetic implications and clinical correlations. *Blood* **109**:259-70.

11 Matutes E, Owusu-Ankomah K, Morilla R, et al. (1994) The immunological profile of B-cell disorders and proposal of a scoring system for the diagnosis of CLL. *Leukemia* **8**:1640-5.

12 Hallek M, German CLL. (2008) Prognostic factors in chronic lymphocytic leukemia. *Ann Oncol* **19**:51-3.

13 Chena C, Arrossagaray G, Scolnik M, et al. (2003) Interphase cytogenetic analysis in Argentinean B-cell chronic lymphocytic leukemia patients: association of trisomy 12 and del(13q14). *Cancer Genet Cytogenet* **146**:154-60.

14 Sotiropoulou G, Pampalakis G, Lianidou E, et al. (2009) Emerging roles of microRNAs as molecular switches in the integrated circuit of the cancer cell. *RNA* **15**:1443-61.

15 Lee Y, Jeon K, Lee JT, et al. (2002) MicroRNA maturation: stepwise processing and subcellular localization. *EMBO J* **21**:4663-70.

16 Gregory RI, Chendrimada TP, Cooch N, et al. (2005) Human RISC couples microRNA biogenesis and post-transcriptional gene silencing. *Cell* **123**:631-40.

17 Calin GA, Croce CM. (2006) Genomics of chronic lymphocytic leukemia microRNAs as new players with clinical significance. *Semin Oncol* **33**:167-73.

18 Calin GA, Dumitru CD, Shimizu M, et al. (2002) Frequent deletions and down-regulation of micro-RNA genes miR15 and miR16 at 13q14 in chronic lymphocytic leukemia. *Proc Natl Acad Sci U S A* **99**:15524-9.

19 Calin GA, Ferracin M, Cimmino A, et al. (2005) A MicroRNA signature associated with prognosis and progression in chronic lymphocytic leukemia. *N Engl J Med* **353**:1793-801.

20 Calin GA, Cimmino A, Fabbri M, et al. (2008) MiR-15a and miR-16-1 cluster functions in human leukemia. Proc Natl Acad Sci U S A **105**:5166-71.

21 Sampath D, Calin GA, Puduvalli VK, et al. (2009) Specific activation of microRNA106b enables the p73 apoptotic response in chronic lymphocytic leukemia by targeting the ubiquitin ligase Itch for degradation. *Blood* **113**:3744-53.

22 Marton S, Garcia MR, Robello C, et al. (2007) Small RNAs analysis in CLL reveals a deregulation of miRNA expression and novel miRNA candidates of putative relevance in CLL pathogenesis. *Leukemia* **22**:330-8.

23 Fulci V, Chiaretti S, Goldoni M, et al. (2007) Quantitative technologies establish a novel microRNA profile of chronic lymphocytic leukemia. *Blood* **109**:4944-51.

24 Costinean S, Zanesi N, Pekarsky Y, et al. (2006) Pre-B cell proliferation and lymphoblastic leukemia/high-

grade lymphoma in E(mu)-miR155 transgenic mice. *Proc Natl Acad Sci U S A* **103**:7024–9.

25 Eis PS, Tam W, Sun L, et al. (2005) Accumulation of miR-155 and BIC RNA in human B cell lymphomas. *Proc Natl Acad Sci U S A* **102**:3627–32.

26 Zenz T, Mohr J, Eldering E, et al. (2009) miR-34a as part of the resistance network in chronic lymphocytic leukemia. *Blood* **113**:3801–8.

27 Stamatopoulos B, Meuleman N, Haibe-Kains B, et al. (2009) microRNA-29c and microRNA-223 down-regulation has in vivo significance in chronic lymphocytic leukemia and improves disease risk stratification. *Blood* **113**:5237–45.

28 Ghosh AK, Shanafelt TD, Cimmino A, et al. (2009) Aberrant regulation of pVHL levels by microRNA promotes the HIF/VEGF axis in CLL B cells. *Blood* **113**:5568–74.

29 Mraz M, Malinova K, Kotaskova J, et al. (2009) miR-34a, miR-29c and miR-17-5p are downregulated in CLL patients with TP53 abnormalities. *Leukemia* **23**:1159–63.

30 Orchard JA, Ibbotson RE, Davis Z, et al. (2004) ZAP-70 expression and prognosis in chronic lymphocytic leukaemia. *Lancet* **363**:105–11.

31 Nemazee D. (2006) Receptor editing in lymphocyte development and central tolerance. *Nat Rev Immunol* **6**:728–40.

32 Market E, Papavasiliou FN. (2003) V(D)J recombination and the evolution of the adaptive immune system. *PLoS Biol* **1**:E16.

33 Volkheimer AD, Weinberg JB, Beasley BE, et al. (2007) Progressive immunoglobulin gene mutations in chronic lymphocytic leukemia: evidence for antigen-driven intraclonal diversification. *Blood* **109**:1559–67.

34 Hamblin TJ, Davis Z, Gardiner A, et al. (1999) Unmutated Ig V(H) genes are associated with a more aggressive form of chronic lymphocytic leukemia. *Blood* **94**:1848–54.

35 Damle RN, Wasil T, Fais F, et al. (1999) Ig V gene mutation status and CD38 expression as novel prognostic indicators in chronic lymphocytic leukemia. *Blood* **94**:1840–7.

36 Schroeder H.W. Jr. Dighiero G. (1994) The pathogenesis of chronic lymphocytic leukemia: analysis of the antibody repertoire. *Immunol Today* **15**:288–94.

37 Qian D, Weiss A. (1997) T cell antigen receptor signal transduction. *Curr Opin Cell Biol* **9**:205–12.

38 Kane LP, Lin J, Weiss A. (2000) Signal transduction by the TCR for antigen. *Curr Opin Immunol* **12**:242–9.

39 Law CL, Sidorenko SP, Chandran KA, et al. (1994) Molecular cloning of human Syk. A B-cell protein-tyrosine kinase associated with the surface immunoglobulin M-B cell receptor complex. *J Biol Chem* **269**:12310–19.

40 Chan AC, Van Oers NS, Tran A, et al. (1994) Differential expression of ZAP-70 and Syk protein tyrosine kinases, and the role of this family of protein tyrosine kinases in TCR signaling. *J Immunol* **152**:4758–66.

41 Chen L, Widhopf G, Huynh L, et al. (2002) Expression of ZAP-70 is associated with increased B-cell receptor signaling in chronic lymphocytic leukemia. *Blood* **100**:4609.

42 Wiestner A, Rosenwald A, Barry TS, et al. (2003) ZAP-70 expression identifies a chronic lymphocytic leukemia subtype with unmutated immunoglobulin genes, inferior clinical outcome, and distinct gene expression profile. *Blood* **101**:4944–51.

43 Crespo M, Bosch F, Villamor N, et al. (2003) ZAP-70 expression as a surrogate for immunoglobulin-variable-region mutations in chronic lymphocytic leukemia. *N Engl J Med* **348**:1764–75.

44 Lin K, Sherrington PD, Dennis M, et al. (2002) Relationship between p53 dysfunction, CD38 expression, and IgV(H) mutation in chronic lymphocytic leukemia. *Blood* **100**:1404–9.

45 Deaglio S, Mallone R, Baj G, et al. (2001) Human CD38 and its ligand CD31 define a unique lamina propria T lymphocyte signaling pathway. *FASEB J* **15**:580–2.

46 Morabito F, Damle RN, Deaglio S, et al. (2006) The CD38 ectoenzyme family: advances in basic science and clinical practice. *Mol Med* **12**:342–4.

47 Deaglio S, Capobianco A, Bergui L, et al. (2003) CD38 is a signaling molecule in B-cell chronic lymphocytic leukemia cells. *Blood* **102**:2146–55.

48 Deaglio S, Vaisitti T, Aydin S, et al. (2006) In-tandem insight from basic science combined with clinical research: CD38 as both marker and key component of the pathogenetic network underlying chronic lymphocytic leukemia. *Blood* **108**:1135–44.

49 Deaglio S, Vaisitti T, Bergui L, et al. (2005) CD38 and CD100 lead a network of surface receptors relaying positive signals for B-CLL growth and survival. *Blood* **105**:3042–50.

50 Dighiero G. (2005) CLL biology and prognosis. *Hematology (Am Soc Hematol Educ Program)* **2005**:278–84.

51 Crowther-Swanepoel D, Wild R, Sellick G, et al. (2008) Insight into the pathogenesis of chronic lymphocytic leukemia (CLL) through analysis of IgVH gene usage and mutation status in familial CLL. *Blood* **111**:5691–3.

52 Landgren O, Kristinsson SY, Goldin LR, et al. (2009) Risk of plasma-cell and lymphoproliferative disorders among 14,621 first-degree relatives of 4,458 patients with monoclonal gammopathy of undetermined significance (MGUS) in Sweden. *Blood* **114**:791–5.

53 Sellick GS, Goldin LR, Wild RW, et al. (2007) A high-density SNP genome-wide linkage search of 206 families identifies susceptibility loci for chronic lymphocytic leukemia. *Blood* **110**:3326–33.

54 Virgilio L, Narducci MG, Isobe M, et al. (1994) Identification of the TCL1 gene involved in T-cell malignancies. *Proc Natl Acad Sci U S A* **91**:12530–4.

55 Bichi R, Shinton SA, Martin ES, et al. (2002) Human chronic lymphocytic leukemia modeled in mouse by targeted TCL1 expression. *Proc Natl Acad Sci U S A* **99**:6955–60.

56 Pekarsky Y, Koval A, Hallas C, et al. (2000) TCL1 enhances Akt kinase activity and mediates its nuclear translocation. *Proc Natl Acad Sci U S A* **97**:3028–33.

57 Laine J, Kunstle G, Obata T, et al. (2000) The proto-oncogene TCL1 is an Akt kinase coactivator. *Mol Cell* **6**:395–407.

58 Herling M, Patel KA, Khalili J, et al. (2006) TCL1 shows a regulated expression pattern in chronic lymphocytic leukemia that correlates with molecular subtypes and proliferative state. *Leukemia* **20**:280–5.

59 Dohner H, Stilgenbauer S, Benner A, et al. (2000) Genomic aberrations and survival in chronic lymphocytic leukemia. *N Engl J Med* **343**:1910–6.

60 Yan XJ, Albesiano E, Zanesi N, et al. (2006) B cell receptors in TCL1 transgenic mice resemble those of aggressive, treatment-resistant human chronic lymphocytic leukemia. *Proc Natl Acad Sci U S A* **103**:11713–8.

61 Schlette E, Tam C, Herling M, et al. (2008) High T-Cell lymphoma breakpoint 1 (TCL1) levels are associated with lack of response and inferior outcome following Fludarabine, Cyclophosphamide, Rituximab (FCR) frontline therapy in patients with chronic lymphocytic leukemia (CLL). *Blood* (Amer J Hematol Annual Meeting) **112**:2086.

62 Lozanski G, Heerema NA, Flinn IW, et al. (2004) Alemtuzumab is an effective therapy for chronic lymphocytic leukemia with p53 mutations and deletions. *Blood* **103**:3278–81.

63 Flinn IW, Neuberg DS, Grever MR, et al. (2007) Phase III trial of fludarabine plus cyclophosphamide compared with fludarabine for patients with previously untreated chronic lymphocytic leukemia: US Intergroup Trial E2997. *J Clin Oncol* **25**:793–8.

64 Frankel AE, Surendranathan A, Black JH, et al. (2006) Phase II clinical studies of denileukin diftitox diphtheria toxin fusion protein in patients with previously treated chronic lymphocytic leukemia. *Cancer* **106**:2158–64.

65 Spaner DE, Masellis A. (2006) Toll-like receptor agonists in the treatment of chronic lymphocytic leukemia. *Leukemia* **21**:53–60.

66 Morton LM, Wang SS, Devesa SS, et al. (2006) Lymphoma incidence patterns by WHO subtype in the United States, 1992–2001. *Blood* **107**:265–76.

67 Tiacci E, Liso A, Piris M, et al. (2006) Evolving concepts in the pathogenesis of hairy-cell leukaemia. *Nat Rev Cancer* **6**:437–48.

68 Baker PK, Pettitt AR, Slupsky JR, et al. (2002) Response of hairy cells to IFN-alpha involves induction of apoptosis through autocrine TNF-alpha and protection by adhesion. *Blood* **100**:647–53.

69 Forconi F, Sahota SS, Raspadori D, et al. (2004) Hairy cell leukemia: at the crossroad of somatic mutation and isotype switch. *Blood* **104**:3312–17.

70 Chang KL, Chen YY, Weiss LM. (1993) Lack of evidence of Epstein-Barr virus in hairy cell leukemia and mono-cytoid B-cell lymphoma. *Hum Pathol* **24**:58–61.

71 Nordstrom M, Hardell L, Linde A, et al. (1999) Elevated antibody levels to Epstein-Barr virus antigens in patients with hairy cell leukemia compared to controls in relation to exposure to pesticides, organic solvents, animals, and exhausts. *Oncol Res* **11**:539–44.

72 Lichtman M, Beutler E, Kipps T, et al. (eds.) (2006) Hairy cell leukemia. In *Williams Hematology* (7th ed.), pp. 1385–93. New York: McGraw-Hill.

73 Anderson KC, Boyd AW, Fisher DC, et al. (1985) Hairy cell leukemia: a tumor of pre-plasma cells. *Blood* **65**:620–9.

74 Yamaguchi M, Machii T, Shibayama H, et al. (1996) Immunophenotypic features and configuration of immunoglobulin genes in hairy cell leukemia-Japanese variant. *Leukemia* **10**:1390–4.

75 Machii T, Yamaguchi M, Inoue R, et al. (1997) Polyclonal B-cell lymphocytosis with features resembling hairy cell leukemia-Japanese variant. *Blood* **89**:2008–14.

76 Cannon T, Mobarek D, Wegge J, et al. (2008) Hairy cell leukemia: current concepts. *Cancer Invest* **26**:860–5.

77 Janckila AJ, Cardwell EM, Yam LT, et al. (1995) Hairy cell identification by immunohistochemistry of tartrate-resistant acid phosphatase. *Blood* **85**:2839–44.

78 Belov L, de la Vega O, dos Remedios CG, et al. (2001) Immunophenotyping of leukemias using a cluster of differentiation antibody microarray. *Cancer Res* **61**:4483–9.

79 Basso K, Liso A, Tiacci E, et al. (2004) Gene expression profiling of hairy cell leukemia reveals a phenotype related to memory B cells with altered expression of chemokine and adhesion receptors. *J Exp Med* **199**:59–68.

80 Bosch F, Campo E, Jares P, et al. (1995) Increased expression of the PRAD-1/CCND1 gene in hairy cell leukaemia. *Br J Haematol* **91**:102530.

81 Liang J, Slingerland JM. (2003) Multiple roles of the PI3K/PKB (Akt) pathway in cell cycle progression. *Cell Cycle* **2**:339–45.

82 Jonsson M, Engstrom M, Jonsson JI. (2004) FLT3 ligand regulates apoptosis through AKT-dependent inactivation of transcription factor FoxO3. *Biochem Biophys Res Commun* **318**:899–903.

83 del Peso L, Gonzalez-Garcia M, Page C, et al. (1997) Interleukin-3-induced phosphorylation of BAD through the protein kinase Akt. *Science* **278**:687–9.

84 Kamiguti AS, Harris RJ, Slupsky JR, et al. (2003) Regulation of hairy-cell survival through constitutive activation of mitogen-activated protein kinase pathways. *Oncogene* **22**:2272–84.

85 Nicolaou F, Teodoridis JM, Park H, et al. (2003) CD11c gene expression in hairy cell leukemia is dependent upon activation of the proto-oncogenes ras and junD. *Blood* **101**:4033–41.

86 Gruber G, Schwarzmeier JD, Shehata M, et al. (1999) Basic fibroblast growth factor is expressed by CD19/CD11c-positive cells in hairy cell leukemia. *Blood* **94**:1077–85.

87 Lentzsch S, Chatterjee M, Gries M, et al. (2004) PI3-K/AKT/FKHR and MAPK signaling cascades are redundantly stimulated by a variety of cytokines and contribute independently to proliferation and survival of multiple myeloma cells. *Leukemia* **18**:1883–90.

88 Kirsch T, Koyama E, Liu M, et al. (2002) Syndecan-3 is a selective regulator of chondrocyte proliferation. *J Biol Chem* **277**:42171–7.

89 Liliemark J. (1997) The clinical pharmacokinetics of cladribine. *Clin Pharmacokinet* **32**:120–31.

90 Piro LD, Ellison DJ, Saven A. (1994) The Scripps Clinic experience with 2-chlorodeoxyadenosine in the treatment of hairy cell leukemia. *Leuk Lymphoma* **14**:121–5.

91 Hagberg H, Lundholm L. (2001) Rituximab, a chimaeric anti-CD20 monoclonal antibody, in the treatment of hairy cell leukaemia. *Br J Haematol* **115**:609–11.

92 Lauria F, Lenoci M, Annino L, et al. (2001) Efficacy of anti-CD20 monoclonal antibodies (Mabthera) in patients with progressed hairy cell leukemia. *Haematologica* **86**:1046–50.

93 Leonard JP, Coleman M, Ketas JC, et al. (2003) Phase I/II trial of epratuzumab (humanized anti-CD22 antibody) in indolent non-Hodgkin's lymphoma. *J Clin Oncol* **21**:3051–9.

94 Leonard JP, Coleman M, Ketas JC, et al. (2004) Epratuzumab,;1; a humanized anti-CD22 antibody, in aggressive non-Hodgkin's lymphoma: phase I/II clinical trial results. *Clin Cancer Res* **10**:5327–34.

95 Riccioni R, Galimberti S, Petrini M. (2007) Hairy cell leukemia. *Curr Treat Options Oncol* **8**:129–134.

96 Kreitman RJ, Wilson WH, Bergeron K, et al. (2001) Efficacy of the anti-CD22 recombinant immunotoxin BL22 in chemotherapy-resistant hairy-cell leukemia. *N Engl J Med* **345**:241–7.

97 Pastan I, Hassan R, FitzGerald DJ, et al. (2006) Immunotoxin therapy of cancer. *Nat Rev Cancer* **6**:559–65.

98 Pastan I, Hassan R, FitzGerald DJ, et al. (2007) Immunotoxin treatment of cancer. *Annu Rev Med* **58**:221–237.

99 Sokol L, Loughran TP, Jr. (2006) Large granular lymphocyte leukemia. *Oncologist* **11**:263–73.

100 Loughran TP, Jr. Starkebaum G. (1987) Large granular lymphocyte leukemia. Report of 38 cases and review of the literature. *Medicine* **66**:397–405.

101 Loughran TP, Jr. (1993) Clonal diseases of large granular lymphocytes. *Blood* **82**:1–14.

102 Lamy T, Loughran TP, Jr. (1999) Current concepts: large granular lymphocyte leukemia. *Blood Rev* **13**:230–40.

103 Lamy T, Loughran TP, Jr. (2003) Clinical features of large granular lymphocyte leukemia. *Semin Hematol* **40**:185–95.

104 Lamy T, Bauer FA, Liu JH, et al. (2000) Clinicopathological features of aggressive large granular lymphocyte leukaemia resemble Fas ligand transgenic mice. *Br J Haematol* **108**:717–23.

105 Nakajima T, Schulte S, Warrington KJ, et al. (2002) T-cell-mediated lysis of endothelial cells in acute coronary syndromes. *Circulation* **105**:570–5.

106 Rossoff LJ, Genovese J, Coleman M, et al. (1997) Primary pulmonary hypertension in a patient with CD8/T-cell large granulocyte leukemia: amelioration by cladribine therapy. *Chest* **112**:551–3.

107 Chen X, Bai F, Sokol L, et al. (2009) A critical role for DAP10 and DAP12 in CD8+ T cell-mediated tissue damage in large granular lymphocyte leukemia. *Blood* **113**:3226–34.

108 Liu JH, Wei S, Lamy T, et al. (2000) Chronic neutropenia mediated by Fas ligand. *Blood* **95**:3219–22.

109 Liu JH, Wei S, Lamy T, et al. (2002) Blockade of Fas-dependent apoptosis by soluble Fas in LGL leukemia. *Blood* **100**:1449–53.

110 Wlodarski MW, O'Keefe C, Howe EC, et al. (2005) Pathologic clonal cytotoxic T-cell responses: nonrandom nature of the T-cell-receptor restriction in large granular lymphocyte leukemia. *Blood* **106**:2769–80.

111 Loughran TP, Jr. Coyle T, Sherman MP, et al. (1992) Detection of human T-cell leukemia/lymphoma virus, type II, in a patient with large granular lymphocyte leukemia. *Blood* **80**:1116–19.

112 Pawson R, Schulz TF, Matutes E, et al. (1997) The human T-cell lymphotropic viruses types I/II are not involved in T prolymphocytic leukemia and large granular lymphocytic leukemia. *Leukemia* **11**:1305–11.

113 Duong YT, Jia H, Lust JA, et al. (2008) Short communication: Absence of evidence of HTLV-3 and HTLV-4 in patients with large granular lymphocyte (LGL) leukemia. *AIDS Res Hum Retroviruses* **24**:1503–5.

114 Hamann D, Baars PA, Rep MH, et al. (1997) Phenotypic and functional separation of memory and effector human CD8+ T cells. *J Exp Med* **186**:1407–18.

115 Sallusto F, Lenig D, Forster R, et al. (1999) Two subsets of memory T lymphocytes with distinct homing potentials and effector functions. *Nature* **401**:708–12.

116 Trimble LA, Kam LW, Friedman RS, et al. (2000) CD3zeta and CD28 down-modulation on CD8 T cells during viral infection. *Blood* **96**:1021–9.

117 Bigouret V, Hoffmann T, Arlettaz L, et al. (2003) Monoclonal T-cell expansions in asymptomatic individuals and in patients with large granular leukemia consist of cytotoxic effector T cells expressing the activating CD94:NKG2C/E and NKD2D killer cell receptors. *Blood* **101**:3198–204.

118 Seder RA, Ahmed R. (2003) Similarities and differences in CD4+ and CD8+ effector and memory T cell generation. *Nat Immunol* **4**:835–42.

119 Mollet L, Fautrel B, Leblond V, et al. (1999) Leukemic CD 3+ LGL share functional properties with their CD 8+ CD 57+ cell counterpart expanded after BMT. *Leukemia* **13**:230–40.

120 Farag SS, Fehniger TA, Ruggeri L, et al. (2002) Natural killer cell receptors: new biology and insights into the graft-versus-leukemia effect. *Blood* **100**:1935–47.

121 Nowakowski GS, Morice WG, Phyliky RL, et al. (2005) Human leucocyte antigen class I and killer immunoglobulin-like receptor expression patterns in T-cell large granular lymphocyte leukaemia. *Br J Haematol* **128**:490–2.

122 Nearman ZP, Wlodarski M, Jankowska AM, et al. (2007) Immunogenetic factors determining the evolution of T-cell large granular lymphocyte leukaemia and associated cytopenias. *Br J Haematol* **136**:237–48.

123 Shah MV, Zhang R, Irby R, et al. (2008) Molecular profiling of LGL leukemia reveals role of sphingolipid signaling in survival of cytotoxic lymphocytes. *Blood* **112**:770–81.

124 Yu J, Liu X, Ye H, et al. (2009) Genomic characterization of the human mitochondrial tumor suppressor gene 1 (MTUS1): 5′ cloning and preliminary analysis of the multiple gene promoters. *BMC Res Notes* **2**:109.

125 Wlodarski MW, Nearman Z, Jankowska A, et al. (2008) Phenotypic differences between healthy effector CTL and leukemic LGL cells support the notion of antigen-triggered clonal transformation in T-LGL leukemia. *J Leukoc Biol* **83**:589–601.

126 Cooray S. (2004) The pivotal role of phosphatidylinositol 3-kinase-Akt signal transduction in virus survival. *J Gen Virol* **85**:1065–76.

127 Richards SJ. (2008) A "pathogenetic" role for CMV in CD4+ LGL proliferations. *Blood* **112**:4367–8.

128 French AR, Yokoyama WM. (2004) Natural killer cells and autoimmunity. *Arthritis Res Ther* **6**:8–14.

129 Sokol L, Agrawal D, Loughran TP. (2005) Characterization of HTLV envelope seroreactivity in large granular lymphocyte leukemia. *Leuk Res* **29**:381–7.

130 Ma BY, Mikolajczak SA, Danesh A, et al. (2005) The expression and the regulatory role of OX40 and 4-1BB heterodimer in activated human T cells. *Blood* **106**:2002–10.

131 Cannons JL, Chamberlain G, Howson J, et al. (2005) Genetic and functional association of the immune signaling molecule 4-1BB (CD137/TNFRSF9) with type 1 diabetes. *J Autoimmun* **25**:13–20.

132 Swa S, Wright H, Thomson J, et al. (2001) Constitutive activation of Lck and Fyn tyrosine kinases in large granular lymphocytes infected with the gamma-herpesvirus agents of malignant catarrhal fever. *Immunology* **102**:44–52.

133 Stevenson GT. (2006) CD38 as a therapeutic target. *Mol Med* **12**:345–6.

134 Isa A, Kasprowicz V, Norbeck O, et al. (2005) Prolonged activation of virus-specific CD8 T cells after acute B19 infection. *PLoS Med* **2**:e343.

135 Sandilands GP, MacPherson SA, Burnett ER, et al. (1997) Differential expression of CD32 isoforms following alloactivation of human T cells. *Immunology* **91**:204–11.

136 Prager E, Staffler G, Majdic O, et al. (2001) Induction of hyporesponsiveness and impaired T lymphocyte activation by the CD31 receptor: ligand pathway in T cells. *J Immunol* **166**:2364–71.

137 Reedquist KA, Ross E, Koop EA, et al. (2000) The small GTPase, Rap1, mediates CD31-induced integrin adhesion. *J Cell Biol* **148**:1151–8.

138 Zehnder JL, Shatsky M, Leung LL, et al. (1995) Involvement of CD31 in lymphocyte-mediated immune responses: importance of the membrane-proximal immunoglobulin domain and identification of an inhibiting CD31 peptide. *Blood* **85**:1282–8.

139 Vivier E, Colonna M. (2005) *Strategies of Natural Killer T cell Recognition and Signaling. Immunobiology of Natural Killer Cell Receptors* (1st ed.), pp. 2–9. Springer-Verlag: Berlin Heidelberg.

140 Loughran TP, Jr. Kidd P, Poiesz BJ. (1994) Familial occurrence of LGL leukaemia. *Br J Haematol* **87**:199–201.

141 Tanaka M, Suda T, Haze K, et al. (1996) Fas ligand in human serum. *Nat Med* **2**:317–22.

142 Lamy T, Liu JH, Landowski TH, et al. (1998) Dysregulation of CD95/CD95 ligand-apoptotic pathway in CD3(+) large granular lymphocyte leukemia. *Blood* **92**:4771–7.

143 Yang J, Epling-Burnette PK, Painter JS, et al. (2008) Antigen activation and impaired Fas-induced death-inducing signaling complex formation in T-large-granular lymphocyte leukemia. *Blood* **111**:1610–6.

144 Schade AE, Powers JJ, Wlodarski MW, et al. (2006) Phosphatidylinositol-3-phosphate kinase pathway activation protects leukemic large granular lymphocytes from undergoing homeostatic apoptosis. *Blood* **107**:4834–40.

145 Zhang R, Shah MV, Yang J, et al. (2008) Network model of survival signaling in large granular lymphocyte leukemia. *Proc Natl Acad Sci U S A* **105**:16308–13.

146 Waldmann TA. (2004) Targeting the interleukin-15/interleukin-15 receptor system in inflammatory autoimmune diseases. *Arthritis Res Ther* **6**:17477.

147 Alekshun TJ, Sokol L. (2007) Diseases of large granular lymphocytes. *Cancer Control* **14**:141–50.

CHAPTER 13
Chronic Lymphocytic Leukemia

Terry Hamblin and Angela Hamblin
Department of Immunohaematology, Cancer Sciences Division, University of Southampton, Southampton, UK

Introduction

Most people begin their article on chronic lympho-cytic leukemia (CLL) with the words "CLL is the commonest leukemia in the Western world". It may be true, but with recent changes in the definition of the disease we cannot be sure. The impression that CLL is getting more common and more benign may be an accident of disease discovery, with more alert physicians recognizing a disease that may or may not be there.

A new heterogeneity in CLL was discovered a decade ago and this has provided a key to the complex pathophysiology and, coincidentally, has important prognostic value. In addition, new treat-ments have become available as well as the means of detecting minimal residual disease. Consequently, we now look at CLL differently. For some patients this will mean never treating their leukemia, but possibly managing late complications; for others, the prospect of a cure, though not without hazard; for yet others, a sequence of treatments and remissions aiming for a balance between benefit and harm, producing the longest possible, good quality life.

Diagnosis

The diagnosis of CLL is superficially easy. For most the only abnormality is the blood count, which shows a lymphocytosis consisting of small round cells consisting of mainly nucleus with little cyto-plasm. The nuclear chromatin is coarsely condensed and nucleoli are not usually visible. Cytoplasm appears as a pale blue rim in Romanowsky stained films. Characteristically there are cells present on the blood film that appear to have burst; these are known as "smudge", "smear", or "basket" cells. An admixture of larger cells is usually seen. Typically, prolymphocytes are present with larger nuclei with less condensed chromatin and a single prominent nucleolus (Plate 13.1).

Very rarely cells with a nuclear cleft are seen, leading to confusion with follicular lymphoma. The term "atypical CLL" has been applied to cases of CLL where the number of prolymphocytes exceeds 10% or where the total of atypical cells including pro-lymphocytes, clefted cells, and plasmacytoid cells exceeds 15% [1]. Although it is a commonly used term, it is not a different disease entity and the term is often used to describe cases of CLL with atypical cell markers. Atypical morphology is often associ-ated with the presence of certain chromosomal abnormalities, particularly trisomy 12 [2].

The definitive diagnosis of CLL relies on the immunophenotype. The cells are monoclonal, assumed by the finding of a single Ig light chain type (either κ or λ) on the surface of the cells, but the quantity of surface Ig is only about 10% of that on normal B-cells. The cells are typically positive for CD5, CD19, and CD23, and negative for FMC7 and surface CD22. The Ig associated molecule CD79b is only weakly positive. The Matutes score [3] utilizes these markers to differentiate CLL from other lym-phoid tumors. In its latest guise, it allocates one point each for positive staining for CD5 and CD23, one

Advances in Malignant Hematology, First Edition. Edited by Hussain I. Saba and Ghulam J. Mufti. © 2011 Blackwell Publishing Ltd.
Published 2011 by Blackwell Publishing Ltd.

point for negative staining with FMC7, and one point each for weak or negative staining for surface Ig and either CD79b or CD22. Most cases of CLL have scores of 4 or 5; those scoring 3 often have "atypical" CLL and those scoring 0–2 have other lymphoid tumors.

The monoclonal antibody FMC7 detects an epitope of CD20 that is obscured by changes in membrane cholesterol metabolism [4]. CD20 is also only relatively weakly expressed on CLL cells compared to other B-cells. There are other antigens that are differentially expressed on CLL cells, including CD43, CD11c, CD25, and very low levels of CD45, but these markers are of less value in distinguishing CLL from other B-cells malignancies than those used in the Matutes score. Flow cytometric examination of CLL cells usually includes CD20 and CD52 in the examining panel since antibodies to these antigens may be used therapeutically.

Monoclonal B-cell lymphocytosis and its effect on the diagnosis of CLL

The apparent incidence of CLL has fluctuated over the years [5] but early stage disease is becoming more common. In the 1950s and 1960s several studies reported incidences in excess of 6 per 100 000, but this was before immunophenotyping when any lymphocytosis over 10×10^9/L was designated CLL. Immunophenotyping has excluded the majority of interlopers and, as a result, the perceived incidence of CLL fell between the 1970s and 1980s. Sgambati et al. [6], reporting on statistics from the National Cancer Institute's Surveillance, Epidemiology and End Results (SEER) Program, described a fall in incidence rates for CLL for white males from 4.2 per 100 000 to 3.2 per 100 000 between 1973 and 1976 while the rate for white females fell from 3.8 to 2.6 over the same period. The rates for those of African American, Hispanic, or Asian origin were much lower.

Relying on individual hematologists rather than death certificates or hospital admissions to record cases will inflate incidences, though this will depend on the enthusiasm of the doctor. Such an exercise in the UK produced an incidence of 5.54 per 100 000 [5]. Changes in guidelines for the diagnosis of CLL have also had an impact on perceived incidence. The latest agreed formulation, published by the International Workshop on CLL (IWCLL) [7], raised the threshold for diagnosis to a B-cell lymphocytosis (rather than a total lymphocytosis) of $>5 \times 10^9$/L and this will undoubtedly reduce the incidence.

In 2002, Rawstron et al. [8], using four-color flow cytometry on blood samples taken for other reasons, discovered that 3.5% of the population over the age of 40 harbors a population of cells immunophenotypically similar to those of CLL. This has been confirmed by others [5]. An International Working Group has designated this condition as monoclonal B-cell lymphocytosis (MBL) and laid down diagnostic criteria (Table 13.1).

Rawstron et al. [9] have reported on the relationship between MBL and CLL. It should be stressed that not all patients with MBL have a lymphocytosis,

Table 13.1 Diagnostic criteria for MBL

---

1 Detection of a monoclonal B-cell population in the peripheral blood with:

  i A kappa:lambda ratio of >3:1 or <0.3:1, or

  ii >25% of B-cells lacking or expressing low levels of surface immunoglobulin, or

  iii A disease-specific immunophenotype.

2 Repeat assessment should demonstrate that the monoclonal B-cell population is stable over a three-month period.

3 Exclusion criteria:

  i Lymphadenopathy or organomegaly, or

  ii Associated autoimmune/infectious disease, or

  iii B-lymphocyte count $>5 \times 10^9$/L, or

  iv Any other feature of a B-lymphoproliferative disorder. However, a paraprotein may be present or associated with MBL and should be evaluated independently.

4 Subclassification:

  i CD5$^+$23$^+$: this is the major subcategory and corresponds to a CLL immunophenotype.

  ii CD5$^+$23$^-$: correlates with moderate levels of CD20 and CD79b expression and with atypical CLL.

  iii CD5$^-$: corresponds to non-CLL lymphoproliferative disease.

---

the B-lymphocyte count could be as low as 0.015×10^9/L. Following up individuals with MBL without a lymphocytosis is unethical and their fate is largely unknown. Among those with a lymphocytosis, follow-up is possible and most are stable over a number of years. He reported that in 28% of these patients there was progressive lymphocytosis and, of these, a quarter required chemotherapy a median of four years after the initial diagnosis. The estimated rate of progression of MBL with lymphocytosis to CLL requiring treatment was 1.1% per year.

Although MBL seldom transforms to CLL, almost all cases of CLL were once MBL. From a large cohort of individuals having regular blood tests Landgren et al. [10] were able to identify 45 patients who developed CLL who had available pre-diagnostic cryopreserved whole blood. Using flow cytometry and molecular techniques they were able to identify an MBL clone in 44 of the specimens.

The new definition of CLL and its relationship to MBL will change clinical practice. Many patients previously designated Stage 0 CLL will be reclassified as MBL. In practice, there will be little point in continuing to follow and perform expensive investigations on patients with a lymphocytosis $<10 \times 10^9$/L.

Etiology, epidemiology and pathobiology

The cause of CLL is unknown. It is more common in males than females, Caucasians than other races, old people than young people, and in families where a first-degree relative already has CLL. Familial cases show the phenomenon of anticipation, where the disease occurs at an earlier age in succeeding generations, but this is probably ascertainment bias; the disease is detected earlier when it is carefully looked for.

Despite extensive searching it is not known whether there is an equivalent normal cell in which the CLL arises. The subject has been extensively discussed by Chiorazzi and Ferrarini [11] but the topic is confused, since CD5 may be both an activation and a lineage marker and, perhaps, by inappro-

priate comparisons with the mouse. It is not certain at what stage in lymphocyte maturation the CLL cell arises, since roughly equal numbers seem to come from a pre- and post-germinal center B-lymphocyte [12, 13]. Diseases originating at these two stages of maturation have vastly different prognoses. However, gene expression profiling suggests that both subtypes are similar, differing from each other by relatively few expressed genes [14]. Such studies also suggest that CLL is very different from other types of lymphoma and that all CLL cells have encountered antigen at some stage in their maturation [15], whether or not they have undergone somatic mutation.

Random use of the 51 different *IGHV* genes would dictate each being used in approximately 2% of cases of CLL, whereas in fact there is a biased usage of V1-69 in the unmutated subset and of V3-23 and V4-34 in the mutated subset. A discovery from Sweden demonstrated that patients whose CLL made use of the V3-21 gene had a poor prognosis whether or not the *IGHV* genes were mutated [16]. Furthermore, a large proportion of the patients whose CLL used V3-21 had strikingly similar sequences for their B-cell receptor (BCR) [17]. The obvious implication is that antigenic stimulation has played a part in the etiology of the leukemia. Subsequently, a new word was coined, "stereotyped," to describe the similarity between BCRs and it was further suggested that over 20% of CLLs [18] used stereotyped BCRs. Patients with low-count MBL rarely demonstrate stereotypy. In a study from Italy only 3.9% of cases expressed a stereotyped BCR [19]. This suggests an important role for antigen engagement in the transformation of MBL to CLL.

Further information on the etiology of CLL has come from attempts to establish a mouse model for the disease [20]. *TCL1* is an oncogene activated by recurrent reciprocal translocations at chromosome segment 14q32.1 in T-cell prolymphocytic leukemia (T-PLL), but TCL1 protein can also be detected at lower levels in CLL cells. A *TCL1* transgenic mouse has been produced that develops a proliferation of polyclonal CD5+ B-cells, starting in the peritoneal cavity at two months, appearing in the spleen at 3–5 months and in the bone marrow at 5–8 months. Monoclonality appears at eight months, first in peritoneal cells and later in other populations. At the age of 13–18 months the mice become visibly ill with enlarged spleens, marked lymphadenopathy and high white cell counts; the blood films show smudge cells, but the predominant cell is a large CD5 + / IgM + lymphocyte; the picture being more characteristic of prolymphocytoid transformation of CLL (CLL/PLL) than of CLL itself. The highest level of TCL1 expression in patients is found in those with unmutated *IGHV* genes, ZAP-70 positivity and the presence of deletions of the long arm of chromosome 11. The question then arises as to whether the TCL1 B-cell lymphoma of mice is not a model of human CLL as a whole, but rather of the more aggressive form with unmutated *IGHV* genes. The leukemia of TCL1 mice uses unmutated *IGHV* genes, and shows a biased use of these genes and stereotyped BCRs.

The extreme differences in geographical variation ought to give us a clue as to etiology. Prevalence rates show a 40-fold difference between white Europeans and North Americans, and Asians, but unlike with other malignancies, Asians migrating to the US retain their low incidence [21]. This suggests a genetic rather than environmental cause, but the disease is similar in Europeans and Asians [22]. The evidence for environmental factors playing a role in the etiology is weak and inconsistent [23]. There was no association with radiation fall-out from the Japanese atomic bombs, but CLL is very rare in Japan, and recently the role of radiation exposure has again surfaced [24].

Somewhere between 5 and 15% of patients have a family history of CLL. Rawstron et al. found a prevalence of unsuspected MBL in 13.5% among 59 first-degree relatives in 21 CLL kindreds [25]. Familial cases of CLL do not differ significantly from sporadic cases [23]. Linkage studies looking at the co-inheritance of genetic markers and CLL have so far been unsuccessful in identifying any genetic defects that make a family member prone to CLL [23].

Searches for single nucleotide polymorphisms (SNP) among candidate genes or molecular pathways have similarly been largely unsuccessful [23], but Raval et al. [26] identified an SNP of the Death-Associated Protein Kinase 1 (*DAPK1)* gene that segregated with the disease in a single large family with CLL and was associated with the downregulation of the enzyme's expression. *DAPK1* is normally silenced by demethylation in sporadic CLL. However, the SNP was found in the germ-line of only one among 263 cases of sporadic CLL from the US and Northern Europe but not among other familial kindreds.

It is likely that no simple genetic defect is responsible for the occurrence of CLL in families, but rather that a large number of components of molecular pathways appear in variant forms that together influence the rates of proliferation and apoptosis of B-lymphocytes.

Clinical and laboratory features

In CLL, the leukemic cells accumulate wherever they normally circulate. Peripheral lymphadenopathy in cervical, axillary, and inguinal regions forms the basis of the clinical staging systems as does enlargement of the spleen and liver. Lymphadenopathy elsewhere may be detected by imaging techniques such as abdominal ultrasound (US) and computerized tomography (CT), but this plays no part in clinical staging. CT scanning in the initial examination of most patients with CLL is unnecessary and can lead to serious mismanagement of patients [27].

Lymphocytic infiltration of the bone marrow can cause anemia and thrombocytopenia, but these may have other causes, such as autoimmunity or hypersplenism, which must be excluded. There is usually no need for bone marrow examination in the initial assessment of patients with CLL.

Two forms of clinical staging are currently used; Rai staging in America [28] and Binet staging in Europe [29]. Details of these systems are given in Table 13.2. Although they differ in detail they both in effect measure tumor mass, and neither measures the pace of disease. Both have prognostic value and both suffer from the same defects (such as using the same threshold hemoglobin value for males and females). Both have stood the test of time and both remain valuable despite the appearance of many new prognostic markers.

Table 13.2 Clinical staging systems in CLL

Rai	Characteristics
Stage 0	Lymphocytosis in blood and bone marrow only
Stage I	Lymphocytosis plus lymphadenopathy
Stage II	Lymphocytosis plus splenomegaly or hepatomegaly
Stage III	Lymphocytosis plus anemia (Hb < 110 g/L)
Stage IV	Lymphocytosis plus thrombocytopenia (platelets < 100×10^9/L)

Binet[a]	Characteristics
Stage A	<3 sites involved, Hb > 100 g/L, platelets > 100×10^9/L
Stage B	≥3 sites involved, Hb > 100 g/L, platelets > 100×10^9/L
Stage C	Hb < 100 g/L or platelets < 100×10^9/L

[a] The Binet system recognizes five sites of involvement: cervical, axillary and inguinal lymph nodes, the liver, and the spleen.

Natural history

Many cases of CLL do not become a clinical problem throughout the lifetime of the patient. The longest survival without treatment that we have found is 52 years. The proportion of patients who progress is unclear owing to many patients with stage 0 disease being reclassified as MBL, but it is still probably a minority. Progression takes the form of increasing lymphadenopathy and splenomegaly. Eventually, normal bone marrow is replaced by CLL cells and anemia, neutropenia, and thrombocytopenia ensue.

There is much confusion about aggressive transformation of CLL [30]. Transformation to acute lymphoblastic leukemia, although reported in the literature, is a myth. Richter's syndrome is now recognized as a rare but regular culmination of CLL. In the largest series of cases, the incidence was 2.8%. It has been accepted that any type of aggressive lymphoma occurring in a patient with CLL may be called Richter's syndrome. Thus, cases of diffuse large B-cell lymphoma, Hodgkin's lymphoma, and even high-grade T-cell lymphoma have received that appellation.

Richter's transformation is often characterized by sudden clinical deterioration and development of systemic symptoms of fever and weight loss. There is usually a rapid enlargement of lymph node masses, especially of retroperitoneal nodes. Hepatomegaly and splenomegaly are common and extranodal disease is often seen. Two types of transformation occur: a true transformation to a clonally related, aggressive lymphoma, and the occurrence of a new, clonally unrelated tumor, perhaps because of diminished immune surveillance. Some of these tumors may be virally induced.

Prolymphocytoid transformation of CLL is often misunderstood. CLL does not transform to PLL; the immunophenotype remains that of CLL and the prolymphocytes do not exceed 55%. Contrary to common perception, half of the cases of CLL/PLL show a stable picture without a progressive increase in prolymphocytes. The prognosis of this group is similar to that of stable CLL without prolymphocytes. In one-third of cases, the increase in prolymphocytes is unsustained, and in less than a fifth there is a definite progression toward a more malignant phase of the disease.

Prognostic indicators

Lymphocyte doubling time

Although clinical stage is a good indicator of prognosis, it really measures tumor bulk and says nothing about rate of progression. In an attempt to measure this dynamic aspect, Montserrat and colleagues analyzed the lymphocyte doubling time (LDT), defined as the time needed to double the peripheral lymphocyte count. Although there was some correlation with clinical stage and the pattern of marrow infiltration, LTD was shown to have independent prognostic significance [31]. Caution must be exercised to exclude other causes for a rise in lymphocyte count such as infection or treatment with corticosteroids.

Serum thymidine kinase

Thymidine kinase (TK) is a cellular enzyme involved in a salvage pathway for DNA synthesis. The cytosolic isoenzyme TK1 is found in the G1/S phase of dividing cells, but is absent in resting cells. Serum TK is related to the number of dividing neoplastic cells and is therefore a measure of proliferation, although a small percentage of dividing cells in a large tumor mass will produce similar levels to a large percentage of dividing cells in a small tumor mass. Serum TK levels have proved useful in assigning prognosis to patients with early-stage CLL [32] and only the fact that it is measured by a radioimmunoassay, unpopular in routine laboratories, prevents it from being widely adopted.

IGHV mutations

B-cell signaling is mediated through the BCR (B-cell antigen receptor), an Ig molecule on the cell surface associated with accessory molecules that facilitate and amplify the signal. Each normal B-cell has a different BCR, designed to engage any possible antigen. This diversity of the Ig heavy chain is programmed by the combination of one from 51 variable (V) region gene segments, one from 27 diversity (D) gene segments, and one from six joining (J) gene segments. Once the lymphocyte has met its designated antigen point mutations in the nucleotide sequence occur and alter the shape of the antibody combining site. Those B-cells with poorly fitting antibody are destined to die; those with the best-fitting antibody survive. By sequencing the Ig genes it is possible, therefore, to tell whether or not somatic mutations have been acquired and therefore whether a lymphocyte has passed through the germinal center where they occur.

Against early dogma, it became clear by the early 1990s that around half the cases of CLL showed evidence of somatic mutation in their Ig heavy chain (*IGHV*) genes. The demonstration that somatic mutations correlated with more benign disease was simultaneously published in mutually confirmatory papers in 1999 [12, 13]. The median survival of patients with unmutated *IGHV* genes was eight years, while that of those with mutated *IGHV* genes was 25 years. An exception to the rule is the tumor that uses the V3-21 gene segment [16]. Whether or not they carry somatic mutations, such cases are aggressive with short survival times.

CD38 expression

Sequencing Ig genes is beyond the capabilities of routine laboratories and surrogate measurements with the same prognostic value have been sought. Surface CD38 expression, detected by flow cytometry, was an early contender [13]. Unfortunately, it soon became clear that, while CD38 is certainly a useful prognostic indicator, individual patients frequently show discordances between CD38 expression and *IGHV* mutations [33]. Hamblin and colleagues estimated that approximately 30% of cases fell into that category, and these had a prognosis intermediate between those who had somatic mutations and were CD38-negative and those who were unmutated and CD38-positive. The same paper also demonstrated that CD38 expression could change during the course of the disease.

Expression of CD38 on the surface of CLL cells is easily measured by flow cytometry. Ideally, the original method should be used [13], but there has been some dispute as to what comprises a positive result for this assay. The original suggestion was to use a 30% threshold. Subsequently, levels of 7% or 5% have been suggested [34, 35]. Applying Youden's index to discover the greatest sensitivity and specificity according to overall survival, a level anywhere between 20 and 30% discriminates equally well [36].

ZAP-70 expression

Gene expression profiles demonstrated only small differences between cases of CLL with mutated and unmutated *IGHV* genes. One group identified 240 genes expressed differently out of 13 868 genes examined [14]. The gene that most distinctly segregated between the two subgroups was that coding for the zeta-associated protein with the molecular weight of 70 kD (ZAP-70), and this was seen as a potential surrogate for *IGHV* mutational analysis.

ZAP-70 is a molecule used to transmit a signal from the T-cell receptor to downstream pathways. Most B-cells lack ZAP-70 and use instead a related tyrosine kinase, Syk, for signal transduction [37]. In most cases of CLL with mutated *IGHV* genes, engagement of the BCR with anti-IgM fails to cause phosphorylation of Syk, while most cases with unmutated *IGHV* genes can signal [38, 39]. It is possible that ZAP-70 inhibits the decay of downstream factors, which would normally terminate the signaling response through Syk [40].

In the initial papers, ZAP-70 expression was shown correctly to predict the *IGHV* mutation status in 93% of cases of CLL. Both ZAP-70 expression and *IGHV* mutational status were equally able to predict time to requirement for treatment [41]. For routine assessment of ZAP-70, a flow cytometry assay is required. This has proved difficult, but at least three different methods have been reported [42–44].

Whereas the assays in the first two papers produced a concordance with *IGHV* gene mutations of over 90%, the concordance of the third, and easier-to-perform, assay was only 77%. This third paper also suggested that ZAP-70 expression added prognostic information that was independent of the effect of *IGHV* gene mutations. Clearly these assays are very dependent on the antibody chosen and the type of fluorochrome, and despite their promise, they have not gained widespread acceptance.

Karyotype

Conventional karyotyping of CLL cells is beyond the capability of most laboratories, but the introduction of interphase FISH has enabled this technique to become a vital part of the evaluation of patients with CLL [45]. There are five common chromosomal abnormalities seen in CLL, four of which have been arranged in a prognostic hierarchy [45, 46].

The most common abnormality, recognized more than 20 years ago and occurring in over 50% of cases, is deletion of part of the long arm of chromosome 13 (del 13q14.3) [47]. Patients with this isolated del 13q14 have a good prognosis, with survival curves that are even better than those with a normal karyotype [45, 46]. Two miRNA genes at 13q14.3, *miR15* and *miR16*, are absent or downregulated in most cases of CLL [48]. As part of normal control of gene expression, *miR-15a* and *miR-16-1* function by targeting multiple oncogenes, including *BCL2*, *MCL1*, *CCND1*, and *WNT3A*, and their absence in CLL appears to be a major factor in preventing apoptosis and progression through the cell cycle [49, 50]. The minimally deleted area on 13q14.3 does not actually include *miR15* and *miR16*, although these genes are deleted in most patients with deletions at 13q14. When the miRNA genes are not deleted the loss of the putative tumor suppressor gene *DLEU2* causes function loss of these genes [51].

Trisomy 12 is the next commonest abnormality, occurring in up to 25% of cases. It is associated with atypical morphology and unmutated *IGHV* genes, when it carries a worse-than-average prognosis [52]. However, those cases associated with mutated *IGHV* genes are often benign. In a study of gene expression profiling, four genes were significantly associated with +12: *HIP1R*, *MYF6*, *P2RY14*, and *CD200* [53]. The overexpressed genes are located on chromosome 12 (*HIP1R*, *MYF6*) but both significantly underexpressed genes (*P2RY14*, *CD200*) reside on the long arm of chromosome 3 pointing to trans-repression in this region. CD200 is generally upregulated in CLL and is thought to play a role in suppressing antitumor immunity [54].

Deletions at 11q23 occur in between 10 and 20% of cases [55] and are associated with a poor prognosis. Patients are typically male and have enlarged abdominal lymph nodes. With newer therapies remission rates are high, but early relapse is typical. Frequently the ataxia telangectasia mutated (ATM) gene is deleted. This gene is involved in the TP53 pathway [56]. Recent studies have indicated that patients can be split into two prognostic groups depending on the mutation status of the remaining ATM allele [57].

Patients with deletions of 17p13 are only part of a larger group with aberrations of the *p53* gene which are detectable in a variety of ways [58–60]. They occur in about 5% of untreated cases, and typically represent those that are unresponsive to modern therapy. Karyotypic evolution occurs [61], and previously treated patients may have up to 30% 17p13 deletions. Patients carrying *p53* aberrations have the worst prognosis of all. Survival of less than two years is commonplace. However, a subgroup of Binet Stage A patients with mutated *IGHV* genes and loss of TP53 may have relatively benign disease [62].

Diverse deletions of part of the long arm of chromosome 6 occur in 6% of cases, almost always as a secondary event. One paper suggests that it has an intermediate prognostic effect and is associated with a high incidence of atypical morphology [63].

Other prognostic factors

Although no other prognostic factor has been widely adopted, there has been no shortage of candidates. A recent review described 10 new prognostic markers derived from gene expression profiling: *TCL1* gene expression, CLLU1 expression, miRNA signature, mRNA signature, and expression of Lipoprotein lipase A, *ADAM29*, *HEM1*, *Septin 10*, *DMD*, and *PEG 10*, and nine others from other sources: VEGF, thrombopoietin, telomere length and activity, CD49d, CD69, FCRL, expression of antiapoptotic genes such as *MCL-1* and the *Bcl-2/Bax* ratio, *MDR1/MDR-3* genes, and *AID* mRNA [64].

How should prognostic factors be used?

Most of the modern prognostic factors were discovered by retrospective analysis of single-center series, but they have now been evaluated by at least four prospective studies. In the CALGB 9712 randomized phase II study of fludarabine and rituximab, given according to two different schedules, there was no difference in response rate among those with different prognostic markers, but significantly shorter median PFS and OS in those with unmutated *IGHV* genes and those with high-risk interphase cytogenetics (del 11q or del 17p) [65]. In a similar Italian study with fludarabine and rituximab, a much shorter PFS was found in patients who were ZAP-70-positive or CD38-positive [66].

In the German CLL4 phase III trial which compared fludarabine (F) with fludarabine plus cyclophosphamide (FC), non-response to FC, poor PFS and OS correlated with deletions of 17p or mutations of *TP53* [67, 68]. This was confirmed by the British CLL4 trial [69, 70], which randomized treatment between F, FC, and chlorambucil. For all treatment groups, a finding of 17p deletion by FISH was associated with non-response and poor PFS and OS. In addition, in a multivariate analysis, unmutated *IGHV* genes, but not expression of either CD38 or ZAP-70, correlated with response, PFS, and OS. There was also an association of del 11q with early relapse.

At present prognostic markers should only be used to direct therapy in the 5% of patients who have 17p deletions. This abnormality is so closely associated with failure to respond to standard therapy that such patients should be treated (preferably in multinational clinical trials) with non-standard agents such as alemtuzumab, high-dose steroids, revlimid, or flavopiridol. There is good evidence that *IGHV* mutational status should be used to help stratify treatments in clinical trials. CD38 expression and/or serum TK might possibly be used in association, but these markers are not yet so completely accepted that they should influence general practice.

Differential diagnosis

Although any peripheral lymphocytosis may be included in the differential diagnosis, in the days of readily available immunophenotyping there are only two conditions that may be seriously confused with CLL: mantle cell lymphoma and splenic marginal zone lymphoma. Small lymphocytic lymphoma is essentially CLL that does not involve the peripheral blood, being confined mainly to lymph nodes, while prolymphocytic leukemia (PLL) is very distinct having >55% CD5 negative circulating prolymphocytes.

Mantle cell lymphoma

In general this is a much more malignant condition than CLL involving lymph nodes, spleen, and bone marrow, and often the peripheral blood. Many patients also have involvement of the colon, a condition known as multiple lymphomatous polyposis. The lymphocytes are of small to medium size with irregular nuclear contours, dispersed nuclear chromatin, and inconspicuous nucleoli. The immunophenotype shows intense surface IgM/IgD, CD5, CD22, and FMC7 positivity but is negative for CD10, CD23, and BCL6. Nuclear cyclin D1 positivity is pathognomonic for the disease. The t(11;14)(q13;q32) between *IGH* and cyclin D1 (*CCND1*) is present in almost all cases and considered the primary genetic event [70].

Mantle cell lymphoma is easily distinguished from CLL on the basis of karyotype and immunophenotype but an indolent form of the disease exists that bears many similarities to CLL with small CLL-like lymphocytes in the blood and marrow and no lymphadenopathy. These cases tend to have mutated *IGHV* genes and long survivals [71].

Splenic marginal zone lymphoma (SMZL)

This is an indolent B-cell malignancy usually involving spleen, bone marrow, and peripheral blood. It often presents as an incidental finding [72]. Previously the term "splenic lymphoma with villous lymphocytes" was used, but it has become evident that the short cytoplasmic projections, which may be either unevenly distributed or more commonly concentrated at one pole of the cell, are not a constant feature of the cell. SMZL cells are small- to intermediate-sized lymphocytes with clumped chromatin and those without villi may have a monocytoid appearance. The immunophenotype is usually distinguishable from that of CLL. CD19, CD20, CD22, CD79b, surface Ig, and FMC7 are all strongly expressed and CD5, CD10, and CD23 are generally absent. However, between 5 and 30% are reported to be CD5 positive. This may cause some confusion with CLL but the other markers are quite distinctly different. There is no distinctive karyotype but trisomy 3 and deletions at 7q are seen quite commonly [73]. The split between mutated and unmutated *IGHV* genes is similar to CLL, but the impact of this marker on prognosis has not been convincingly established. A paraprotein is found in the serum of approximately a third of patients and 10% show autoimmune phenomena. The majority of patients have splenomegaly. Many patients require no treatment for many years, and for most the first-line treatment is splenectomy. It is probable that the same types of immunochemotherapy that are effective in CLL will be effective in SMZL, but there are no clinical trial data to establish this.

Small lymphocytic lymphoma (SLL)

The term SLL is used for cases of CLL that have evidence of lymphadenopathy but fewer than 5×10^9/L peripheral blood lymphocytes. Such patients should be managed in the same way as patients with CLL. It is a mistake to manage them as if they were just another type of low-grade lymphoma.

Management of CLL

There is no evidence that early treatment of asymptomatic patients benefits them, although the trials that have been done used simple alkylating agents and treated all comers without regard to prognosis. It may well be that a more selective approach with more effective therapy would be of benefit and this is currently being investigated. The current advice is that patients who are asymptomatic (i.e., Rai Stage 0 and some Stage I and II patients, and Binet Stage A and some Stage B patients) should be managed by watchful waiting until the criteria for treatment in Table 13.3 are met [7].

When treatment is recommended, the choice of therapy has hitherto been between an alkylating agent (such as chlorambucil or cyclophosphamide) and a purine analog (such as fludarabine, cladribine, or pentostatin) and, more recently, a combination of the two. Although early trials suggested that purine analogs were more effective than alkylating agents, they are rather more toxic and by increasing the dose of alkylating agent, response rates are similar to those of purine analogs and toxicity is still less [69]. Combinations of the two increase response rates and lengths of remissions, though toxicity is increased still further [68, 69]. However, until recently no initial treatment has been shown to be preferable to any other in terms of OS, probably because salvage therapy is so effective. Justification for accepting PFS as a surrogate end point in clinical trials rests on the assumption that being in remission produces a better QOL than being in relapse. In a disease like CLL where so many people are asymptomatic and a course of treatment can produce a long-lasting toxicity such as T-cell immunodeficiency, the effectiveness of treatment needs to be weighed very carefully against toxicity.

The German CLL 8 study, which compared the combination of fludarabine and cyclophosphamide (FC) with the same combination with the addition of rituximab (FCR) in 817 untreated patients, found that at three years, 87% were alive in the FCR arm,

Table 13.3 IWCLL indications for treatment

At least one of the following criteria should be met:

1 Evidence of progressive marrow failure as shown by the development of worsening of anemia and/or thrombocytopenia.

2 Massive (at least 6 cm below the left costal margin) or progressive or symptomatic splenomegaly.

3 Massive nodes (at least 10 cm in longest diameter) or progressive or symptomatic lymphadenopathy.

4 Progressive lymphocytosis with an increase of more than 50% in a two-month period or a lymphocyte doubling time (LDT) of less than six months. LDT can be obtained by linear regression extrapolation of absolute lymphocyte counts obtained at intervals of two weeks over an observation period of two to three months. In patients with initial lymphocyte counts of $<30 \times 10^9$/L, LDT should not be used as a single treatment indicator. Other factors such as infection, vaccination, or treatment with corticosteroids that induce a rapid rise in lymphocyte count should be excluded.

5 Autoimmune hemolytic anemia or thrombocytopenia that is poorly responsive to corticosteroids or other standard therapy.

6 Constitutional symptoms defined as one of the following:

• Unintentional weight loss of 10% or more during the previous six months,

• Significant fatigue (ECOG PS 2 or worse; inability to work or perform usual activities),

• Fevers higher than 38°C for two weeks or more without other evidence of infection,

• Night sweats for more than one month without evidence of infection.

Neither hypogammaglobulinemia nor paraproteinemia is an indication for treatment. Very high leukocyte counts do not cause the symptoms associated with leukocyte aggregates that are seen in patients with other types of leukemia and therefore are not an indication for treatment.

---

compared with 83% in the FC arm (p = 0.01). This is the first time that a randomized clinical trial has shown that any first-line treatment extends overall survival over its comparator. As further evidence of its superiority, the complete response rate was more than doubled and the non-responder rate halved by the addition of the monoclonal antibody Median progression-free survival was 51.8 months in the FCR group compared with 32.8 months in the FC group (p < 0.0001) [74]. This study has led to FCR becoming established as the first-line therapy in most countries in the Western world. The questions now to be answered are: (1) Can FCR be safely given to the majority of patients? (2) Is FCR sufficient for all patients? (3) Is FCR needed for all patients?, and (4) Can FCR be afforded?

Can FCR be given safely?

According to SEER statistics, the average age at presentation for CLL is 72 [6]. Clinical trials seldom include many patients over 70. Only 10% of the patients included in the CLL 8 trial were over 70 [74]. We must await full publication for a complete analysis of this trial, but we do have documentation of a large, non-randomized, phase II trial of FCR in patients with CLL that was performed at the M.D. Anderson Cancer Center [75]. In this trial, 300 patients were treated every four weeks for a planned total of six courses of FCR (rituximab 375–500 mg/m^2 on day 1, fludarabine 25–30 mg/m^2 daily, cyclophosphamide 250–300 mg/m^2 daily on days 1 to 3 of each course and days 2 to 4 for the first course only). The patients were followed up for a median of six years, and the complete response rate was 72% – far higher than for previous treatments such as FC (35%) or fludarabine alone (29%). Just under half of those in CR had no detectable residual disease and the median time to progression was 80 months, with a projected 60% PFS at six years. This result must be seen in context: the patients in this study were relatively young; the median age was 57 years, and only 14% were aged 70 years or older. Patients over the age of 70 years were significantly less likely to complete the optimum six cycles of therapy and to achieve complete remission. It is co-morbidities rather than age that limit the use of FCR. The use of fludarabine is restricted by renal impairment and reduced bone marrow reserve combines with the long-term T-lymphocytopenia caused by fludarabine to generate a 10% risk of serious or opportunistic infections during the first year of remission. Late occurring neutropenia (19% after the completion of therapy, 28% after the recovery of blood counts) is particularly challenging.

For patients with co-morbidities a less toxic treatment may be required. Chlorambucil is still the prime choice for such patients, but trials of its use with rituximab are under way.

Is FCR sufficient for all patients?

Chromosomal studies have revealed that patients with 11q or 17p deletions have a particularly poor prognosis [45]. The addition of rituximab to FC seems to push those with 11q deletions back into the standard-risk group [74], but those with 17p deletions remain refractory to treatment. Once this group requires treatment, it is probably better to avoid FCR and embark on a different treatment protocol involving alemtuzumab, high-dose corticosteroids, revlimid, or flavopiridol [75, 76].

Even those patients who respond to FCR eventually relapse, and salvage therapy for these is difficult. Consideration is being given to treatment to eliminate residual disease following the achievement of a complete remission with either alemtuzumab or stem cell allograft [75–77]. Both options are hazardous and timing of such interventions is critical. Maintenance rituximab has proved successful in the management of follicular lymphoma in remission, and trials in CLL are under way [75].

Is FCR needed for all patients?

A subgroup of patients with mutated *IGHV* genes undoubtedly requires treatment and yet has a better prognosis than the group with unmutated *IGHV*

genes when treated with either FC or FCR [69, 74]. Some of these patients will be so close to the end of their natural lifespan that the extra toxicity of FCR compared to chlorambucil will not be thought worth it. On the other hand, younger patients might well find the prospect of FCR encouraging.

Is FCR affordable?

The very high cost of rituximab compared to other agents will put FCR out of the reach of patients in most countries of the world. For them the FC combination is probably the best option. Generic "rituximab" may well be available shortly in some developing countries.

Current areas of research in therapy

Well over 100 clinical trials are currently taking place in CLL with many more agents in the pre-clinical phase of developments [78]. Following the success of monoclonal antibodies in the treatment of lymphoma several monoclonals apart from rituximab are jockeying for position in the treatment of CLL, including alemtuzumab, the anti-CD20 antibodies ofatumumab and veltuzumab (as well as others with only numbers to identify them), the anti-CD23 antibody, lumiliximab, the anti-CD74 antibody, milatuzumab, as well as antibodies against CD22, CD25, CD40, CD200, and VEGF, HLA-DRβ and transferrin receptor, some of which are linked to toxins or isotopes. Several kinase inhibitors are being tested including dasatinib, sunitinib, sorafenib, and staurosporin; other agents like oblimersen and obatoclax target bcl-2. Nucleoside analogs such as clofarabine, nelarabine, and acadesine show some promise, as do topoisomerase inhibitors like mitoxantrone. There is a range of immunomodulatory agents including lenalidomide and thalidomide, and demethylating agents, proteosome inhibitors, heat shock protein inhibitors, histone deacetylase inhibitors, DNA repair inhibitors, and many others less well defined.

The old East German alkylating agent bendamustine is enjoying a new lease of life since its chemical structure resembles the purine analogs. Whether it shares activity with purine analogs is less certain. It may be that researchers are taking the opportunity to give an alkylating agent in a larger dose.

The place of stem cell transplantation in CLL therapy is incompletely defined [79]. Autografting probably cures no one, but does produce very prolonged remissions, especially in patients with mutated *IGHV* genes. Standard allografts are too toxic to be contemplated except in very young patients. Allografts following reduced intensity conditioning are currently being explored, and seem capable of producing cures in patients whose disease is refractory to other treatments. However, there is no agreement on which conditioning regimen should be used or which patients should be accepted into a program. The majority of patients are probably too old to contemplate this treatment which is best employed in those under 65 years of age. While many would be willing to apply the treatment to all with TP53 disorders, others would prefer it to be demonstrated that such patients were refractory to standard treatment first. Unfortunately, randomized controlled clinical trials are scarce in transplant units, but a careful phase 2 study from Germany does give us extra information. Of 90 patients under the age of 65 enrolled on the basis of refractoriness to a fludarabine-containing regimes or relapse with one year, or progressive disease with unfavorable genetic features (del 11q, del 17p, and/or unmutated *IGVH* status) the four-year actuarial survival was 65%. The non-relapse mortality was 23% and the event-free survival was 42%. Multivariate analysis demonstrated that uncontrolled disease at the time of transplant and the use of alemtuzumab for *in vivo* T-cell depletion had an adverse effect on event-free and overall survival [80].

Complications of CLL and its treatment

Autoimmunity

Autoimmunity is a common complication of CLL, but it principally affects the formed elements of the blood [30]. By far the most common manifestation is warm-antibody hemolytic anemia which occurs in about 15% of cases, mainly in progressive disease. CLL is the commonest known cause of autoimmune hemolytic anemia (AHA). The mechanism is obscure but may relate to CLL cells acting as antigen-presenting cells and presenting irregular epitopes to the immune system. Treatment with fludarabine (though not with FC or FCR) is known to trigger episodes of hemolysis that are severe and difficult to control. The mechanism of this seems to be the greater suppression of regulatory T-cells compared to helper T-cells.

Autoimmune thrombocytopenia is much rarer, occurring in around 1% of patients (often with AHA as Evans' syndrome), and autoimmune neutropenia and pure red cell aplasia are even rarer. Non-hemic autoimmunity does occur but is very uncommon. Cases of glomerulonephritis have been triggered by fludarabine, as have some cases of the blistering skin disease, paraneoplastic pemphigus. CLL cells secrete very little Ig and, therefore, conditions that are caused by the secreted Ig having autoantibody activity such as cold agglutination syndrome or acquired angioedema may be examples of other types of lymphoma being mistaken for CLL.

Treatment of AHA should be with prednisolone 1mg/kg. If this fails to control the hemolysis or if reduction of the corticosteroid dose to a safe level for long-term therapy cannot be achieved then the CLL should be treated, but autoimmunity is not in itself an indication for treatment of the tumor.

Immunodeficiency

All patients with CLL have a degree of immunodeficiency [81]. The most obvious manifestation is hypogammaglobulinemia which is present in up to 85% of patients. Infection is the major cause of death in between a quarter and a half of patients. The common bacterial infections are very prevalent, but reactivation of latent viruses, particularly herpes zoster and herpes simplex, occurs in about a third of patients. This clearly points to a T-cell defect. Paradoxically, the numbers of circulating T-cells are increased in most patients, though not in patients who have never encountered cytomegalovirus (CMV). A large proportion of CD8+ T-cells are directed against CMV peptides. It is not clear to what extent the T-cell defect in CLL is related to latent CMV infection and how much to the presence of the CLL itself.

Treatment with purine analogs or alemtuzumab leads to profound T-cell depletion. In the case of fludarabine, CD4+ T-cells are reduced to the levels seen in AIDS and do not recover for two years. Treatment with alemtuzumab requires monitoring for CMV reactivation which warrants early treatment with antivirals.

Intravenous Ig infusions are the chief remedy for hypogammaglobulinemia, though they have no effect on low levels of IgA or IgM. Several clinical trials have demonstrated reduction of mild and moderate bacterial infections but no decrease in mortality. One study estimated that the cost of one quality-adjusted-life-year (QALY) was US$6 million. My own practice is to confine treatment to patients whose serum IgG is <300 mg/dl and who have had at least two bacterial infections in a 12-month period. A dose of 250 mg/kg every four weeks is recommended.

Following treatment with either alemtuzumab or a purine analog, prophylaxis against *Pneumocystis jirovecii* is normally given with cotrimoxazole 960 mg on alternate days continued for a minimum of six months after stopping therapy, although some authorities recommend monitoring the count of CD4+ T-cells and continuing the cotrimoxazole until the count is $<0.2 \times 10^9$/L. In patients with a history of herpes simplex or herpes zoster prophylaxis with aciclovir should also be given. In some patients with particular risk factors such as previous systemic fungal infection, severe and prolonged neutropenia, the use of high-dose steroids and several previous rounds of immunosuppressive therapy, antifungal prophylaxis is also indicated. The choice of drug is fluid and any recommendation here will probably be out of date before publication.

As a general rule, it is not safe to use live vaccines in CLL patients (see Box 13.1). Recently, there has been a difference of opinion about the varicella/zoster vaccine, which is recommended by vaccinologists but forbidden by CLL specialists. There have been no trials of its safety in CLL patients and it is, therefore, best avoided. Vaccines are seldom efficacious in CLL. Even Stage 0 patients have very poor responses. In general, antibody responses to vaccines have been weak. Protein vaccines have produced weak to moderate responses in up to 50% of patients, chiefly in early-stage patients with normal serum Ig levels, but responses to polysaccharide

---

Box 13.1 Vaccination in CLL.

Vaccines that should be avoided in CLL
BCG
MMR
Poliomyelitis (oral)
Rotavirus
Typhoid (oral)
Vaccinia
Varicella-zoster
Yellow fever
Vaccines that are permissible
Anthrax
Cholera (oral)
Diphtheria
Haemophilus influenzae type b
Hepatitis A
Hepatitis B
Influenza
Menningococcus
Pertussis
Pneumococcus
Poliomyelitis (injection)
Rabies
Tetanus
Tick-borne encephalitis
Typhoid (injection)

---

vaccines have been virtually zero. The problem of poor response to polysaccharide vaccines can be partially overcome by conjugation to protein antigens. In the case of haemophilus, conjugation to tetanus toxoid is effective. For pneumococcal vaccines, conjugation to diphtheria CRM197 carrier protein produces a more effective vaccine capable of eliciting antibody responses in 40% of patients with CLL, most effectively in Binet Stage A patients.

References

1 Bennett JM, Catovsky D, Daniel MT, et al. (1989) Proposals for the classification of chronic (mature) B and T lymphoid leukaemias. French-American-British (FAB) Cooperative Group. *J Clin Pathol* **42**:567–84.

2 Matutes E, Oscier D, Garcia-Marco-J, et al. (1996) Trisomy 12 defines a group of CLL with atypical morphology: correlation between cytogenetic, clinical and laboratory features in 544 patients. *Brit J Haem* **92**:382–8.

3 Moreau EJ, Matutes E, A'Hern RP, et al. (1997) Improvement of the chronic lymphocytic leukemia scoring system with the monoclonal antibody SN8 (CD79b). *Am J Clin Pathol* **108**:378–82.

4 Polyak MJ, Ayer LM, Szczepek AJ, Deans JP. (2003) A cholesterol-dependent CD20 epitope detected by the FMC7 antibody. *Leukemia* **17**:1384–9.

5 Hamblin TJ. (2009) Just exactly how common is CLL? *Leuk Res* **33**:1452–3.

6 Sgambati MT, Linet MS, Devesa SS. (1991) Chronic lymphocytic leukemia: epidemiological, familial, and genetic aspects. In Cheson BD (ed.) *Chronic Lymphoid Leukemias* (2nd ed.), pp. 33–62. Marcel Dekker: New York.

7 Hallek M, Cheson BD, Catovsky D, et al. (2008) Guidelines for the diagnosis and treatment of chronic lymphocytic leukemia: a report from the International Workshop on Chronic Lymphocytic Leukemia updating the National Cancer Institute-Working Group 1996 guidelines. *Blood* **111**:5446–56.

8 Rawstron AC, Green MJ, Kuzmicki A, et al. (2002) Monoclonal B lymphocytes with the characteristics of "indolent" chronic lymphocytic leukemia are present in 3.5% of adults with normal blood counts. *Blood* **100**:635–9.

9 Rawstron AC, Bennett FL, O'Connor SJM, et al. (2008) Monoclonal B-cell lymphocytosis and chronic lymphocytic leukemia. *N Engl J Med* **359**:575–83.

10 Ladgren O, Albitar M, Wanlong M, et al. (2009) B cell clones as early markers for Chronic Lymphocytic Leukemia. *N Engl J Med* **360**:659–67.

11 Chiorazzi N, Ferrarini M. (2008) Origin and nature of chronic lymphocytic leukemia B cells. In O'Brien Sand Gribben JG (eds.) *Chronic Lymphocytic Leukemia*, pp. 1–18. Informa Healthcare: New York.

12 Hamblin TJ, Davis Z, Gardiner A, Oscier DG, Stevenson FK. (1999) Unmutated Ig V(H) genes are associated with a more aggressive form of chronic lymphocytic leukemia. *Blood* **94**:1848–54.

13 Damle RN, Wasil T, Fais F, et al. (1999) Ig V gene mutation status and CD38 expression as novel prognostic indicators leukemia. *Blood* **94**:1840–47.

14 Rosenwald A, Alizadeh AA, Widhopf G, et al. (2001) Relation of gene expression phenotype to immunoglobulin mutation genotype in B cell chronic lymphocytic leukemia. *J Exp Med* **194**:1639–47.

15 Klein U, Tu Y, Stolovitzky GA, et al. (2001) Gene expression profiling of B cell chronic lymphocytic leukemia reveals a homogeneous phenotype related to memory B cells. *J Exp Med* **194**:1625–38.

16 Tobin G, Thunberg U, Johnson A, et al. (2002). Somatically mutated Ig V(H)3-21 genes characterize a new subset of chronic lymphocytic leukemia. *Blood* **99**:2262–64.

17 Tobin G, Thunberg U, Johnson A, et al. (2003) Chronic lymphocytic leukemias utilizing the VH3-21 gene display highly restricted Vlambda2-14 gene use and homologous CDR3s: implicating recognition of a common antigen epitope. *Blood* **101**:4952–7.

18 Stamatopoulos K, Belessi C, Moreno C, et al. (2007) Over 20% of patients with chronic lymphocytic leukemia carry stereotyped receptors: pathogenic implications and clinical correlations. *Blood* **109**:259–70.

19 Dagklis A, Fazi C, Sala C, et al. (2009) The immunoglobulin gene repertoire of low count CLL-like MBL is different from CLL: diagnostic implications for clinical monitoring. *Blood* **114**:26–32.

20 Hamblin TJ. (2009) The TCL1 mouse as a model for chronic lymphocytic leukemia. *Leuk Res* doi: 10.1016/j.leukres.2009.08.004 (accessed August 20, 2009).

21 Pan JWY, Cook LS, Scwartz SM, Weiss NS. (2002) Incidence of leukaemia in Asian migrants to the United States and their descendants. *Cancer Causes Control* **13**:791–5.

22 Irons RD, Le A, Bao L. et al. (2009) Characterization of chronic lymphocytic leukemia/small lymphocytic lymphoma (CLL/SLL) in Shanghai, China: Molecular and cytogenetic characteristics, IgV gene restriction and hypermutation patterns. *Leuk Res* **33**;1599–603.

23 Goldin LR, Slager SL. (2007) Familial CLL: genes and environment. *Hematology* **1**:339–45.

24 Hamblin TJ. (2008) Have we been wrong about ionizing radiation and chronic lymphocytic leukemia? *Leuk Res* **32**:523–5.

25 Rawstron AC, Yuille MR, Fuller J, et al. (2002) Inherited predisposition to CLL is detectable as subclinical monoclonal B-lymphocyte expansion. *Blood* **100**:2289–90.

26 Raval A, Tanner SM, Byrd JC, et al. (2007) Downregulation of death-associated protein kinase 1 (DAPK1) in chronic lymphocytic leukemia. *Cell* **129**:879–90.

27 Dighiero G, Hamblin TJ. (2008) Chronic lymphocytic leukaemia. *Lancet* **371**:1017–29.

28 Rai KR, Sawitsky A, Cronkite ER, et al. (1975) Clinical staging of chronic lymphocytic leukemia. *Blood* **46**:219–34.

29 Binet J-L, Leporier M, Dighiero G, et al. (1977) A clinical staging system for chronic lymphocytic leukemia. *Cancer* **40**:855–64.

30 Hamblin TJ. (2007) Aggressive transformations and paraneoplastic complications of chronic lymphocytic leukemia. In Sekeres MA, Kalaycio ME, Bolwell BJ (eds.) *Clinical Malignant Hematology*, pp. 251–64. McGraw-Hill Professional: New York.

31 Montserrat E, Sanchez-Bisono J, Vinolas N and Rozman C. (1986) Lymphocyte doubling time in chronic lymphocytic leukaemia: analysis of its prognostic significance. *Brit J Haematol* **62**:567–75.

32 Hallek M, Langenmayer I, Nerl C, et al. (1999) Elevated serum thymidine kinase levels identify a subgroup at high risk of disease progression in early, non-smoldering chronic lymphocytic leukemia. *Blood* **93**:1732–7.

33 Hamblin TJ, Orchard JA, Ibbotson RE, et al. (2002) CD38 expression and immunoglobulin variable region mutations are independent prognostic variables in chronic lymphocytic leukemia, but CD38 expression may vary during the course of the disease. *Blood* **99**:1023–9.

34 Krober A, Seiler T, Benner A, et al. (2002) V(H) mutation status, CD38 expression level, genomic aberrations, and survival in chronic lymphocytic leukemia. *Blood* **100**:1410–6.

35 Thornton PD, Gustolisi G, Morilla R, et al. (2001) CD38 as a prognostic indicator in B-CLL. *Leuk Lymphoma* **42** (Suppl 1): 35–6.

36 Hamblin TJ, Orchard JA, Gardiner A, et al. (2000) Immunoglobulin V genes and CD38 expression in CLL. *Blood* **95**:2455–7.

37 Hamblin AD, Hamblin TJ. (2005) Functional and prognostic role of ZAP-70 in CLL. *Expert Opin Ther Targets* **9**:1165–78.

38 Chen L, Widhopf G, Huynh L, et al. (2002) Expression of ZAP-70 is associated with increased B-cell receptor signaling in chronic lymphocytic leukemia. *Blood* **100**:4609–14.

39 Lanham S, Hamblin T, Oscier D, et al. (2003) Differential signaling via surface IgM is associated with VH gene mutational status and CD38 expression in chronic lymphocytic leukemia. *Blood* **101**:1087–93.

40 Gobessi S, Laurenti L, Longo PG, et al. (2007) ZAP-70 enhances B-cell receptor signaling in spite of absent or inefficient tyrosine kinase activation in chronic lymphocytic leukemia and lymphoma B-cells. *Blood* **109**:2032–9.

41 Wiestner A, Rosenwald A, Barry T, et al. (2003) ZAP-70 expression identifies a chronic lymphocytic leukemia subtype with unmutated immunoglobulin genes, inferior clinical outcome and distinct gene expression profile. *Blood* **101**:4944–51.

42 Crespo M, Bosch F, Villamor N, et al. (2003) ZAP-70 expression as a surrogate for immunoglobulin-variable region mutations in chronic lymphocytic leukemia. *N Engl J Med* **348**:1764–75.

43 Orchard JA, Ibbotson RE, Davis Z, et al. (2004) ZAP-70 expression by flow cytometry is a good prognostic marker in CLL and a potential surrogate for immunoglobulin VH gene mutations. *Lancet* **363**:105–11.

44 Rassenti LZ, Huynh L, Toy TL, et al. (2004) ZAP-70 compared with immunoglobulin heavy-chain gene mutation status as a predictor of disease progression in chronic lymphocytic leukemia. *N Engl J Med* **351**:893–901.

45 Dohner H, Stilgenbauer S, Benner A, et al. (2000) Genomic aberrations and survival in chronic lymphocytic leukemia. *N Engl J Med* **343**:1910–6.

46 Juliusson G, Oscier DG, Fitchett M, et al. (1990) Prognostic subgroups in B-cell chronic lymphocytic leukemia defined by specific chromosomal abnormalities. *N Engl J Med* **323**:720–4.

47 Fitchett M, Griffiths MJ, Oscier DG, et al. (1987) Chromosome abnormalities involving band 13q14 in hematologic malignancies. *Cancer Genet Cytogenet* **24**:43–50.

48 Calin GA, Liu CG, Shimizu M, et al. (2004) MicroRNA profiling reveals distinct signatures in B-cell chronic lymphocytic leukemia. *Proc Natl Acad Sci U S A* **101**:11755–60.

49 Cimmino A, Callin GA, Fabbri M, et al. (2005) miR-15 and miR-16 induce apoptosis by targeting BCL2. *Proc Natl Acad Sci U S A* **102**:13944–9.

50 Aqeilan RI, Calin GA, Croce CM. (2010) miR-15a and miR-16-1 in cancer: discovery, function and future perspectives. *Cell Death Differ* **17**:215–20.

51 Lerner M, Harada M, Loven J, et al. (2009) *DLEU2*, frequently deleted in malignancy, functions as a critical host gene of the cell cycle inhibitory microRNAs miR-15a and miR-16-1. *Exp Cell Res* **315**:2941–52.

52 Oscier DG, Matutes E, Copplestone A, et al. (1997) Prognostic factors in stage A chronic lymphocytic leukaemia; the importance of atypical lymphocyte

morphology and abnormal karyotype for disease progression in stage A CLL. *Brit J Haematol* **98**:934–9.

53 Porpaczy E, Bilban M, Heinze G, et al. (2009) Gene expression signature of chronic lymphocytic leukaemia with Trisomy 12. *Eur J Clin Invest* **39**:568–75.

54 Kretz-Rommel A, Qin F, Dakappagari N, et al. (2007) CD200 expression on tumor cells suppresses antitumor immunity: new approaches to cancer immunotherapy. *J Immunol* **178**:5595–605.

55 Dohner H, Stilgenbauer S, James M, et al. (1997) 11q deletions identify a new subset of B-cell chronic lymphocytic leukemia characterized by extensive nodal involvement and inferior prognosis. *Blood* **89**:2516–22.

56 Lin K, Sherrington PD, Dennis M, et al. (2002) Relationship between p53 dysfunction, CD38 expression, and IgV(H) mutation in chronic lymphocytic leukemia. *Blood* **100**:1404–9.

57 Austen B, Powell JE, Alvi A, et al. (2005) Mutations in the ATM gene lead to impaired overall and treatment-free survival that is independent of IGVH mutation status in patients with B-CLL. *Blood* **106**:3175–82.

58 Dohner H, Fischer K, Bentz M, et al. (1995) p53 gene deletion predicts for poor survival and non-response to therapy with purine analogs in chronic B-cell leukemias. *Blood* **85**:1580–9.

59 Oscier DG, Gardiner AC, Mould SJ, et al. (2002) Multivariate analysis of prognostic factors in CLL:Clinical stage, IGVH gene mutational status, and loss or mutation of the p53 gene are independent prognostic factors. *Blood* **100**:1177–84.

60 Krober A, Seller T, Benner A, et al. (2002) VH mutation status, CD38 expression level, genomic aberrations, and survival in chronic lymphocytic leukemia. *Blood* **100**:1410–16.

61 Shanafelt TD, Witzig TE, Fink SR, et al. (2006) Prospective evolution during long-term follow-up of patients with untreated early stage chronic lymphocytic leukemia. *J Clin Oncol* **24**:4634–41.

62 Best OG, Gardiner AC, Davis ZA, et al. (2009) A subset of Binet stage A CLL patients with TP53 abnormalities and mutated IGHV genes have stable disease. *Leukemia* **23**:212–4.

63 Cuneo A, Rigolin GM, Bigoni R, et al. (2004) Chronic lymphocytic leukemia with 6q- shows distinct haematological features and intermediate prognosis. *Leukemia* **18**:476–483.

64 Codony C, Crespo N, Abrisqueta P, Montserrat E, Bosch F. (2009) Gene expression profiling in chronic lymphocytic leukaemia. *Best Pract Res Clin Haematol* **22**:211–22.

65 Byrd JC, Gribben JG, Peterson BL, et al. (2006) Select high-risk features predict earlier progression following chemo-immunotherapy with fludarabine and rituximab in chronic lymphocytic leukemia: justification for risk-adapted therapy. *J Clin Oncol* **24**:437–43.

66 Del Poeta G, Del Principe MI, Consalvo MA, et al. (2005) The addition of rituximab improves clinical outcome in untreated patients with ZAP-70 negative chronic lymphocytic leukemia. *Cancer* **104**:2743–52.

67 Zenz T, Eichhorst B, Busch R, et al. (2010) TP53 mutation and survival in chronic lymphocytic leukemia. *J Clin Oncol* **28**:4773–9.

68 Eichhorst BF, Busch R, Hopfinger G, et al. (2006) Fludarabine plus cyclophosphamide versus fludarabine alone in first-line therapy of younger patients with chronic lymphocytic leukemia. *Blood* **107**:885–91.

69 Catovsky D, Richards S, Matutes E, et al. (2007) Assessment of fludarabine plus cyclophosphamide for patients with chronic lymphocytic leukemia (the LRF CLL4 trial): a randomised controlled trial. *Lancet* **370**:230–9.

70 Oscier DG, Wade R, Davis Z, et al. (2010) Prognostic factors identified three risk groups in the UK LRF CLL4 trial, independent of treatment allocation. *Haematologica* **95**:1705–12.

71 Swerdlow SH, Campo E, Seto M, Muller-Hermelink HK. (2008) Mantle cell lymphoma. In Swerdlow SH, Campo E, Harris NL, et al. (eds.) *WHO Classification of Tumours of Haematopoietic and Lymphoid Tissues* (4th ed.), pp. 229–32. IARC: Lyon.

72 Orchard J, Garand R, Davis Z, et al. (2003) A subset of t(11;14) lymphoma with mantle cell features displays mutated *IgV$_H$* genes and includes patients with good prognosis, non-nodal disease. *Blood* **101**:4975–81.

73 Oscier D, Owen R, Johnson S. (2005) Splenic marginal zone lymphoma. *Blood Rev* **19**:39–51.

74 Hallek M, Fischer K, Fingerle-Rowson-G, et al. (2010) Addition of rituximab to fludarabine, and cyclophosphamide, in patients with chronic lymphocytic leukaemia: a randomized, open label, phase 3 trial. *Lancet* **376**:1164–74.

75 Hamblin TJ. (2009) Fludarabine, Cyclophosphamide and Rituximab: No country for old men? *Nat Clin Pract Oncol* **6**:130–131.

76 Robak T. (2010) How to improve treatment outcome in chronic lymphocytic leukemia? *Leuk Res* **34**:272–5.

77 Pleyer L, Egle A, Hartmann TN, Greil R. (2009) Molecular and cellular mechanisms of CLL: novel therapeutic approaches. *Nat Rev Clin Oncol* **6**:405–18.

78 Byrd JC, Awan F, Lin TS, Grever MR. (2008) New therapies in chronic lymphocytic leukemia. In O'Brien S and Gribben JG (eds.) *Chronic Lymphocytic Leukemia,* pp. 165–84. Informa Healthcare: New York.

79 Gribben JG. (2008) Stem cell transplantation in CLL. In O'Brien S and Gribben JG (eds.) *Chronic Lympho-cytic Leukemia,* pp. 185–200. Informa Healthcare: New York.

80 Dreger P, Dohner H, Ritgen M, et al. (2010) Allogeneic stem cell transplantation provides durable disease control in poor risk chronic lymphocytic leukemia: long-term clinical and MRD results of the German CLL Study Group CLL3X trial. *J Clin Oncol* **28**:4473–9.

81 Hamblin AD, Hamblin TJ. (2008) The immunodeficiency of chronic lymphocytic leukaemia. *British Medical Bulletin* **87**:49–62.

CHAPTER 14

Acute Lymphoblastic Leukemia

Susan O'Brien, Stefan Faderl, Deborah Thomas and Hagop M. Kantarjian
Department of Leukemia, University of Texas M.D. Anderson Cancer Center, Houston, TX, USA

Epidemiology and etiology

Acute lymphoblastic leukemia (ALL) is a common malignancy in children, where it constitutes about 80% of all childhood leukemias and 25% of all childhood cancers. In contrast, it represents less than 3% of malignancies in adults [1]. ALL is more frequent among Caucasians [2]. In most cases no etiology can be established. The peak age of development of childhood cases, an association of ALL with industrialized or affluent societies and in urban areas, and the occasional clustering of childhood ALL have led to two interrelated hypotheses: population-mixing and delayed infection [3, 4]. The former hypothesis suggests that clusters of ALL arise when non-immune individuals are exposed to common infections after population-mixing with carriers. The latter hypothesis proposes that individuals from affluent environments with a prenatally acquired preleukemic clone and low exposure to infections early in life are predisposed to aberrant responses to common infections at an age when increased lymphoid proliferation is occurring [5–8].

Clinical presentation and laboratory abnormalities

Signs and symptoms of ALL include fatigue, constitutional symptoms, easy bruising or bleeding, dyspnea, dizziness, and infections. Less than 10% of patients have symptomatic CNS involvement at diagnosis, although the frequency is higher in patients with mature B-cell ALL (Burkitt's leukemia/lymphoma). T-lineage ALL with a mediastinal mass can cause stridor and wheezing, pericardial effusions, and superior vena cava syndrome. Testicular involvement occurs predominantly in infant and adolescent boys. Except for mature B-cell ALL, involvement of the gastrointestinal tract is uncommon. Table 14.1 summarizes the features of patients with adult ALL presenting to a tertiary referral center [9].

Morphology and cytochemistry

Morphologic evaluation, accompanied by cytochemical stains, is the initial step in diagnosis and has been the basis for the French-American-British (FAB) classification of ALL [10].

Although no cytochemical stain is diagnostic for ALL, the key cytochemical feature of ALL is lack of myeloperoxidase (MPO) and non-specific esterase (NSE) activity. Terminal deoxynucleotidyl transferase (TdT) is a useful marker to distinguish between reactive versus malignant lymphocytosis. L3 ALL is usually TdT-negative. The World Health Organization (WHO) *Classification of Neoplastic Diseases of the Hematopoietic and Lymphoid Tissues* stresses the importance of immunologic and cytogenetic-molecular features over morphologic characteristics [11].

Immunophenotyping

Most cases of ALL (70–85%) are of B lineage [12]. They can be divided into: (1) pre-pre-B ALL (pro-B ALL), (2) early pre-B (common ALL), (3) pre-B ALL,

Advances in Malignant Hematology, First Edition. Edited by Hussain I. Saba and Ghulam J. Mufti. © 2011 Blackwell Publishing Ltd. Published 2011 by Blackwell Publishing Ltd.

Table 14.1 Features of adult acute lymphocytic leukemia at presentation (N=770)

Characteristic	Variable
Median age, yrs	40.5
Range	13–92
≥60 yrs (%)	21
ECOG performance status >2 (%)	5
Organ involvement (%)	
Lymphadenopathy	32
Splenomegaly	25
Hepatomegaly	16
Median WBC (x 10^9/L)	7.7
Range	(0.2–669.6)
WBC >30 × 10^9/L (%)	24
Chemistry abnormalities (%)	
↑ Lactic dehydrogenase	50
Creatinine ≥1.3 mg/dL	14
Bilirubin ≥1.3 mg/dL	11
Immunophenotype (%)	
Precursor B	60
Mature B	12
T-cell	14
Other (null, biphenotypic)	14
Myeloid marker positive (%)	49
Karyotype (%)	
Diploid	26
Ph-positive	19
t(8;14); t(8;2); t(8;22)	6
Hyperdiploid	7
Hypodiploid	3
Risk assignment (%)	
Standard	20
High	80

Data from Wolfraim et al. [25].

Table 14.2 Immunophenotypic classification of ALL

	Positive surface markers
B lineage	
pro-B (pre-pre-B)	TdT, CD19, CD79a, CD22
early pre-B (common)	TdT, CD19, CD79a, CD10
pre-B	TdT, CD19, CD79a, CD10, cIg
mature B	CD19, CD20, CD10$^+$, CD22, CD79a, sIg
T lineage	
pro-T	TdT, CCD3, +/– CD2, CD3, CD7
common T	TdT, CCD3, CD2, CD5, CD7, CD4, CD8, CD1a
mature T	CD3, CD2, CD5, CD7, CD4 or CD8, +/– TdT

and (4) mature B ALL (Table 14.2). Pre-pre-B-ALL blasts express CD19, CD79a, or CD22, but no other B-cell antigens. CD19-positive, CD10-negative, cytoplasmic immunoglobulin-negative B-lineage ALL with myeloid marker coexpression is common in infants with ALL, and is typically associated with t(4;11), *MLL* gene rearrangement, and a poor prognosis. Common ALL (cALL, early pre-B ALL) is the most frequent immunophenotype. It is characterized by expression of CD10 (common ALL antigen, CALLA) and is a common immunophenotype in Philadelphia chromosome (Ph)-positive ALL. Pre-B-ALL blasts express TdT, HLA-DR, CD19, CD79a, and cytoplasmic Ig. A proportion of pre-B-ALL cases are associated with the translocation t(1;19). Mature B-cell-ALL (Burkitt's leukemia) blasts express surface immunoglobulin (sIg, usually IgM), are clonal for κ or λ light chains, and lack expression of TdT. About half are CD10-positive, which may be associated with a better prognosis. Expression of CD20 is ubiquitous in mature B-cell ALL, whereas it occurs in only about 35 to 50% of other ALL subtypes.

T-cell ALL accounts for 15 to 20% of cases [13] and, similar to B-lineage ALL, can be stratified into subtypes based on different stages of intrathymic differentiation (Table 14.2). T-cell ALL expresses various levels of CD1a, CD2, CD3, CD4, CD5, CD7, and CD8. CD7 is the most sensitive T-cell marker, but lacks specificity because cases of AML or NK cell leukemia may be CD7-positive. Cytoplasmic CD3 (cCD3) is the most lineage-specific marker for T-cell differentiation. Mature T-cell ALL expresses both surface CD3 (sCD3) and cCD3, CD2 and either CD4 or CD8 but not both. Earlier stages of differentiation (precursor T-cell ALL corresponding to a "prothymocyte" or "immature thymocyte" type) express cCD3 but not sCD3. sCD3- and CD7-positive T-cell ALL suggests a poor prognosis. T-cell ALL with the lack of CD1a and CD8 expression (in association with low expression of CD5 and frequent coexpression of myeloid-associated markers CD13 and CD33) appears to be especially aggressive [14].

Coexpression of myeloid-associated antigen is common (15 to 50% in adult ALL; 5 to 35% in children), and does not necessarily indicate bilineage leukemia. Myeloid-associated marker expression is more frequent in ALL with t(9;22), t(4;11), and t(12;21) with *TEL-AML1* fusion, and is usually absent in mature B-cell ALL. Myeloid-associated marker expression has no prognostic significance, but is useful to distinguish leukemic cells from normal lymphoid progenitor cells, enhancing detection of minimal residual leukemia.

Cytogenetic and molecular abnormalities

Identification of cytogenetic and molecular abnormalities (Figure 14.1) [15–19] provides pathobiological insights, serves as targets for drug development, and furnishes prognostic information, which has been translated into risk-adapted therapies [18, 19].

Numerical abnormalities

Numerical chromosome abnormalities are prognostically more useful in children, although the biological basis of their prognostic relevance remains undefined. Hypodiploidy defines a karyotype with less than 46 chromosomes. Among hypodiploid cases, only those with <44 chromosomes have a worse prognosis, especially cases with near-haploidy or its multiplication.

Hyperdiploidy is defined by chromosome numbers of more than 46. It is more common in children than in adults (~25% vs. 5%) [20, 21]. Hyperdiploid blasts from patients with ALL have been shown to accumulate more methotrexate and methotrexate polyglutamate, and to be more sensitive to other drugs such as mercaptopurine, thioguanine, cytarabine, and L-asparaginase. This may further explain why response duration and survival are better for patients with hyperdiploid chromosomes.

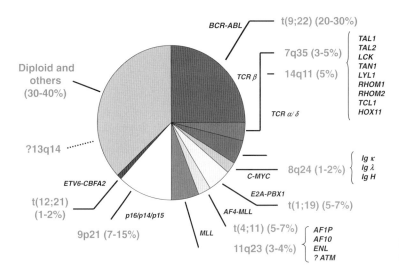

Figure 14.1 Cytogenetic abnormalities in adult ALL.

Structural abnormalities
Translocation t(9;22)
The Philadelphia chromosome (Ph), a translocation between the long arms of chromosome 9 and 22, t(9;22)(q34;q11), is the most common abnormality in adult ALL (15 to 30%), but is rare in children (<5%). At the molecular level, the *BCR* gene on chromosome 22q11 is fused to the *ABL* gene on 9q34. The chimeric *BCR-ABL* gene is translated into hybrid BCR-ABL oncoproteins of different sizes and molecular weights depending on the breakpoint location within *BCR*. Whereas p210$^{BCR-ABL}$ is the most frequent oncoprotein in CML, p190$^{BCR-ABL}$ occurs in 60–80% of patients with Ph-positive ALL. Patients with Ph-positive ALL are typically older, present with higher white blood cell and blast counts, and have a pre-B-cell immunophenotype; the cells often coexpress myeloid antigens. Ph-positive ALL used to be one of the subtypes with the worst long-term disease-free survival; however, use of BCR-ABL tyrosine kinase inhibitors (reviewed below), in conjunction with chemotherapy, has dramatically improved outcomes in recent times.

Translocation t(12;21) and del(12p)
ETV6 (*TEL*) is a transcription-regulating gene of the Ets family of transcription factors. Fused to *RUNX1* (*AML1*, *CBFA2*) on chromosome 21q22, it forms a fusion protein with the ability to alter both self-renewal and differentiation capacity. Using molecular assays, the cryptic translocation is found in up to 30% of children with ALL, making it the most frequently occurring cytogenetic-molecular abnormality in pediatric pre-B ALL. This cytogenetic-molecular abnormality, however, is rare in adults. *ETV6-RUNX1*-positive ALL has been associated with an excellent outcome in children.

Del(9p21)
Abnormalities of 9p21 occur in up to 15% of patients with ALL. The blasts are predominantly of T-cell lineage. The prognosis in these patients is generally unfavorable; the disease is characterized by higher rates of relapse and shorter survival. The prognostic associations are stronger in children and are less well defined in adult ALL.

MLL rearrangements (11q23)
The mixed lineage leukemia gene *MLL* (*ALL-1, HRX, HTRX1*) on 11q23 is frequently involved in reciprocal rearrangements with genes located on chromosomes 4q21, 9p22, 19p13, 1p32, and many others. The fusion of *MLL* with *AF4* on chromosome 4q21 is a frequent abnormality in infant ALL, accounting for up to 85% of cases, but is detected in only 3 to 8% of adults [22]. Adults with this translocation tend to be older, have higher white blood cell counts and organomegaly; sites such as the CNS are involved more frequently. The constellation of CD10-negative, cytoplasmic immunoglobulin-positive myeloid antigen expressing pre-B ALL has a high *MLL* rearrangement rate [23]. The prognosis of *MLL* leukemias is poor in infants and adults but is intermediate in children over one year of age [24].

E2A rearrangements (19p13)
The two known translocations with *E2A* rearrangements on chromosome 19p13 are t(1;19)(q23;p13) and t(17;19)(q21;p13). Translocation t(1;19) is associated with pre-B ALL phenotype expressing cytoplasmic Ig. The frequency in childhood ALL is around 3% in whites and 12% in blacks; it is uncommon (<3%) in adults. Translocation t(17;19) is a rarer variant associated with hypercalcemia and DIC at diagnosis and has a generally poor outcome.

8q24 rearrangements
The *C-MYC* gene, located on 8q24, is involved in one of the three translocations with kappa or lambda Ig light chain locus in mature B ALL: (1) The t(8;14) (q24;q32), occurs most commonly (80%), and juxtaposes C-MYC to the Ig heavy chain (IgH) gene locus on 14q32; (2) t(8;22)(q24;q11), occurs in about 15% of B-ALL patients and involves the Ig lambda gene locus on 22q11; and (3) t(2;8) (p12;q24)], which is the least frequent translocation and involves the Ig kappa gene locus on 2p12.

T-cell receptor (TCR) gene rearrangements
TCR gene rearrangements define the majority of cytogenetic abnormalities in T-lineage ALL. Genes for T-cell receptors are located on chromosomes

14q11 (TCR α/δ), 7q15 (TCR γ), and 7q35 (TCR δ). Although no specific cytogenetic abnormality can be linked to a specific clinical subtype of T-lineage ALL, a number of distinct chromosomal translocations have been identified. The clinical relevance of the translocations depends on the partner genes involved. In most cases, partner genes are deregulated and come under the influence of promoter/enhancer regions of *TCRs* [21].

Other molecular abnormalities

More than 50% of cases of T-cell ALL have activating mutations that involve *NOTCH1*, a gene encoding a transmembrane receptor that regulates normal T-cell development [25].This genetic abnormality was associated with a favorable prognosis in one study of childhood T-cell ALL [26].

Gene expression microarrays

Microarray technology has been used to establish gene expression profiles that further distinguish subtypes of ALL, to stratify patients according to risk and response, identify genetic markers associated with drug sensitivity and resistance pathways, and provide useful insights into pathogenesis and biology of ALL [14, 27–29]. Although the possibilities of gene expression profiling are very intriguing, issues related to reproducibility, statistical significance, and practical application need to be resolved before gene expression profiling is ready for clinical use. The emergence of proteomics also raises questions about the significance of gene expression versus protein expression profiles.

Epigenetic alterations in ALL

Aberrant methylation of promoter-associated CpG islands and silencing of genes related to the tumor phenotype is an important step in the process of malignant transformation of cells [30]. Epigenetic silencing of cancer-related genes is common in ALL at diagnosis and relapse where abnormal methylation patterns are found in up to 80% of patients [31]. Recently, the interplay between methylation changes and organization of histone complexes has become a focus of attention, not least because many drugs (e.g., DNA methyltransferase inhibitors, HDAC inhibitors) are now available to target these various aspects of epigenetic alterations.

The therapy of ALL

Starting in the 1960s, researchers at St Jude Children's Research Hospital were highly successful with combination therapies of all available antileukemia drugs that were delivered in a sequence of extended courses of therapy [32]. Therapeutic strategies in adult ALL have been patterned after the pediatric regimens using the same basic principles: induction therapy followed by early intensification and consolidation, CNS-directed treatment, and a prolonged maintenance phase (Figure 14.2). Given

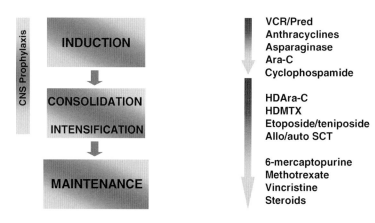

R I S K – O R I E N T E D   T H E R A P Y

Figure 14.2 Principles of ALL therapy.

the high remission rates with these regimens, the focus of current ALL programs is concentrated on improvement of remission duration and survival of adult patients, and to improvement in QOL in pediatric patients. Validation of subtype-specific prognostic models and development of risk-adapted and targeted therapy designs have become the major objectives of clinical trials.

Prognostic factors

Information from morphological assessment, immunophenotyping, karyotype analysis, molecular genetics and, increasingly, measurements of minimal residual disease (MRD), have contributed to a more comprehensive risk-stratification of patients. For example, gene expression analysis in T-lineage ALL has shown that high expression of *ERG* and *HOX11L2* are unfavorable features and associations with other molecular markers have been established [33–35].

Monitoring of MRD after induction and during consolidation has emerged as one of the most powerful predictors of relapse and has been useful to further stratify standard-risk patients [36, 37]. The German Multicenter Study Group for Adult Acute Lymphoblastic Leukemia (GMALL) prospectively monitored 196 standard-risk ALL patients at up to nine time-points in the first year of therapy with quantitative polymerase chain reaction [36]. MRD was predictive for relapse and, according to the rapidity of eradication of MRD or persistence of MRD over time, three risk groups could be defined with a three-year relapse risk varying between 0% (low-risk group) to 94% (high-risk group).

Other factors with impact on prognosis have been identified (e.g., time to platelet recovery during induction, expression of drug resistance markers, pharmacogenetics). Their validation in the context of prognostic models is still lacking [38–40].

Induction therapy

Vincristine, corticosteroids, and a third agent (anthracyclines in adults and asparaginase in children) have long been the backbone of ALL induction therapy. No difference in outcome has been established based on the type of anthracycline.

Additional drugs have become part of ALL induction and intensification cycles. These include cytarabine, methotrexate, cyclophosphamide, L-asparaginase and less frequently, etoposide, teniposide, m-amsacrine, or other agents. Although improved CR rates beyond the expected 90% is difficult, intensification of induction and early consolidation has demonstrated a positive impact on remission duration and survival; this effect has been stronger for specific subtypes. Cytarabine and cyclophosphamide have increased response rates and DFS in T-cell ALL [41]. Given the poorer tolerance of L-asparaginase in adults, it has been used less often in those patients, although large randomized pediatric ALL trials have demonstrated improved survival rates when L-asparaginase was given throughout the remission and/or post-remission phase [42, 43]. The most commonly used form of asparaginase is derived from *E.coli*; its major limitation is development of hypersensitivity reactions and its poor tolerability in adults. Pegasparaginase is a modified form of *E.coli* asparaginase with a longer serum half-life and reduced risk of hypersensitivity reactions; several studies have been reported in adults [44–46]. Fractionation of cyclophosphamide and high doses of methotrexate have improved the outcome in mature B-cell ALL [47].

Recently, monoclonal antibodies have been included in ALL induction programs. Most experience exists with the anti-CD20 chimeric antibody rituximab. Expression of CD20 has been associated with a higher relapse rate in adult patients with pre-B ALL [48], although the association of outcome with CD20 expression remains disputed in children [49]. Several studies have shown improvement in prognosis with chemotherapy plus rituximab combinations, especially in mature B-cell ALL where CD20 expression is ubiquitous [50, 51].

Steroids are a standard part of ALL induction and prednisone or prednisolone is the most commonly used steroid, particularly during the maintenance phase. Compared to prednisone and prednisolone, dexamethasone has shown better *in vitro* antileukemic activity and achievement of higher drug levels in the cerebrospinal fluid (CSF). Using a dose of 6 mg or 6.5 mg/m^2 throughout therapy, the Children Oncology Group and UK MRC randomized trials demonstrated a significant reduction in isolated CNS relapse and a significant improvement of EFS [52, 53]. On the other hand, a smaller study from the Tokyo Children's Cancer Study Group including 231 children with standard- and intermediate-risk ALL showed no difference between dexamethasone (8 mg/m^2 during induction and 6 mg/m^2 during intensifications) and prednisolone (60 mg/m^2 and 40 mg/m^2, respectively) [54].

Given the intensity of induction combinations, supportive care has become an important part of ALL therapy. The rationale for hematopoietic growth factors includes shortening of the duration of myelosuppression and myelosuppression-associated infectious complications. In addition, rapid recovery of the marrow following chemotherapy allows timely administration of dose-intense treatment regimens [55]. Three randomized adult trials have demonstrated advantages of using hematopoietic growth factors such as G-CSF [56–58]. In a pediatric randomized trial, G-CSF treatment had limited clinical utility [59]. The role of erythropoietic growth factors in the decrease of transfusion requirements is being studied.

Post-remission therapy

Post-remission therapy consists of an intensified consolidation followed by maintenance therapy, and stem cell transplantation (STC) for some patients. Following the experience in children with ALL, an intensification of post-remission therapy has improved outcome, particularly in patients with high-risk disease. However, there is no consensus on the optimal type or duration of consolidation. Consolidation programs typically consist of a repetition of the induction sequence or rotational programs including additional agents, which may benefit particular ALL subtypes.

Most maintenance schedules include 6-mercaptopurine, methotrexate, and monthly pulses of vincristine and prednisone, and extend over two to three years. Further intensifications during maintenance are being studied, but remain investigational. Maintenance therapy has become subset-specific: it is of little value in mature B-cell ALL as these patients relapse within the first year of remission and rarely later; tyrosine kinase inhibitors (TKIs)

have become an integral component in Ph-positive ALL; and other T-cell-specific drugs such as nelarabine are being studied in T-lineage ALL.

SCT has improved outcome for patients with high-risk ALL in first CR. Although there has been resistance to use SCT for standard-risk patients in CR1, recent reports suggest that the benefit of SCT extends to some standard-risk patients, possibly based on MRD levels or other features not captured by traditional prognostic markers.

The LALA94 study focused on a risk-adapted post-remission strategy and the role of allogeneic SCT in ALL [60]. A total of 922 patients were divided into standard-risk, high-risk, Ph-positive, and CNS-positive. All patients received a four-week induction and then either post-remission chemotherapy (standard-risk group) or allogeneic SCT (all other risk groups) if an HLA-identical sibling was identified. Autologous SCT was offered to patients without a donor, or patients were randomized between autologous SCT and chemotherapy in the absence of Ph- or CNS-positive disease. The study showed better disease-free survival for high-risk ALL patients transplanted in first CR. Autologous transplant did not confer a significant benefit over chemotherapy.

The Groupe Ouest-Est d'Etude des Leucémies et Autres Maladies du Sang (GOELAMS) has evaluated the impact of allogeneic SCT for high-risk patients in first CR versus delayed autologous SCT for patients without matched donors and those older than 50 years [61]. On an ITT analysis for patients younger than 50 years, six-year overall survival was significantly improved with allogeneic SCT compared with autologous SCT (75% vs. 40%, p = 0.0027).

The MRC UKALLXII/ECOG E2993 trial attempted to determine if allogeneic SCT was beneficial for all suitable adult patients and if a single autologous SCT could be as effective as post-remission chemotherapy [62]. The study enrolled 1929 patients between 15 and 59 years of age. All patients who had an HLA-matched sibling donor were assigned to receive an allogeneic SCT, whereas those who did not or were over age 55 were randomized to receive an autologous SCT versus chemotherapy. All patients received induction chemotherapy and intensification with high-dose methotrexate. High-risk was defined as age >35 years, leukocytosis ($\geq 30 \times 10^9$/L for

B-lineage and 100×10^9/L for T-lineage) and Ph ALL. The CR rate was 90% and five-year survival was 43% for all patients. The following results emerged: (1) survival at five years was 53% for Ph-negative patients with a donor, versus 45% for those without a donor (p = 0.02); (2) five-year survival for Ph-negative standard-risk patients was superior for patients with a donor compared to those without (62% vs. 52%; p = 0.02); (3) five-year survival for high-risk patients was not significantly different whether patients had a donor or not (41% vs. 35%; p = 0.2). In this group, transplant-related toxicity prevented a better outcome and abrogated the effect of a reduction in relapse rate; (4) post-remission chemotherapy resulted in superior event-free and overall survival when compared to autologous SCT (p = 0.02 and 0.03, respectively).

Although a broader role of allogeneic SCT for patients with ALL in first CR is now emerging, optimal timing remains challenging. Novel therapies (e.g., TKIs for Ph ALL) may affect outcome requiring a reassessment of SCT in some of the risk groups. Non-myeloablative SCT has been successfully used in older or debilitated patients. The major impediment for SCT remains the fact that less then 30% of patients have a matched sibling donor. Much work has been invested in improving transplants from partially matched related donors, matched unrelated donors (MUD), and umbilical cord blood (UCB). Bishop et al. evaluated outcomes with autologous SCT and MUD SCT in 260 adult patients in CR1 or CR2. Although treatment-related mortality was higher with MUD SCT, relapse risk was lower and five-year leukemia-free and overall survival rates were similar (37% vs. 39%, 38% vs. 39%, respectively) [63]. Similar results have been reported by other groups.

CNS prophylaxis

CNS involvement is rare at diagnosis (<5% in children and <10% in adults). However, in the absence of CNS prophylaxis, CNS disease occurs in 40–50% of patients and was a major obstacle to cure. CNS relapse can occur as isolated CNS disease, following marrow recurrence, or concomitantly with a marrow or testicular relapse or both. As CNS relapse confers a poor prognosis irrespective of the intensity

of retreatment (with the possible exception of late CNS relapses) effective CNS prophylaxis is important [64, 65].

Risk factors for CNS involvement include younger age, T-lineage and mature B-cell ALL immunophenotype, a high white blood cell count, and the presence of blasts in cerebrospinal fluid at diagnosis. Expression of CD7, CD56, and interleukin-15 were found to have prognostic implications with regard to extramedullary manifestions of ALL. Elevated serum LDH levels and a high proliferative index ($S + G_2M > 14\%$) proved to be sensitive predictors of the risk of CNS disease.

Therapeutic modalities for CNS prophylaxis include intrathecal (IT) chemotherapy (methotrexate, cytarabine, steroids), high-dose systemic chemotherapy (methotrexate, cytarabine, L-asparaginase, dexamethasone, 6-thioguanine), and craniospinal irradiation (XRT). Combined triple modality IT therapy is more effective for CNS control than IT methotrexate alone, but carries a higher risk of treatment-related CNS morbidity and unexpectedly was associated with an increased risk of bone marrow and testicular relapse in one randomized trial [66]. One explanation for this paradoxical finding is that an "isolated" CNS relapse may in fact be an early manifestation of systemic relapse, and that better CNS control favors leukemic relapse in other sites at a later time. Several studies in children and adults have demonstrated that IT therapy is equivalent to craniospinal XRT, so that the role of cranial XRT has become controversial. Adverse effects of XRT can be severe and disabling leading to seizures, dementia, and intellectual dysfunction, as well as other complications such as multiple endocrinopathies and growth retardation in children. CNS prophylaxis based on high-dose systemic therapy alone is not sufficient.

Pharmacogenetics and mechanisms of drug resistance

By affecting pharmacodynamics, the cytogenetic-molecular characteristics of leukemic cells can influence treatment outcome [67]. For example, hyperdiploidy cases accumulate higher intracellular methotrexate polyglutamates because they have extra copies of the gene encoding reduced folate carrier, an active transporter of methotrexate. Blasts with a t(12;21) and *ETV6-RUNX1* fusion are more sensitive to asparaginase. Cells harboring *MLL* rearrangements have increased sensitivity to cytarabine, possibly by overexpression of cellular cytarabine receptors.

In addition to acquired genetic abnormalities, an association between germ-line genetic characteristics (involving genes encoding drug-metabolizing enzymes, transporters, and drug targets) and drug metabolism and sensitivity to chemotherapy is being recognized as well [68]. Rocha et al. [69] determined whether ALL outcome was related to 16 genetic polymorphisms affecting the pharmacodynamics of antileukemic agents. They found that, among 130 children with high-risk disease, the glutathione *S*-transferase (*GSTM1*) non-null genotype had a higher risk of relapse, which was further increased by the thymidylate synthetase (*TYMS*) 3/3 genotype. Homozygosity for the triple-tandem repeat polymorphism of the thymidylate synthase gene has been associated with increased levels of the enzyme, and with inferior outcome in children with ALL in another study as well. Other polymorphisms of relevance in response to ALL therapy involve the methylenetetrahydrofolate reductase (*MTHFR*) and thiopurine methyltransferase (*TPMT*) gene. It is noteworthy that in some cases, polymorphisms cause increased sensitivity to drugs and may predict for a higher probability of side effects (including second cancers) as much as higher sensitivity and improved outcome. Interestingly, pharmacogenetics of bone marrow mesenchymal cells can also affect treatment outcome, for example high levels of asparagine synthetase can protect ALL cells from asparaginase treatment [70]. Most of these studies have been conducted in children with ALL and knowledge about pharmacokinetic variables and how they contribute to outcome in adult ALL remains sparse.

Minimal residual disease (MRD)

In children and adults relapse is thought to result from residual leukemia cells, which persist following achievement of a morphologic and cytogenetic remission, but remain undetectable by conventional methods such as microscopy and cytochemical stains. A number of sensitive techniques have been developed including multicolor flow cytometry and and polymerase chain reaction (PCR) assays. Detection of residual leukemia cells depends on identification of unique leukemia cell markers. For flow cytometry, aberrant expression of surface marker combinations can be followed, whereas for PCR, leukemia-specific fusions genes (e.g., *BCR-ABL, MLL-AF4, ETV6-RUNX1*) or patient-specific junctional regions of rearranged immunoglobulin and T-cell receptor genes constitute appropriate markers [71, 72].

Many studies in both children and adults have provided convincing evidence for the usefulness of MRD monitoring to assess relapse risk [73, 74]. High levels of MRD at the end of induction therapy, persistently high levels during consolidation and maintentance, and continuous increases of MRD levels at any point, are associated with a high risk of relapse [75]. Whereas more adults have higher levels of MRD at the completion of induction, and the relapse risk is higher even with low levels of MRD compared to children, continuous MRD assessment over several time-points has proved predictive for relapse in adult patients as well.

Assessment of MRD status has been included in a number of recent studies to decide about intensification of post-remission therapy. Several questions still remain: (1) What is a clinically relevant threshold of residual disease upon which clinical decisions should be based? (2) Which are the most appropriate time points to measure MRD following induction, and how do they change in the context of the specific treatment administered? (3) Does intervention based on a molecular relapse improve outcome, and if so, do response criteria need to be modifed to include molecular responses? and (4) How reproducible are MRD assays and how reliably can MRD data from different institutions be compared? In this respect some progress of standardization has been made through initiatives such as Europe Against Cancer (EAC) and BIOMED [76]. Finally, the conundrum remains that some patients with residual disease will never relapse, whereas not all molecular responders are safe from disease recurrence.

Salvage therapy

Prognosis of adult patients with relapsed ALL remains poor. In the MRC UKALLXII/ECOG 2993 study, overall survival at five years after relapse was only 7% [77]. Factors predicting better outcome (indicating five-year survival rates of 11–12%) included age younger than 20 years and remission durations of more than two years. Although there is no standard approach to salvage therapy, there is general consensus that allogeneic SCT should be offered in this situation. For patients who have achieved a second remission, long-term leukemia-free survival rates of 14 to 43% have been reported with subsequent SCT.

For many patients SCT is not an option because of lack of a suitable donor, comorbid conditions (e.g., infections, poor performance status), or uncontrollable disease. Most non-transplant salvage attempts are modeled after patterns familiar from front-line therapy. Direct comparisons of various regimens are difficult because of differences in patient characteristics, prior drug exposure and sensitivity, number of salvage attempts, variations in dose and schedule of agents, the use of SCT as consolidation in some patients, and not least because of the overall poor outcome.

Exploration of new agents for ALL therapy remains important [78]. Rituximab, a chimeric monoclonal antibody targeting the cell surface protein CD20, has been combined with chemotherapy to improve outcome in subsets of patients with ALL. The role of alemtuzumab, a humanized CD52-directed monoclonal antibody, in CD52-positive ALL and in combination with chemotherapy in aggressive T-lymphocytic malignancies is being explored. Other monoclonal antibodies are in earlier stages of their clinical assessment.

Clofarabine is a new generation purine nucleoside modeled after fludarabine and cladribine, but with a different mechanism of action and spectrum of activity [79]. In a phase II trial of clofarabine in 61 pediatric patients with relapsed or refractory ALL, 30% responded. Median remission duration for children who did not proceed to SCT was six weeks, but sustained remissions for up to 64 weeks have been reported in some patients. Clofarabine was approved by the FDA for children with ALL relapse

in December of 2004. Nelarabine is a soluble prodrug of 9-β-D-arabinofuranosylguanine (ara-G) with activity predominantly in relapsed T-lineage lymphoid malignancies and approved by the FDA for this indication in October 2005. Response rates of 33% and up to 41% have been achieved in a group of 121 children and 39 adults with relapsed T-lineage leukemia/lymphoma, respectively [80, 81]. Neurotoxicity is the major toxicity of nelarabine, which is both dose- and schedule-dependent. Of interest are other established compounds that have been modified to achieve more advantageous pharmacokinetic properties such as pegylated asparaginase, liposomal doxorubicin, or liposomal vincristine. Experience of 52 patients who have been treated with liposomal vincristine on two different studies demonstrated an overall response rate of 21% with another 23% of the patients achieving hematologic improvement [82]. A larger multicenter study of liposomal vincristine in ALL relapse is ongoing.

Disease subtypes

Ph-positive ALL

Historically, Ph-positive ALL had the worst survival rates with standard chemotherapy and, being much more frequent in adults than children, contributed to some degree to the overall worse prognosis of adult patients. It has long been assumed that chemotherapy alone is insufficient to cure Ph-positive ALL and SCT is required. In one of the largest prospective studies to date by the International ALL Trial Group, 167 patients with Ph-positive ALL received either a matched related SCT (n = 49), a matched unrelated donor transplant (n = 23), an autologous SCT (n = 7), or continued with chemotherapy alone (n = 77) [83]. Although the treatment-related mortality was higher with SCT (37% for matched sibling transplants, 43% for matched unrelated donor transplants, 14% with autologous SCT, 8% with chemotherapy), the risk of relapse at five years was lower with allogeneic SCT (29%) compared with autologous SCT/chemotherapy (81%). Likewise, the five-year survival probability was 43% with allogeneic SCT, and 19% with autologous SCT or chemotherapy. Experience with alternative stem cell sources (unrelated, haploidentical, umbilical cord) is more limited. Comparisons of antileukemic activity remain difficult due to the retrospective nature and small and heterogeneous patient populations in most studies.

Since the discovery of imatinib and several newer generation TKIs an array of new treatment possibilities in Ph-positive ALL have become available. Imatinib competitively binds to the ATP binding site of BCR-ABL and inhibits autoactivation of the oncoprotein as well as phosphorylation of downstream intracellular proteins. Imatinib has single agent activity in Ph-positive ALL with hematologic response rates ranging from 20 to 30%, but response durations are short; thus many investigators have combined imatinib with multiagent chemotherapy [84–87]. The group at MDACC combined imatinib with hyper-CVAD. Of the 54 patients with a median age of 51 years (range 17 to 84 years) treated, 93% achieved a complete remission with a median time to response of 21 days. The complete molecular response rate based on nested PCR was 52%. Survival at three years did not differ

depending on whether or not patients received a SCT (63% vs. 56%). Outcome was superior to hyper-CVAD alone: three-year overall survival rates were 55% versus 15% (p < .001) [84]. (Figure 14.3) There is a general consensus that imatinib is more effective when started early during induction and when given concurrently with and subsequent to induction and consolidation rather than alternating with chemotherapy [87].

Dasatinib and nilotinib are two second-generation TKIs, which are more potent than imatinib in *in vitro* models; they have activity against most imatinib-resistant kinase domain mutations. Both have shown efficacy in imatinib-resistant Ph-positive ALL [88, 89].

Mature B ALL (Burkitt's leukemia)

Mature B-cell ALL is a rare entity and predominates in children. The difference between the ALL variety and its lymphoma counterpart is mostly semantic. A diagnosis of ALL is made when the marrow blasts exceed 25% in the absence of significant extramedullary disease. Conventional ALL therapy is not

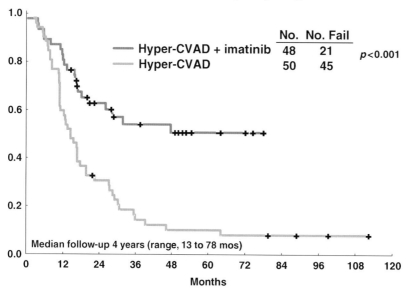

Figure 14.3 Survival in *de novo* Philadelphia chromosome positive ALL with hyper-CVAD and imatinib compared to historical data with hyper-CVAD alone.

successful. Only adaptation of short-course intensive therapy protocols has substantially improved prognosis of these patients. Complete remission rates now exceed 80%, with two-year DFS rates of 60 to 80%. Relapses are rare after the first year. Intensive early prophylactic intrathecal therapy in addition to intensive systemic administration of methotrexate and cytarabine, significantly reduced the systemic and CNS relapse rates [90, 91].

Thomas et al. combined hyper-CVAD with rituximab to treat 31 newly diagnosed patients with mature B-ALL or lymphoma and a median age of 46 years (29% older than 60 years) [90]. The overall CR rate was 86%. The three-year overall survival and disease-free survival rates were 89% and 88%, respectively.

Treatment of HIV-related mature B-cell ALL/lymphoma remains challenging [92, 93]. Short-course, intensive ALL protocols have proved more effective for these patients than conventional lymphoma therapies such as CHOP. Using the same regimen of hyper-CVAD with rituximab in combination with highly active antiretroviral treatment (HAART), a complete remission rate of 92% has been reported with nearly 50% of the patients living longer than two years from diagnosis.

Summary

Progress in the understanding of the biology of ALL and refinements of prognostic systems have led to increasingly sophisticated therapy. Patients with mature B-cell ALL do best with short-term dose-intensive therapies, whereas outcome in T-cell ALL has improved with the addition of cyclophosphamide and cytarabine. Treatment for Ph-positive ALL should include TKIs, ideally from the start and probably best maintained for years thereafter. The role of transplantation has been modified according to better and more predictable risk stratification. Transplantation should be considered in first remission in high-risk patients without prohibitively serious comorbidities, or any patients beyond a first remission.

The key to improving prognosis of ALL, especially for adult patients, lies in continuously defining the many subtypes of ALL. Elaboration of the biologic characteristics will lead to more accurate risk stratification. Treatment programs in ALL are complex and will continue to be. Although development of new drugs and agents is vital, to understand modes of action and pharmacokinetic properties of existing drugs and to know how to include new agents remains an ongoing challenge.

References

1 Jemal A, Siegel R, Ward E, et al. (2006) Cancer statistics. *CA Cancer J Clin* **56**:106–30.

2 Wartenberg D, Groves FD, Adelman AS. (2008) Acute lymphoblastic leukemia: Epidemiology and etiology. In Estey EH, Faderl S, Kantarjian H (eds.) *Acute Leukemias* (1st ed.), pp. 77–93. Springer: Berlin.

3 Kinlen LJ. (2004) Infections and immune factors in cancer: the role of epidemiology. *Oncogene* **23**:6341–8.

4 Greaves MF. (2006) Infection, immune responses and etiology of childhood leukaemia. *Bat Rev Cancer* **6**:193–203.

5 Greaves MF, Maia AT, Wiemels, JL, Ford AM. (2003) Leukemia in twins: lessons in natural history. *Blood* **102**:2321–33.

6 Wiemels JL, Cazzaniga G, Daniotti M. (1999) Prenatal origin of acute lymphoblastic leukaemia in children. *Lancet* **354**:1499–1503.

7 Hong D, Gupta R, Ancliff P, et al. (2008) Initiating and cancer-propagating cells in *TEL-AML1*-associated childhood leukemia. *Science* **319**:336–9.

8 Pui CH, Robison L, Look AT. (2008) Acute lymphoblastic leukemia. *Lancet* **371**:1030–43.

9 Kantarjian HM, Thomas D, O'Brien S, et al. (2004) Long-term follow-up results of hyperfractionated cyclophosphamide, vincristine, doxorubicin, and dexamethasone (Hyper-CVAD), a dose-intensive regimen, in adult acute lymphocytic leukemia. *Cancer* **101**:2788–801.

10 Bennett JM, Catovsky D, Daniel MT, et al. (1981) The morphologic classification of acute lymphoblastic leukemia: concordance among observers and clinical correlations. *Br J Haematol* **47**:553–61.

11 Jaffe ES, Harris NL, Stein H, Vardiman JW (eds.) (2000) *World Health Organization Classification of Tumours: Pathology and Genetics of Tumours of Haematopoietic and Lymphoid Tissues*, pp. 111–87. IARC: Lyon.

12 Huh YO, Ibrahim S. (2000) Immunophenotypes in adult acute lymphoblastic leukemia. Role of flow cytometry in diagnosis and monitoring of disease. *Hematol Oncol Clin North Am* **14**:1251–65.

13 Pui C-H, Sandlund JT, Pei D, et al. (2003) Results of therapy for acute lymphoblastic leukemia. *JAMA* **290**:2001–7.

14 Coustan-Smith E, Mullighan CG, Onciu M, et al. (2009) A new biologic subtype of very high risk acute lymphoblastic leukemia. *Lancet Oncol* **10**:47–156.

15 Faderl S, Kantarjian HM, Talpaz M, Estrov Z. (1998) Clinical significance of cytogenetic abnormalities in adult acute lymphoblastic leukemia. *Blood* **91**: 3995–4019.

16 Wetzler M, Dodge RK, Mrozek K, et al. (1999) Prospective karyotype analysis in adult acute lymphoblastic leukemia: The Cancer and Leukemia Group B experience. *Blood* **93**:383.

17 Mancini M, Scappaticci D, Cimino G, et al. (2005) A comprehensive genetic classification of adult acute lymphoblastic leukemia (ALL): analysis of the GIMEMA 0496 protocol. *Blood* **105**:3434–41.

18 Pui CH, Williams WE. (2006) Treatment of acute lymphoblastic leukemia. *N Engl J Med* **354**:166–78.

19 Moorman AV, Harrison CJ, Buck GA, et al. (2007) Karyotype is an independent prognostic factor in adult acute lymphoblastic leukemia (ALL): analysis of cytogenetic data from patients treated on the Medical Research Council (MRC) UKALLXII/Eastern Cooperative Oncology Group (ECOG) 2993 trial. *Blood* **109**:3189–97.

20 Faderl S, Albitar M. (2000) Insights into the biologic and molecular abnormalities in adult acute lymphocytic leukemia. *Hematol Oncol Clin North Am* **14**:1267–88.

21 Pui CH, Relling MV, Downing Jr., (2004) Acute lymphoblastic leukemia. *N Engl J Med* **350**:1535–48.

22 Pieters R, Schrappe M, De Lorenzo, et al. (2007) A treatment protocol for infants younger than 1 year with acute lymphoblastic leukemia (Interfant-99): an observational study and a multicentre randomized trial. *Lancet* **370**:240–50.

23 Gleissner B, Goekbuget N, Rieder H, et al. (2005) CD10⁻ pre-B acute lymphoblastic leukemia (ALL) is a distinct high-risk subgroup of adult ALL associated with a high frequency of *MLL* aberrations: results of the German Multicenter Trials for Adult ALL (GMALL). *Blood* **106**:4054–6.

24 Pui C-H, Gaynon PS, Boyett JM, et al. (2002) Outcome of treatment in childhood acute lymphoblastic leukaemia with rearrangements of the 11q23 chromosomal region. *Lancet* **359**:1909–15.

25 Wolfraim LA, Fernandez TM, Mamura M, et al. (2004) Loss of Smad3 in acute T-cell lymphoblastic leukemia. *N Engl J Med* **351**:552–9.

26 Breit S, Stanulla M, Flohr T, et al. (2006) Activating *NOTCH1* mutations predict favorable early treatment response and long-term outcome in childhood precursor T-cell lymphoblastic leukemia. *Blood* **108**:1151–7.

27 Mullighan CG, Goorha S, Radtke I, et al. (2007) Genome-wide analysis of genetic alterations in acute lymphoblastic leukaemia. *Nature* **446**:758–64.

28 Fine BM, Stanulla M, Schrappe M, et al. (2004) Gene expression patterns associated with recurrent chromosomal translocations in acute lymphoblastic leukemia. *Blood* **103**:1043–9.

29 Holleman A, Cheok MH, den Boer ML, et al. (2004) Gene-expression patterns in drug-resistant acute lymphoblastic leukemia cells and response to treatment. *N Engl J Med* **351**:533–42.

30 Issa JP. (2007) DNA methylation as a therapeutic target in cancer. *Clin Cancer Res* **13**:1634–7.

31 Garcia-Manero G, Daniel J, Smith TL, et al. (2002) DNA methylation of multiple promoter-associated CpG islands in adult acute lymphoblastic leukemia. *Clin Cancer Res* **8**:2217–24.

32 George P, Hernandez K, Hustu O, et al. (1968) A study of "total therapy" of acute lymphocytic leukemia in children. *J Pediatr* **72**:399–408.

33 Asnafi V, Buzyn A, Thomas X, et al. (2005) Impact of TCR status and genotype on outcome in adult T-cell acute lymphoblastic leukemia, a LALA-94 study. *Blood* **105**:3072–8.

34 Baldus CD, Burmeister T, Martus P, et al. (2006) High expression of the ETS transcription factor ERG predicts adverse outcome in acute T-lymphoblastic leukemia in adults. *J Clin Oncol* **24**:4714–20.

35 Baldus CD, Martus P, Burmeister T, et al. (2007) Low ERG and BAALC expression identifies a new subgroup of adult acute T-lymphoblastic leukemia with a highly favorable outcome. *J Clin Oncol* **25**:3739–45.

36 Brüggemann M, Raff T, Flohr T, et al. (2006) Clinical significance of minimal residual disease quantification in adult patients with standard-risk acute lymphoblastic leukemia. *Blood* **107**:1116–23.

37 Holowiecki H, Krawczyk-Kulis M, Giebel S, et al. (2007) Minimal residual disease status is the most important predictive factor in adults with acute lymphoblastic leukemia. Prospective, multicenter PALG 4-2002 MRD Study. *Blood* **110**:830.

38 Faderl S, Thall PF, Kantarjian HM, Estrov Z. (2002) Time to platelet recovery predicts outcome of patients with de novo acute lymphoblastic leukaemia who have achieved a complete remission. *Br J Haematol* **117**:869–74.

39 Casale F, D'Angelo V, Addeo R, et al. (2004) P-glycoprotein 170 expression and function as an adverse independent prognostic factor in childhood acute lymphoblastic leukemia. *Oncol Rep* **12**:1201–7.

40 Aplenc R, Lange B. (2004) Pharmacogenetic determinants of outcome in acute lymphoblast leukaemia. *Br J Haematol* **125**:421–34.

41 Kantarjian HM. (2001) Adult acute lymphoblastic leukemia. Future research directions. *Hematol Oncol Clin North Am* **15**:207–11.

42 Nachman JB, Sather HN, Sensel MG, et al. (1998) Augmented post-induction therapy for children with high-risk acute lymphoblastic leukemia and a slow response to initial therapy. *N Engl J Med* **338**:1663–71.

43 Pession A, Valsecchi MG, Masera G, et al. (2005) Long-term results of a randomized trial on extended use of high-dose L-asparaginase for standard risk acute lymphoblastic leukemia. *J Clin Oncol* **28**:7161–7.

44 Graham ML. (2003) Pegaspargase: a review of clinical studies. *Advanced Drug Delivery Reviews* **55**:1293–302.

45 Wetzler M, Sanford BL, Kurtzberg J, et al. (2007) Effective asparagine depletion with pegylated asparaginase results in improved outcomes in adult acute lymphoblastic leukemia, Cancer and Leukemia Group B Study 9511. *Blood* **109**:4164–7.

46 Douer D, Yampolsky H, Cohen LJ, et al. (2007) Pharmacodynamics and safety of intravenous pegaspargase during remission induction in adults aged 55 years or younger with newly diagnosed acute lymphoblastic leukemia. *Blood* **109**:2744–50.

47 Hoelzer D, Ludwig W-D, Eckhard E, et al. (1996) Improved outcome in adult B-cell acute lymphoblastic leukemia *Blood* **87**:495–508.

48 Thomas DA, O'Brien S, Jorgensen JL, et al. (2009) Prognostic significance of CD20 expression in adults with de novo precursor B-lineage acute lymphoblastic leukemia. *Blood* **113**:6330–7.

49 Jeha S, Behm F, Pei D, et al. (2006) Prognostic significance of CD20 expression in childhood B-cell precursor acute lymphoblastic leukemia. *Blood* **108**:3302–4.

50 Attias D, Weitzman S. (2008) The efficacy of rituximab in high-grade pediatric B-cell lymphoma/leukemia, a review of available evidence. *Curr Opin Pediatr* **20**:17–22.

51 Thomas DA, Faderl S, O'Brien S, et al. (2006) Chemoimmunotherapy with hyper-CVAD plus rituximab for the treatment of adult Burkitt and Burkitt-type lymphoma or acute lymphoblastic leukemia. *Cancer* **106**:1569–80.

52 Bostrom BC, Sensel MR, *Sather HN et al.* (2003) Dexamethasone versus prednisone and daily oral versus weekly intravenous mercaptopurine for patients with standard-risk acute lymphoblastic leukemia, a report from the Children's Cancer Group. *Blood* **101**:3809–17.

53 Mitchell CD, Richards SM, Kinsey SE, et al. (2005) Benefit of dexamethasone compared with prednisolone for childhood acute lymphoblastic leukaemia, results of the UK Medical Research Council ALL97 randomized trial. *Br J Haematol* **129**:734–45.

54 Igarashi S, Manabe A, Ohara A, et al. (2005) No advantage of dexamethasone over prednisolone for the outcome of standard- and intermediate-risk childhood acute lymphoblastic leukemia in the Tokyo Children's Cancer Study Group L95-14 protocol. *J Clin Oncol* **23**:6489–98.

55 Smith TJ, Khatcheressian J, Lyman GH, et al. (2006) 2006 update of recommendations for the use of white blood cell growth factors, an evidence-based clinical practice guideline. *J Clin Oncol* **24**:3187–205.

56 Ottmann OG, Hoelzer D, Gracien E, et al. (1995) Concomitant granulocyte colony-stimulating factor and induction chemoradiotherapy in adult acute lymphoblastic leukemia, a randomized phase III trial. *Blood* **86**:444–50.

57 Geissler K, Koller E, Hubmann E, et al. (1997) Granulocyte colony-stimulating factor as an adjunct to induction chemotherapy for adult acute lymphoblastic leukemia: a randomized phase III study. *Blood* **90**:590–6.

58 Larson RA, Dodge RK, Linker CA, et al. (1998) A randomized controlled trial of filgrastim during remission induction and consolidation chemotherapy for adults with acute lymphoblastic leukemia, CALGB study 9111. *Blood* **92**:1556–64.

59 Pui C-H, Bouett JM, Hughes WT, et al. (2007) Human granulocyte colony-stimulating factor after induction

chemotherapy in children with acute lymphoblastic leukemia. *N Eng J Med* **336**:1781–7.

60 Thomas X, Boiron J-M, Huguet F, et al. (2004) Outcome of treatment in adults with acute lymphoblastic leukemia, analysis of the LALA-94 trial. *J Clin Oncol* **22**:4075–86.

61 Hunault M, Harousseau J-L, Delain M, et al. (2004) Better outcome of adult acute lymphoblastic leukemia after early genoidentical allogenetic bone marrow transplantation (BMT) than after late high-dose therapy and autologous BMT: a GOELAMS trial. *Blood* **104**:3028–37.

62 Goldstone AH, Richards SM, Lazarus HM, et al. (2008) In adults with standard-risk acute lymphoblastic leukemia (ALL) the greatest benefit is achieved from a matched sibling allogeneic transplant in first complete remission (CR) and an autologous transplant is less effective than conventional consolidation/maintenance chemotherapy in all patients: final results of the International ALL Trial (MRC UKALLXII/ECOG E2993). *Blood* 111: 1827–33.

63 Bishop MR, Logan Br, Gandham S. et al. (2008) Long-term outcomes of adults with acute lymphoblastic leukemia after autologous or unrelated donor bone marrow transplantation: a comparative analysis by the National Marrow Donor Program and Center for International Blood and Marrow Transplant Research. *Bone Marrow Transplant* **18**:41: 635–42.

64 Pui CH. (2006) Central nervous system disease in acute lymphoblastic leukemia, prophylaxis and treatment. *Hematology (Am Soc Hematol Educ Program)* **2006**:142–6.

65 Lazarus HM, Richards SM, Chopra R, et al. (2006) Central nervous system involvement in adult acute lymphoblastic leukemia at diagnosis, results from the international ALL trial MRC UKALLXII/ECOG E2993. *Blood* **108**:465–72.

66 Matloub Y, Lindemulder S, Gaynon PS, et al. (2006) Intrathecal triple therapy decreases central nervous system relapse but fails to improve event-free survival when compared to intrathecal methotrexate: results of the Children's Cancer Group (CCG) 1952 study for standard-risk acute lymphoblastic leukemia. A report from the Children's Oncology Group. *Blood* **108**:1165–73.

67 Pui CH, Relling MV, Evans WE. (2003) Role of pharmacogenomics and pharmacodynamics in the treatment of acute lymphoblastic leukemia. *Best Pract Res Clin Haematol* **15**:741–56.

68 Evans WE, Relling MV. (2004) Moving towards individualized medicine with pharmacogenomics. *Nature* **429**:464–8.

69 Rocha JCC, Cheng C, Liu W, et al. (2005) Pharmacogenetics of outcome in children with acute lymphoblastic leukemia. *Blood* **105**:4752–8.

70 Iwamoto S, Mihara K, Downing JR, et al. (2007) Mesenchymal cells regulate the response of acute lymphoblastic leukemias to asparaginase. *J Clin Invest* **117**:1049–57.

71 Stanulla M, Cario G, Meissner B, et al. (2007) Integrating molecular information into treatment of childhood acute lymphoblastic leukemia – a perspective from the BFM Study Group. *Blood Cells Mol Dis* **39**:160–3.

72 Diguiseppe JA. (2007) Acute lymphoblastic leukemia, diagnosis and detection of minimal residual disease following therapy. *Clin Lab Med* **27**:533–49.

73 Raff T, Gökbuget N, Lüschen S, et al. (2007) Molecular relapse in adults standard-risk ALL patients detected by prospective MRD monitoring during and after maintenance treatment, data from the GMALL 06/99 and 07/03 trials. *Blood* **109**:910–15.

74 Cavé H, van der Werf J, Suciu S, et al. (1998) Clinical significance of minimal residual disease in childhood acute lymphoblastic leukemia. *N Engl J Med* **339**:591–8.

75 Pui C-H, Campana D, Evans WE. (2001) Childhood acute lymphoblastic leukemia, current status and future perspectives. *Lancet Oncol* **2**:597–607.

76 Gabert J, Beillard E, van der Velden VH, et al. (2003) Standardization and quality control studies of "real-time" quantitative reverse transcriptase polymerase chain reaction of fusion gene transcripts for residual disease detection in leukemia: A Europe Against Cancer program. *Leukemia* **17**:2318–57.

77 Fielding AK, Richards SM, Chopra R, et al. (2007) Outcome of 609 adults after relapse of acute lymphoblastic leukemia (ALL) an MRC UKALLXII/ECOG 2993 study. *Blood* **109**:944–50.

78 Pui C-H, Jeha S. (2007) New therapeutic strategies for the treatment of acute lymphoblastic leukaemia. *Nat Rev Drug Discov* **6**:149–65.

79 Jeha S, Kantarjian H. (2007) Clofarabine for the treatment of acute lymphoblastic leukemia. *Expert Rev Anticancer Ther* **7**:113–18.

80 Berg SL, Blaney SM, Devidas M, et al. (2005) Phase II study of nelarabine (compound 506U78) in children and young adults with refractory T-cell malignancies: a

report from the Children's Oncology Group. *J Clin Oncol* **23**:3376–82.

81 DeAngelo DJ, Yu D, Johnson JL, et al. (2007) Nelarabine induces complete remissions in adults with relapsed or refractory T-lineage acute lymphoblastic leukemia or lymphoblastic lymphoma: Cancer and Leukemia Group B study 19801. *Blood* **109**:5136–42.

82 Thomas DA, Kantarjian HM, Stock W, et al. (2007) Safety and efficacy of Marqibo (vincristine sulfate liposomes injection, OPTISOME™) for the treatment of adults with relapsed or refractory acute lymphocytic leukemia (ALL). *Blood* **110**:263.

83 Fielding AK, Rowe JM, Richards SM, et al. (2009) Prospective outcome data on 267 unselected adult patients with Philadelphia chromosome-positive acute lymphoblastic leukemia confirms superiority of allogeneic transplantation over chemotherapy in the pre-imatinib era, results from the International ALL Trial MRC UKALLXII/ECOG2993. *Blood* **113**:4489–96.

84 Thomas DA, Kantarjian HM, Ravandi F, et al. (2007) Long-term follow-up after frontline therapy with the Hyper-CVAD and imatinib mesylate regimen in adults with Philadelphia (Ph) positive acute lymphocytic leukemia (ALL). *Blood* **110**:10.

85 Yanada M, Takeuchi J, Sugiura I, et al. (2006) High complete remission rate and promising outcome by combination of imatinib and chemotherapy for newly diagnosed BCR-ABL-positive acute lymphoblastic leukemia, a phase II study by the Japan Adult Leukemia Study Group. *J Clin Oncol* **20**:460–6.

86 de Labarthe A, Rousselot P, Huguet-Rigal F, et al. (2007) Imatinib combined with induction or consolidation chemotherapy in patients with de novo Philadelphia chromosome-positive acute lymphoblastic leukemia, results of the GRAAPH-2003 study. *Blood* **109**:1408–13.

87 Wassmann B, Pfeifer H, Goekbuget N, et al. (2006) Alternating versus concurrent schedules of imatinib and chemotherapy as front-line therapy for Philadelphia-positive acute lymphoblastic leukemia (Ph+ ALL). *Blood* **108**:1469–77.

88 Ottmann O, Dombret H, Martinelli G, et al. (2007) Dasatinib induces rapid hematologic and cytogenetic responses in adult patients with Philadelphia chromosome positive acute lymphoblastic leukemia with resistance or intolerance to imatinib, interim results of a phase II study. *Blood* **110**: 2309–15.

89 Kantarjian H, Giles F, Wunderle L, et al. (2007) Nilotinib in imatinib-resistant CML and Philadelphia chromosome-positive ALL. *N Engl J Med* **354**: 2542–51.

90 Di Nicola M, Carlo-Stella C, Mariotti J, et al. (2004) High response rate and manageable toxicity with an intensive, short-term chemotherapy programme for Burkitt's lymphoma in adults. *Br J Haematol* **126**:815–20.

91 Thomas DA, Faderl S, O'Brien S, et al. (2006) Chemoimmunotherapy with hyper-CVAD plus rituximab for the treatment of adult Burkitt and Burkitt-type lymphoma or acute lymphoblastic leukemia. *Cancer* **106**:1569–80.

92 Cortes J, Thomas D, Rios A, et al. (2002) Hyperfractionated cyclosphosphamide, vincristine, doxorubicin, and dexamethasone and highly active antiretroviral therapy for patients with acquired immunodeficiency syndrome-related Burkitt lymphoma/leukemia. *Cancer* **94**:1492–9.

93 Hoffmann C, Wolf E, Wyen C, et al. (2006) AIDS-associated Burkitt or Burkitt-like lymphoma, short intensive polychemotherapy is feasible and effective. *Leuk Lymphoma* **47**:1872–80.

CHAPTER 15

Large Granular Lymphocyte Leukemia

Xin Liu and Thomas P. Loughran, Jr.
Penn State Hershey Cancer Institute, Penn State University, Hershey, PA, USA

Introduction

LGL leukemia was initially described as a clonal expansion of malignant LGL marked by increased numbers of circulating LGL and infiltration in marrow, liver, spleen, and lung [1]. Both T-cell and NK-cell LGL leukemia subtypes can manifest as indolent or aggressive disorders, distinguished by sustained LGL, clonal origin of leukemic LGL, and characteristic immunophenotype. Indolent T-cell LGL leukemia has a favorable prognosis and it is the most common subtype, representing approximately 85% of all cases diagnosed in Western countries. This entity is more frequently diagnosed in older individuals. The aggressive type of NK-cell LGL leukemia typically occurs in younger individuals, with median age at diagnosis of 39 years and with a higher prevalence in Asia and South America. This subtype usually is a very aggressive and fatal illness with poor outcome [2].

Normal LGL development and maturation

LGL represent 10–15% of the total peripheral blood mononuclear cells in normal adults and are characterized by abundant cytoplasm with azurophilic granules and eccentric nuclei (Plate 15.1) [3, 4]. The majority of these cells (85%) are derived from the CD3$^-$ natural killer (NK)-cell lineage, and a minority is derived from the CD3$^+$ T-cell lineage (15%). T-cell LGL is post-thymic, antigen-primed,

cytotoxic CD8$^+$ T-lymphocytes. NK-cell LGL belongs to the innate immune system with the capability of non-major histocompatibility complex (MHC)-restricted cytotoxicity.

T-lymphocytes originate from hematopoietic stem cells in the bone marrow, then migrate to the thymus, where they undergo somatic rearrangements of the V, D, and J elements of their T-cell receptor (TCR) genes [5]. The TCR is a heterodimer consisting of two polypeptides, which are usually α and β chains. A minority of T-cells express a related receptor composed of γ and δ chains [6]. During T-cell maturation in the thymus, after the developing T-cell has rearranged the β and α chain, it expresses both CD4 and CD8 cell surface markers. The interaction of TCRs with antigens bound to MHC molecules causes the double-positive T-cell to develop into either the CD4$^+$ helper T-cell or cytotoxic CD8$^+$ T-cell (CTL) lineage [7, 8]. The primary role of CTL is to eradicate viral infections. This involves the synthesis of lytic molecules such as perforin and granzymes, which cause direct lysis and death of target cells infected by viruses [9]. In addition, effector cytotoxic T-cells express Fas ligand, a member of the tumor necrosis factor receptor family. Fas ligand can bind Fas, which broadly distributes in normal tissue, and initiate apoptosis in the target cell through this pathway [10].

NK cells, like T-cells, develop from a common precursor. NK cells share many properties with cytotoxic T-cells, including the expression of lytic molecules, the expression of CD8, and the expression of NK receptors and Fas ligand [11, 12]. However,

Advances in Malignant Hematology, First Edition. Edited by Hussain I. Saba and Ghulam J. Mufti. © 2011 Blackwell Publishing Ltd.
Published 2011 by Blackwell Publishing Ltd.

NK-cell LGL do not express CD3 or have rearranged TCR. Without the prior antigen stimulation and clonal expansion, NK cells kill target cells, including viral-infected cells and tumor cells, in a non-MHC-restricted fashion [13].

Etiology and pathogenesis

The etiology of LGL leukemia has not been elucidated. Chronic activation by exogenous antigens such as virus or endogenous autoantigen has been implicated as an initial stimulus leading to an expansion of LGL [14, 15]. It has also been suggested that T-cell LGL leukemia could represent an autoimmune disorder caused by chronic antigenic stimulation, leading to extreme expansion of only one clone of CD8$^+$ cytotoxic T-cells [16, 17]. An association of T-cell LGL leukemia with several different autoimmune conditions supports this hypothesis. Seroindeterminate reactivity against HTLV-I envelope epitope BA21 has been described in approximately 50% of patients with CD3$^+$ and 73% of patients with CD3$^-$ LGL leukemia [18]. Human T-cell leukemia virus II (HTLV-II) sequences have been detected in two patients with indolent T-cell LGL leukemia [19, 20]. However, most patients with LGL leukemia are not infected with prototypical members of the HTLV family, including HTLV-I, HTLV-II, or bovine leukemia virus (BLV) [21, 22]. Epstein-Barr virus (EBV) is implicated in the pathogenesis of aggressive NK-cell leukemia [23].

Of note, LGL leukemia often does not behave as a typical malignancy; instead, leukemic LGL appear to retain some physiologic properties of normal LGL and resemble an exaggerated response to a putative immunodominant antigen [17]. One of the hypotheses postulates that the initial events in the pathogenesis of LGL leukemia may involve an underlying immune response to exogenous antigens, for example, sustained viral infections.

The malignant T-cell LGL population, which arises from a single cell, has the same TCR gene rearrangement pattern. Southern blotting and polymerase chain reaction (PCR) are the two methods most commonly used for confirmation of clonality [24]. A panel of monoclonal antibodies can also be used against the variable domain of the β chain as a new clonality technique in T-cell malignancies [25]. In addition, the antigen-specific portion of the T-cell receptor (TCR), the variable β (VB)-chain complementarity-determining region 3 (CDR3), can serve as a molecular signature of a T-cell clone in T-cell LGL leukemia patients [17]. By contrast, leukemic NK LGL has TCR genes in a non-rearranged germ-line position. In the past, cytogenetic abnormalities and clonality studies based on the X-chromosome inactivation pattern (XCIP) were the only methods available for confirmation of the clonal origin of the NK-cell population [26]. Aberrant expression of a new class of NK-cell receptors, killer cell immunoglobulin-like receptors (KIRs), has been reported in some patients with LGL leukemia [27]. Specifically, leukemic NK LGL cells had high levels of activating receptors and a loss of inhibitory receptors [28], suggesting a potential use of KIR expression as clonality markers for NK-cell LGL leukemia.

Clinical manifestations

T-cell LGL leukemia are found in the elderly, with an average age at initial examination of approximately 60 years [29, 30]. Males and females are equally affected. The average time from appearance of symptoms to diagnosis of T-cell LGL leukemia is 37 months [31]. A median survival of more than 10 years is typical for patients with T-cell LGL leukemia [32, 33]. Approximately two-thirds of the patients with indolent T-cell LGL leukemia develop fever, recurrent bacterial infections, fatigue, and weight loss during the course of their disease, while another one-third of the patients are asymptomatic. Mild to moderate splenomegaly is seen in 20–60% of patients [29, 30]. Diffuse infiltration of red splenic pulp with preservation of sinuses and white pulp cords is characteristic of T-cell LGL leukemia [34]. Hepatomegaly is less common, with an incidence of <20% [29–31]. Pulmonary artery hypertension (PAH) is an unusual presentation of this disease [35].

Laboratory investigation demonstrates that neutropenia, often severe, is the most common feature and present in 60 to 85% of symptomatic patients at initial examination [3, 33, 36]. Up to 50% of patients are diagnosed based on the detection of asymptomatic cytopenias with an absolute neutrophil count of less than 500/μl [33]. Bone marrow infiltration or hypersplenism is not responsible for the degree of cytopenias; whereas dysregulated Fas/Fas ligand pathways as well as elevated level of cytokines such as tumor necrosis factor α and interferon γ, which are known to inhibit erythropoeisis, may contribute to cytopenias in LGL leukemia [29,30, 37].

Anemia with a hemoglobin level <11 g/dL is found in approximately half of the patients with T-cell LGL leukemia [36]. Approximately 20% of patients require transfusions. Coombs-positive autoimmune hemolytic anemia is diagnosed only in rare cases [38]. Pure red cell aplasia (PRCA) characterized by hypoproliferative anemia and the absence of mature erythroid precursors in normocellular marrow occurs in 8–19% of patients [36]. Thrombocytopenia ($<150 \times 10^9$/L) presents in about 20% of patients [3]. However, severe thrombocytopenia requiring transfusions is rare [32]. The peripheral blood smear displays a large number of granular lymphocytes in most patients (Plate 15.1), although patients usually have either a normal absolute lymphocyte count or a mild lymphocytosis [36]. The number of circulating granular lymphocytes is elevated, with an absolute LGL count greater than 2000/μl (normal range 200–400/μl) [29, 39]. However, 25–30% patients with T-cell LGL leukemia may display a smaller population (<500/μl) of circulating LGL [3]. In these cases, a bone marrow biopsy/aspirate may be helpful for evaluation. Examination of the marrow may reveal discrete interstitial and sinusoidal infiltration with clonal populations of LGL [30]. Notably, the number of circulating LGL or degree of bone marrow infiltration often does not correlate with cytopenias or systemic symptoms [2, 40].

Most LGL leukemia patients have a normal karyotype while less than 10% exhibit karyotypic abnormalities, including deletions of chromosomes 6 and 5q, trisomies of chromosomes 3, 8 and 14, and inversions of 12p and 14q [1, 41, 42].

Similar to chronic T-cell LGL leukemia, chronic NK-cell LGL leukemia is a disease with an indolent course. Forty percent of patients with this disease present with cytopenias, cutaneous vasculitis, peripheral neuropathy, and splenomegaly, while 60% are asymptomatic [43].

Both aggressive NK-cell and aggressive T-cell LGL leukemia are acute illnesses, with B symptoms including fever, night sweats, and weight loss, and lymphocytosis, hepatosplenomegaly, lymphadenopathy, severe anemia and thrombocytopenia, and hemophagocytic syndrome. Death can be measured in days to weeks following onset [36, 44, 45].

LGL leukemia cells have a mature T- or NK-cell immunophenotype [36]. CD57 is a 110-kDa glycoprotein found on NK cells and activated effector CD8$^+$ T-cells. It is a characteristic marker for LGL leukemia [46]. The NK-cell marker CD56 is often detected in aggressive NK-cell LGL leukemia [47]. Therefore, patients with T-cell LGL leukemia present with a typical phenotype of CD3$^+$/CD8$^+$/CD57$^+$/CD16$^+$/TCRαβ [43]. Furthermore, weaker expression of CD5 and/or CD7 can be useful in differentiating the malignant T-cell LGL population from normal T-lymphocytes [48]. Uncommon immunophenotypic variants such as CD3$^+$/CD4$^+$/CD8$^+$/CD57$^+$/TCRαβ, CD3$^+$/CD4$^+$/CD8$^-$/CD57$^+$/TCRαβ, and CD3$^+$/CD4$^-$/CD8$^-$/CD57$^+$/TCRγδ might also be associated with indolent T-cell LGL leukemia [30, 36]. In contrast, patients with NK-cell LGL leukemia, no matter whether chronic or acute form, display a distinct immunophenotype of CD3$^-$/CD16$^+$/CD56$^+$ [43].

The most common autoimmune disorder associated with T-cell LGL leukemia is rheumatoid arthritis, which manifests in about 25–33% of patients [29, 30]. A significant proportion of patients (40–60%) with T-cell LGL leukemia present with immunologic abnormalities, including seropositivity for rheumatoid factor, elevated levels of β2-microglobulin or lactate dehydrogenase, antinuclear antibodies, polyclonal hypergammaglobulinemia, circulating immune complexes, antineutrophil and antiplatelet antibodies, as well as positive direct antiglobulin test (anti-Coombs) [3, 30, 36]. A rare autoimmune clinical entity, Felty syndrome, which is characterized by the triad of rheumatoid arthritis, neutropenia, and splenomegaly, closely resembles T-cell LGL leukemia with rheumatoid arthritis [49]. Both diseases have a significantly higher frequency of expression of the HLA-DR4 haplotype than matched healthy controls, suggesting that they may represent a clinical spectrum of the identical disorder [49]. Case reports of patients with LGL leukemia associated with Sjögren's syndrome, systemic lupus erythematosis, and Hashimoto's thyroiditis have also been reported [3, 50, 51]. Myelodysplasia (MDS) and paroxysmal nocturnal hemoglobinuria (PNH) often overlap with T-cell LGL leukemia, which may favor an immune basis for this disease [52, 53].

Diagnosis

Diagnosis of T-cell LGL leukemia is based on the following criteria: (1) $CD3^+$ and $CD57^+$ cells >300/µl or $CD8^+$ cells >650/µl in peripheral blood, and (2) evidence for clonal T-cell receptor gene rearrangement based on positive flow cytometric analysis, T-cell receptor TCR-Vβ chain PCR, or by Southern blot analysis (Figure 15.1).

Diagnosis of NK-cell LGL leukemia is based on the following criteria: $CD56^+$ or $CD16^+$ NK cells

>750/µl in peripheral blood lasting for more than six months (Figure 15.1).

Differential diagnosis

Non-leukemic LGL proliferations may be transient or chronic. Transient (<6 months) and chronic (>6 month) expansions of LGL are two benign conditions in the spectrum of disorders of LGL [30]. Transient reactive populations of LGL have been detected in patients with viral infections, autoimmune diseases, and malignancies, post-splenectomy patients and in patients after allogeneic bone marrow transplantation and solid organ transplantation [50, 54–60]. Additionally, patients with chronic myeloid leukemia (CML) and Philadelphia chromosome (Ph) + acute lymphoblastic leukemia (ALL), also manifest a marked expansion of LGL after receiving dasatinib, a broad-spectrum tyrosine kinase inhibitor [61]. The reactive LGL are either polyclonal with expression of the T-cell ($CD3^+$) immunophenotype or NK cells. Of note, the TCR clonality *per se* is not a necessary indication of malignancy [58]. Thus,

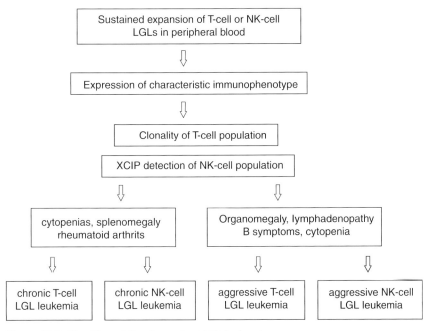

Figure 15.1 Algorithm of the diagnosis of LGL leukemia.

clinical follow-up is important before assigning a diagnosis of LGL leukemia to individuals with LGL features and a monoclonal CD8$^+$ lymphocytosis. LGL count usually normalizes spontaneously or within six months with treatment of the underlying condition. In the absence of a clonal marker, clinical presentation is the most important factor available for the differential diagnosis of these two conditions. Patients with chronic expansion of NK-cell LGL and systemic symptoms or infiltration of the bone marrow, spleen, or liver could be appropriately classified in the category of chronic NK-cell leukemia. Asymptomatic patients might be given a diagnosis of benign chronic NK-cell lymphocytosis.

Therapeutic algorithm

The majority of patients with T-cell or NK-cell LGL leukemia have a clinically indolent course with a median survival time over 10 years. The most common indications for therapy include recurrent infections, severe neutropenia, symptomatic anemia or thrombocytopenia, symptomatic splenomegaly, and severe B symptoms [30]. First-line, single-agent therapy with low-dose methotrexate (10 mg/m^2 per week), cyclophosphamide (50–100mg orally daily), and cyclosporine A (5–10 mg/kg per day) can control symptoms and cytopenias in approximately 50–60% of patients [62–64], but this approach is not curative. Although 60–70% of patients with T-cell LGL leukemia require therapy during the course of their disease, 30% of patients need only watchful follow-up [36, 65]. It is recommended that four months of treatment be given before a decision is made to change to an alternative agent because of no response. Responders usually require indefinite therapy to prevent relapses; however, durable remission can be achieved with only a short course of treatment in some patients. Therapy with low-dose methotrexate can control both LGL leukemia and rheumatoid arthritis [36, 66]. Cyclosporine A is sometimes used as an initial therapy; however, toxicities of long-term treatment are greater in older patients as compared to the side effects of methotrexate or cyclophosphamide. After the achievement of the best response, the dose of cyclosporine

A should be tapered down to obtain the lowest effective maintenance dose [43]. Corticosteroids appear less effective than methotrexate, cyclosporine A, or cyclophosphamide as a monotherapy. However, their combination with these drugs may improve B symptoms and hematologic features [30]. Hematopoietic growth factors (G-CSF, GM-CSF) have also been used successfully as first-line monotherapy for neutropenia or as a supportive treatment together with immunosuppressive therapy [67, 68]. It is noteworthy that correction of cytopenias with therapy may be achieved without alleviation of the clone, which often is resistant to therapy. On the other hand, complete normalization of the neutrophil count is not necessary for improvement of symptoms [69, 70].

Patients who fail first-line therapy may benefit from second-line monotherapy with nucleoside analogs, including fludarabine, 2'-deoxycoformycine, and 2-chloroxyadenosine [71, 72]. The high intensity of CD52 expression on malignant LGL supports the potential efficacy of utilization of targeted therapy with a humanized anti-CD52 antibody (alemtuzumab) in T-LGL leukemia patients [73]. CD2 is expressed on mature T-cells and NK cells. Siplizumab, a humanized monoclonal antibody to CD2, was being tested in phase I clinical trials in patients with relapsed/refractory CD2$^+$ T-cell lymphoma/leukemia, including T-cell LGL leukemia. However, the trial was terminated when EBV-related lymphoproliferative disease was identified in patients following siplizumab therapy, probably due to the ability of siplizumab to deplete both T- and NK cells without affecting B-cells in these patients [74]. Improvement of pulmonary artery pressure and erythroid differentiation was reported in a phase II clinical trial using a farnesyltransferase inhibitor, tipifarnib, in an NK-cell LGL leukemia patient with pulmonary artery hypertension (PAH) [75]. This study was based on work showing that constitutively activated Ras is a survival pathway in leukemic LGL [76]. Both autologous and allogeneic hematopoietic stem cell transplantation have been rarely used in younger patients with T-cell LGL leukemia refractory to conventional therapy [77].

Notably, the involvement of the spleen occurs in many patients with T-cell LGL leukemia [29, 30].

Clinically, splenectomy can be beneficial in relieving the gastrointestinal-related symptoms of nausea, early satiety, and pain related to splenomegaly [78]. In addition, removal of enlarged spleens could have a favorable impact on refractory and symptomatic cytopenias [38, 78, 79]. However, the procedure is not curative.

Aggressive T-cell/NK-cell LGL leukemia usually has a rapid progressive course and is refractory to conventional chemotherapy, with a median survival time of two months. Induction chemotherapy with an intensive ALL-like regimen followed by allogeneic SCT has been used with curative intent in a limited number of cases [78].

Conclusions

Since the discovery of LGL leukemia more than 20 years ago, the progress in laboratory and clinical research has led to a further understanding of the biology and prognosis of this rare disease. LGL leukemia is not a single disease but rather a diverse spectrum of clinical conditions, in regard to etiologies, biologic behaviors, and prognoses. Patients with indolent T-cell or NK-cell LGL leukemia often have a favorable prognosis, with median survival time over 10 years. By contrast, patients with aggressive T-cell or NK-cell LGL leukemia have poor outcomes. Both indolent and aggressive conditions can present with similar cell morphologies and immunophenotypes; therefore, the differential clinical presentations between two groups are the most important prognostic predictors for patients. The elucidation of the etiopathogenesis and characterization of new specific molecular targets in this disease will facilitate the development of more advanced and less toxic therapeutics for LGL leukemia patients.

References

1 Loughran TP, Jr., Kadin ME, Starkebaum G, et al. (1985) Leukemia of large granular lymphocytes: association with clonal chromosomal abnormalities and autoimmune neutropenia, thrombocytopenia, and hemolytic anemia. *Ann Intern Med* **102**:169–75.

2 Alekshun TJ, Sokol L. (2007) Diseases of large granular lymphocytes. *Cancer Control* **14**:141–50.

3 Lamy T, Loughran TP. (1998) Large granular lymphocyte leukemia. *Cancer Control* **5**:25–33.

4 Timonen T, Ortaldo JR, Herberman RB. (1981) Characteristics of human large granular lymphocytes and relationship to natural killer and K cells. *J Exp Med* **153**:569–82.

5 Alt FW, Blackwell TK, DePinho RA, Reth MG, Yancopoulos GD. (1986) Regulation of genome rearrangement events during lymphocyte differentiation. *Immunol Rev* **89**:5–30.

6 Strominger JL. (1989) Developmental biology of T cell receptors. *Science* **244**:943–50.

7 Kingston R, Jenkinson EJ, Owen JJ. (1985) A single stem cell can recolonize an embryonic thymus, producing phenotypically distinct T-cell populations. *Nature* **317**:811–3.

8 Kisielow P, Leiserson W, Von Boehmer H. (1984) Differentiation of thymocytes in fetal organ culture: analysis of phenotypic changes accompanying the appearance of cytolytic and interleukin 2-producing cells. *J Immunol* **133**:1117–23.

9 Spaeny-Dekking EH, Hanna WL, Wolbink AM, et al. (1998) Extracellular granzymes A and B in humans: detection of native species during CTL responses in vitro and in vivo. *J Immuno* **160**:3610–6.

10 Hanabuchi S, Koyanagi M, Kawasaki A, et al. (1994) Fas and its ligand in a general mechanism of T-cell-mediated cytotoxicity. *Proc Natl Acad Sci USA* **91**:4930–4.

11 Clement MV, Haddad P, Soulie A, et al. (1990) Involvement of granzyme B and perforin gene expression in the lytic potential of human natural killer cells. *Res Immunol* **141**:477–89.

12 Arase H, Arase N, Saito T. (1995) Fas-mediated cytotoxicity by freshly isolated natural killer cells. *J Exp Med* **181**:1235–8.

13 Moretta L, Bottino C, Pende D, et al. (2002) Human natural killer cells: their origin, receptors and function. *Eur J Immunol* **32**:1205–11.

14 Zambello R, Trentin L, Facco M, et al. (1995) Analysis of the T cell receptor in the lymphoproliferative disease of granular lymphocytes: superantigen activation of clonal CD3$^+$ granular lymphocytes. *Cancer Res* **55**:6140–5

15 Epling-Burnette PK, Loughran TP, Jr., (2003) Survival signals in leukemic large granular lymphocytes. *Semin Hematol* **40**:213–20.

16 O'Keefe CL, Plasilova M, Wlodarski M, et al. (2004) Molecular analysis of TCR clonotypes in LGL: a clonal model for polyclonal responses. *J Immunol* **172**:1960–9.

17 Wlodarski MW, O'Keefe C, Howe EC, et al. (2005) Pathologic clonal cytotoxic T-cell responses: nonrandom nature of the T-cell-receptor restriction in large granular lymphocyte leukemia. *Blood* **106**:2769–80.

18 Loughran TP, Jr., Hadlock KG, Yang Q, et al. (1997) Seroreactivity to an envelope protein of human T-cell leukemia/lymphoma virus in patients with CD3⁻ (natural killer) lymphoproliferative disease of granular lymphocytes. *Blood* **90**:1977–81.

19 Loughran TP, Jr., Coyle T, Sherman MP, et al. (1992) Detection of human T-cell leukemia/lymphoma virus, type II, in a patient with large granular lymphocyte leukemia. *Blood* **80**:1116–9.

20 Loughran TP, Jr., Hadlock KG, Perzova R, et al. (1998) Epitope mapping of HTLV envelope seroreactivity in LGL leukaemia. *Br J Haematol* **101**:318–24.

21 Perzova RN, Loughran TP, Dube S, et al. (2000) Lack of BLV and PTLV DNA sequences in the majority of patients with large granular lymphocyte leukaemia. *Br J Haematol* **109**:64–70.

22 Pawson R, Schulz TF, Matutes E, Catovsky D. (1997) The human T-cell lymphotropic viruses types I/II are not involved in T prolymphocytic leukemia and large granular lymphocytic leukaemia. *Leukemia* **11**:1305–11.

23 Hart DN, Baker BW, Inglis MJ, et al. (1992) Epstein-Barr viral DNA in acute large granular lymphocyte (natural killer) leukemic cells. *Blood* **79**:2116–23.

24 Ryan DK, Alexander HD, Morris TC. (1997) Routine diagnosis of large granular lymphocytic leukaemia by Southern blot and polymerase chain reaction analysis of clonal T cell receptor gene rearrangement. *Mol Pathol* **50**:77–81.

25 van den Beemd R, Boor PP, van Lochem EG, et al. (2000) Flow cytometric analysis of the Vbeta repertoire in healthy controls. *Cytometry* **40**:336–45.

26 Wong KF, Zhang YM, Chan JK. (1999) Cytogenetic abnormalities in natural killer cell lymphoma/leukaemia – is there a consistent pattern? *Leuk Lymphoma* **34**:241–50.

27 Zambello R, Semenzato G. (2003) Natural killer receptors in patients with lymphoproliferative diseases of granular lymphocytes. *Semin Hematol* **40**:201–12.

28 Epling-Burnette PK, Painter JS, Chaurasia P, et al. (2004) Dysregulated NK receptor expression in patients with lymphoproliferative disease of granular lymphocytes. *Blood* **103**:3431–9.

29 Lamy T, Loughran TP, Jr., (1999) Current concepts: large granular lymphocyte leukemia. *Blood Rev* **13**:230–40.

30 Lamy T, Loughran TP, Jr., (2003) Clinical features of large granular lymphocyte leukemia. *Semin Hematol* **40**:185–95.

31 Herling M, Khoury JD, Washington LT, et al. (2004) A systematic approach to diagnosis of mature T-cell leukemias reveals heterogeneity among WHO categories. *Blood* **104**:328–35.

32 Dhodapkar MV, Li CY, Lust JA, Tefferi A, Phyliky RL. (1994) Clinical spectrum of clonal proliferations of T-large granular lymphocytes: a T-cell clonopathy of undetermined significance? *Blood* **84**:1620–7.

33 Rose MG, Berliner N. (2004) T-cell large granular lymphocyte leukemia and related disorders. *Oncologist* **9**:247–58.

34 Osuji N, Matutes E, Catovsky D, Lampert I, Wotherspoon A. (2005) Histopathology of the spleen in T-cell large granular lymphocyte leukemia and T-cell prolymphocytic leukemia: a comparative review. *Am J Surg Pathol* **29**:935–41.

35 Rossoff LJ, Genovese J, Coleman M, Dantzker DR. (1997) Primary pulmonary hypertension in a patient with CD8/T-cell large granulocyte leukemia: amelioration by cladribine therapy. *Chest* **112**:551–3.

36 Loughran TP, Jr., (1993) Clonal diseases of large granular lymphocytes. *Blood* **82**:1–14.

37 Liu JH, Wei S, Lamy T, et al. (2000) Chronic neutropenia mediated by fas ligand. *Blood* **95**:3219–22.

38 Gentile TC, Loughran TP, Jr., (1996) Resolution of autoimmune hemolytic anemia following splenectomy in CD3⁺ large granular lymphocyte leukemia. *Leuk Lymphoma* **23**:405–8.

39 Loughran TP, Jr., Starkebaum G. (1987) Clinical features in large granular lymphocytic leukemia. *Blood* **69**:1786.

40 Sood R, Stewart CC, Aplan PD, et al. (1998) Neutropenia associated with T-cell large granular lymphocyte leukemia: long-term response to cyclosporine therapy despite persistence of abnormal cells. *Blood* **91**:3372–8.

41 Oshimi K, Yamada O, Kaneko T, et al. (1993) Laboratory findings and clinical courses of 33 patients with granular lymphocyte-proliferative disorders. *Leukemia* **7**:782–8.

42 Wong KF, Chan JC, Liu HS, Man C, Kwong YL. (2002) Chromosomal abnormalities in T-cell large granular lymphocyte leukaemia: report of two cases and review of the literature. *Br J Haematol* **116**:598–600.

43 Sokol L, Loughran TP, Jr., (2006) Large granular lymphocyte leukemia. *Oncologist* **11**:263–73.

44 Ruskova A, Thula R, Chan G. (2004) Aggressive natural killer-cell leukemia: report of five cases and review of the literature. *Leuk Lymphoma* **45**:2427–38.

45 Gentile TC, Uner AH, Hutchison RE, et al. (1994) CD3$^+$, CD56$^+$ aggressive variant of large granular lymphocyte leukemia. *Blood* **84**:2315–21.

46 Melenhorst JJ, Brummendorf TH, Kirby M, Lansdorp PM, Barrett AJ. (2001) CD8$^+$ T cells in large granular lymphocyte leukemia are not defective in activation- and replication-related apoptosis. *Leuk Res* **25**:699–708.

47 Loughran TP, Jr., (1999) CD56$^+$ hematologic malignancies. *Leuk Res* **23**:675–6.

48 Lundell R, Hartung L, Hill S, Perkins SL, Bahler DW. (2005) T-cell large granular lymphocyte leukemias have multiple phenotypic abnormalities involving pan-T-cell antigens and receptors for MHC molecules. *Am J Clin Pathol* **124**:937–46.

49 Starkebaum G, Loughran TP, Jr., Gaur LK, Davis P, Nepom BS. (1997) Immunogenetic similarities between patients with Felty's syndrome and those with clonal expansions of large granular lymphocytes in rheumatoid arthritis. *Arthritis Rheum* **40**:624–6.

50 Sampalo Lainz A, Lopez-Gomez M, Jimenez-Alonso J. (1995) Proliferation of large granular lymphocytes in patients with systemic lupus erythematosus. *Rev Clin Esp* **195**:373–9.

51 Molad Y, Okon E, Stark P, Prokocimer M. (2001) Sjogren's syndrome associated T cell large granular lymphocyte leukemia: a possible common etiopathogenesis. *J Rheumatol* **28**:2551–2.

52 O'Malley DP. (2007) T-cell large granular leukemia and related proliferations. *Am J Clin Pathol* **127**:850–9.

53 Huh YO, Medeiros LJ, Ravandi F, et al. (2009) T-cell large granular lymphocyte leukemia associated with myelodysplastic syndrome: a clinicopathologic study of nine cases. *Am J Clin Pathol* **131**:347–56.

54 Gorochov G, Debre P, Leblond V, et al. (1994) Oligoclonal expansion of CD8$^+$ CD57$^+$ T cells with restricted T-cell receptor beta chain variability after bone marrow transplantation. *Blood* **83**:587–95.

55 Halwani F, Guttmann RD, Ste-Croix H, Prud'homme GJ. (1992) Identification of natural suppressor cells in long-term renal allograft recipients. *Transplantation* **54**:973–7.

56 Smith PR, Cavenagh JD, Milne T, et al. (2000) Benign monoclonal expansion of CD8+ lymphocytes in HIV infection. *J Clin Pathol* **53**:177–81.

57 Schwab R, Szabo P, Manavalan JS, et al. (1997) Expanded CD4$^+$ and CD8$^+$ T cell clones in elderly humans. *J Immunol* **158**:4493–9.

58 Rossi D, Franceschetti S, Capello D, et al. (2007) Transient monoclonal expansion of CD8$^+$/CD57$^+$ T-cell large granular lymphocytes after primary cytomegalovirus infection. *Am J Hematol* **82**:1103–5.

59 Mohty M, Faucher C, Vey N, et al. (2002) Features of large granular lymphocytes (LGL) expansion following allogeneic stem cell transplantation: a long-term analysis. *Leukemia* **16**:2129–33.

60 Kelemen E, Gergely P, Lehoczky D, et al. (1986) Permanent large granular lymphocytosis in the blood of splenectomized individuals without concomitant increase of in vitro natural killer cell cytotoxicity. *Clin Exp Immunol* **63**:696–702.

61 Mustjoki S, Ekblom M, Arstila TP, et al. (2009) Clonal expansion of T/NK-cells during tyrosine kinase inhibitor dasatinib therapy. *Leukemia* **23**:1398–405.

62 Loughran TP, Jr., Kidd PG, Starkebaum G. (1994) Treatment of large granular lymphocyte leukemia with oral low-dose methotrexate. *Blood* **84**:2164–70.

63 Battiwalla M, Melenhorst J, Saunthararajah Y, et al. (2003) HLA-DR4 predicts haematological response to cyclosporine in T-large granular lymphocyte lymphoproliferative disorders. *Br J Haematol* **123**:449–53.

64 Matrai Z, Lelkes G, Milosevits J, Paldine HP, Pecze K. (1997) T-cell large granular lymphocytic leukemia associated with pure red cell aplasia, successfully treated with cyclophosphamide. *Orv Hetil* **138**:2075–80.

65 Pandolfi F, Loughran TP, Jr., Starkebaum G, et al. (1990) Clinical course and prognosis of the lymphoproliferative disease of granular lymphocytes. *A multicenter study. Cancer* **65**:341–8.

66 Bowman SJ, Sivakumaran M, Snowden N, et al. (1994) The large granular lymphocyte syndrome with rheumatoid arthritis. Immunogenetic evidence for a broader definition of Felty's syndrome. *Arthritis Rheum* **37**:1326–30.

67 Lamy T, LePrise PY, Amiot L, et al. (1995) Response to granulocyte-macrophage colony-stimulating factor (GM-CSF) but not to G-CSF in a case of agranulocytosis

associated with large granular lymphocyte (LGL) leukemia. *Blood* **85**:3352–3.

68 Weide R, Heymanns J, Koppler H, et al. (1994) Successful treatment of neutropenia in T-LGL leukemia (T gamma-lymphocytosis) with granulocyte colony-stimulating factor. *Ann Hematol* **69**:117–9.

69 Gabor EP, Mishalani S, Lee S. (1996) Rapid response to cyclosporine therapy and sustained remission in large granular lymphocyte leukemia. *Blood* **87**: 1199–200.

70 Bargetzi MJ, Wortelboer M, Pabst T, et al. (1996) Severe neutropenia in T-large granular lymphocyte leukemia corrected by intensive immunosuppression. *Ann Hematol* **73**:149–51.

71 Mercieca J, Matutes E, Dearden C, MacLennan K, Catovsky D. (1994) The role of pentostatin in the treatment of T-cell malignancies: analysis of response rate in 145 patients according to disease subtype. *J Clin Oncol* **12**:2588–93.

72 Sternberg A, Eagleton H, Pillai N, et al. (2003) Neutropenia and anaemia associated with T-cell large granular lymphocyte leukaemia responds to fludarabine with minimal toxicity. *Br J Haematol* **120**:699–701.

73 Osuji N, Del Giudice I, Matutes E, et al. (2005) CD52 expression in T-cell large granular lymphocyte leukemia – implications for treatment with alemtuzumab. *Leuk Lymphoma* **46**:723–7.

74 O'Mahony D, Morris JC, Stetler-Stevenson M, et al. (2009) EBV-related lymphoproliferative disease complicating therapy with the anti-CD2 monoclonal antibody, siplizumab, in patients with T-cell malignancies. *Clin Cancer Res* **15**:2514–22.

75 Epling-Burnette PK, Sokol L, Chen X, et al. (2008) Clinical improvement by farnesyltransferase inhibition in NK large granular lymphocyte leukemia associated with imbalanced NK receptor signaling. *Blood* **112**:4694–8.

76 Epling-Burnette PK, Bai F, Wei S, et al. (2004) ERK couples chronic survival of NK cells to constitutively activated Ras in lymphoproliferative disease of granular lymphocytes (LDGL). *Oncogene* **23**:9220–9.

77 Toze CL, Shepherd JD, Connors JM, et al. (2000) Allogeneic bone marrow transplantation for low-grade lymphoma and chronic lymphocytic leukemia. *Bone Marrow Transplant* **25**:605–12.

78 Subbiah V, Viny AD, Rosenblatt S, et al. (2008) Outcomes of splenectomy in T-cell large granular lymphocyte leukemia with splenomegaly and cytopenia. *Exp Hematol* **36**:1078–83.

79 Coad JE, Matutes E, Catovsky D. (1993) Splenectomy in lymphoproliferative disorders: a report on 70 cases and review of the literature. *Leuk Lymphoma* **10**:245–64.

CHAPTER 16

Hairy Cell Leukemia

Kevin T. Kim, Darren S. Sigal and Alan Saven
Division of Hematology/Oncology, Scripps Clinic, La Jolla, CA, USA

Introduction and history

Hairy cell leukemia (HCL) is a rare chronic B-cell lymphoproliferative disorder, characterized by pancytopenia, splenomegaly, and the presence of hairy cells in the peripheral blood, bone marrow, and spleen. Ewald first used the term "leukämische reticuloendotheliose" in a case of acute leukemia that later became associated with HCL [1]. In 1958, Bouroncle et al. distinguished leukemic reticuloendotheliosis as a separate hematologic and pathologic entity [2]. In 1966, Schrek et al. coined the term "hairy cells" to describe abnormal mononuclear cells with irregular cytoplasmic projections [3].

Epidemiology

HCL accounts for 2–3% of all adult leukemias in the US, with an annual incidence of 600 new patients. HCL typically afflicts middle-aged Caucasian males, with a male to female ratio ranging from 4:1 to 7:1. HCL has not been reported in children, and it presents at a median age of 52 years. There is a higher reported incidence in Ashkenazi Jews [4].

Etiology/pathogenesis

There is no known cause for HCL. A higher incidence of HCL has been reported in patients with prior exposure to organic solvents or radiation [4, 5]. There are conflicting studies regarding the possible etiologic role of Epstein-Barr in the development of HCL [6, 7].

Reports of familial HCL demonstrate that some cases are associated with specific HLA haplotypes [8, 9]. However, there are no common HLA haplotypes detected in random cases of patients with HCL [8]. Clonal chromosomal abnormalities occur in up to 67% of HCL patients, with chromosome 5 being most commonly involved [10, 11]. Other abnormalities described include monoallelic deletions and mutations of p53 and BCL-6 [12–14].

The normal counterpart of the hairy cell remains speculative. However, immunologic studies in HCL demonstrate that hairy cells are of B-lymphocyte lineage. Hairy cells possess Ig heavy and light chain gene rearrangements, which occur during B-cell development [15]. Hairy cells also express the pan B-cell antigens CD19, CD20, and CD22 [16]. In more than 90% of cases, hairy cells display light chain restricted surface Ig [17, 18].

Ontologically, hairy cells are between activated mature B-cells and plasma cells. HCL, along with other B-cell neoplasms such as large cell and immunoblastic lymphomas that represent later stages in B-cell development, show an elevated expression of the c-src proto-oncogene. In contrast, neoplastic cells of early and intermediate stages of B-cell maturation (acute lymphoblastic leukemia/lymphoma and chronic lymphocytic leukemia) show low levels of c-src proto-oncogene expression [19]. Hairy cells strongly express the plasma cell-associated antigen (PCA-1) and respond to known triggers of B-cell activation and differentiation, further supporting

Advances in Malignant Hematology, First Edition. Edited by Hussain I. Saba and Ghulam J. Mufti. © 2011 Blackwell Publishing Ltd.
Published 2011 by Blackwell Publishing Ltd.

the hypothesis that hairy cells represent late-stage, pre-plasma cell B-lymphocytes [20].

Initial comparisons suggested that the monocytoid B-lymphocyte was the normal counterpart to the hairy cell. Hairy cells in the involved spleen have an immunophenotype that is virtually identical to that of reactive and neoplastic monocytoid B-lymphocytes [21]. Another study comparing 42 cases of HCL and 24 cases of monocytoid B-cell lymphoma showed similar immunophenotypes, with CD103 being expressed more commonly in HCL [22].

There are key differences between monocytoid cells and hairy cells that argue against a direct relationship. First, monocytoid cells are tartrate-resistant acid phosphatase (TRAP) negative and express IgM heavy chain, in contrast to hairy cells which are TRAP positive and predominantly express IgG [23]. Second, histological and immunohistochemical analyses of reactive monocytoid B-cells point to monocytoid B-cell lymphoma as their neoplastic counterpart [24], making it unlikely to have two distinct neoplasms arising from one normal cell type. Finally, the lack of Tac and PCA-1 on monocytoid B-cells, and the absence of anti-muscle-specific actin on hairy cells, are important differences [21, 22].

Therefore, despite evidence linking the monocytoid B-cells and hairy cells, the true cell of origin of HCL remains elusive. Machii et al. proposed the term "hairy B-cell lymphoproliferative disorder" – characterized in four patients by the presence of splenomegaly, lymphocytosis, abnormal lymphocytes with round nuclei, abundant pale cytoplasm and long microvilli on their surfaces, and polyclonal overexpression of IgG – as the benign counterpart of HCL [25].

Clinical features

HCL typically has an insidious onset, characterized by pancytopenia, splenomegaly, and circulating hairy cells. Twenty-six percent of patients were reported to be asymptomatic when HCL was diagnosed on routine blood tests or as an incidental finding on physical examination [26]. Another 27% of patients reportedly presented with fatigue

and weakness [26, 27]. Atypical infections with organisms such as Mycobacterium kansasii, Aspergillus, Pneumocystis carinii, and Cryptococcus neoformans, as well as typical infections were the initial symptom in 29% of patients [26, 27]. Sixteen percent of patients had bleeding complications, usually presenting with ecchymoses or petechiae [26, 27]. Severe hemorrhage is rare and is likely to be a result of platelet dysfunction and low platelet counts [26]. In 25% of patients, symptomatic splenomegaly with abdominal fullness and early satiety was present at diagnosis. Splenomegaly is an almost universal finding in HCL and its absence should point to another diagnosis [12]. Hepatomegaly is found in 50% of patients [2, 26, 27]. Clinically significant lymphadenopathy is rare.

HCL patients have an increased risk of both hematologic and solid organ malignancies. These malignancies tend to be aggressive with median survivals of 8.8 months [28].

Laboratory features

Peripheral blood

Pancytopenia was reported to be present in 79% of patients in a study of 211 patients by Flandrin et al. [26]. Neutropenia is seen in over 75% of patients and monocytopenia is common. Anemia is normochromic and normocytic. The percentage of circulating hairy cells varies widely from 0 to 99%. Hairy cells are mononuclear cells with an eccentric or central nucleus. The nucleus may be round or bilobed. The cells have a variable amount of blue-gray cytoplasm and characteristic projections on the surface (see Plate 16.1).

Bone marrow

The classic "fried egg" appearance results from the abundant hairy cell cytoplasm separating the monotonous nuclei, which are round to oval, or spindle-shaped (see Plate 16.2). Hairy cell infiltration of the marrow may be focal or diffuse. Marrow aspiration may be difficult or impossible due to the insoluble fibronectin matrix laid down by the hairy cells [12, 29].

Spleen, liver, and lymph nodes

Splenomegaly is found in 90% of patients. Grossly the spleen has a dark red, smooth surface. Cut sections reveal "red cell lakes" or pseudosinuses, which are blood-filled sinuses lined by hairy cells and filled with erythrocytes and leukocytes [27, 30]. Microscopic examination shows the hairy cells filling the red pulp cords and sinuses, and displacing the white pulp, which is normally rich in T- and B-lymphocytes.

Massive hepatomegaly is rare. Mild to moderate enlargement is found in 50% of patients. Hairy cells infiltrate the sinusoids and portal tracts, and rarely involve the liver parenchyma. There is usually no disruption of the liver architecture.

Lymphadenopathy is generally clinically insignificant but is found in up to 35% of patients. Bulky internal lymphadenopathy can occur. Lymph nodes may be focally or diffusely involved by the hairy cells.

Cytochemistry

Hairy cell cytoplasm stains strongly for TRAP due to the presence of isoenzyme 5 acid phosphatase, which confers tartrate resistance [31]. TRAP stain is not very sensitive since highly variable percentages of hairy cells may be TRAP positive [32]. It has also been found that TRAP positivity is seen in CLL, Hodgkin lymphoma, normal B-lymphocytes, and even myeloid cells [33].

Immunophenotype

Hairy cells express the pan B-cell antigens CD19, CD20, CD22, and HLA-DR [16, 34, 35]. Co-expression of CD11c, CD25, and CD103 is virtually diagnostic of HCL (see Figure 16.1). CD103 has the

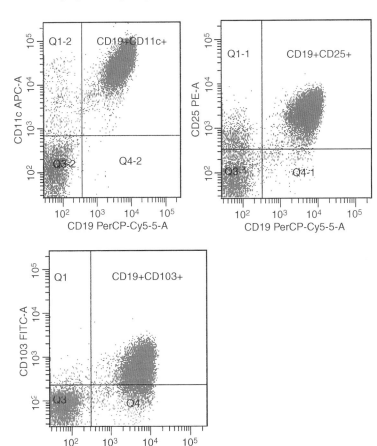

Figure 16.1 The characteristic immunophenotypic profile of hairy cell leukemia with expression of CD11c (bright), CD25, and CD103.

highest sensitivity and specificity for HCL [36]. Twenty-six percent of cases show weak expression of CD10 and 5% of cases demonstrate weak expression of CD5 [16]. Flow cytometry is able to detect hairy cells present in less than 1% of peripheral blood lymphocytes.

Immunohistochemistry

Routine fixation and processing of bone marrow biopsy specimens destroys the majority of antigens used in detecting circulating hairy cells found in the peripheral blood [37]. However, L26 (CD20 antibody) and DBA.44 can be used to stain hairy cells in paraffin sections of bone marrow [22, 38]. They are fixative-resistant monoclonal antibodies that are sensitive, but not specific, for hairy cells.

Differential diagnosis (see Table 16.1)

Splenic lymphoma with villous lymphocytes (SLVL) is a marginal zone lymphoma that presents with splenomegaly and cytopenias. Patients frequently have an absolute lymphocytosis and an elevated monoclonal protein. SLVL cells express CD11c and CD25, but rarely CD103 [39, 40]. These cells are TRAP negative. In contrast to hairy cells that have circumferential cytoplasmic projections, projections on SLVL cells are more polar.

B-cell prolymphocytic leukemia (PLL) presents with splenomegaly and extreme lymphocytosis with a median lymphocyte count of 350×10^9/L [41]. Anemia and thrombocytopenia are common findings. PLL cells have a centrally located nucleus with condensed chromatin and a large nucleolus [32].

Table 16.1 Hairy cell leukemia differential diagnosis

	HCL	HCL-variant	Splenic lymphoma with villous lymphocytes	B-prolymphocytic leukemia
Morphology				
Cytoplasmic projections	Circumferential serrated border and small villi	Broad-based long projections	Small, polar villi	Circumferential small, thin-based diffuse villi
Nucleus	Eccentric or central ± mall nucleolus	Central ± small nucleolus	± prominent nucleoli	Central with large, single nucleolus
TRAP	Strong	Weak	Weak	Weak
Monocytopenia	Yes	No	No	No
Lymphocytosis at presentation	No	Yes	Usually yes	Yes
Flow cytometry				
CD22	Strong	Strong	Strong	Strong
CD11c	Strong	Strong	Weak	Strong
CD25	Strong	Absent	Weak	Absent
CD103	Strong	Weak	Absent	Absent

HCL-variant is a rare disorder that shares features of HCL and PLL. Patients present with splenomegaly and an elevated WBC. Monocytopenia and neutropenia are invariably absent [42, 43]. HCL-variant cells morphologically resemble PLL cells and have cytoplasmic projections. They express CD11c but usually not CD25 and have variable TRAP staining [43, 44]. HCL-variant has a more aggressive course and generally does not respond as well to typical HCL therapies [43, 45].

Treatment

Indications for treatment

Treatment for HCL is appropriate if significant neutropenia (neutrophil count $<1.0 \times 10^9$/L), anemia (Hgb < 10 g/dL) and/or thrombocytopenia (platelet count $<100 \times 10^9$/L) is present, or if a patient has recurrent infections or symptomatic splenomegaly [46]. Otherwise, watchful waiting is indicated since the early institution of treatment confers no advantage in terms of response or survival. If treatment is warranted, therapeutic options include splenectomy, interferon, pentostatin, cladribine, rituximab, and the experimental immunotoxin BL22 (see Tables 16.2 and 16.3).

Treatments of historical interest
Splenectomy

The therapeutic value of splenectomy in HCL has been well recognized since the description of HCL as a distinct entity. Catovsky described 28 patients with HCL and cytopenias involving two or more cell lines who had undergone splenectomy [32]. Sixty-one percent of the patients achieved a complete remission (CR), defined as Hgb >11 g/dL, neutrophil count $>1.0 \times 10^9$/L and platelet count $>100 \times 10^9$/L, with an overall response rate of 93%. Achieving CR

Table 16.2 Initial purine analog treatments

Treatment	Dose	CR	PR	ORR	OS
Pentostatin					
Spiers [59]	5 mg/m^2 IV on d 1-2 Q 2 wks	59%	37%	96%	all alive at >1 to >375 days
Kraut [60]	4 mg/m^2 IV Q 2 wks	87%	4%	91%	NR
Cassileth [61]	5 mg/m^2 IV on d 1-2 Q 2 wks	64%	20%	84%	all alive at 31–60 mos
Grever [62]	4 mg/m^2 IV Q 2 wks	76%	3%	79%	median OS not reached at 57 mos
Flinn [63]	4 mg/m^2 IV Q 2 wks	NR	NR	NR	90% at 5 yrs
Else [64]	4 mg/m^2 IV Q wk $\times$ 4 then Q 2 wks	81%	15%	96%	96% at 10 yrs
Cladribine					
Saven [46]	0.085–0.1 mg/kg/d IV $\times$ 7 d	91%	7%	98%	96% at 48 mos
Hoffman [66]	0.1 mg/kg/d IV $\times$ 7 d	76%	24%	100%	95% at 55 mos
Tallman [67]	0.1 mg/kg/d IV $\times$ 7 d	80%	18%	98%	86% at 4 yrs
Goodman [68]	0.1 mg/kg/d IV $\times$ 7 d	95%	5%	100%	97% at 108 mos
Chadha [69]	0.1 mg/kg/d IV $\times$ 7 d	79%	21%	100%	87% at 12 yrs

Table 16.3 Treatment at relapse

Treatment	Author	Dose	CR	PR	ORR
Cladribine					
	Goodman [68]	0.1 mg/m^2/d IV × 7 d	75%	8%	83%
	Chadha [69]	0.1 mg/m^2/d IV × 7 d	52%	30%	82%
Pentostatin					
	Saven [46]	NR	43%	43%	86%
Rituximab					
	Hagberg [74]	375 mg/m^2 IV Q wk × 4	55%	9%	64%
	Nieva [75]	375 mg/m^2 IV Q wk × 4	13%	13%	26%
	Thomas [76]	375 mg/m^2 IV Q wk × 8	53%	27%	80%
BL22					
	Kreitman [77]	0.2 to 0.4 mg Q 3wk × 16	69%	12%	81%

appeared to be important in that all patients in PR relapsed, whereas only half of patients in CR relapsed with a longer interval to relapse. Golomb et al. described 65 patients with HCL who underwent splenectomy and showed a 65% overall response rate and a 68% five-year OS [47]. Interestingly, response to splenectomy did not correlate with spleen weight. Acutely ill HCL patients with severe infections were successfully treated with splenectomy, achieving a rapid neutrophil increment [48]. In a large retrospective study, patients with HCL who had splenectomy had a statistically significantly longer OS compared to patients who had not undergone splenectomy (median survival not reached at 96 months and 20 months, respectively) [49]. Splenectomy is now principally of historic interest only, given the dramatic effectiveness of systemic treatments in HCL.

Interferon alpha

Quesada et al. first described the efficacy of interferon alpha (IFN) in seven patients with HCL [50]. The exact mechanism of action is unknown, but it exerts a potent antiproliferative effect on lymphoma cell lines *in vitro*, and it may induce differentiation of malignant cells [50]. IFN is generally used in HCL patients with active infections where purine analogs are contraindicated because of immunosuppression. There are two formulations of IFN, 2a and 2b, which are identical except at amino acid 23. IFN alpha 2a is given as 3 million units daily for six months then three times weekly for another six months. IFN alpha 2b is given as 2 million units three times weekly for 12 months. Although CR is rare, PR is achieved in 57 to 70% [51–54]. Some reported lower response rates in splenectomized patients whereas others reported no differences [51, 53]. IFN therapy can maintain responses during treatment, but relapses occur once therapy is discontinued. Golomb et al. demonstrated that duration of IFN therapy does not influence the clinical course after treatment is discontinued, and retreatment with IFN at relapse is just as effective as the initial treatment with IFN [55]. IFN is not used as primary treatment in HCL because of the vast superiority of purine analogs in the treatment of HCL.

Newer treatments

Pentostatin

Spiers and Parekh first reported the use of pentostatin in two patients with HCL and observed resolution of splenomegaly and pancytopenia within four weeks of treatment [56]. Pentostatin (deoxycoformycin) is a natural product of *streptomyces antibioticus*, and it is a tight binding, irreversible inhibitor of adenosine deaminase (ADA). ADA is an enzyme that catalyzes the deamination of adenosine to inosine and deoxyadenosine to deoxyinosine. Accumulation of deoxyadenosine triphosphate as the result of ADA inhibition induces DNA strand breaks and lymphocytotoxicity. Congenital deficiency of ADA results in the disease "Severe Combined Immunodeficiency Disorder" (SCID). Similarly, the therapeutic administration of pentostatin to inhibit ADA results in potent immunodeficiency. There is a profound decrease in all lymphocyte subpopulations with T-cells being more affected than B-cells or NK cells [57, 58]. CD4+ cells rapidly decrease to low levels, usually <100/μL and persist at low levels during the treatment period and for up to one year after discontinuation of therapy [57]. There is an accompanying loss of immune function with peripheral blood cells showing a decreased ability to respond to mitogens (phytohemagglutinin and concanavalin A) and alloantigens [57].

Spiers et al. treated 27 HCL patients with pentostatin at 5 mg/m^2 for two days every two weeks and showed 59% CR and 37% PR [59]. Pentostatin was equally effective in previously untreated patients and patients who had undergone splenectomy and/or IFN beforehand. In another study of 23 HCL patients, pentostatin was given at 4 mg/m^2 every two weeks [60]. Twenty patients achieved bone marrow documented CRs at a median of 5.4 months. The median duration of CR was 12.6 months. There were no opportunistic or fatal infections. Cassileth et al. treated 50 HCL patients with pentostatin at 5 mg/m^2 for two days every two weeks and demonstrated 64% CR and 20% PR [61]. After 35 months of follow-up, 4 of 32 patients who had achieved CR relapsed and 2 of 10 patients who had achieved PR relapsed. A randomized comparison of pentostatin and IFN showed superior CR and relapse-free survival with pentostatin [62]. However, the difference in OS was not statistically significant, possibly as the result of the crossover design of the study. The same investigators showed that, during long-term follow-up for a median 9.3 years, five-year OS was 90% and the estimated 10-year OS was 81% [63]. In 87 patients who were initially treated with IFN, the OS was similar to that of patients who were initially treated with pentostatin. Else et al. demonstrated an excellent 10-year OS of 96% in 185 patients treated with pentostatin with median follow-up of 12.5 years [64].

Cladribine

Cladribine (2-chlorodeoxyadenosine) is an ADA-resistant purine analog. It selectively accumulates as the 5′-triphosphate derivative in cells rich in deoxycytidine kinase. The cytotoxic activity of cladribine is independent of cell division.

Piro et al. at Scripps Clinic first described the activity of cladribine in 12 patients with HCL [65]. Seven patients had undergone a prior splenectomy, and five patients had received IFN. Cladribine was given as a single course at a dose of 0.1 mg/kg/day continuous IV infusion for seven days. Eleven patients achieved CR and one patient achieved a PR. The total leukocyte count decreased a few days after the infusion was begun with a rapid decline in the number of circulating hairy cells. Normalization of complete blood counts and clearance of hairy cells in the bone marrow were observed within eight weeks after the initiation of therapy. Fever occurred in seven patients during or immediately after the infusion, but no infections were documented. Subsequent studies confirmed this excellent response to cladribine. Hoffman et al. reported that treatment with cladribine resulted in 76% CR and 24% PR [66]. The relapse-free survival was 80% and OS was 95% at median follow-up of 55 months. Tallman et al. treated 52 patients with cladribine and achieved CR in 80% and PR in 18% with four-year PFS of 72% and OS of 86% [67].

Investigators at Scripps Clinic reported an update of 209 patients who had at least seven years of follow-up [68]. Ninety-five percent of the patients achieved CR, and the overall response rate was 100%. The median duration of the first response was 98 months, and it was significantly longer for those patients who had achieved CR versus PR (99 months versus 37 months, respectively). Thirty-seven percent of the patients relapsed after a median time of 42 months. Chadha et al. at Northwestern University showed a 12-year PFS of 54% and an OS of 87% [69].

Similar to pentostatin, cladribine suppresses the immune system for a prolonged period. Seymour et al. reported that, in 40 HCL patients who responded to cladribine, CD4+ count was 743/μL before treatment and 139/μL after treatment [70]. There was one opportunistic infection documented. CD4+ count remained lower than baseline at a median of 23 months after therapy, and the median time to reach a CD4+ count of 365/μL (lower limit of normal range) was 40 months. Others have reported remarkably similar median nadir CD4+ counts of 128/μL and 126/μL, respectively [71, 72]. CD8+ count also decreased significantly; however, it normalized within three months, whereas the CD4+ count required one to two years to normalize [71]. Despite prolonged suppression of the CD4+ count, delayed infections are uncommon and usually are *herpes zoster* reactivations [46]. Neutropenic fever during cladribine treatment is common, occurring in 42% of patients [73]. The use of filgrastim did not confer any benefit in terms of number of febrile patients, number of febrile days, or frequency of admission for antibiotics [73].

The risk of second malignancies was increased in cladribine-treated patients, with the observed-to-expected ratio of developing a second malignancy as compared with the National Cancer Institute SEER Program data being 2.03 [68].

Relapsed disease
Purine analogs
A second course of cladribine still has activity in patients who relapse after an initial course of cladribine. Goodman et al. demonstrated 75% CR and 8% PR in patients receiving a second course of

cladribine at relapse [68]. The median duration of second response was 35 months. Chadha et al. also showed good efficacy of cladribine used at relapse, with 12 of 23 patients who had relapsed after cladribine achieving a CR after a second course of cladribine and seven patients achieving a PR [69]. There appears to be no cross-resistance between pentostatin and cladribine despite similar mechanism of action. Seven patients who relapsed after cladribine received pentostatin, and three patients achieved CR and three patients achieved PR [46].

Rituximab
Rituximab is a monoclonal antibody directed against CD20. Hairy cells strongly express CD20. Hagberg et al. first showed activity of rituximab in HCL, with 6 of 11 patients achieving CR [74]. Nieva et al. treated 24 patients who relapsed after cladribine with rituximab (375 mg/m^2 weekly for four doses) and showed 13% CR and 13% PR [75]. Thomas et al. demonstrated a higher response rate when rituximab was given weekly at the same dose for eight weeks [76]. Of 15 patients who relapsed after pentostatin or cladribine, 53% of the patients achieved CR, and the overall response rate was 80%.

Anti-CD22
BL22 is a recombinant immunotoxin containing an anti-CD22 variable domain fused to truncated *Pseudomonas* exotoxin. Investigators at the National Cancer Institute treated 16 patients who were resistant to cladribine with BL22 in a dose-escalation trial [77]. BL22 was administered by IV infusion every other day for three doses. Eleven patients achieved CR and two patients achieved PR. Two patients developed hemolytic uremic syndrome which was completely reversible.

Scripps clinic treatment algorithm
Initial therapy includes the purine analogs pentostatin and cladribine. In actively infected patients requiring therapy, interferon alpha and splenectomy are therapeutic options; however, they are generally of historical interest only. If a

patient relapses, the indications for salvage therapy are the same as that for initial therapy. At Scripps Clinic, if a relapse occurs more than 18 months following a first course of cladribine, a second course of cladribine or pentostatin is recommended. However, if the relapse occurs within 18 months, the patient has a hypoplastic bone marrow, has had a prior severe opportunistic infection, then we generally recommend non-purine analog treatments, such as interferon, rituximab, splenectomy, or BL22 on study (see Figure 16.2). Alternative treatment schemes are also possible at relapse. Patients relapsing within 18 months of initial therapy and without a hypoplastic marrow can be treated with the alternative purine analog. In addition, single agent rituximab can be administered to patients relapsing 18 months after initial therapy, instead of rechallenging with a purine analog.

Minimal residual disease

Despite the effectiveness of the purine analogs in treating HCL, relapses occur in the majority of patients. Minimal residual disease (MRD) may predict patients who will relapse after a treatment with cladribine. Wheaton et al. studied bone marrow biopsies from 39 patients with HCL in morphologic CR three months after receiving a course of cladribine [78]. They detected MRD by immunohistochemistry (IHC) using the monoclonal antibodies anti-CD20, anti-CD45RO, and DBA.44. Five of 39 patients had MRD detectable by IHC that was not evident by routine H & E staining, and two patients relapsed at one- and two-year follow-up, respectively. In contrast, only 2 of 27 patients with no MRD had relapsed at a median follow-up of two years. To improve upon the eradication of MRD, Ravandi et al. treated 13 patients with a course of cladribine followed by eight weekly doses of rituximab [79]. MRD assessed by flow cytometry (FC) and consensus primer polymerase chain reaction (PCR) was evident in 85% and 45% of the patients, respectively, after the treatment with cladribine. After the completion of rituximab, MRD assessed by FC and PCR was eradicated in 92% and 92% of the

patients, respectively. This demonstrated that the eradication of MRD in HCL is feasible. However, it did not address whether the eradication of MRD leads to a reduced risk of clinical relapse.

Sigal et al. evaluated 19 patients at Scripps Clinic who were in continuous complete hematologic remission (CHR) after a single course of cladribine [80]. The median time from diagnosis was 18 years and the median time from cladribine was 16 years. MRD was assessed in the bone marrow by IHC using CD20, DBA.44, TRAP and annexin, multiparameter FC and consensus primer PCR. Three patients had morphologic evidence of hairy cells in the bone marrow by IHC. Seven patients had evidence of MRD in the bone marrow by FC and PCR, whereas nine patients had no evidence of MRD. This suggested that a single course of cladribine can induce very long-term eradication of MRD and may potentially be curative in some patients. In addition, patients with MRD or even morphologic disease may have a prolonged period of CHR. This questions the clinical significance of adding rituximab to cladribine in an attempt to eliminate MRD.

Summary and recommendations

HCL is an indolent malignant disorder characterized by cytopenias, splenomegaly, and hairy cells in the peripheral blood and bone marrow. Patients may be asymptomatic or may present with symptomatic splenomegaly or recurrent infections. HCL is diagnosed by identifying hairy cells morphologically and flow cytometry by the identification of lymphocytes demonstrating the co-expression of CD11c, CD25, and CD103. Treatment is only indicated if there are significant cytopenias or symptoms. Standard front-line therapy includes the purine analogs cladribine or pentostatin. At relapse, several options are available (see "Scripps Clinic treatment algorithm" and Figure 16.2). Purine nucleoside analogs have dramatically altered the natural history of HCL. Patients treated with cladribine or pentostatin can now anticipate a dramatic response rate and a prolonged period of remission.

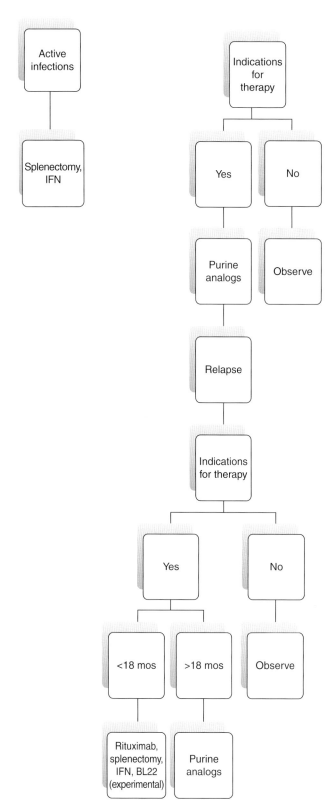

Figure 16.2 Algorithm for treatment at Scripps Clinic.

Acknowledgement

We thank Dr. Robert Sharpe, Department of Pathology, Scripps Clinic, La Jolla, CA, for providing Plates 16.1 Plates 16.2, and Figure 16.1 as well as their legends.

References

1 Ewald O. (1923) Die leukämische reticuloendotheliose. *Deutsches Arch Klin Med* **142**:222–8.

2 Bouroncle BA, Wiseman BK, Doan CA. (1958) Leukemic reticuloendotheliosis. *Blood* **13**:609–30.

3 Schrek R, Donnelly WJ. (1966) "Hairy" cells in blood lymphoreticular neoplastic disease and "flagellated" cells of normal lymph nodes. *Blood* **27**:199–211.

4 Oleske D, Golomb HM, Farber MD, Levy PS. (1985) A case-control inquiry into the etiology of hairy cell leukemia. *Am J Epidemiol* **121**:675–83.

5 Stewart DJ, Keating MJ. (1980) Radiation exposure as a possible etiologic factor in hairy cell leukemia (leukemic reticuloendotheliosis). *Cancer* **46**:1577–80.

6 Wolf BC, Martin AW, Neiman RS, et al. (1990) The detection of Epstein-Barr virus in hairy cell leukemia cells by in situ hybridization. *Am J Pathol* **136**:717–23.

7 Chang KL, Chen YY, Weiss LM. (1993) Lack of evidence of Epstein-Barr virus in hairy cell leukemia and monocytoid B-cell lymphoma. *Hum Pathol* **24**:58–61.

8 Colovic MD, Jankovic GM, Wiernik PH. (2001) Hairy cell leukemia in first cousins and review of the literature. *Eur J Haemotol* **67**:185–8.

9 Wylin RF, Greene MH, Palutke M, et al. (1982) Hairy cell leukemia in three siblings: an apparent HLA-linked disease. *Cancer* **49**:538–42.

10 Haglund U, Juliusson G, Stellan B, Gahrton G. (1994) Hairy cell leukemia is characterized by clonal chromosome abnormalities clustered to specific regions. *Blood* **83**:2637–45.

11 Sambani C, Trafalis DT, Mitsoulis-Mentzikoff C, et al. (2001) Clonal chromosome rearrangements in hairy cell leukemia: personal experience and review of literature. *Cancer Genet Cytogenet* **129**:138–44.

12 Villianatou K, Brito-Babapulle V, Matutes E, Atkinson S, Catovsky D. (1999) p53 gene deletion and trisomy 12 in hairy cell leukemia and its variant. *Leuk Res* **23**:1041–5.

13 König EA, Kusser WC, Day C, et al. (2000) p53 mutations in hairy cell leukemia. *Leukemia* **14**:706–11.

14 Capello D, Vitolo U, Pasqualucci L, et al. (2000) Distribution and pattern of BCL-6 mutations throughout the spectrum of B-cell neoplasia. *Blood* **95**:651–9.

15 Korsmeyer SJ, Greene WC, Cossman J, et al. (1983) Rearrangement and expression of immunoglobulin genes and expression of Tac antigen in hairy cell leukemia. *Proc Natl Acad Sci U S A* **80**:4522–6.

16 Robbins BA, Ellison DJ, Spinosa JC, et al. (1993) Diagnostic application of two-color flow cytometry in 161 cases of hairy cell leukemia. *Blood* **82**:1277–87.

17 Golomb HM, Davis S, Wilson C, Vardiman J. (1982) Surface immunoglobulins on hairy cells of 55 patients with hairy cell leukemia. *Am J Hematol* **12**:397–401.

18 Burns GF, Cawley JC, Worman CP, et al. (1978) Multiple heavy chain isotypes on the surface of the cells of hairy cell leukemia. *Blood* **52**:1132–47.

19 Lynch SA, Brugge JS, Fromowitz F, et al. (1993) Increased expression of the src proto-oncogene in hairy cell leukemia and a subgroup of B-cell lymphomas. *Leukemia* **7**:1416–22.

20 Anderson KC, Boyd AW, Fisher DC, et al. (1985) Hairy cell leukemia: a tumor of pre-plasma cells. *Blood* **65**:620–9.

21 Burke JS, Sheibani K. (1987) Hairy cells and monocytoid B lymphocytes: are they related? *Leukemia* **1**:298–300.

22 Stroup R, Sheibani K. (1992) Antigenic phenotypes of hairy cell leukemia and monocytoid B-cell lymphoma: an immunohistochemical evaluation of 66 cases. *Hum Pathol* **23**:172–7.

23 Traweek ST, Sheibani K, Winberg CD, et al. (1989) Monocytoid B-cell lymphoma: its evolution and relationship to other low-grade B-cell neoplasms. *Blood* **73**:573–8.

24 Plank L, Hansmann ML, Fischer R. (1993) The cytological spectrum of the monocytoid B-cell reaction: recognition of its large cell type. *Histopathology* **23**:425–31.

25 Machii T, Yamaguchi M, Inoue R, et al. (1997) Polyclonal B-cell lymphocytosis with features resembling hairy cell leukemia-Japanese variant. *Blood* **89**: 2008–14.

26 Flandrin G, Sigaux F, Sebahoun G, Bouffette P. (1984) Hairy cell leukemia: clinical presentation and follow-up of 211 patients. *Semin Oncol* **11**:458–71.

27 Turner A, Kjeldsberg CR. (1978) Hairy cell leukemia: a review. *Medicine (Baltimore)* **57**:477–99.

28 Kampmeier P, Spielberger R, Dickstein J, et al. (1994) Increased incidence of second neoplasms in patients treated with interferon alpha 2b for hairy cell leukemia: a clinicopathologic assessment. *Blood* **83**:2931–8.

29 Burthem J, Cawley JC. (1994) The bone marrow fibrosis of hairy-cell leukemia is caused by the synthesis and assembly of a fibronectin matrix by the hairy cells. *Blood* **83**:497–504.

30 Nanba K, Soban EJ, Bowling MC, Berard CW. (1977) Splenic pseudosinuses and hepatic angiomatous lesions. Distinctive features of hairy cell leukemia. *Am J Clin Pathol* **67**:415–26.

31 Li CY, Yam LT, Lam KW. (1970) Studies of acid phosphatase isoenzymes in human leukocytes demonstration of isoenzyme cell specificity. *J Histochem Cytochem* **18**:901–10.

32 Catovsky D. (1977) Hairy-cell leukaemia and prolymphocytic leukaemia. *Clin Haematol* **6**:245–68.

33 Drexler HG, Gaedicke G, Minowada J. (1985) Isoenzyme studies in human leukemia-lymphoma cells lines. II. Acid phosphatase. *Leuk Res* **9**:537–48.

34 Falini B, Schwarting R, Erber W, et al. (1985) The differential diagnosis of hairy cell leukemia with a panel of monoclonal antibodies. *Am J Clin Pathol* **83**:289–300.

35 Hsu SM, Yang K, Jaffe ES. (1983) Hairy cell leukemia: a B cell neoplasm with a unique antigenic phenotype. *Am J Clin Pathol* **80**:421–8.

36 Visser L, Shaw A, Slupsky J, et al. (1989) Monoclonal antibodies reactive with hairy cell leukemia. *Blood* **74**:320–5.

37 Thaler J, Denz H, Dietze O, et al. (1989) Immunohistological assessment of bone marrow biopsies from patients with hairy cell leukemia: changes following treatment with alpha-2-interferon and deoxycoformycin. *Leuk Res* **13**:377–83.

38 Hounieu H, Chittal SM, al Saati T, et al. (1992) Hairy cell leukemia. Diagnosis of bone marrow involvement in paraffin-embedded sections with monoclonal antibody DBA. 44. *Am J Clin Pathol* **98**:26–33.

39 Troussard X, Valensi F, Duchayne E, et al. (1996) Splenic lymphoma with villous lymphocytes: clinical presentation, biology and prognostic factors in a series of 100 patients. Groupe Français d'Hématologie Cellulaire (GFHC). *Br J Haematol* **93**:731–6.

40 Matutes E, Morilla R, Owusu-Ankomah K, Houlihan A, Catovsky D. (1994) The immunophenotype of splenic lymphoma with villous lymphocytes and its relevance to the differential diagnosis with other B-cell disorders. *Blood* **83**:1558–62.

41 Galton DA, Goldman JM, Wiltshaw E, et al. (1974) Prolymphocytic leukaemia. *Br J Haematol* **27**:7–23.

42 Cawley JC, Burns GF, Hayhoe FG. (1980) A chronic lymphoproliferative disorder with distinctive features: a distinct variant of hairy-cell leukaemia. *Leuk Res* **4**:547–59.

43 Sainati L, Matutes E, Mulligan S, et al. (1990) A variant form of hairy cell leukemia resistant to alpha-interferon: clinical and phenotypic characteristics of 17 patients. *Blood* **76**:157–62.

44 Catovsky D, O'Brien M, Melo JV, Wardle J, Brozovic M. (1984) Hairy cell leukemia (HCL) variant: an intermediate disease between HCL and B prolymphocytic leukemia. *Semin Oncol* **11**:362–9.

45 Tetreault SA, Robbins BA, Saven A. (1999) Treatment of hairy cell leukemia-variant with cladribine. *Leuk Lymphoma* **35**:347–54.

46 Saven A, Burian C, Koziol JA, Piro LD. (1998) Long-term follow-up of patients with hairy cell leukemia after cladribine treatment. *Blood* **92**:1918–26.

47 Golomb HM, Vardiman JW. (1983) Response to splenectomy in 65 patients with hairy cell leukemia: an evaluation of spleen weight and bone marrow involvement. *Blood* **61**:349–52.

48 Mintz U, Golomb HM. (1979) Splenectomy as initial therapy in twenty-six patients with leukemic reticuloendotheliosis (hairy cell leukemia). *Cancer Res* **39**:2366–70.

49 Jansen J, Hermans J. (1981) Splenectomy in hairy cell leukemia: a retrospective multicenter analysis. *Cancer* **47**:2066–76.

50 Quesada JR, Reuben J, Manning JT, Hersh EM, Gutterman JU. (1984) Alpha interferon for induction of remission in hairy-cell leukemia. *N Engl J Med* **310**:15–18.

51 Quesada JR, Hersh EM, Manning J, et al. (1986) Treatment of hairy cell leukemia with recombinant alpha-interferon. *Blood* **68**:493–7.

52 Ratain MJ, Golomb HM, Vardiman JW, et al. (1988) Relapse after interferon alfa-2b therapy for hairy cell leukemia: analysis of prognostic variables. *J Clin Oncol* **6**:1714–21.

53 Berman E, Heller G, Kempin S, et al. (1990) Incidence of response and long-term follow-up in patients with hairy cell leukemia treated with recombinant interferon alfa-2a. *Blood* **75**:839–45.

54 Golomb HM, Jacobs A, Fefer A, et al. (1986) Alpha-2 interferon therapy of hairy cell leukemia: a multicenter study of 64 patients. *J Clin Oncol* **4**:900–5.

55 Golomb HM, Ratain MJ, Fefer A, et al. (1988) Randomized study of the duration of treatment with interferon alfa-2b in patients with hairy cell leukemia. *J Natl Cancer Inst* **80**:369–73.

56 Spiers ASD, Parekh SJ, Bishop MB. (1984) Hairy-cell leukemia: induction of complete remission with pentostatin (2′-deoxycoformycin). *J Clin Oncol* **2**:1336–42.

57 Urba WJ, Baseler MW, Kopp WC, et al. (1988) Deoxycoformycin-induced immunosuppression in patients with hairy cell leukemia. *Blood* **73**:38–46.

58 Kraut EH, Neff JC, Bouroncle BA, Gochnour D, Grever MR. (1990) Immunosuppressive effects of pentostatin. *J Clin Oncol* **8**:848–55.

59 Spiers ASD, Moore D, Cassileth PA, et al. (1987) Remissions in hairy cell leukemia with pentostatin (2′-deoxycoformycin). *N Engl J Med* **316**:825–30.

60 Kraut EH, Bouroncle BA, Grever MR. (1989) Pentostatin in the treatment of advanced hairy cell leukemia. *J Clin Oncol* **7**:168–72.

61 Cassileth PA, Cheuvart B, Spiers ASD, et al. (1991) Pentostatin induces durable remissions in hairy cell leukemia. *J Clin Oncol* **9**:243–6.

62 Grever M, Kopecky K, Foucar MK, et al. (1995) Randomized comparison of pentostatin versus interferon alfa-2a in previously untreated patients with hairy cell leukemia: an intergroup study. *J Clin Oncol* **13**:974–82.

63 Flinn IW, Kopecky KJ, Foucar MK, et al. (2000) Long-term follow-up of remission duration, mortality, and second malignancies in hairy cell leukemia patients treated with pentostatin. *Blood* **96**:2981–6.

64 Else M, Ruchlemer R, Osuji N, et al. (2005) Long remissions in hairy cell leukemia with purine analogs. *Cancer* **104**:2442–8.

65 Piro LD, Carrera CJ, Carson DA, Beutler E. (1990) Lasting remissions in hairy cell leukemia induced by a single infusion of 2-chlorodeoxyadenosine. *N Engl J Med* **322**:1117–21.

66 Hoffman MA, Janson D, Rose E, Rai KR. (1997) Treatment of hairy cell leukemia with cladribine: response, toxicity, and long-term follow-up. *J Clin Oncol* **15**:1138–42.

67 Tallman MS, Hakimian D, Rademaker AW, et al. (1996) Relapse of hairy cell leukemia after 2-chlorodeoxyadenosine: long-term follow up of the Northwestern University experience. *Blood* **88**:1954–9.

68 Goodman GR, Burian C, Koziol JA, Saven A. (2003) Extended follow-up of patients with hairy cell leukemia after treatment with cladribine. *J Clin Oncol* **21**:891–6.

69 Chadha P, Rademaker AW, Mendiratta P, et al. (2005) Treatment of hairy cell leukemia with 2-chlorodeoxyadenosine (2-CdA): long-term follow-up of the Northwestern University experience. *Blood* **106**: 241–6.

70 Seymour JF, Kurzrock R, Freireich EJ, Estey EH. (1994) 2-chlorodeoxyadenosine induces durable remissions and prolonged suppression of CD4+ lymphocyte counts in patients with hairy cell leukemia. *Blood* **83**:2906–11.

71 Juliusson G, Lenkei R, Liliemark J. (1994) Flow cytometry of blood and bone marrow cells from patients with hairy cell leukemia: phenotype of hairy cells and lymphocyte subsets after treatment with 2-chlorodeoxyadenosine. *Blood* **83**:3672–81.

72 Estey EH, Kurzrock R, Kantarjian HM, et al. (1992) Treatment of hairy cell leukemia with 2-chlorodeoxyadenosine (2-CdA). *Blood* **79**:882–7.

73 Saven A, Burian C, Adusumalli J, Koziol J. (1999) Filgrastim for cladribine-induced neutropenic fever in patients with hairy cell leukemia. *Blood* **93**:2471–7.

74 Hagberg H, Lundholm L. (2001) Rituximab, a chimaeric anti-CD20 monoclonal antibody, in the treatment of hairy cell leukemia. *Br J Haematol* **115**:609–11.

75 Nieva J, Bethel K, Saven A. (2003) Phase II study of rituximab in the treatment of cladribine-failed patients with hairy cell leukemia. *Blood* **102**:810–13.

76 Thomas DA, O'Brien S, Bueso-Ramos C, et al. (2003) Rituximab in relapsed or refractory hairy cell leukemia. *Blood* **102**:3906–11.

77 Kreitman RJ, Wilson WH, Bergeron K, et al. (2001) Efficacy of the anti-CD22 recombinant immunotoxin BL22 in chemotherapy-resistant hairy cell leukemia. *N Engl J Med* **345**:241–7.

78 Wheaton S, Tallman MS, Hakimian D, Peterson L. (1996) Minimal residual disease may predict bone marrow relapse in patients with hairy cell leukemia treated with 2-chlorodeoxyadenosine. *Blood* **87**: 1556–60.

79 Ravandi F, Jorgensen JL, O'Brien S, et al. (2006) Eradication of minimal residual disease in hairy cell leukemia. *Blood* **107**:4658–62.

80 Sigal D, Sharpe RW, Burian C, Saven A. (2008) Potential curability of cladribine in selected patients with hairy cell leukemia. Proceedings of ASCO. *J Clin Oncol* **26**:18010.

CHAPTER 17

Molecular Basis of B-cell Lymphomas

Elizabeth M. Sagatys, Eduardo M. Sotomayor and Jianguo Tao

Department of Oncological Sciences and Experimental Therapeutics Program, and Department of Malignant Hematology,
H. Lee Moffitt Cancer Center and Research Institute, Tampa, FL, USA

Introduction

The recently revised WHO classification (2008) uses a multiparameter approach to classify B-cell lymphomas. Clonal B-cell lymphoproliferative disorders are classified, in part, based on the normal cell stage they resemble. To understand how B-cell lymphomas develop, it is important to understand normal B-cell development from the progenitor B-cell to memory B-cell or plasma cell. The major types of B-cell lymphomas can be tied to their stage of maturation. B-lymphoblastic leukemia/lymphoma arises from the precursor B-cell in the bone marrow. Mantle cell lymphoma arises from the pre-germinal center cells of the periphery. Follicular lymphoma, Burkitt's lymphoma, some diffuse large B-cell lymphomas (DLBCL), and Hodgkin lymphomas arise from germinal center cells. Marginal zone and MALT lymphomas, lymphoplasmablastic lymphoma, chronic lymphocytic leukemia/small lymphocytic lymphoma, some diffuse large B-cell lymphomas, and plasma cell myeloma arise from post-germinal center cells [1]. Regarding the mechanisms of lymphomagenesis, the development of lymphomas can be placed into three broad categories: (1) enhanced cell growth and proliferation, (2) apoptosis inhibition, and (3) impaired differentiation. In this chapter, we will therefore describe the molecular basis of B-cell development and how aberrations at different stages can lead to B-cell malignancies.

Precursor B-cell development

Immunoglobulin rearrangement

B-cell development begins in the bone marrow. There, progenitor B-cells undergo Ig variable (V_H), diversity (D_H), and joining (J_H) genes rearrangement and the subsequent expression of surface Ig. $V_H D_H J_H$ rearrangements have recently been tied to Ikaros expression by early B-cell precursors. Ikaros is a Kruppel-like zinc finger transcription factor that plays an important role in B-cell lineage determination and Ig heavy chain (IgH) rearrangement [2].

Ig $V_H D_H J_H$ rearrangement is a multistep process. In immature B-cell precursors, there is initial rearrangement of the D_H and J_H gene segments with V_H rearrangement completing the process in the early pre-B-cell stage. This rearrangement is initiated by recombination-activating genes (RAG1 and RAG2) [3, 4]. Cleavage sites in the Ig gene associated with RAG have been shown to be involved in chromosomal translocations such as t(14;18) and t(11;14) [3]. The finished Ig heavy chain has the V_H D_H J_H regions, in addition to complementary-determining regions (CDR) and framework regions (FR). The CDRs, particularly CDR3, are critical in antigen recognition [5]. Among the 123 V_H segments, 79 are pseudogenes, leaving the remaining 44 genes functional [6]. Of the 27 D_H segments, 25 have been demonstrated to be involved in antibody production. The V_H and D_H gene segments can be

Advances in Malignant Hematology, First Edition. Edited by Hussain I. Saba and Ghulam J. Mufti. © 2011 Blackwell Publishing Ltd.
Published 2011 by Blackwell Publishing Ltd.

divided into seven families based on high-sequence homology [5]. The V_H3 family is the largest group and V_H6 family is the closest to the D_HJ_H loci [6, 7]. Six of the nine J_H segments are functional [8]. Further changes in the Ig genes, such as isotype switching and somatic hypermutation, occur as the lymphocytes mature into memory B-cells or plasma cells [9].

Based on the assumption that all of the segments, including pseudogenes, have an equal chance of being selected in recombination, there should not be a predilection for particular gene segments to be involved in the development of a neoplastic clone. This hypothesis has been demonstrated to be true for most of the lymphomas, with the exception of B-acute lymphoblastic leukemia (B-ALL) [10–12]. B-ALL demonstrates an increased rearrangement with V_H6 family genes, which as mentioned earlier are closest to the D_HJ_H loci [13]. There was also overrepresentation of J_H regions J_H4, J_H5, and J_H6 [11]. Based on these finding, Mortuza et al. postulate that the rate of V_H expression is proportional to its proximity to the J_H locus [11]. Loss of additional recombinations between the V_H genes and the D_HJ_H loci may be seen during leukemogenesis [11].

Pax-5

Pax-5 is a B-cell lineage-specific activator protein that is initially expressed early in B-cell development. It is consistently expressed throughout B-cell maturation, until lost in plasma cells. Pax-5 maintains B-cell differentiation by activating B-cell specific genes and inhibiting non-B-lineage genes [14, 15]. Pax-5 has many roles in B-cell development, including lineage commitment, differentiation, and adhesion and migration of mature B-cells [14]. While the exact mechanism is unknown, transcription factors E2A and EBF1 have been identified as possible candidates for Pax-5 activation [16, 17]. EBF1 is involved in methylation of the CD79a gene promoter region; however, there does not appear to be a role for EBF1-initiated methylation in Pax-5 regulation [18]. Pax-5 activity is directly regulated by B-lymphocyte-induced maturation protein 1 (BLIMP1) [19]. Among the many roles of Pax-5, it is involved in

inhibiting X-box binding protein 1 (XBP1), a plasma cell differentiation regulator [20]. By inhibiting Pax-5, BLIMP1 allows for the activation of XBP1 and subsequent plasma cell differentiation [21].

Pre-germinal center differentiation and proliferation

If precursor B-cells are the infants and post-germinal center B-cells are the mature adults, then pre-germinal center B-cells would be the prepubescent adolescents. These B-cells have moved from the bone marrow and now reside in the interfollicular areas and mantle zones of lymph nodes. When presented with antigen stimulation, these B-cells can progress into the so-called extrafollicular B-blast (EBB) [1]. EBB can mature into short-lived plasma cells that secrete IgM or may move into the germinal center to become a centroblast [1]. Memory B-cells found in the marginal zone can also develop from EBB. These lymphocytes lack Ig somatic hypermutation [1].

The prototypic pre-germinal center neoplasm is mantle cell lymphoma (MCL). MCL is an intermediate grade B-cell lymphoma with co-expression of CD19 and CD5 with stronger CD20 expression than seen in CLL. The defining characteristic of MCL is the demonstration of cyclin D1 expression [22]. Increased cell cycling and defective apoptosis and DNA repair mechanisms can lead to MCL.

Cyclin D1 is a protein produced by the gene BCL-1. Cyclin D1 production is upregulated in MCL most commonly by a translocation between BCL-1 on chromosome 11 and the IgH gene [23, 24]. While it is certainly important in the development of MCL, cyclin D1 by itself is not sufficient to cause lymphoma [25]. MCL in the absence of cyclin D1 remains a controversial diagnosis. However, recent data does suggest that other cyclins, particularly cyclins D2 and D3, are capable of replacing cyclin D1 and being involved in the molecular pathogenesis of MCL [26].

Cyclin D1 acts on many different intracellular pathways during the development of MCL. Cyclin D1 is complexed with cyclin-dependent kinase (CDK) 4/6 and promotes the phosphorylation of

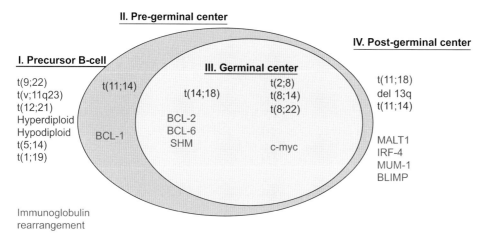

Figure 17.1 Common translocations and molecular markers in B-cell lymphomas. Ig rearrangement occurs in the bone marrow during precursor B-cell development. B-ALL, which arises in the bone marrow, has many associated translocations. The most common are listed. In the pre-germinal center, increased expression of BCL-1 due to the translocation t(11;14) can lead to mantle cell lymphoma (MCL). The translocation t(11;14) has also been found in plasma cell myeloma. Somatic hypermutation (SHM) occurs in the germinal center, which is formed with the help of BCL-6. Follicular lymphoma is associated with aberrant expression of BCL-2. Burkitt's lymphoma, another follicle center cell origin lymphoma, is associated with an increase in c-myc due to translocations with either the heavy chain or light chain Ig genes. In the post germinal center, as BCL-6 levels decrease BLIMP1 levels increase leading to plasma cell differentiation. IRF4/MUM1 is increased in plasma cells by the activation of the NF-kB pathway. Extranodal marginal zone lymphoma is associated with t(11;18) with MALT1 expression.

retinoblastoma (Rb). Through the phosphorylation of Rb, the transcription factor E2F is released, allowing the cell to progress from G1 to S phase [22]. E2F also plays a role in p53 stabilization by increasing the production of p14ARF. P14ARF inhibits the degradation of p53 by MDM2 [27]. P53 can lead to increased levels of p21 and, as such, to increased apoptosis. Normal p53 function is dependent on the ataxia telangiectasia mutated (ATM) gene. ATM gene abnormalities have been detected in 40–75% of MCL [28, 29]. Several other genetic alterations have been described in MCL, including homozygous deletions of INK4a/ARF, microdeletions of Rb1 gene, and overexpression of CDK4 genes [27, 30, 31]. The effects of genes such as p27KIP1 and p16INK4, which act on the retinoblastoma (Rb) gene pathway, are downregulated by cyclin D1 [22, 32]. P16INK4 normally acts to suppress the cyclin D1/CDK4/6 complex. P27KIP1 complexed with p21 acts to inhibit another cell cycle progression complex cyclinE/CDK2 [22, 31].

Germinal center differentiation and proliferation

B-cells that have been exposed to antigens can move into the primary follicle and form a germinal center. This antigen exposure results in the Ig heavy and light chain variable regions undergoing somatic hypermutation (SHM). Normal centroblasts lose the ability to express BCL-2 and are susceptible to apoptosis. As such, centroblasts are marked for apoptosis unless they are saved by positive selection [33]. It is thought that germinal center B-cells have suppressed the NF-kB pathway leading to decreased expression of antiapoptotic genes BCL-2, BCL-X$_L$, and A1. When a lymphocyte is chosen for positive selection, there is activation of the NF-kB pathway leading to an increased expression of these antiapoptotic genes [34–36]. Germinal center-derived lymphomas are derived by Ig transformation from either variable region gene recombination (i.e., BCL-2-IgH), somatic hypermutation (i.e., BCL-6 in DLBCL, c-myc in endemic Burkitt's lymphoma), or class switching (i.e., c-myc in sporadic Burkitt's lymphoma) [37].

BCL-2

BCL-2 is an antiapoptotic protein coded by a gene found on chromosome 18. The BCL-2-IgH rearrangement has been identified in follicular center cell-derived tumors such as follicular lymphoma and some diffuse large B-cell lymphomas. BCL-2 has an area in the major breakpoint region that allows for cleavage by RAG nucleases that are also involved in Ig rearrangement [38]. When placed adjacent to the IgH locus, BCL-2 expression is increased and overrides the pro-apoptotic tendencies of the centroblasts [39].

BCL-2-IgH translocation alone does not appear to be sufficient to cause lymphoma. This translocation has been demonstrated in non-neoplastic B-cells and in transgenic mice, where BCL-2 is controlled by Eμ [35, 39, 40]. Additional genetic alterations appear to be necessary for the development of lymphoma.

BCL-6 and immunoglobulin somatic hypermutation

Expression of BCL-6 is necessary for the formation of germinal centers [41, 42]. Centroblasts express this suppressor of B-cell activation and terminal differentiation. Once B-cells enter the germinal center, they are able to undergo rapid division and Ig somatic hypermutation (SHM). SHM is mediated by activation-induced cytosine deaminase (AID) and is key in the development of polyclonal B-cells in normal germinal centers [43]. BCL-6 inhibits the previously discussed BLIMP1, preventing plasma cell differentiation [44, 45]. P27KIP1, an inhibitor of cyclin-dependent kinases which induces senescence, is also suppressed by BCL-6 [44]. This could be the explanation as to why BCL-6 is able to facilitate cell division in normal germinal centers.

AID has been shown to be capable of damaging genes that contain SHM hotspot sequences [46]. Potential oncogenes such as BLK, SYK, PIM, RHOH, PAX5, and MYC have been shown to be mutated by AID-dependent mechanisms [43, 47]. Like BCL-2,

BCL-6 has been shown to not be solely responsible for the development of lymphomas when a study on expression of BCL-6 failed to induce germinal center cell lymphomas in the absence of AID and SHM [47].

BCL-6 can repress DNA repair mechanisms by inhibiting transcription of ataxia telangiectasia and Rad3-related genes (ATR) [48]. ATR is important in DNA damage sensing and repair [43]. In addition to ATR repression, BCL-6 can also inhibit other key DNA repair genes such as CHEK1, TP53, and CDKN1A [49–51]. It is thought that this sustained DNA repair repression leads to lymphomagenesis by allowing for additional genetic alterations [43].

As the B-cell matures into memory B-cells or plasma cells, BCL-6 expression is decreased. BLIMP1 is able to inhibit BCL-6, blocking B-cell gene expression and proliferation genes [52]. This facilitates plasma cell differentiation. Other physiologic mediators of BCL-6 downregulation are CD40 and signal transducer and activator of transcription 5 (STAT5) [43]. CD40 expression is upregulated as B-cells exit the germinal centers. CD40 acts on the NF-kB pathway by inducing interferon regulatory factor 4 (IRF4) [53]. The IRF4-NF-kB pathway is capable of further suppressing BCL-6 expression [43]. STAT5 can bind to the exon1 and intron 1 of BCL-6 and directly repress BCL-6 expression [54].

C-myc

C-myc is a transcription factor involved in enhancing cell growth and proliferation. The enhanced proliferation allows for increased selectable B-cells in germinal centers. C-myc can be translocated to either the Ig heavy or light chain (t(8;14), t(2,8), or t(8,22)). This class-switching Ig transformation is seen in sporadic Burkitt's lymphomas and some DLBCL [37]. AID has been shown to be involved in c-myc upregulation [55]. Endemic Burkitt's lymphoma and some DLBCL demonstrate somatic hypermutation of the c-myc gene, thereby altering its function as a transcription factor [37, 56, 57].

Dysregulated c-myc has oncogenic roles as both a transcriptional regulator and as an inducer of genomic instability [58]. Genomic instability is thought to be due to a non-transcription role of myc on DNA replication [59]. Mutations in myc can lead to a decreased expression of BCL2 interacting mediator (BIM). BIM normally acts to bind and inactivate BCL-2 [60, 61]. When BIM is decreased, BCL-2 expression can result in activation of antiapoptotic mechanisms.

Post-germinal center differentiation and proliferation

As the mature B-cells exit the germinal center they can take two pathways: becoming either a memory B-cell or a plasma cell. Prototypic post-germinal center cell neoplasms are marginal zone lymphoma, small lymphocytic lymphoma/chronic lymphocytic leukemia, and plasmacytoma [1]. The memory B-cells and plasma cells that have traveled through the germinal center have Ig somatic hypermutation, unlike the memory B-cells that are derived from pre-germinal center B-cells [1]. As the lymphocytes travel from the germinal center into the perifollicular area, there is a change from the proliferation of the germinal center to the final differentiation to the post-germinal center. This is accomplished by the downregulation of BCL-6 by interferon regulatory factor 4/multiple myeloma oncogenes 1 (IRF4/MUM1) [53].

IRF4/MUM1
CD40 has been associated with decreasing the levels of BCL-6 in cells exiting the germinal center. As CD40 expression increases there is activation of the NF-kB pathway. One target of the NF-kB pathway is IRF4 [43]. As previously mentioned, IRF4 is capable of decreasing BCL-6 expression further and is involved in terminal differentiation and apoptosis [62].

MUM1 is a myeloma-associated oncogene that is activated by the translocation t(6;14)(p25;q32) with the IgH and is found in 20% of myeloma [63, 64]. MUM1 levels are highest in plasma cells and activated T-cells [65]. It is believed that overexpression of IRF4/MUM1 may lead to tumorigenesis [65].

BLIMP1
Plasma cells are derived from post-germinal center lymphocytes with an increase in the previously discussed BLIMP1. In addition to inhibiting Pax-5, BLIMP1 is able to block other mature B-cell functions including SHM, and represses c-myc, inhibiting cell cycling. Plasma cells do not typically undergo cell cycling [52, 66]. BLIMP1 and BCL-6 have a double-negative regulatory effect as rising BLIMP1 levels decrease BCL6 levels in B-lymphocytes and, conversely rising BCL-6 levels decreases BLIMP1 levels [66].

Antigen stimulation
Since post-germinal center B-cells and plasma cells are able to migrate to other tissues, they tend to return to the sites of antigen stimulation. As such, plasma cells return to the bone marrow, MALT lymphocytes return to the gastrointestinal tract and splenic marginal zone cells return to the spleen [67]. Post-germinal center-derived lymphomas are commonly associated with antigen stimulation. MALT lymphomas, both marginal zone type are associated with *Helicobacter pylori* infection and may respond early on to *H. pylori* eradication therapy [68]. Splenic marginal zone lymphomas have been associated with hepatitis C and have demonstrated response to interferon alpha therapy [69].

Conclusions

As the molecular mechanisms involved in B-cell lymphomagenesis are unveiled, novel therapeutic approaches are being developed. Through an understanding of these molecular principles, novel targeted approaches have been translated into the clinical arena. For instance, proteosome inhibitors such as bortezomib have shown antitumor activity in a variety of B-cell malignancies through inhibition of the survival NF-kB pathway [70]. BCL-2 inhibitors by inducing B-cell apoptosis are showing promise as therapeutic agents in B-cell tumors [71]. In addition, inhibitors of BCL-6 that would target only survival functions could be of great benefit and are currently in development [43]. Finally, cell-cycle inhibitors such as CDK-inhibitors and cyclin D1 inhibitors might prove to be of therapeutic value in B-cell malignancies characterized by a high proliferation index such as mantle cell lymphoma. Needless to say, a continued effort to better understand the complex molecular pathogenesis of B-cell malignancies would pave the way for the next generation of novel molecularly based therapeutic approaches against these tumors.

References

1 Jaffe ES, Harris NL, Stein H, et al. (2008) Introduction and overview of the classification of the lymphoid neoplasms. In Swerdlow SH, Campo E, Harris NL,et al. (eds.) *WHO Classification of Tumours of Haematopoietic and Lymphoid Tissues* (4th ed.), pp. 158–66. Lyon: IARC.

2 Reynaud D, Demarco IA, Reddy KL, et al. (2008) Regulation of B cell fate commitment and immunoglobulin heavy-chain gene rearrangements by Ikaros. *Nat Immunol* **9**:927–36.

3 Shaffer AL, Rosenwald A, Staudt LM. (2002) Lymphoid malignancies: the dark side of B-cell differentiation. *Nat Rev Immunol* **2**:920–32.

4 Fugmann SD, Lee AI, Shockett PE, Villey IJ, Schatz DG. (2000) The RAG proteins and V(D)J recombination: complexes, ends, and transposition. *Annu Rev Immunol* **18**:495–527.

5 Li A, Rue M, Zhou J, et al. (2004) Utilization of Ig heavy chain variable, diversity, and joining gene segments in children with B-lineage acute lymphoblastic leukemia: implications for the mechanisms of VDJ recombination and for pathogenesis. *Blood* **103**:4602–9.

6 Matsuda F, Ishii K, Bourvagnet P, et al. (1998) The complete nucleotide sequence of the human immunoglobulin heavy chain variable region locus. *J Exp Med* **188**:2151–62.

7 Cook GP, Tomlinson IM. (1995) The human immunoglobulin VH repertoire. *Immunol Today* **16**:237–42.

8 Ravetch JV, Siebenlist U, Korsmeyer S, Waldmann T, Leder P. (1981) Structure of the human immunoglobulin mu locus: characterization of embryonic and rearranged J and D genes. *Cell* **27**:583–91

9 Rui L, Goodnow CC. (2006) Lymphoma and the control of B cell growth and differentiation. *Curr Mol Med* **6**:291–308.

10 Davidkova G, Pettersson S, Holmberg D, Lundkvist I. (1997) Selective usage of VH genes in adult human B lymphocyte repertoires. *Scand J Immunol* **45**:62–73.

11 Mortuza FY, Moreira IM, Papaioannou M, et al. (2001) Immunoglobulin heavy-chain gene rearrangement in adult acute lymphoblastic leukemia reveals preferential usage of J(H)-proximal variable gene segments. *Blood* **97**:2716–26.

12 Brezinschek HP, Brezinschek RI, Lipsky PE. (1995) Analysis of the heavy chain repertoire of human peripheral B cells using single-cell polymerase chain reaction. *J Immunol* **155**:190–202.

13 Coyle LA, Papaioannou M, Yaxley JC, et al. (1996) Molecular analysis of the leukaemic B cell in adult and childhood acute lymphoblastic leukaemia. *Br J Haematol* **94**:685–93.

14 Delogu A, Schebesta A, Sun Q, et al. (2006) Gene repression by Pax5 in B cells is essential for blood cell homeostasis and is reversed in plasma cells. *Immunity* **24**:269–81.

15 Schebesta A, McManus S, Salvagiotto G, et al. (2007) Transcription factor Pax5 activates the chromatin of key genes involved in B cell signaling, adhesion, migration, and immune function. *Immunity* **27**:49–63.

16 Bain G, Maandag EC, Izon DJ, et al. (1994) E2A proteins are required for proper B cell development and initiation of immunoglobulin gene rearrangements. *Cell* **79**:885–92.

17 Lin H, Grosschedl R. (1995) Failure of B-cell differentiation in mice lacking the transcription factor EBF. *Nature* **376**:263–7.

18 Decker T, Pasca di Magliano M, McManus S, et al. (2009) Stepwise activation of enhancer and promoter regions of the B cell commitment gene Pax5 in early lymphopoiesis. *Immunity* **30**:508–20.

19 Lin KI, Angelin-Duclos C, Kuo TC, Calame K. (2002) Blimp-1-dependent repression of Pax-5 is required for differentiation of B cells to immunoglobulin M-secreting plasma cells. *Mol Cell Biol* **22**:4771–80.

20 Reimold AM, Ponath PD, Li YS, et al. (1996) Transcription factor B-cell lineage-specific activator protein regulates the gene for human X-box binding protein 1. *J Exp Med* **183**:393–401.

21 Reimold AM, Iwakoshi NN, Manis J, et al. (2001) Plasma cell differentiation requires the transcription factor XBP-1. *Nature* **412**:300–7.

22 Swerdlow SH, Campo E, Seto M, Muller-Hermelink HK. (2008) Mantle cell lymphoma. In Swerdlow SH,

Campo E, Harris NL, et al. (eds.) *WHO Classification of Tumours of Haematopoietic and Lymphoid Tissues* (4th ed.). Lyon: IARC.

23 Li JY, Gaillard F, Moreau A, et al. (1999) Detection of translocation t(11;14)(q13;q32) in mantle cell lymphoma by fluorescence in situ hybridization. *Amer J Path* **154**:1449–52.

24 Rosenberg CL, Wong E, Petty EM, et al. (1991) PRAD1, a candidate BCL1 oncogene: mapping and expression in centrocytic lymphoma. *Proc Natl Acad Sci. USA* **88**:9638–42.

25 Smith MR. (2008) Mantle cell lymphoma: advances in biology and therapy. *Curr Opin Hematol* **15**:415–21.

26 Fu K, Weisenburger DD, Greiner TC, et al. (2005) Cyclin D1-negative mantle cell lymphoma: a clinico-pathologic study based on gene expression profiling. *Blood* **106**:4315–21.

27 Hernandez L, Bea S, Pinyol M, et al. (2005) CDK4 and MDM2 gene alterations mainly occur in highly proliferative and aggressive mantle cell lymphomas with wild-type INK4a/ARF locus. *Cancer Res* **65**:2199–206.

28 Camacho E, Hernandez L, Hernandez S, et al. (2002) ATM gene inactivation in mantle cell lymphoma mainly occurs by truncating mutations and missense mutations involving the phosphatidylinositol-3 kinase domain and is associated with increasing numbers of chromosomal imbalances. *Blood* **99**:238–44.

29 Schaffner C, Idler I, Stilgenbauer S, Dohner H, Lichter P. (2000) Mantle cell lymphoma is characterized by inactivation of the ATM gene. *Proc Natl Acad Sci USA* **97**:2773–8.

30 Pinyol M, Bea S, Pla L, et al. (2007) Inactivation of RB1 in mantle-cell lymphoma detected by nonsense-mediated mRNA decay pathway inhibition and microarray analysis. *Blood* **109**:5422–9.

31 Pinyol M, Hernandez L, Cazorla M, et al. (1997) Deletions and loss of expression of p16INK4a and p21Waf1 genes are associated with aggressive variants of mantle cell lymphomas. *Blood* **89**:272–80.

32 Jares P, Campo E, Pinyol M, et al. (1996) Expression of retinoblastoma gene product (pRb) in mantle cell lymphomas. Correlation with cyclin D1 (PRAD1/CCND1) mRNA levels and proliferative activity. *Amer J Pathol* **148**:1591–600.

33 MacLennan IC. (1994) Germinal centers. *Annu Rev Immunol* **12**:117–39.

34 Craxton A, Chuang PI, Shu G, Harlan JM, Clark EA. (2000) The CD40-inducible Bcl-2 family member A1 protects B cells from antigen receptor-mediated apoptosis. *Cell Immunol* **200**:56–62.

35 Liu Y, Hernandez AM, Shibata D, Cortopassi GA. (1994) BCL2 translocation frequency rises with age in humans. *Proc Natl Acad Sci USA* **91**:8910–4.

36 Tuscano JM, Druey KM, Riva A, et al. (1996) Bcl-x rather than Bcl-2 mediates CD40-dependent centrocyte survival in the germinal center. *Blood* **88**:1359–64.

37 Kuppers R, Klein U, Hansmann ML, Rajewsky K. (1999) Cellular origin of human B-cell lymphomas. *New Engl J Med* **341**:1520–9.

38 Raghavan SC, Swanson PC, Wu X, Hsieh CL, Lieber MR. (2004) A non-B-DNA structure at the Bcl-2 major breakpoint region is cleaved by the RAG complex. *Nature* **428**:88–93.

39 McDonnell TJ, Korsmeyer SJ. (1991) Progression from lymphoid hyperplasia to high-grade malignant lymphoma in mice transgenic for the t(14; 18). *Nature* **349**:254–6.

40 Strasser A, Harris AW, Cory S. (1993) E mu-bcl-2 transgene facilitates spontaneous transformation of early pre-B and immunoglobulin-secreting cells but not T cells. *Oncogene* **8**:1–9.

41 Dent AL, Shaffer AL, Yu X, Allman D, Staudt LM. (1997) Control of inflammation, cytokine expression, and germinal center formation by BCL-6. *Science* **276**:589–92.

42 Ye BH, Cattoretti G, Shen Q, et al. (1997) The BCL-6 proto-oncogene controls germinal-centre formation and Th2-type inflammation. *Nat Genet* **16**:161–70.

43 Ci W, Polo JM, Melnick A. (2008) B-cell lymphoma 6 and the molecular pathogenesis of diffuse large B-cell lymphoma. *Curr Opin Hematol* **15**:381–90.

44 Shaffer AL, Yu X, He Y, et al. (2000) BCL-6 represses genes that function in lymphocyte differentiation, inflammation, and cell cycle control. *Immunity* **13**:199–212.

45 Vasanwala FH, Kusam S, Toney LM, Dent AL. (2002) Repression of AP-1 function: a mechanism for the regulation of Blimp-1 expression and B lymphocyte differentiation by the B cell lymphoma-6 proto-oncogene. *J Immunol* **169**:1922–9.

46 Liu M, Duke JL, Richter DJ, et al. (2008) Two levels of protection for the B cell genome during somatic hypermutation. *Nature* **451**:841–5.

47 Pasqualucci L, Bhagat G, Jankovic M, et al. (2008) AID is required for germinal center-derived lymphomagenesis. *Nat Genet* **40**:108–12.

48 Ranuncolo SM, Wang L, Polo JM, et al. (2008) BCL6-mediated attenuation of DNA damage sensing triggers growth arrest and senescence through a p53-dependent pathway in a cell context-dependent manner. *J Biol Chem* **283**:22565–72.

49 Phan RT, Dalla-Favera R. (2004) The BCL6 proto-oncogene suppresses p53 expression in germinal-centre B cells. *Nature* **432**:635–9.

50 Ranuncolo SM, Polo JM, Melnick A. (2008) BCL6 represses CHEK1 and suppresses DNA damage pathways in normal and malignant B-cells. *Blood Cells, Molecules & Diseases* **41**:95–9.

51 Phan RT, Saito M, Basso K, Niu H, Dalla-Favera R. (2005) BCL6 interacts with the transcription factor Miz-1 to suppress the cyclin-dependent kinase inhibitor p21 and cell cycle arrest in germinal center B cells. *Nat Immunol* **6**:1054–60.

52 Lin Y, Wong K, Calame K. (1997) Repression of c-myc transcription by Blimp-1, an inducer of terminal B cell differentiation. *Science* **276**:596–9.

53 Saito M, Gao J, Basso K, et al. (2007) A signaling pathway mediating downregulation of BCL6 in germinal center B cells is blocked by BCL6 gene alterations in B cell lymphoma. *Cancer Cell* **12**:280–92.

54 Walker SR, Nelson EA, Frank DA. (2007) STAT5 represses BCL6 expression by binding to a regulatory region frequently mutated in lymphomas. *Oncogene* **26**:224–33.

55 Klein U, Dalla-Favera R. (2008) Germinal centres: role in B-cell physiology and malignancy. *Nat Rev Immunol* **8**:22–33.

56 Pasqualucci L, Neumeister P, Goossens T, et al. (2001) Hypermutation of multiple proto-oncogenes in B-cell diffuse large-cell lymphomas. *Nature* **412**:341–6.

57 Hoang AT, Lutterbach B, Lewis BC, et al. (1995) A link between increased transforming activity of lymphoma-derived MYC mutant alleles, their defective regulation by p107, and altered phosphorylation of the c-Myc transactivation domain. *Mol Cell Biol* **15**:4031–42.

58 Vafa O, Wade M, Kern S, et al. (2002) c-Myc can induce DNA damage, increase reactive oxygen species, and mitigate p53 function: a mechanism for oncogene-induced genetic instability. *Molecular Cell* **9**:1031–44.

59 Dominguez-Sola D, Ying CY, Grandori C, et al. (2007) Non-transcriptional control of DNA replication by c-Myc. *Nature* **448**:445–51.

60 Hemann MT, Bric A, Teruya-Feldstein J, et al. (2005) Evasion of the p53 tumour surveillance network by tumour-derived MYC mutants. *Nature* **436**:807–11.

61 Yano T, Sander CA, Clark HM, et al. (1993) Clustered mutations in the second exon of the MYC gene in sporadic Burkitt's lymphoma. *Oncogene* **8**:2741–8.

62 Teng Y, Takahashi Y, Yamada M, et al. (2007) IRF4 negatively regulates proliferation of germinal center B cell-derived Burkitt's lymphoma cell lines and induces differentiation toward plasma cells. *Euro J Cell Biol* **86**:581–9.

63 Iida S, Rao PH, Butler M, et al. (1997) Deregulation of MUM1/IRF4 by chromosomal translocation in multiple myeloma. *Nat Genet* **17**:226–30.

64 Yoshida S, Nakazawa N, Iida S, et al. (1999) Detection of MUM1/IRF4-IgH fusion in multiple myeloma. *Leukemia* **13**:1812–6.

65 Ponzoni M, Arrigoni G, Doglioni C. (2007) New transcription factors in diagnostic hematopathology. *Adv Anat Pathol* **14**:25–35.

66 Shaffer AL, Lin KI, Kuo TC, et al. (2002) Blimp-1 orchestrates plasma cell differentiation by extinguishing the mature B cell gene expression program. *Immunity* **17**:51–62.

67 Butcher EC. (1990) Warner-Lambert/Parke-Davis Award lecture. Cellular and molecular mechanisms that direct leukocyte traffic. *Amer J Pathol* **136**:3–11.

68 Morgner A, Miehlke S, Fischbach W, et al. (2001) Complete remission of primary high-grade B-cell gastric lymphoma after cure of Helicobacter pylori infection. *J Clin Oncol* **19**:2041–8.

69 Hermine O, Lefrere F, Bronowicki JP, et al. (2002) Regression of splenic lymphoma with villous lymphocytes after treatment of hepatitis C virus infection. *New Engl J Med* **347**:89–94.

70 Adams J. (2002) Preclinical and clinical evaluation of proteasome inhibitor PS–341 for the treatment of cancer. *Curr Opin Chem Biol* **6**:493–500.

71 Letai A, Bassik MC, Walensky LD, et al. (2002) Distinct BH3 domains either sensitize or activate mitochondrial apoptosis, serving as prototype cancer therapeutics. *Cancer Cell* **2**:183–92.

CHAPTER 18

Non-Hodgkin Lymphomas

Nathan Fowler and Peter McLaughlin
Department of Lymphoma/Myeloma, University of Texas M.D. Anderson Cancer Center, Houston, TX, USA

Epidemiology and incidence

The non-Hodgkin lymphomas (NHL) are a heterogeneous group of B- and T-cell malignancies primarily involving the lymphoid system. The classification and diagnosis of NHL has evolved over the past several decades; the World Health Organization (WHO) currently recognizes over 30 different subtypes of the disease (see partial list in Table 18.1) [1]. The incidence of NHL increased markedly from 1970 until 1990, but appears to have slowed over the past two decades. It is estimated that over sixty thousand patients with NHL will be diagnosed in the US in 2009, representing 4% of all newly diagnosed malignancies [2]. NHL is the fifth leading cause of cancer mortality. The disease appears to have a geographic variation between subtypes, although the disparity observed in different populations is poorly understood. For instance, there is a seven-fold difference in the incidence of follicular lymphoma between the US and Asia [3]. Conversely, in Asia a higher percentage of NHL are T-cell types. For certain rare lymphomas, the geographic pattern of incidence is partially understood: in Japan and parts of the Caribbean, adult T-cell leukemia/lymphoma (ATLL) is prevalent in association with HTLV-1 infection; and classical Burkitt's lymphoma (BL) was first described in the malaria belt of Africa, in conjunction with Epstein-Barr virus (EBV) infection. Nasal NK/T-cell lymphoma occurs at disproportionately high rates in Asia and parts of Central and South America. Among Hodgkin lymphoma (HL) cases, the nodular sclerosis subtype is more commonly seen in the West,

whereas the mixed cellularity subtype is more common in developing countries; patterns of EBV infection play a role in some cases of HL, too.

NHL is generally a disease of older adults, with the diagnosis much more common after age 40 and peaking in the sixth decade of life. Due to advances in therapy as well as supportive care, the number of patients living extended periods following the diagnosis is increasing, and it is estimated that over half a million patients are currently living in the US with NHL. The reality of a cure remains possible in a subset of patients. Due to an evolving and better understanding of the biology of the disease, and to the subsequent development of newer targeted agents, this potentially curable subset is likely increasing.

Etiological clues

Not surprisingly, there is evidence that immune dysregulation, either from chronic stimulation or from immunosuppression, may play a key role in the development of some lymphomas. It has long been recognized that patients with significant immunosuppression, either from primary or secondary conditions, are at increased risk for the disease. The level of immunosuppression may play a role in the evolution of NHL: following solid organ transplantation, early aggressive immunosuppression appears to correlate with increased lymphoma risk. In addition, withdrawal of immunosuppression in organ transplant patients can lead to disease regression [4]. Patients with HIV are at highest risk

Advances in Malignant Hematology, First Edition. Edited by Hussain I. Saba and Ghulam J. Mufti. © 2011 Blackwell Publishing Ltd. Published 2011 by Blackwell Publishing Ltd.

Table 18.1 Major lymphoma subtypes

Precursor lymphoid neoplasms

(B- and T-lymphoblastic leukemic/lymphoma)

Mature B-cell neoplasms

  Chronic lymphocytic leukemia/small lymphocytic lymphoma

  Hairy cell leukemia

  Marginal zone lymphoma

    (splenic; nodal; extranodal/MALT)

  Lymphoplasmacytic

  Follicular lymphoma

  Mantle cell lymphoma

  Diffuse large B-cell lymphoma

  Primary mediastinal LBCL

  Burkitt's lymphoma

  "Unclassifiable", with features of DLBCL and:

    (a) BL, or (b) Hodgkin lymphoma

Mature T- and NK cell neoplasms

  Adult T-cell leukemia/lymphoma

  Extranodal NK/T-cell lymphoma, nasal type

  Hepatosplenic T-cell lymphoma

  Mycosis fungoides and Sézary syndrome

  Primary cutaneous CD30-positive T-cell disorders

  Peripheral T-cell lymphoma, NOS

  Angioimmunoblastic T-cell lymphoma

  Anaplastic large cell lymphoma:

    (2 distinct types: ALK-positive and ALK-negative)

Hodgkin lymphoma

Immunodeficiency-associated disorders

Histocytic and dendritic cell neoplasms

MALT: mucosa-associated lymphoid tissue; NOS: not otherwise specified; BL: Burkitt's lymphoma; LBCL: large B-cell lymphoma

of developing NHL when their immunosuppression is severe, and the advent of HAART (highly active antiretroviral therapy) appears to have mitigated some of this risk [5].

Chronic immune stimulation likely plays a role in lymphomagenesis. Several viral and bacterial infectious agents have been linked to the development of lymphoma. Nearly all cases of post-transplant lymphoma and a large portion of HIV-associated lymphomas have been linked to unrestrained proliferation of EBV-infected lymphocytes [4, 5]. Nearly 100% of HIV-associated CNS lymphomas and 95% of the African endemic form of BL are associated with EBV co-infection. Other viruses implicated in the development of NHL include hepatitis C in B-cell lymphoma, HTLV-1 in ATLL, and HHV-8 in HIV-associated body cavity lymphoma [6]. The link between *H. pylori* infection and gastric marginal zone B-cell lymphomas (MZL) of mucosa-associated lymphoid tissue (MALT) is well established. Removal of the antigenic drive through treatment of the underlying bacterial infection can lead to disease remission in many patients with gastric MALT lymphoma [7]. MZL of the skin have been associated with *Borrelia bergdorferi* [7]. The causal relationship between extranodal MZL of other organs and infection is less understood and remains an area of ongoing investigation.

Autoimmune diseases such as Crohn's disease, rheumatoid arthritis, celiac disease, systemic lupus, Sjögren's syndrome, and Felty's syndrome have an increased incidence of lymphoma. While the drugs used in the treatment of these diseases may increase overall lymphoma risk, there is likely a contributory relationship between the patient's underlying immune dysregulation and the development of the NHL.

Despite these clues, the majority of patients with newly diagnosed NHL have no identifiable risk factors or family history of the disease.

Cytogenetics and molecular genetics

Molecular pathways of note

Exciting advances in our knowledge of the biology of the lymphomas are covered in greater detail elsewhere in this textbook. Several basic aspects will be covered briefly here, with emphasis on issues that can have a bearing on clinical decision making.

It has long been known that there are characteristic cytogenetic abnormalities in many lymphomas. It is notable but not surprising that immunoglobulin heavy chain (IgH) gene translocations are commonly involved in several B-cell lymphomas. Nearly all cases of BL are associated with the c-myc translocation. In over 80% of cases, this occurs between the myc gene and IgH gene t(8;14). Translocation of c-myc is not exclusive to BL; it can be seen in a minority of diffuse large B-cell lymphomas (DLBCL) and multiple myelomas [8].

In follicular lymphoma (FL), bcl-2 gene rearrangement is common. One clinical spin-off of this knowledge is the utilization of polymerase chain reaction (PCR) technology to monitor for subclinical residual disease in FL patients. Knowledge about bcl-2 has also led to therapeutic developments such as antisense oligonucleotide therapy, which can oppose the antiapoptotic and chemo-resistance effects of overexpression of Bcl-2, occurring in many lymphomas as well as other malignancies.

In a subset of DLBCL, dysregulation of bcl-6 is a hallmark. Insights into the key role of bcl-6 in B-cell development within the germinal center have led to the development of small molecule peptides that may soon be suitable for clinical trial testing [9]. Other cytogenetic findings are correlated with molecular genetic abnormalities in Table 18.2.

Gene expression profiling (GEP) has provided a wealth of information that correlates with clinical outcomes. Recent large GEP studies suggest that survival following diagnosis can be predicted by biologic differences among lymphomas at the time of diagnosis. In FL, immune response signatures correlate with survival independently of clinical prognostic variables, indicating a major role for non-neoplastic cells such as T-cells and follicular dendritic cells (FDC) in determining outcome [10]. In DLBCL too, gene expression signatures can identify DLBCL subsets with different prognoses [11]. At times DLBCL and BL can be difficult to distinguish, and GEP may someday help make this distinction.

These and other GEP findings are provocative and enlightening, but GEP is a research tool, not a

Table 18.2 Characteristic cytogenetic abnormalities in non-Hodgkin lymphoma

Lymphoma type	Translocation	Oncogene
Follicular	t(14;18)	bcl-2
Mantle cell	t(11;14)	Cyclin D1
Diffuse large B-cell	3q27	bcl-6
Burkitt's	t(8;14)	c-myc
T-cell ALCL	t(2;5)	NPM/ALK
Lymphoplasmacytic	t(9;14)	PAX-5
MALT	t(11;18)	API2/MALT1
	t(1;14)	and others
	and others	

T-cell ALCL: T-cell anaplastic large cell lymphoma; MALT: mucosa-associated lymphoid tissue

standard evaluation technique. Even so, the resultant insights can or may be translated to clinical practice, for instance through the use of immunohistochemistry staining algorithms in DLBCL that may approximate the GEP findings. Promising therapeutic insights may be forthcoming from GEP studies too, for example by improving our understanding of the role of the NF-κB pathway in lymphoma, or the potential for inhibitors of the protein kinase C (PKC) pathway [12, 13].

Classification and diagnosis of non-Hodgkin lymphoma

Lymphoma subtypes can be correlated with phases of normal lymphocyte differentiation as illustrated for B-cell lymphomas in Figure 18.1.

The evolution of lymphoma classifications is a rich literature. Early purely morphological schemes (e.g., that of Rappaport) gave way to ones that integrated lymphocyte biology and phenotype information, for example, those of Lukes and Collins, Karl Lennert from the Kiel group, and the Revised European-American Lymphoma (REAL) schemes. Increasingly, clinical and molecular biology information has been

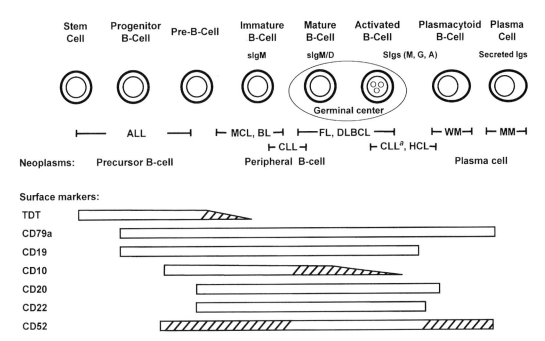

Figure 18.1 Normal B-cell differentiation and marker expression, and corresponding B-cell malignancies.
[a]CLL identified twice because there are two subtypes, defined by immunoglobulin gene mutation status.
SIg: surface immunoglobulin; ALL: acute lymphoblastic leukemia (B-lymphoblastic leukemia/lymphoma); MCL: mantle cell lymphoma; BL: Burkitt's lymphoma; CLL: chronic lymphocytic leukemia/small lymphocytic leukemia; FL: follicular lymphoma; DLBCL: diffuse large B-cell lymphoma; HCL: hairy cell leukemia; WM: Waldenström's macroglobulinemia (lymphoplasmacytic lymphoma); MM: multiple myeloma
(Adapted from Harris et al. (2001) In Jaffe et al. (eds.) *Pathology and Genetics of Tumours and Haematopoietic Tumours and Lymphoid Tissues.* Lyon: IARC.)

integrated [1, 14, 15]. The clinical thumbnail sketches of the Working Formulation (WF) are exemplary, although dated [14]. The inclusion of a commentary section with dissenting opinions among the co-authors in the WF report is entertaining and enlightening. The current World Health Organization (WHO) system is now in its second iteration [1].

Phenotype information is fundamental in the WHO classification system, starting with the basic distinction between B- and T-cell lymphomas. Ancillary immunostains are often important, for example, cyclin D1 staining if mantle cell lymphoma (MCL) is a consideration. Estimation of the proliferative fraction with a stain such as Ki-67 can also be useful. In some cases, fluorescence in situ hybridization (FISH) studies for suspected gene rearrangements (e.g., c-myc) can provide important supplemental information.

The WHO classification, unlike the REAL schema and others, uses the term "follicular" to designate the germinal center phenotype (e.g., CD10-positive) rather than lymph node architecture [1]. In older systems, it was the follicular architecture that was shown to correlate compellingly with clinical outcome. The WHO scheme emphasizes the need to estimate the extent of follicular architecture in the report. However, a somewhat unfortunate consequence of the use of the word "follicular" in the WHO scheme is that cytology samples can be diagnosed as "FL" despite the lack of any information about lymph node architecture.

Vexing classification issues persist. For instance, the largest category among T-cell lymphomas is an acknowledged heterogeneous entity designated "peripheral T-cell lymphoma, not otherwise specified" (PTCL, NOS). Two other lymphoma categories are identified as "unclassifiable", but are in fact quite precisely defined: one with features overlapping between DLBCL and BL, and the other between DLBCL and HL [1].

Many entities can be subdivided. FL can be graded (1, 2, 3a, 3b) based on the proportion of small and large lymphoma cells in a biopsy. FL grade 3b, which is characterized by sheets of large cells, is biologically and clinically more similar to DLBCL than to the indolent types of FL [1]. DLBCL can be subdivided based on clinical features, morphology, and other criteria including molecular profile if data is available.

The importance of the clinical presentation in determining lymphoma subtype is notable for several entities. The biopsy alone is insufficient to define primary mediastinal large B-cell lymphoma (PMLBCL). PMLBCL is sometimes defined in a self-fulfilling way, restricted only to Stage I–II presentations in the mediastinum. Other literature on PMLBCL includes Stage III–IV cases if the dominant and primary site is the mediastinum [16]. Likewise, the clinical features need to be taken into account to categorize the spectrum of disease that includes the benign entity lymphomatoid papulosis, and the T-cell lymphomas primary cutaneous anaplastic large cell lymphoma (ALCL), or even some cases of mycosis fungoides (MF).

The importance of the lymph node (or other) biopsy, and ancillary tests

With the increasing sophistication of technologies to assess biopsy material, the importance of obtaining adequate and representative tissue deserves emphasis. It has been shown that small amounts of tissue can lead to misclassification of lymphoma, which can have devastating consequences in treatment decisions. It is advisable to anticipate the possible need for ancillary testing.

Presentation and natural history of NHL

NHLs have varied clinical presentations. Patients with indolent disease can present with chronic, slowly developing lymphadenopathy, or with progressive splenomegaly and cytopenias. Patient survival is generally measured in years, and treatment can be deferred in some cases. In contrast, patients with aggressive NHL often present with an acute process including massive and rapid nodal growth, and threatened organ function. Without prompt and effective treatment, the process can be life-threatening within months or even weeks. An overview of outcomes for four major categories of B-cell lymphomas is shown in Table 18.3 [17].

Table 18.3 Survival and failure-free survival of major B-cell lymphomas

Lymphoma type	% Survival:		% Failure-free:	
	2-Yr	5-Yr	2-Yr	5-Yr
MALT	90	80	75	65
FL	85	70	65	45
DLBCL	55	45	50	45
MCL	65	25	30	10

MALT: mucosa-associated lymphoid tissue; FL: follicular lymphoma; DLBCL: diffuse large B-cell lymphoma; MCL: mantle cell lymphoma
(Adapted from Armitage et al. [17].)

Prognostic models have been developed that stratify patients better than the Ann Arbor staging system. For DLBCL, the International Prognostic Index (IPI) stratifies patients based upon age, lactate dehydrogenase (LDH), number of extranodal sites, performance status, and age [18]. Similar tools have been developed and validated in other lymphoma subtypes including FL (FLIPI, F2) and HL (IPS) [19–21]. Table 18.4 portrays features common to the various prognostic models.

Current staging techniques are directed at detecting all sites of nodal and extranodal involvement. Staging recommendations vary depending on a lymphoma's propensity to involve a specific organ system. In nearly all cases, CT imaging of the neck, chest, abdomen, and pelvis, and a bone marrow exam is recommended. In order to further clarify and highlight the differences in presentation and staging between different lymphoma subtypes, the subsequent discussion will be divided into the following subtypes: indolent NHL, aggressive NHL, and highly aggressive NHL.

Indolent NHL
Follicular lymphoma
FL often has a subtle presentation, with painless swelling noted in one or more lymph node stations. If the disease occurs in the abdomen, nodes can grow

Table 18.4 Similar features in different lymphoma prognostic models

| | Aggressive lymphoma | Follicular lymphoma | | Hodgkin lymphoma |
	IPI [18]	FLIPI [19]	FLIPI-2 [20]	IPS [21]
Age	Y ($\geq$60)	Y ($\geq$60)	Y ($\geq$60)	Y ($\geq$45)
Stage	Y (>III–IV)	Y (>III–IV)	†	Y (>IV)
LDH	Y	Y	†	
PS	Y ($\geq$2)	†	†	
E sites	Y ($\geq$2)	†	†	†
LN sites		Y (>4)	†	
Hgb		Y ($\leq$12)	Y ($\leq$12)	Y ($\leq$10.5)
B2m	†	†	Y	
Marrow	†	†	Y	
Bulk*	†		Y	
WBC				Y$^\Delta$
% lymphs				Y$^\Delta$
Gender		†		Y
Albumin	†	†		Y

Y: Yes, factor is in model (relevant cut-off level in parenthesis); IPI: International Prognostic Index; FLIPI: Follicular Lymphoma Prognostic Index; IPS: International Prognostic Score; E: extranodal; LN: lymph node
* Bulk defined variably. In FLIPI-2: 6 cm maximum diameter. In IPI: $\geq$10 cm
† Significant factor in univariate analysis but not included +/or fell out of model in multivariate analysis
Δ In IPS, hematologic adverse features include leukocytosis (WBC $\geq$15 000) and lymphopenia (ALC <600, or lymphs <8%)

quite large, leading to symptoms from increased tumor bulk and local organ compression. The diagnosis is often delayed due to the slow onset of disease and the ability of nodes to wax and wane without treatment. Most patients are diagnosed with multiple sites of involvement; using conventional staging techniques, approximately 70–80% of patients are found to have Stage III or IV disease [17, 20, 21]. In Stage I patients, PCR analysis of the peripheral blood or bone marrow is frequently positive for cells with bcl-2 gene rearrangement, suggesting that even in Stage I cases, FL is likely a systemic disease [22, 23]. As tumor burden increases, patients can experience constitutional B symptoms such as night sweats, fevers, and weight loss. The presence of B symptoms has been associated with a worse prognosis, and correlates with increased levels of inflammatory proteins such as C-reactive protein and cytokines such as interleukin-6 [24, 25].

Although FL generally originates in lymph nodes, it can involve nearly any organ system. Common sites of extranodal involvement include first and foremost the bone marrow, but also the GI tract and skin. Cutaneous FLs often present with localized disease, but can recur at distant cutaneous sites following local therapy. Involvement of the CNS by FL is rare.

The natural progression and survival following diagnosis of FL is heterogeneous and can include transformation into DLBCL. The median survival is in the order of 8–10 years but some patients will survive 15–20 years, while 10–15% will have a rapidly fatal course and die within one year of diagnosis. Biologic and clinical models have been developed to help predict outcomes in FL. Variations in the length of survival and time to disease progression can be predicted by the FLIPI prognostic model which was created and validated in trials from the pre-rituximab era [19].

Marginal zone lymphoma

The three categories of MZL (nodal, mucosa-associated, and splenic marginal zone) have different clinical presentations. Patients with nodal MZL have a presentation similar to FL, with most patients experiencing painless swelling in one or more lymph nodes. Stage III or IV disease is common. Splenic

MZL often presents with symptoms of moderate to massive splenomegaly, such as abdominal fullness, early satiety, and bloating [7]. Cytopenias are often noted, even when the marrow is minimally involved due to splenic sequestration. When bone marrow is extensively involved, peripheral lymphocyte counts can be elevated. Nodal involvement is variable, and splenomegaly is occasionally the only radiographic abnormality.

The most common sites of MALT lymphoma are the gastric mucosa, parotid and salivary glands, skin, lungs, conjunctiva, intestinal tract, thyroid, and breast [7]. Gastric MALT lymphoma can present with ulcer symptoms such as nausea and dyspepsia. Endoscopy often reveals ulcerations, erythema, and occasional nodular areas in the gastric mucosa. Lymphoepithelial lesions on biopsy are characteristic, and up to 90% of patients will be positive for an underlying infection with *H. pylori* [26]. Gastric MALT is commonly localized to the stomach or has lymphatic spread limited to peri-gastric nodal chains. The presentation of non-gastric MALT lymphoma is variable. Patients often present with localized symptoms related to a space-occupying lesion in the involved organ.

Small lymphocytic lymphoma

Small lymphocytic lymphoma (SLL) is often considered the nodal counterpart of chronic lymphocytic leukemia (CLL), and is part of the same entity in the WHO classification [1]. The presentation is similar to other indolent lymphomas, with slow progression of peripheral lympadenopathy. The staging evaluation commonly identifies SLL cells in the bone marrow or peripheral blood. However, in contrast to CLL, the peripheral lymphocyte count is usually only slightly elevated or normal, with the diagnosis of SLL generally reserved for patients with lymphocyte counts less than 5000/μL [26]. In SLL as in CLL, Richter's syndrome can occur with transformation into aggressive DLBCL.

Aggressive NHL
Diffuse large B-cell lymphoma

DLBCLs are the most common subtype of NHL, making up over 30% of newly diagnosed cases. The disease often presents in the sixth decade of life, although variants such as primary mediastinal large cell lymphoma usually present earlier, between 30 and 40 years of age. Unlike most indolent lymphomas, limited Stage disease at diagnosis is common, with 30–40% of patients presenting with Stage I or II disease [14, 17]. At diagnosis, the presence of B symptoms or an elevated serum LDH are not uncommon. The onset of symptoms can be rapid.

Primary mediastinal (thymic) large B-cell lymphoma (PMLBCL) is recognized as a distinct clinicopathologic entity. PMLBCL has a distinct gene expression profile that in part resembles that seen in classical HL [27, 28]. PMLBCL typically occurs in younger patients and is more common in females. Most patients have disease limited to the chest. Bone marrow involvement is rare. Symptoms occur secondary to an enlarging compressive thoracic mass with chest pain, shortness of breath, and possible superior vena cava syndrome at diagnosis [16]. One-third of patients can have pericardial and/or pleural effusions [29].

Mantle cell lymphoma

MCL can have a varied initial presentation and clinical course, and typically presents with advanced stage disease with involvement of multiple nodal sites. Splenomegaly is seen in up to 40% of patients and marrow involvement is common. The most common extranodal site is the gastrointestinal tract; up to 90% of patients will have GI involvement with extensive workup [30]. Overt "polyposis coli" presentations are rare but dramatic, with symptoms that can include diarrhea and melena.

T-cell lymphoma

Most T-cell lymphomas share features common to other lymphomas, including frequent involvement of lymph nodes, the liver, the spleen, and the bone marrow. The most common variant is an admittedly heterogeneous group known as peripheral T-cell lymphoma, type not otherwise specified (PTCL, NOS) [1, 31].

Mycosis fungoides (MF) is predominantly a cutaneous disease. A separate TNM-based staging system is used for MF, which emphasizes the extent of skin involvement, and which integrates the less frequent manifestations of lymph node spread, organ involvement, or blood involvement. The leukemic phase of MF (Sézary syndrome) is notable in that it can occur in the absence of obvious bone marrow infiltration.

Several other T-cell lymphomas also have skin manifestations, including the cutaneous variant of ALCL, and ATLL. In the most severe leukemic (acute) phase of ATLL, hypercalcemia is also a common feature. For some T-cell lymphomas, the typical presentation of the disease is captured in the name of the entity, including hepatosplenic T-cell lymphoma and enteropathy-associated T-cell lymphoma, the latter of which involves the GI tract and is often associated with celiac disease.

ALCL cases that are positive for anaplastic lymphoma kinase (ALK) expression are biologically fascinating; ALK is a potential therapeutic target [32]. The t(2;5)(p23;q35) translocation and numerous variants are a characteristic feature of ALK-positive ALCL.

Patients with angioimmunoblastic T-cell lymphoma (AITL) often present with extensive lymphadenopathy, hepatosplenomegaly, skin rash, and constitutional symptoms. Several additional distinctive features can occur that are indicative of immune dysregulation, including hypergammaglobulinemia and Coombs-positive hemolytic anemia. The lymph node pathology often includes a polyclonal plasma cell infiltrate and EBV-positive B cells. Another common pathologic feature, as suggested by the name AITL, is vascular hyperplasia. The frequent expression in AITL of the chemokine CXCL13 is a clue that AITL derives from follicular helper T cells [33].

Extranodal NK/T-cell lymphoma, nasal type is a distinct pathologic entity that is commonly associated with EBV infection. The disease is predominately diagnosed in Asian, Central and South American countries, but is occasionally seen in other parts of the world. The tumor typically occurs in the midline nasal region, and is often locally aggressive, with invasion of surrounding tissues including the orbit, bone, and sinus cavity common at presentation. Prompt diagnosis and treatment are essential due to the critical location of the tumor and its propensity for local destruction.

Highly aggressive lymphoma
Burkitt's lymphoma

BL is a highly aggressive B-cell malignancy typically characterized by a rapid proliferation rate and the translocation of myc (8q24). The classic morphology is that of a diffuse infiltration of intermediate-sized B-cells with high nuclear-to-cytoplasmic ratio and a "starry sky" appearance [34]. Typically Ki-67 staining will be positive in 90–100% of cells. In cases with high proliferation rates and atypical morphology, the distinction between DLBCL and BL can be difficult. Recent molecular studies have demonstrated that BL has a unique gene expression signature. In these reports, the signature was also present in a significant number of patients previously diagnosed with DLBCL, highlighting the inconsistency of current diagnostic techniques [35, 36].

Patients with BL often present with symptoms of a rapidly enlarging abdominal mass and B symptoms. Clinical workup of newly diagnosed patients includes a tissue biopsy with immunohistochemical and cytogenetic analysis. Further workup should include a lumbar puncture with flow cytometric analysis, and testing of HIV status. Bone marrow involvement is found in up to 70% of patients, and leptomeningeal spread is common [34]. Serum LDH is often elevated and electrolyte abnormalities can be present.

T-lymphoblastic leukemia/lymphoma

T-lymphoblastic leukemia/lymphoma (T-LBL) is a disease of adolescents and young adults. Over half of patients present with a mediastinal mass, often with associated symptoms that can include overt superior vena cava obstruction. There is a high risk for leptomeningeal spread. Marrow involvement is frequent; the spectrum of this disease overlaps with T-ALL.

Treatment – an overview

There are multiple management options for patients with newly diagnosed NHL; the decision is influenced by the classification of disease, the presentation, and other features. Patients with aggressive disease require prompt intensive therapy, while patients with indolent NHL can sometimes be observed for a while without treatment. The treatment of NHL underwent a major advance with the development of combination chemotherapy regimens utilizing agents with different mechanisms of action. The use of combination regimens, often in conjunction with radiation and biologic therapy, has become the treatment of choice for most patients with NHL. Most regimens combine agents of various classes to overcome drug resistance and minimize overlapping toxicity as described in Table 18.5.

Radiation therapy

Lymphomas are mostly radiosensitive diseases, even at relatively modest doses in the range of 30–45 Gy. Hence, when the presentation is localized (Stage I–II), radiation therapy (RT) can play an important role. That role in aggressive lymphoma and HL is usually in conjunction with or after chemotherapy. In indolent lymphoma, RT alone can be employed in appropriate circumstances. The inherent sensitivity of lymphoma to RT, coupled with the frequency of Stage III–IV disease, has provided the impetus for the development of techniques that can deliver RT systemically, that is, radioimmunotherapy (RIT) [37]. The role of RIT in conjunction with chemotherapy is an area of considerable current interest. RT can also be employed in other settings of multicentric advanced stage lymphoma, for example, total body electron beam RT for some cases of MF; total lymphoid irradiation approaches for some Stage III FL cases; and total body irradiation (TBI) which is sometimes employed in the context of myeloablative preparative programs in SCT approaches. The latter scenario is another possible setting for the use of RIT [38].

Biologic therapy

Recent progress in the understanding of the pathways that contribute to lymphoma cell survival, and resistance to cell death, has led to the identification of multiple targets for drug therapy. These discoveries have contributed to the development of several new classes of drugs, including monoclonal antibodies targeting lineage-specific antigens and receptors, and small molecules that inhibit intracellular signaling pathways. The identification of stable

Table 18.5 Common chemotherapy variants

Backbone	Acronym	Agents	Typical disease utilization	Front-line or salvage
Alkylating Agent:	–	Chlorambucil (±prednisone)	Indolent lymphoma	Both
	COP/CVP [80]	Cyclophosphamide, vincristine, prednisone	Indolent Lymphoma	Both
Cyclophosphamide and doxorubicin[b]:	CHOP [81]	COP agents, plus doxorubicin	DLBCL; indolent lymphoma	Both
	EPOCH [91]	CHOP agents, plus etoposide	DLBCL; MCL; AIDS-related lymphoma	Mainly front-line
	MACOP B [86]	CHOP agents, plus methotrexate and bleomycin	DLBCL	Front-line
Intensified cyclophosphamide and doxorubicin programs:	Hyper-CVAD [55]	CHOP agents (intensified), plus cytarabine and methotrexate	MCL; Burkitt's lymphoma	Mainly front-line
	CODOX-M and IVAC [92]	CHOP (without prednisone) and methotrexate, ifosfamide, etoposide	Burkitt's lymphoma	Front-line
	ACVBP [98]	CHOP agents (intensified, with vindesine instead of vincristine), and bleomycin, methotrexate, ifosfamide, etoposide, and cytarabine	DLBCL	Front-line
Nucleoside analog-based programs[b]:	FND [83]	Fludarabine, mitoxantrone, dexamethasone	Indolent lymphoma	Both
	FCM [99]	Fludarabine, cyclophosphamide, mitoxantrone	Indolent lymphoma; MCL	Both
	PCR[a] [100]	Pentostatin, cyclophosphamide, rituximab	Indolent lymphoma; CLL	Both

(Continued)

Table 18.5 (*Continued*)

Backbone	Acronym	Agents	Typical disease utilization	Front-line or salvage
Regimens that may be non-cross-resistant with CHOP[b]:	DHAP [101]	Dexamethasone, cytarabine, cisplatin	Mainly aggressive lymphoma	Salvage
	ICE [94]	Ifosfamide, mesna, carboplatin, etoposide	Mainly aggressive lymphoma	Salvage
	MINE [95]	Mesna, ifosfamide, mitoxantrone, etoposide	Indolent and aggressive lymphoma	Salvage
	R-GemOX[a] [96]	Rituximab, gemcitabine, oxaliplatin	Mainly aggressive lymphoma	Salvage
	TTR [97]	Toptecan, paclitaxel, rituximab	Mainly aggressive lymphoma	Salvage

[a] Some regimens developed in the rituximab era; virtually all others can be given in conjunction with rituximab, for example, the R-CHOP regimen
[b] Variants include:
For CHOP: CHOP-14 (shortened interval)
For MACOP-B: M-BACOD
For DHAP: ESHAP (with etoposide), or ASHAP (with doxorubicin)
For FCM: FC (no mitoxantrone)

antigenic targets such as CD20 on the B-cell surface, combined with the development of hybridoma and recombinant engineering technology for production of chimeric and fully humanized antibodies, has allowed monoclonal antibody therapy to become integrated into the majority of regimens for newly diagnosed and relapsed B-cell lymphoma [39].

A major emphasis of current research is to identify and target mechanisms that are known to be dysregulated in NHL, such as cell cycle and growth regulatory pathways, programmed cell death pathways, intracellular protein assembly/degradation pathways, de-repression of tumor suppressor genes though epigenetic approaches (e.g., hypomethylating agents and histone deacetylase (HDAC) inhibitors), and targeting of the immune microenvironment through immunomodulatory drugs (IMiDs).

Stem cell transplant
Front-line therapy
The use of hematopoietic SCT as part of front-line therapy for NHL remains an area of active study. Although phase II trials in patients with high-risk DLBCL suggested a potential benefit to transplant as part of initial therapy, results have been conflicting and randomized trials have failed to confirm this benefit [40]. Similarly, studies using SCT in first remission for patients with indolent lymphoma have shown a benefit in event-free survival (EFS), but no change in OS [41]. In general, SCT for B-cell lymphoma is currently not recommended as first-line therapy outside of a clinical trial. A notable exception is MCL, in which an SCT in first remission is commonly employed. Recent trials have investigated incorporating SCT into front-line therapy in T-cell and CNS lymphoma, and phase II trials have demonstrated impressive results [42, 43].

Salvage therapy
High-dose therapy followed by autologous SCT has been more extensively investigated in relapsed NHL. Its benefit is well established and is considered the treatment of choice for patients with relapsed chemosensitive aggressive NHL. The PARMA trial, a large randomized international study, showed a benefit in both five-year EFS (46% vs. 12%) and OS (53% vs. 32%), in patients with DLBCL

who were assigned to autologous SCT versus chemotherapy alone, respectively [44]. The benefit of autologous SCT is limited for patients whose DLCBL is refractory or progressive following salvage therapy [45].

SCT in patients with relapsed indolent disease is probably the most effective salvage therapy option available, although many patients will still relapse following therapy, and toxicity is an issue, including secondary malignancies [40, 46].

Allogeneic SCT in the management of relapsed indolent lymphoma shows promise. Although early trials demonstrated significant toxicity, the increasing use of reduced intensity conditioning regimens has led to decreased treatment-related mortality. A recent trial in patients with relapsed FL using a non-myeloablative conditioning regimen with fludarabine, cyclophosphamide, and rituximab showed an eight-year OS and PFS of 85% and 83% respectively [47]. Allogeneic transplant is also under investigation for relapsed MCL following failure of primary therapy and for patients with aggressive NHL who fail or are ineligible for autologous SCT.

Management of non-Hodgkin lymphoma subtypes

Indolent lymphomas
Follicular lymphoma
Due to the prolonged natural history of FL and the variable clinical course, no single standard of care has emerged for untreated patients. Although the course is often marked by long remissions, most patients with advanced disease ultimately relapse and die of the malignancy. Multiple treatment options exist for patients with newly diagnosed disease, ranging from observation only to a variety of combined chemo-immunotherapy regimens. Observation only is often a valid approach for patients with advanced stage disease who are asymptomatic. Without treatment, a minority of patients will have temporary spontaneous remissions since the disease often follows an indolent prolonged course. Early intervention has historically not been shown to prolong survival, so the decision to treat and the regimen of choice is often based

upon tumor burden, disease-associated symptoms and the patient's co-morbid conditions [48]. Untreated FL has excellent response rates to both single agents and combined chemo-immunotherapy regimens. Several key trials in indolent lymphoma are reviewed in Table 18.6.

The vast majority of patients with advanced stage disease will relapse following primary therapy. Multiple salvage regimens are available with response rates ranging from 40–90% (Table 18.5). While the general rule of thumb when deciding upon salvage regimens is to choose non-cross-resistant agents, many patients will respond to retreatment with the induction regimen.

Using current staging techniques, 20–30% of patients with FL will be diagnosed with early stage disease [17]. Patients with Stage I and II disease represent a unique subset of FL, in that prolonged remissions and possible cure can be attained following primary therapy. Involved field radiotherapy will result in long-term remissions in nearly half of all newly diagnosed patients. The 10-year OS in most studies approaches 50–70% [49]. Efforts to incorporate combined modality approaches into front-line treatment may provide a benefit in long-term outcomes through the eradication or suppression of occult systemic disease [50].

The development of prognostic tools such as the FLIPI identifies patients who are more likely to have a poor outcome [19]. In a study by Buske et al., patients with high-risk FLIPI scores had a two-year time to treatment failure (TTF) of 67% versus 90% and 92% for intermediate- and low-risk groups, respectively [51]. Despite these findings, no standard of care has yet emerged to stratify treatment regimens based upon the level of pretreatment risk.

Marginal zone lymphoma

The treatment recommendations and natural history of nodal MZL are similar to those for FL. Asymptomatic patients with minimal disease can often be observed closely without intervention. Treatment regimens for patients with advanced stage disease are similar to those used for FL. Splenic

Table 18.6 Trials of note in indolent lymphoma

Author, year, ref.	% FL	Regimen(s)	% CR	% PR	% FFS (@time)	% Surv (@time)
A. Randomized						
Marcus et al. 2005 [80]	100	CVP	10	47	23 (3-yr)	85 (30 mo)
		R-CVP	41	40	52	89
Hiddemann et al. 2005 [81]	100	CHOP	17	73	50 (3-yr)	89 (2-yr)
		R-CHOP	20	77	75	96
Zinzani et al. 2004 [82]	100	FM → R	68	28	63 (3-yr)	94 (3-yr)
		CHOP → R	42	56		
Tsimberidou et al. 2002 [83]	79	FND	79	18	41 (3-yr)	84 (3-yr)
		ATT	87	10	50	82
Morschhauser et al. 2008 [84]	100	Various	–	–	25 (3-yr)	–
		Various → RIT	–	–	47	–
B. Notable						
Press et al. 2006 [85]	100	CHOP → RIT	69	22	67 (5-yr)	87 (5-yr)

Abbreviations, see Table 18.5, plus: ATT: alternating triple therapy; RIT: radioimmunotherapy

MZL is a distinct pathologic subtype that often presents with disease limited to the spleen and bone marrow. As in nodal MZL, observation is an adequate management choice in patients who are asymptomatic. In patients with significant cytopenias or symptoms from splenomegaly, local therapy is often effective. Splenectomy, or splenic radiotherapy in ineligible patients, will often provide relief from disease symptoms [7]. Systemic therapy options are similar to other indolent lymphomas. Single agent rituximab has been shown to have impressive activity [7, 52].

MZL of MALT type often presents with localized extranodal disease. The stomach is most commonly involved in approximately 30% of patients. In cases of gastric MALT, *H. pylori* infection is detected in 90% of cases. Eradication of the organism through antibiotic therapy in patients with Stage IE disease will lead to disease regression in over two-thirds of patients [7]. The results of early restaging should be interpreted carefully, as disease regression can be gradual, and complete remission may take up to one year following antibiotic treatment. Patients who are *H. pylori* negative or do not respond to antibiotic therapy can be treated with local radiotherapy with excellent results. Treatment recommendations for patients with extensive disease follows those of FL, with multiple combined chemo-immunotherapy regimens demonstrating overall response rates greater than 80% [53]. Non-gastric MALT makes up the remaining 70% of new cases. The prognosis is generally excellent. Radiation therapy is often the treatment of choice in patients with localized disease. Patients with extensive disease requiring therapy will often respond to regimens similar to other indolent lymphomas [7].

Small lymphocytic lymphoma

Patients with SLL are often asymptomatic when diagnosed, and the disease typically follows an indolent course. The diagnosis of limited stage disease is rare. Similar to the other indolent lymphomas, patients can be observed and no evidence supports a survival benefit with early treatment. Purine analog-containing combinations are often the treatment of choice, and studies suggest a benefit in PFS when compared to traditional alkylator-based regimens [54]. Rituximab has limited single agent activity in SLL, but rituximab's inclusion in combination with chemotherapy appears to improve response rates. Currently available combination regimens are not curative, and novel agents and combinations are being explored. Recent studies with allogeneic transplantation appear promising. Clinical trial participation is encouraged, especially in patients with relapsed or refractory disease.

Aggressive lymphomas
Diffuse large B-cell lymphoma

DLBCL accounts for the majority of aggressive B-cell lymphomas. As noted in Table 18.7, many of the most influential clinical trials in aggressive lymphoma have focused mainly on DLBCL. DLBCL can be subdivided based on: anatomic site of presentation (e.g., primary CNS, primary cutaneous "leg type," or primary effusion lymphoma); phenotype or molecular profile (e.g., CD5-positive, or activated B-cell (ABC) type); or morphologic or other features. The pace of the disease and the onset of symptoms can be quick. The disease is detected with limited stage in about one-third of cases. In some cases, notably those of extranodal origin sites such as the thyroid, an underlying MALT lymphoma component is sometimes detected. The selection of therapy for DLBCL is based on the presenting stage and other prognostic factors. The most commonly used prognostic model for aggressive lymphomas is the IPI, which was based largely on DLBCL cases, all treated in the pre-rituximab era [18].

Immuno-chemotherapy such as R-CHOP is the backbone of therapy for most DLBCL cases. In localized disease settings, radiation therapy (RT) can play a role. In high-risk situations (IPI ≥3), therapy more intensive than R-CHOP has been explored, but there is ongoing controversy about the role, timing, and impact of intensified therapy. With some DLBCL presentations, the risk of CNS relapse is sufficiently high to warrant intrathecal chemoprophylaxis. Examples include testicular and paraspinal presentation, patients with multiple extranodal sites, and patients with concurrent HIV infection.

Table 18.7 Trials of note in aggressive lymphoma

Author, year, ref.	% DLBCL	Regimen(s)	% CR	% PR	% FFS (@time)	% Surv (@time)
A. Randomized						
Fisher et al. 1993 [86]	81	CHOP	44	36	41	54
		MACOP-B	51	32	41 (3-yr)	50 (3-yr)
		M-BACOD	48	34	46 (3-yr)	52 (3-yr)
		ProMACE-CytaBoM	56	31	46 (3-yr)	50 (3-yr)
Pfreundschuh et al. 2006 [87]	100	CHOP-like	68	–	59 (3-yr)	84 (3-yr)
		R-CHOP-like	86	–	79	93
Feugier et al. 2005 [88]	100	CHOP	63	6	29 (5-yr)	45 (5-yr)
		R-CHOP	75	8	47	58
Pfreundschuh et al. 2008 [89]	80	CHOP-14x6	68	7	42	68
		CHOP-14x8	72	4	53 (3-yr)	66 (3-yr)
		R-CHOP-14x6	78	4	66	78
		R-CHOP-14x8	76	3	63	72
B. Large-scale, notable						
Cabanillas et al. 1998 [90]	89	ATT	79	18	~58 (3-yr)	61 (3-yr)
Wilson et al. 2008 [91]	100	R-EPOCH	94	4	79 (5-yr)	80 (5-yr)
Mead et al. 2002 [92]	0 (BL trial)	CODOX-M and IVAC	76	10	65 (2-yr)	73 (2-yr)
Thomas et al. 2006 [93]	0 (BL trial)	R-h-CVAD	86	11	80 (3-yr)	89 (3-yr)
Romaguera et al. 2005 [55]	0 (MCL trial)	R-h-CVAD	87	10	64 (3-yr)	85 (3-yr)
C. Salvage Regimens						
Moskowitz et al. 1999 [94]	72	ICE	24	42	33 (3-yr)	25 (3-yr)
Rodriguez et al. 1995 [95]	56	MINE-ESHAP	48	21	20 (2-yr)	47 (2-yr)
El Gneoui et al. 2007 [96]	72	R-Gem Ox	50	33	43 (2-yr)	66 (2-yr)
Younes et al. 2001 [97]	81	Topotecan + paclitaxel	12	36	<25 (1-yr)	–

Abbreviations, see Table 18.5, plus: ATT: alternating triple therapy; DLBCL: diffuse large B-cell lymphoma; BL: Burkitt's lymphoma; MCL: mantle cell lymphoma

Mantle cell lymphoma

MCL represents only about 7% of lymphomas, but it has been the focus of attention because of its relatively recent recognition, its generally poor outlook with standard therapy, its unique biology, and the promising therapeutic options that have become available which target biological pathways that are dysregulated in MCL. Limited-stage MCL is infrequent. A slow clinical pace is occasionally seen, but most commonly, prompt institution of intensive therapy is appropriate. Modest therapy such as CHOP has typically resulted in low CR rates and short-duration control of disease. SCT in first remission has been extensively pursued [40]. Intensive non-SCT approaches have also been used, notably the hyper-CVAD regimen (fractionated cyclophosphamide, vincristine, doxorubicin, and dexamethasone, alternating with high-dose methotrexate and cytarabine) [55].

Notable successes have been reported in treating recurrent MCL with bortezomib (a proteasome inhibitor), and temsirolimus (an mTOR inhibitor). Conversely, results have been disappointing with flavopiridol (a cyclin-dependent kinase inhibitor) to date, although its potential favorable interaction with other agents is noteworthy [56]. The utility of such agents in MCL, in which there is dysregulation of relevant cell growth and proliferation pathways (cyclin D1; Pl3K/AKT/mTOR; NFκB), fosters hope that "targeted" therapies may soon result in more effective and hopefully less toxic therapy for MCL and many other malignancies.

T-cell lymphoma

T-cell lymphomas are a heterogeneous group of diseases and are less common than B-cell NHL. Treatment is less well studied and most regimens have been adapted from the B-cell NHL literature. Outcomes following systemic therapy are generally poor.

Peripheral T-cell lymphoma (PTCL), type not otherwise specified (NOS), is a WHO-defined heterogeneous subgroup of nodal and extranodal T-cell lymphomas [1]. Treatment recommendations traditionally are similar to those for DLBCL, with most patients receiving CHOP-like regimens without rituximab. Results following standard therapy are inferior to those seen in DLBCL, with five-year OS ranging between 38–41% [57]. The use of SCT as consolidation therapy has been explored, with several retrospective trials showing five-year disease-free survival ranging from 63–79% for patients transplanted in first complete remission (CR1) [58]. Results should be interpreted with caution, as the ability to attain a complete remission to primary therapy is a powerful prognostic marker, so the role of selection bias must be considered.

Anaplastic large cell lymphoma (ALCL) is a CD30 positive T-cell lymphoma with two WHO variants, defined by the presence or absence of the anaplastic lymphoma kinase (ALK) gene translocation and ALK protein expression. Although the two variants have similar phenotypic and morphologic characteristics, they likely represent two biologically distinct entities [1]. ALK-positive ALCL is more common in younger patients and has a favorable prognosis when compared to ALK-negative cases following treatment with conventional anthracycline-containing regimens such as CHOP. While intensive regimens have been employed in children, CHOP-like therapy is most commonly employed in adults. CD30 is a therapeutic target, and anti-CD30 naked and conjugated antibodies are currently in clinical trials.

NK/T-cell lymphoma, nasal type has an aggressive clinical course and has historically been associated with poor survival. The tumor is extremely radiosensitive. However, despite response rates greater than 80% to radiotherapy, over 50% of patients with limited stage disease will ultimately relapse [59]. A combined modality approach utilizing local radiotherapy with anthracycline-based chemotherapy is recommended. The timing of radiotherapy may also influence outcome. A recent Chinese study suggests that radiotherapy given prior to chemotherapy results in improved OS [60]. Chemotherapy is the treatment of choice for patients with disseminated disease. The use of L-asparaginase-containing regimens and SCT has shown promise in the salvage setting [59].

Mycosis fungoides is a cutaneous lymphoma of mature T-cells. The disease generally has a prolonged natural history with a relapsing and remitting course. Treatment is aimed at alleviating cutaneous symptoms and will often result in temporary remissions, but is rarely curative. The tumor typically responds to multiple modalities of therapy including topical steroids, radiation, topical chemotherapy, and phototherapy. Initial systemic therapy often involves the use of immunomodulating drugs and biologic therapy. In cases of advanced or refractory disease chemotherapeutics such as gemcitabine and liposomal doxorubicin have shown activity [61].

Highly aggressive lymphoma
Burkitt's lymphoma

Prompt diagnosis and initiation of treatment of BL is essential. Due to the high risk of tumor lysis, electrolyte abnormalities should be corrected, including aggressive prophylaxis with allopurinol or rasburicase. Bicarbonate infusion should be started prior to therapy [62]. BL was previously associated with poor outcomes following standard regimens such as CHOP [63]. The use of dose-intense regimens such as those developed for acute lymphoblastic leukemia (ALL) have dramatically improved outcomes. The NCI developed CODOX-M/IVAC regimen (cyclophosphamide, vincristine, doxorubicin, and high-dose methotrexate alternating with ifosfamide, etoposide, and high dose cytarabine, along with intrathecal methotrexate and cytarabine) demonstrated cure rates of 90% in children and young adults, albeit with significant toxicity [64]. Subsequent modified versions of this protocol have been published with reduced toxicity and cure rates of approximately 64% [65]. The M.D. Anderson Cancer Center published results using a pediatric ALL regimen hyper-CVAD (cyclophosphamide, vincristine, doxorubicin, and dexamethasone) alternating with methotrexate and cytarabine for adults with BL showing prolonged complete remission rates of 57% [66]. The addition of rituximab to this combination improved the three-year OS to 89% [67]. Newer regimens show promise, and in a recent study of 23 patients with and without HIV at the National Institute of Health, the dose-adjusted EPOCH-R (etoposide, prednisone, vincristine, cyclophosphamide, doxorubicin, with rituximab and intrathecal methotrexate) regimen demonstrated a durable complete response rate at 28 months of 100% [68]. Due to the high risk of leptomeningeal spread, all patients should receive intrathecal chemoprophylaxis as part of their initial therapy.

Late effects of treatment

Due to the indolent nature of several NHLs, as well as the possibility of cure in patients with localized and/or aggressive NHL, an understanding of the late effects of treatment is essential for the practicing clinician. Commonly encountered late toxicities associated with treatment for NHL include secondary malignancies, delayed or prolonged organ toxicity, and late effects on reproductive capability.

Secondary malignancies

Secondary malignancies are clearly a very serious late complication of therapy for lymphoma. Defining the etiology of secondary malignancies is difficult as patients with lymphoma likely are inherently susceptible to develop a secondary cancer. Due to the young age at diagnosis, and the high curability of HL, the risk of secondary malignancies in HL survivors has been well studied. Retrospective studies have shown that HL survivors are at an overall increased risk for second malignancies when compared to the general population, with relative risks ranging between 4 to 18 depending on the length of follow-up [69]. In NHL, the risk of a secondary malignancy appears to be lower. Many of the secondary cancers that occur following therapy for NHL are hematologic, including therapy-associated myelodysplastic syndrome and acute leukemia [70, 71]. The two- to eight-fold increase in risk appears to be related to alkylating agents and plateaus at 10–15 years after therapy [71].

Patients treated with radiation as a single modality or in combination with chemotherapy are at increased risk of a secondary malignancy within the radiation field. Common secondary solid tumors developing after therapy for NHL include lung cancer, breast cancer, thyroid cancer, gastrointestinal cancers, and sarcomas [72, 73]. The risk appears to be related to cumulative doses of radiation received and the length of follow-up. The breast cancer risk following radiation is greatest in young women, with relative risks between 6 and 17 in patients treated before age 30 [72]. Unlike the risk of secondary leukemias, the risk for a secondary solid tumor does not plateau, and studies have shown increased relative risks up to 25 years following therapy [73]. With advances in imaging and radiation techniques that have resulted in smaller and more precise radiation dosing, the risk of secondary solid tumors will likely decrease. Chemotherapeutics can also increase the risk of secondary solid tumors, for instance, alkylating agents have been associated with an increased risk of lung cancer [74]. This risk appears to be independent to the risk associated with radiotherapy.

Secondary organ toxicity

Secondary organ toxicity can occur during treatment, as well as years following the completion of therapy. The most common organs affected include the lungs, kidneys, and heart. Pulmonary toxicity is associated with both radiation and chemotherapy including bleomycin, gemcitabine, and others. Bleomycin-induced pulmonary fibrosis is most common following doses of more than 200 to 400 U/m^2 [75].

Acute and delayed cardiotoxicity can occur after radiotherapy or chemotherapy, notably anthracyclines. Systolic dysfunction is the most common abnormality. The risk of cardiotoxicity appears to be dose-dependent and increases proportionally in a non-linear fashion with the total dose of anthracyclines given (1–5% up to 550 mg/m^2, 30% at 600 mg/m^2, and 50% at 1 g/m^2) [76]. Risk factors reported to be associated with the development of anthracycline cardiomyopathy include age at treatment initiation (<18 yr and >65 yr), associated hypertension or pre-existing cardiac disease, and associated mediastinal radiation [76]. Mediastinal radiotherapy has been associated with coronary artery disease, pericarditis, valvular disease, cardiomyopathy, and arrhythmias.

Infertility

The late effects on reproductive ability following treatment for NHL are less well studied than for HL, largely due to the older age of NHL patients. In younger women with aggressive NHL treated with CHOP, the rate of gonadal dysfunction is quite low. In a study of 36 young women (ages 17–40) treated with CHOP or CHOP-like regimens, all but two resumed menstrual cycles in the first complete remission [77]. In a European meta-analysis of late non-neoplastic events following therapy for NHL, the cumulative incidence of infertility at 15 years in women less than 40 years old was 29% [78]. The rate of gonadal dysfunction rises with age and subsequent lines of salvage therapy. Although the impact is variable, fertility can be preserved even after high-dose chemotherapy with stem cell support. In men the incidence of infertility appears to be lower, although in a study of young survivors of aggressive NHL, all male patients tested had some degree of oligospermia or azoospermia [79].

References

1 Swerdlow S, Campo E, Harris NL,et al. (eds) (2008) *WHO Classification of Tumours of Haematopoeitic and Lymphoid Tissue* (4th ed.). Lyon: IARC.

2 Jemal A, Siegel R, Ward E, et al. (2008) Cancer statistics, 2008. *CA Cancer J Clin* **58**:71–96.

3 Anderson JR, Armitage JO, Weisenburger DD, et al. (1998) Epidemiology of the non-Hodgkin's lymphomas: Distributions of the major subtypes differ by geographic locations. *Ann Oncol* **9**:717–20.

4 Bakker N, van Imhoff G. (2007) Post-transplant lymphoproliferative disorders: From treatment to early detection and prevention? *Haematologica* **92**: 1447–50.

5 Volberding PA, Baker KR, Levine AM. (2003) Human immunodeficiency virus hematology. *Hematology (Am Soc Hematol Educ Program)* **2003**:294–313.

6 Pagano J. (2002) Viruses and lymphomas. *N Engl J Med* **347**:78–9.

7 Kahl B, Yang D. (2008) Marginal zone lymphomas: Management of nodal, splenic, and MALT NHL. *Hematology (Am Soc Hematol Educ Program)* **2008**:359–64.

8 Campanero M. (2008) Mechanisms involved in Burkitt's lymphoma tumor formation. *Clin Transl Oncol* **10**:250–5.

9 Abramson JS, Shipp M. (2005) Advances in the biology and therapy of diffuse large B-cell lymphoma: Moving toward a molecularly targeted approach. *Blood* **106**:1164–74.

10 Dave S, Wright G, Tan B, et al. (2004) Prediction of survival in follicular lymphoma based on molecular features of tumor-infiltrating immune cells. *N Engl J Med* **351**:2159–69.

11 Rosenwald A, Wright G, Chan WC, et al. (2002) The use of molecular profiling to predict survival after chemotherapy for diffuse large-B-cell lymphoma. *N Engl J Med* **346**:1937–47.

12 Davis RE, Brown KD, Siebenlist U, et al. (2001) Constitutive nuclear factor B activity is required for survival of activated B cell-like diffuse large B-cell lymphoma cells. *J Exp. Med* **194**:1861–74.

13 Shipp M, Ross K, Tamayo P, et al. (2002) Diffuse large B-cell lymphoma outcome prediction by gene-expression profiling and supervised machine learning. *Nat Med* **8**:68–74.

14 Non-Hodgkin's lymphoma pathologic classification project. (1982) National Cancer Institute sponsored study of classification of non-Hodgkin's lymphomas: Summary and description of working formulation for clinical usage. *Cancer* **49**:2112–35.

15 Harris NL, Jaffe ES, Stein H, et al. (1994) A revised European-American classification of lymphoid neoplasm: A proposal from the International Lymphoma Study Group. *Blood* **84**:1361–92.

16 Johnson PM, Davies AJ. (2008) Primary mediastinal B-cell lymphoma. *Hematology (Am Soc Hematol Educ Program)* **2008:**349–58.

17 Armitage JO, Weisenburger DD. (1998) New approach to classifying non-Hodgkin's lymphomas: Clinical features of the major histologic subtypes. Non-Hodgkin's Lymphoma Classification Project. *J Clin Oncol* **16**:2780–95.

18 Shipp MA, Harrington DP, Anderson JR, et al. (1993) A predictive model for aggressive non-Hodgkin's lymphoma. The International Non-Hodgkin's Lymphoma Prognostic Factors Project. *N Engl J Med* **329**:987–94.

19 Solal-Céligny P, Roy P, Colombat P, et al. (2004) Follicular Lymphoma International Prognostic Index. *Blood* **104**:1258–64.

20 Federico M, Bellei M, Marcheselli L, et al. (2009) Follicular Lymphoma International Prognostic Index 2: A new prognostic index for follicular lymphoma developed by the International Follicular Lymphoma Prognostic Factor Project. *J Clin Oncol* **27**:4555–62.

21 Hasenclever D, Diehl V. (1998) A prognostic score for advanced Hodgkin's disease. *N Engl J Med* **339**:1506–14.

22 Plancarte F, López-Guillermo A, Arenillas L, et al. (2005) Follicular lymphoma in early stages: High risk of relapse and usefulness of the Follicular Lymphoma International Prognostic Index to predict the outcome of patients. *Eur J Haematol* **76**:58–63.

23 Ha CS, Cabanillas F, Lee MS, et al. (1997) Serial determination of the bcl-2 gene in the bone marrow and peripheral blood after central lymphatic irradiation for Stages I–III follicular lymphoma: A preliminary report. *Clin Cancer Res* **3**:215–19.

24 Legouffe E, Rodriguez C, Picot MC, et al. (1998) C-reactive protein serum level is a valuable and simple prognostic marker in non-Hodgkin's lymphoma. *Leuk Lymphoma* **31**:351–7.

25 Seymour JF, Talpaz M, Cabanillas F, et al. (1995) Serum interleukin-6 levels correlate with prognosis in diffuse large-cell lymphoma. *J Clin Oncol* **13**:575–82.

26 Kahl BS. (2003) Update: Gastric MALT lymphoma. *Curr Opin Oncol* **15**:347–52.

27 Hofmann WJ, Momburg F, Moller P. (1988) Thymic medullary cells expressing B lymphocyte antigens. *Hum Pathol* **19**:1280–7.

28 Savage K, Monti S, Kutok J, et al. (2003) The molecular signature of mediastinal large B-cell lymphoma differs from that of other diffuse large B-cell lymphomas and shares features with classical Hodgkin lymphoma. *Blood* **102**:3871–9.

29 Van Besien K, Kelta M, Bahaguna P. (2001) Primary mediastinal B-cell lymphoma: A review of pathology and management. *J Clin Oncol* **19**:1855–64.

30 Romaguera JE, Medeiros LF, Hagemeister FB, et al. (2003) Frequency of gastrointestinal involvement and its clinical significance in mantle cell lymphoma. *Cancer* **97**:586–91.

31 Rüdiger T, Weisenburger DD, Anderson JR, et al. (2002) Peripheral T-cell lymphoma (excluding anaplastic large-cell lymphoma): Results from the Non-Hodgkin's Lymphoma Classification Project. *Ann Oncol* **13**:140–9.

32 Chiarle R, Voena C, Ambrogio C, et al. (2008) The anaplastic lymphoma kinase in the pathogenesis of cancer. *Nat Rev Cancer* **8**:11–23.

33 Mourad N, Mounier N, Brière J, et al. (2008) Clinical, biologic, and pathologic features in 157 patients with angioimmunoblastic T-cell lymphoma treated within the Groupe d'Etude des Lymphomes de l'Adulte (GELA) trials. *Blood* **111**:4463–70.

34 Perkins AS, Friedberg JW. (2008) Burkitt's lymphoma in adults. *Hematology* **2008**:341–8.

35 Hummel M, Bentink S, Berger H, et al. (2006) A biologic definition of Burkitt's lymphoma from transcriptional and genomic profiling. *N Engl J Med* **354**:2419–30.

36 Dave SS, Fu K, Wright GW, et al. (2006) Molecular diagnosis of Burkitt's lymphoma. *N Engl J Med* **354**:2431–42.

37 Morschhauser F, Radford J, Van Hoof A, et al. (2008) Phase III trial of consolidation therapy with yttrium-90–ibritumomab tiuxetan compared with no additional therapy after first remission in advanced follicular lymphoma. *J Clin Oncol* **26**:5156–64.

38 Gopal AK, Rajendran JG, Gooley TA, et al. (2007) High-dose [^{131}I] tositumomab (anti-CD20) radioimmunotherapy and autologous hematopoietic stem-cell transplantation for adults ≥60 years old with relapsed or refractory B-cell lymphoma. *J Clin Oncol* **25**:1396–1402.

39 Cheson B, Leonard J. (2008) Monoclonal antibody therapy for B-cell non-Hodgkin's lymphoma. *N Engl J Med* **359**:613–26.

40 Wrench D, Gribben J. (2008) Stem cell transplantation for non-Hodgkin's lymphoma. *Hematol Oncol Clin N Am* **22**:1051–79.

41 Deconinck E, Foussard C, Milpied N, et al. (2005) High-dose therapy followed by autologous purged stem-cell transplantation and doxorubicin-based chemotherapy in patients with advanced follicular lymphoma: A randomized multicenter study by GOELAMS. *Blood* **105**:3817–23.

42 Rodríguez J, Conde E, Gutiérrez A, et al. (2007) Frontline autologous stem cell transplantation in high-risk peripheral T-cell lymphoma: a prospective study from The Gel-Tamo Study Group. *Eur J Haematol* **79**:32–8.

43 Illerhaus G, Marks R, Ihorst G, et al. (2006) High-dose chemotherapy with autologous stem cell transplantation and hyperfractionated radiotherapy as first-line treatment of primary CNS lymphoma. *J Clin Oncol* **24**:3865–70.

44 Philip T, Guglielmi C, Hagenbeek A, et al. (1995) Autologous bone marrow transplantation as compared with salvage chemotherapy in relapses of chemotherapy-sensitive non-Hodgkin's lymphoma. *N Engl J Med* **333**:1540–5.

45 Gribben JG, Goldstone AH, Linch DC, et al. (1989) Effectiveness of high-dose combination chemotherapy and autologous bone marrow transplantation for patients with non-Hodgkin's lymphomas who are still responsive to conventional-dose therapy. *J Clin Oncol* **7**:1621–9.

46 Rohatiner A, Nadler L, Davies A, et al. (2007) Myeloablative therapy with autologous bone marrow transplantation for follicular lymphoma at the time of second or subsequent remission: Long-term follow-up. *J Clin Oncol* **25**:2554–9.

47 Khouri I, McLaughlin P, Saliba R, et al. (2008) Eight-year experience with allogeneic stem cell transplantation for relapsed follicular lymphoma after non-myeloablative conditioning with fludarabine, cyclophosphamide, and rituximab. *Blood* **111**:5530–6.

48 Czuczman MS. (2006) Controversies in follicular lymphoma: "Who, what, when, where, and why?" *(Not necessarily in that order!)* *Hematology* **2006**:303–10.

49 Mac Manus MP, Hoppe RT. (1996) Is radiotherapy curative for stage I and II low-grade follicular lymphoma? Results of a long-term follow-up study of patients treated at Stanford University. *J Clin Oncol* **14**:1282–90.

50 Seymour JF, Pro B, Fuller L, et al. (2003) Long-term follow-up of a prospective study of combined modality therapy for Stage I–II indolent non-Hodgkin's lymphoma. *J Clin Oncol* **21**:2115–22.

51 Buske C, Hoster E, Dreyling M, et al. (2006) Brief report: The Follicular Lymphoma International Prognostic Index (FLIPI) separates high-risk from intermediate- or low-risk patients with advanced-stage follicular lymphoma treated front-line with rituximab and the combination of cyclophosphamide, doxorubicin, vincristine, and prednisone (R-CHOP) with respect to treatment outcome. *Blood* **108**:1504–8.

52 Kalpadakis C, Pangalis G, Vassilakopoulos T, et al. (2008) Rituximab monotherapy is the treatment of choice of splenic marginal zone lymphoma (SMZL). *Ann Oncol* **19**:Abstract No. 367.

53 Morgner A, Schmelz R, Thiede C, et al. (2007) Therapy of gastric mucosa associated lymphoid tissue lymphoma. *World J Gastroenterol* **13**:3554–66.

54 Leporrier M, Chevret S, Cazin B, et al. (2001) Randomized comparison of fludarabine, CAP, and CHOP in 938 previously untreated stage B and C chronic lymphocytic leukemia patients. *Blood* **98**:2319–25.

55 Romaguera JE, Fayad L, Rodriguez MA, et al. (2005) High rate of durable remissions after treatment of newly diagnosed aggressive mantle cell lymphoma with rituximab plus hyper-CVAD alternating with rituximab plus high-dose methotrexate and cytarabine. *J Clin Oncol* **23**:7013–23.

56 O'Connor OA. (2007) Mantle cell lymphoma: Identifying novel molecular targets in growth and survival pathways. *Hematology* **2008**:270–6.

57 Foss F. (2009) Treatment approaches for aggressive T-cell lymphomas. *ASCO Educational Book* **2009**:480–5.

58 Horwitz SM. (2008) Novel therapies and role of transplant in the treatment of peripheral T-cell lymphomas. *Hematology* **2008**:289–96.

59 Liang R. (2009) Advances in the management and monitoring of extranodal NK/T-cell lymphoma, nasal type. *Br J Haematol* **147**:13–21.

60 Huang M, Jiang Y, Liu W, et al. (2008) Early or up-front radiotherapy improved survival of localized extranodal NK/T-cell lymphoma, nasal-type in the upper aerodigestive tract. *Int J Radiat Oncol Biology Physics* **70**:166–74.

61 Horwitz S, Olsen E, Duvic M, et al. (2008) Review of the treatment of mycosis fungoides and Sézary syndrome: A stage-based approach. *JNCCN* **6**:436–42.

62 Yustein J, Dang C. (2007) Biology and treatment of Burkitt's lymphoma. *Curr Opin Hematol* **14**:375–81.

63 Smeland S, Blystad AK, Kvaloy SO, et al. (2004) Treatment of Burkitt's/Burkitt-like lymphoma in adolescents and adults: A 20-year experience from the Norwegian Radium Hospital with the use of three successive regimens. *Ann Oncol* **15**:1072–8.

64 Magrath I, Adde M, Shad A, et al. (1996) Adults and children with small noncleaved-cell lymphoma have a similar excellent outcome when treated with the same chemotherapy regimen. *J Clin Oncol* **14**:925–34.

65 Lacasce A, Howard O, Lib S, et al. (2004) Modified Magrath regimens for adults with Burkitt and Burkitt-like lymphomas: Preserved efficacy with decreased toxicity. *Leuk Lymphoma* **45**:761–7.

66 Thomas DA, Cortes J, O'Brien S, et al. (1999) Hyper-CVAD program in Burkitt's-type adult acute lymphoblastic leukemia. *J Clin Oncol* **17**:2461–70.

67 Thomas DA, Faderl S, O'Brien S, et al. (2006) Chemoimmunotherapy with hyper-CVAD plus rituximab for the treatment of adult Burkitt and Burkitt-type lymphoma or acute lymphoblastic leukemia. *Cancer* **106**:1569–80.

68 Dunleavy K, Little, RF, Pittaluga S, et al. (2008) A prospective study of dose-adjusted (DA) EPOCH with rituximab in adults with newly diagnosed Burkitt lymphoma: a regimen with high efficacy and low toxicity. *Ann Oncol* **19**:iv83.

69 Adams M, Constine L, Lipshultz S. (2006) Late effects of therapy for Hodgkin's lymphoma. *JNCCN* **3**:249–57.

70 Travis LB, Curtis RE, Stovall M, et al. (1994) Risk of leukemia following treatment for non-Hodgkin's lymphoma. *J Natl Cancer Inst* **86**:1450–7.

71 Mudie NY, Swerdlow AJ, Higgins CD, et al. (2006) Risk of second malignancy after non-Hodgkin's lymphoma: A British Cohort Study. *J Clin Oncol* **24**: 1568–74.

72 van Leeuwen FE, Klokman WJ, Veer MB, et al. (2000) Long-term risk of second malignancy in survivors of Hodgkin's disease treated during adolescence or young adulthood. *J Clin Oncol* **18**:487–97.

73 Bhatia S, Yasui Y, Robison LL, et al. (2003) High risk of subsequent neoplasms continues with extended follow-up of childhood Hodgkin's disease: Report from the Late Effects Study Group. *J Clin Oncol* **21**:4386–94.

74 Travis LB, Gospodarowicz M, Curtis RE, et al. (2002) Lung cancer following chemotherapy and radiotherapy for Hodgkin's disease. *J Natl Cancer Inst* **94**:182–92.

75 Horning SJ, Adhikari A, Rizk N, et al. (1994) Effect of treatment for Hodgkin's disease on pulmonary function: Results of a prospective study. *J Clin Oncol* **12**:297–305.

76 Carver JR, Shapiro C, Ng A, et al. (2007) American Society of Clinical Oncology clinical evidence review on the ongoing care of adult cancer survivors: Cardiac and pulmonary late effects. *J Clin Oncol* **25**:3991–4008.

77 Elis A, Tevet A, Yerushalmi R, et al. (2006) Fertility status among women treated for aggressive non-Hodgkin's lymphoma. *Leuk Lymphoma* **47**:623–7.

78 Moser E, Noordijk E, Carde P, et al. (2005) Late non-neoplastic events in patients with aggressive non-Hodgkin's lymphoma in four randomized European Organization for Research and Treatment of Cancer Trials. *Clin Lymphoma Myeloma* **6**:122–30.

79 Haddy T, Adde M, McCalla J, et al. (1998) Late effects in long-term survivors of high-grade non-Hodgkin's lymphomas. *J Clin Oncol* **16**:2070–9.

80 Marcus R, Imrie K, Belch A, et al. (2005) CVP chemotherapy plus rituximab compared with CVP as first-line treatment for advanced follicular lymphoma. *Blood* **105**:1417–23.

81 Hiddemann W, Kneba M, Dreyling M, et al. (2005) Frontline therapy with rituximab added to the combination of cyclophosphamide, doxorubicin, vincristine, and prednisone (CHOP) significantly improves the outcome for patients with advanced-stage follicular lymphoma compared with therapy with CHOP alone: Results of a prospective randomized study of the German Low-Grade Lymphoma Study Group. *Blood* **106**:3725–32.

82 Zinzani P, Pulsoni A, Perrotti A, et al. (2004) Fludarabine plus mitoxantrone with and without rituximab versus CHOP with and without rituximab as front-line treatment for patients with follicular lymphoma. *J Clin Oncol* **100**:2654–61.

83 Tsimberidou A, McLaughlin P, Younes A, et al. (2002) Fludarabine, mitoxantrone, dexamethasone (FND) compared with an alternating triple therapy (ATT)

regimen in patients with Stage IV indolent lymphoma. *Blood* **100**:4351–7.

84 Morschhauser F, Radford J, Van Hoof A, et al. (2008) Phase III trial of consolidation therapy with yttrium-90–ibritumomab tiuxetan compared with no additional therapy after first remission in advanced follicular lymphoma. *J Clin Oncol* **10**:5156–64.

85 Press OW, Unger JM, Braziel R, et al. (2006) Phase II trial of CHOP chemotherapy followed by tositumomab/iodine I-131 tositumomab for previously untreated follicular non-Hodgkin's lymphoma: Five-year follow-up of Southwest Oncology Group Protocol S9911. *J Clin Oncol* **24**:4143–9.

86 Fisher RI, Gaynor ER, Dahlberg S, et al. (1993) Comparison of a standard regimen (CHOP) with three intensive chemotherapy regimens for advanced non-Hodgkin's lymphoma. *N Engl J Med* **328**:1002–6.

87 Pfreundschuh M, Trümper L, Österborg A, et al. (2006) CHOP-like chemotherapy plus rituximab versus CHOP-like chemotherapy alone in young patients with good-prognosis diffuse large-B-cell lymphoma: A randomised controlled trial by the MabThera International Trial (MInT) Group. *Lancet Oncol* **7**:379–91.

88 Feugier P, Van Hoof A, Sebban C, et al. (2005) Long-term results of the R-CHOP study in the treatment of elderly patients with diffuse large B-cell lymphoma: a study by the Groupe d'Etude des Lymphomes de l'Adulte. *J Clin Oncol* **23**:4117–26.

89 Pfreundschuh M, Schubert J, Ziepert M, et al. (2008) Six versus eight cycles of bi-weekly CHOP-14 with or without rituximab in elderly patients with aggressive CD20+ B-cell lymphomas: A randomized controlled trial (RICOVER-60). *Lancet Oncol* **9**:105–16.

90 Cabanillas F, Rodriguez-Diaz Pavon J, Hagemeister FB, et al. (1998) Alternating triple therapy for the treatment of intermediate grade and immunoblastic lymphoma. *Ann Oncol* **9**:511–18.

91 Wilson WH, Dunleavy K, Pittaluga S, et al. (2008) Phase II Study of dose-adjusted EPOCH and rituximab in untreated diffuse large B-cell lymphoma with analysis of germinal center and post-germinal center biomarkers. *J Clin Oncol* **26**:2717–24.

92 Mead GM, Sydes MR, Walewski J, et al. (2002) An international evaluation of CODOX-M and CODOX-M alternating with IVAC in adult Burkitt's lymphoma: results of United Kingdom Lymphoma Group LY06 study. *Ann Oncol* **13**:1264–74.

93 Thomas DA, Faderl S, O'Brien S, et al. (2006) Chemoimmunotherapy with hyper-CVAD plus rituximab for the treatment of adult Burkitt and Burkitt-type lymphoma or acute lymphoblastic leukemia. *Cancer* **106**:1569–80.

94 Moskowitz CH, Bertino JR, Glassman JR, et al. (1999) Ifosfamide, carboplatin, and etoposide: A highly effective cytoreduction and peripheral-blood progenitor-cell mobilization regimen for transplant-eligible patients with non-Hodgkin's lymphoma. *J Clin Oncol* **17**:3776–85.

95 Rodriguez MA, Cabanillas FC, Velasquez W, et al. (1995) Results of a salvage treatment program for relapsing lymphoma: MINE consolidated with ESHAP. *J Clin Oncol* **13**:1734–41.

96 El Gnaoui T, Dupuis J, Belhadj K, et al. (2007) Rituximab, gemcitabine and oxaliplatin: An effective salvage regimen for patients with relapsed or refractory B-cell lymphoma not candidates for high-dose therapy. *Ann Oncol* **18**:1363–8.

97 Younes A, Preti HA, Hagemeister FB, et al. (2001) Paclitaxel plus topotecan treatment for patients with relapsed or refractory aggressive non-Hodgkin's lymphoma. *Ann Oncol* **12**:923–7.

98 Tilly H, Lepage E, Coiffer B, et al. (2003) Intensive conventional chemotherapy (ACVBP regimen) compared with standard CHOP for poor-prognosis aggressive non-Hodgkin lymphoma. *Blood* **102**:4284–9.

99 Anderson V, Perry C. (2007) Fludarabine: A review of its use in non-Hodgkin's lymphoma. *Drugs* **67**:1633–55.

100 Samaniego F, Fanale M, Pro B, et al. (2008) Pentostatin, cyclophosphamide, and rituximab (PCR) achieve high response rates in indolent B-cell lymphoma without prolonged myelosuppression. *Blood* **112**:835.

101 Witzig T, Geyer S, Kurtin P, et al. (2008) Salvage chemotherapy with rituximab DHAP for relapsed non-Hodgkin lymphoma: A phase II trial in the North Central Cancer Treatment Group. *Leuk Lymphoma* **49**:1074–80.

CHAPTER 19
Hodgkin Lymphoma

Michael Crump
University of Toronto and Division of Medical Oncology and Hematology, Princess Margaret Hospital, Toronto, Canada

Epidemiology

Hodgkin lymphoma (HL) typically represents approximately 8% of lymphomas in adults and 35% in children. Recent data from 12 Surveillance Epidemiology and End Results (SEER) databases in the US show that the incidence of HL is about 3.3 per 100 000 in men and 2.6 per 100 000 in women using World Health Organization (WHO) criteria for diagnosis of lymphoid malignancies [1]. Data from North America and Europe show no consistent trend in incidence over the last two decades suggesting that no important new causes of Hodgkin lymphoma have been introduced on a population level during this time. An evaluation of mortality from Hodgkin lymphoma mortality in Europe showed a decline in age-standardized mortality from 1.42/100 000 in 1980–1989 to 1.17 in 2002–2004 [2]. This decrease was more pronounced in countries in Central and Eastern Europe where mortality fell from 1.42 in 1980–1984, to 0.76 in 2000–2004. It is unlikely that changes in lymphoma classification could account for such a large decrease, and these changes are attributed to improvements in systemic therapy over the last two decades [3]. Overall mortality from HL declined from 0.82/100 000 in 1990–1994 to 0.49 in 2000–2004; a change of 40% in all 27 countries represented in the European Union.

It has been recognized for more than 40 years that Epstein Barr virus (EBV) plays a fundamental role at least in some cases of HL [4] (Table 19.1). An increased incidence of HL after infectious mononucleosis has been reported in several studies. EBV is not, however, uniformly present in all cases of HL and is less frequently seen in HL in young adults, the population for which the association with infectious mononucleosis is strongest [5]. It has been reported that infectious mononucleosis-associated lymphomas occurred about three years after EBV infection, and that infectious mononucleosis is associated only with EBV-positive HL. A relationship between certain HLA class I antigens and HL risk after EBV infection has been described, perhaps due to failure of presentation of immunogenic EBV peptides [6]. There are reports that EBV + HL is associated with a better outcome [7], and it may be that EBV-positive and EBV-negative HL have different underlying etiologies.

The incidence of HL is higher in Western countries and shows a bimodal age distribution, with a peak between the ages of 15 and 34, and a second increase after age 60. In developing countries, where the seroprevalence of EBV in the population is generally greater, there is no bimodal distribution and the incidence of HL increases with age.

Increasingly attention has been focused on genetic factors that predispose to the development of lymphomas, including HL. The striking increase in risk for monozygotic twins of patients with HL, with no observed increased risk for dizygotic twins, provided the initial evidence supporting an underlying genetic susceptibility [8]. It has been shown in a number of studies that the risk of HL is higher among first-degree relatives of individuals with cancer. For example, data from the Swedish Cancer Registry suggested that a family history of chronic lymphocytic leukemia or non-HL in a first-degree relative was associated with

Advances in Malignant Hematology, First Edition. Edited by Hussain I. Saba and Ghulam J. Mufti. © 2011 Blackwell Publishing Ltd. Published 2011 by Blackwell Publishing Ltd.

Table 19.1 Differential diagnosis of Hodgkin lymphoma from other large cell lymphomas

Marker	CHL	NLPHL	TCRBCL	ALCL, ALK-
CD 30	+	−	−	+
CD 15	+/−	−	−	−
CD 45	−	+	+	+/−
CD 20	−/+	+	+	−
Ig	−	+/−	+/−	−
PAX5	+	+	+	−
CD 2	−	−	−	−/+
CD 3	−	−	−	+/−
EMA	−	+/−	+/−	+/−
LMP1	+/−	−	−	−

CHL: classical Hodgkin lymphoma; NLPHL: nodular lymphocyte predominant Hodgkin lymphoma; TCRBCL: T-cell-rich large B-cell lymphoma; ALCL, ALK-: anaplastic large T-cell lymphoma, ALK protein negative; + all cases are positive; +/−majority of cases positive;−/+ minority of cases positive; -all cases are negative (Modified from Stein H et al. (2008) In WHO Classification of Tumours of Haematopoietic and Lymphoid Tissues, pp. 326–9. Lyon: IARC.).

a two-fold relative risk of HL [9]. Concordance in a family history of HL increased four-fold among those with a first-degree relative who had HL; however, no increased risk of HL was seen in first-degree relatives of patients with Waldenström's macroglobulinemia or lymphoplasmacytic lymphoma. Overall, about 1–1.5% of patients with HL will have a family history of another type of lymphoma. Relative risk of HL is about 2.4 for first-degree relatives of a patient with chronic lymphocytic leukemia, 3.1 for those with a first-degree relative with HL, and 1.4 for other types of non-HL. Long-term treatment outcome for patients with a family history of HL does not seem to be any different from those without a family history [10].

Polymorphisms in a number of genes associated with immune response have been linked with an increased risk of lymphoma (reviewed in [11]).

Individuals with a personal history of autoimmune disorders such as rheumatoid arthritis or immune thrombocytopenic purpura, as well as a family history of certain autoimmune conditions, are at higher risk for HL [12]. Polymorphisms in DNA nucleotide excision repair genes may increase the risk of HL [13]. Other studies evaluating common polymorphisms in immune response genes have highlighted the relationship between polymorphisms in the IL6 gene and HL. Polymorphisms in the IL10 promoter have been observed with an increased frequency in those developing non-HL and has not been reported in those with HL [14].

Treatment of limited stage Hodgkin lymphoma

The long-term outcome of patients with HL with limited extent of disease at diagnosis, defined as Stage I and II using the Ann Arbor Staging Classification, has repeatedly been shown to be excellent. It is recognized that different prognostic groups exist within the population of patients with localized HL. Prospective clinical trials have defined favorable and unfavorable patient populations using somewhat different, but overlapping criteria (Table 19.2). Occasionally, patients with B symptoms or bulky mediastinal or other masses are treated in a similar fashion to those with advanced Ann Arbor stage disease. The prognostic factors described by Hasenclever and Diehl [15] that define outcome in patients with advanced stage disease (age >45, male sex, Stage IV, low serum albumin, anemia, lymphopenia or leukocytosis) do not appear to provide any additional prognostic information in those with limited stage HL [16].

The principle of treating involved and adjacent apparently uninvolved nodal areas became the standard of care in the radiotherapeutic approach to HL in the 1960s, and along with the fundamental observation about the relationship between dose and in-field recurrence rate, led to the development of the first curative treatment strategies (Table 19.3) [17, 18]. Although cure rates of over 80% can be achieved with subtotal nodal (STNI or "extended field") radiation, several trials have established that

Table 19.2 Prognostic groupings for Stage I/II Hodgkin lymphoma

Clinical trials group	Favorable (or Early)	Unfavorable (or Intermediate)
GHSG	Stage IA, IB, IIA: Without any of - bulky mediastinal mass - extranodal disease - ESR $\geq$50 (A), $\geq$30 (B) - $\geq$3 nodal regions involved	Stage IA, IB, IIA: With one of - bulky mediastinal mass - extranodal disease - ESR $\geq$50 (A), $\geq$30 (B) - $\geq$3 nodal regions Stage IIB[a] with one of: - ESR $\geq$50 (A), $\geq$30 (B) - $\geq$3 nodal regions
EORTC	Stage I/II: Without any of - bulky mediastinal mass - age >50 - ESR $\geq$50 (A), $\geq$30 (B) - $\geq$4 nodal regions involved	Stage I/II: With any of - bulky mediastinal mass - age >50 - ESR $\geq$50 (A), $\geq$30 (B) - $\geq$4 nodal regions
NCIC-CTG	Stage IA and IIA[b] With all of the following - LP or NS histology - age <40 - ESR <50 - <4 nodal regions involved	Stage IA and IIA[b] With any of the following - MC or LD histology - age $\geq$40 - ESR $\geq$50 - $\geq$4 nodal regions involved

[a] Stage IIB with bulky mediastinal mass or extranodal disease is considered advanced stage in GHSG trials
[b] Presence of bulky mediastinal mass ineligible for the NCIC-CTG HD6 trial
GHSG: German Hodgkin's Study Group; EORTC: European Organization for Research and Treatment of Cancer; NCIC-CTG: National Cancer Institute of Canada Clinical Trials Group (Modified from Tsang RW et al. (2006) *Curr Probl Cancer* 30:107–58.)

combination chemotherapy followed by radiation (combined modality therapy, CMT) results in superior disease control and OS compared to radiotherapy alone. A comparison by the Southwest Oncology Group (SWOG) of doxorubicin and vinblastine followed by STNI to STNI alone showed an improvement in PFS at three years (93% vs. 81%) favoring

CMT; long-term follow-up evaluating possible difference in OS is awaited [19]. The German Hodgkin Study Group (GHSG) HD7 trial comparing two cycles of ABVD (Appendix) followed by extended field radiation to radiotherapy alone showed an improvement from the addition of chemotherapy in freedom from treatment failure (FFTF) at seven

Table 19.3 Definition of radiation fields for Hodgkin lymphoma

Definition	Size of field
Involved nodal	Initially involved nodes
Involved field	Initially involved nodal regions; cervical, supraclavicular, axilla, mediastinum, para-aortic (spleen, iliac, inguinal)
Extended field	Initially involved and contiguous nodal regions
Mantle field	Bilateral cervical ($\pm$ postauricular), supraclavicular, infraclavicular, axillary nodes and mediastinum + hilar nodes
Subtotal nodal	Mantle + para-aortic (+ spleen)
Inverted Y	Para-aortic iliac + inguinal nodes
Total nodal	Mantle + inverted Y

years (88% vs. 67%), due to a higher relapse rate among patients receiving radiotherapy alone (22% vs. 3%) [20]. Patients in this trial had none of the risk factors defined by the GHSG (large mediastinal mass, massive splenic involvement, extranodal involvement, high ESR, three or more lymph node areas). The European Organization for Research and Treatment of Cancer (EORTC) and Groupe d'Etude des Lymphomes de l'Adulte (GELA) reported superior five-year EFS in patients with favorable HL receiving three cycles of MOPP-ABV plus involved field radiation (98% vs. 74%) compared to patients receiving STNI, and improved 10-year OS (97% vs. 92%; p<0.001) [21].

Although the delivery of radiation to clinically or radiologically uninvolved but adjacent nodal areas may reduce the risk of subsequent relapse, it has long been appreciated that such extended radiotherapy fields are associated with increased short-term and long-term toxicity, including a high rate of second malignancies. With the advent of effective chemotherapy to eradicate subclinical or microscopic disease outside the radiation field, a number of trials were undertaken to evaluate the use of radiation delivered to clinically or radiologically defined sites of disease (involved field radiotherapy, IFRT). Mature results of the Milan Cancer Institute trial of four cycles of ABVD followed by either IFRT or STNI report similar long-term FFTF (94% and 94%) and OS (94% and 96%) [22]. A study from the GHSG in unfavorable early stage HL randomized patients to 30 Gy extended field or 30 Gy involved field (both with additional 10 Gy to sites of bulky disease) following COPP-ABVD chemotherapy. FFTF was similar in patients receiving extended field (86%) or involved field (84%) radiation, as was OS at five years (91% vs. 92%) [23]. Hematologic and gastrointestinal toxicity was more frequent in the EF arm as were secondary neoplasms (4.5% vs. 2.8%) although the latter difference was not statistically significant. Further reduction in the exposure of normal tissues to radiation can be accomplished by the use of involved nodal radiation (INRT) [24], a concept that is currently undergoing evaluation in controlled trials. Although no randomized trials have been reported, preliminary data in patients with limited stage HL suggest that local control may be similar when INRT is part of combined modality therapy [25] when pre-chemotherapy nodes are <5 cm. Additional follow-up of these trials will be important to determine whether a reduction in radiation field size leads to a decrease in long-term morbidity and mortality from cardiovascular disease and second cancers, discussed below.

Randomized trials have also established the optimum chemotherapy regimen and number of cycles in the combined modality treatment approach to early stage HL. In the EORTC H.7 trial, EBVP for six cycles followed by IFRT resulted in superior 10-year EFS (88% vs. 78%) compared to STNI, but no difference in OS. In unfavorable patients, 10-year EFS was significantly worse with EBVP compared to MOPP/ABV (68% vs. 88%), as was OS (79% vs. 87%; p = 0.018) [26]. A second study by the EORTC in unfavorable patients randomized to ABVD versus MOPP showed an improvement in freedom from progression at six years in favor of ABVD, 88% versus 76%, and a non-significant improvement in OS, 91% versus 85% [27]. Similar to trials of MOPP-containing therapy in advanced stage HL, MOPP had significantly greater hematologic and gonadal toxicity than ABVD, although significant decreases in pulmonary function tests were observed more frequently with ABVD.

To this point in time, these trials in limited stage HL, both favorable and unfavorable, establish two to four cycles of ABVD followed by IFRT as the treatment of choice for patients with limited stage HL [28, 98]. Newer treatment regimens currently being tested in limited stage patients, such as Stanford V or BEACOPP (Appendix), are discussed below.

There is considerable interest in identifying patient subsets where radiotherapy can be omitted, in an effort to reduce toxicity without compromising disease control. A number of important trials have recently been reported, testing chemotherapy alone to treatment including radiation. A single-centre trial randomized 150 patients to subtotal nodal irradiation or observation after six cycles of ABVD chemotherapy [29]. This study, which also included patients with Stage IIIA disease, showed no improvement in PFS or OS from the addition of radiation.

A larger trial by the NCIC Clinical Trials Group and the ECOG randomized patients with Stage IA and IIA HL without bulky mediastinal disease, to receive a treatment strategy that included extended field radiation or ABVD alone. The final end point of this trial, which evaluates the impact of treatment regimen on control of HL and mortality from late complications of radiotherapy, is 12-year OS [30]. Patients without risk factors (Table 19.2) received either mantle and upper abdominal radiation, or ABVD for four cycles (those with a complete response (CR) after two cycles) or six cycles (those with a partial response (PR) after two cycles). Patients with any risk factor received two cycles of ABVD followed by extended field radiation, or four to six cycles of ABVD as above. This trial showed superior five-year freedom from progression in patients allocated to radiotherapy (93% vs. 87%; $p = 0.006$) but at the time of reporting, no difference in OS. In a subset analysis, patients in the ABVD arm who obtained a complete response after two cycles of chemotherapy had a particularly favorable outcome compared to patients who had less than a complete response (freedom from progression 95% vs. 81%; $p = 0.007$) [30]. Functional imaging

with Gallium or fluorodeoxyglucose positron emission tomography (FDG-PET) was not used to evaluate response in this study.

It is clear that patients with favorable HL treated with combined modality therapy including ABVD have a very low likelihood of disease recurrence. To date, the relapse rate in the German HD7 trial comparing involved to extended field therapy is only 4% [23]; in GHSG HD10 comparing two or four cycles of ABVD and 20 or 30 Gy IFRT, the relapse rate is 5% [31], and in the NCIC trial described above it was 7%. It has been shown that relapses following chemotherapy alone occur in sites of previous disease, which would have been encompassed by an involved or extended radiation field had CMT been used [32, 33]. The long-term outcome of patients who relapse after brief chemotherapy and radiotherapy are significantly worse than those who relapse after radiation alone, due to the ability of combination chemotherapy in the latter patient population to produce second complete remissions and durable FFTF. The long-term outcome for patients who relapse after doxorubicin-based CMT is relatively poor: five-year freedom from second treatment failure (FF2F) was 52% and OS was 67% in one recent report. Prognostic factors at the time of relapse – the presence of anemia, complete remission <1 year, and advanced disease stage – are important predictors of long-term outcome of patients relapsing after combined modality therapy [31]. Currently, patients who relapse after anthracycline-based chemotherapy, even for limited stage disease, are usually referred for high-dose therapy with stem cell support.

In light of this, and the fact that long-term follow-up of randomized trials of treatment omitting radiotherapy is not yet available, discussions with patients regarding treatment options need to proceed cautiously. Treatment with chemotherapy alone potentially offers good disease control and equivalent OS with potentially less late radiation-induced toxicity. On the other hand, patients must understand that the risk of disease recurrence is higher without radiotherapy. For those patients who relapse, second-line treatment will include high-dose therapy and stem cell support, with the attendant risk of gonadal toxicity and an increased risk of secondary acute leukemia and solid tumors [34].

Therapy of advanced-stage Hodgkin lymphoma

In the two decades that followed the introduction of the MOPP regimen (mechlorethamine, vincristine, procarbazine, prednisone) in 1964, the mortality rate for HL decreased by 65% [35]. Long-term follow-up of patients treated with this regimen demonstrated that half the patients were alive and in remission a median of more than 15 years from the end of treatment. Substantial numbers of patients – 19% of those in CR in the original NCI study – died of intercurrent illnesses including acute leukemia, and most long-term survivors suffered from permanent sterility [36]. The numerous controlled trials that demonstrated the superiority of ABVD over MOPP are now of historical interest [37]. ABVD, until recently, has been the regimen of choice for the treatment of advanced stage HL following controlled trials and observational studies that confirm the following: ABVD is as effective as alternating regimens, has less mucosal, hematologic, and infectious toxicity, appears to be free of long-term leukemogenic risk, and fertility appears to be preserved in both men and women [38, 39]. Standard therapy for advanced stage HL and patients with Stage II disease with risk factors, is six to eight cycles of ABVD at full dose; treatment on time every two weeks occasionally requires growth factor support, especially for elderly patients or those with comorbidities, but treatment without granulocyte colony-stimulating factor (G-CSF) despite significant treatment-day neutropenia is feasible and safe [40, 41]. Nevertheless, long-term survivors previously demonstrated abnormalities in pulmonary and cardiac function, and up to 30% of patients are forced to discontinue bleomycin because of acute bleomycin lung toxicity [42]. Bleomycin lung toxicity is a particularly important cause of morbidity and mortality in elderly patients treated with ABVD.

In the 1990s, a number of new regimens were introduced based on empiric observations and modeling chemotherapy response. The seven-drug Stanford V regimen (doxorubicin, vinblastine, mechlorethamine, vincristine, bleomycin, etoposide, prednisone) is administered over 12 weeks and was designed to reduce exposure to chemotherapy agents with the greatest potential for organ toxicity, especially doxorubicin, mechlorethamine, and bleomycin; and includes involved field radiation to sites of tumor bulk greater than 5 cm, limiting exposure to the lung and pericardium [43]. An initial pilot study from Stanford reported five-year freedom from progression of 89% and OS 96%, in the 142 patients with Stage III or IV disease, or locally extensive mediastinal lymphoma. These results were subsequently confirmed in a trial by the ECOG involving 45 patients treated in multiple centers: freedom from progression was 85% and OS 96% [44].

Encouraged by these results, randomized trials were initiated in North America and Europe comparing Stanford V to conventional doxorubicin-based regimens such as ABVD (Table 19.4). The importance of the inclusion of radiotherapy in the treatment of advanced stage HL has been

Table 19.4 Recent randomized trials of novel regimens in advanced HL

N patients CR (%)		Progression (%)	5y FFTF (%)	OS (yr)
EscBEACOPP [48]	466	96	2	87	91 (5)
BEACOPP	469	88	8	76	88
COPP-ABVD	260	85	10	69	83
ABVD [96]	99	70	12	65	84 (5)
BEACOPP	98	81	2	78	92
COPP-EBV-CAD	98	69	10	71	91
ABVD [46]	122	89	8	85	90
Stanford V[a]	107	76	13	73	82
MOPP-EBV-CAD	106	94	0	94	88
ABVD [97]	261	67	5	76	90 (5)
Standford V[a]	259	57	6	74	92

[a] Note that radiation was received by 73% of patients in the Stanford V arm in the UK trial [97] and 66% of patients in the Intergruppo Italiano Linfomi trial [46], compared to 91% in the original report of this regimen from Stanford [43]
CR: complete response rate; FFTF: freedom from treatment failure; OS: overall survival

questioned, since earlier studies suggested no improvement in disease control and potentially inferior long-term survival. More recent data using regimens equivalent to ABVD suggest no advantage to the addition of consolidation radiation compared to additional cycles of chemotherapy or no further treatment [45]. The Intergruppo Italiano Linfomi (GISL) compared ABVD to Stanford V and the nine-drug regimen MOPP-EBV-CAD in a three-arm trial involving 355 patients [46]. Those who responded to chemotherapy received radiation to sites of previous bulky disease. The protocol gave the option to omit radiotherapy in cases where complete response had been achieved. Seventy-six patients in the ABVD arm, 50 in the MOPP-EBV-CAD arm, and only 71 patients in the Stanford V arm received radiotherapy, a point for which this study has been criticized since radiation is integral to the Stanford V regimen. At five years, FFTF and OS were inferior for patients in the Stanford V arm. A second trial performed by the ECOG and the National Cancer Institute of Canada Clinical Trials Group, randomized patients with advanced HL to either ABVD or Stanford V. The latter arm included mandated radiotherapy as originally described in the phase II study from Stanford; enrolment is complete, but results of the trial are not yet available.

The German Hodgkin's Study Group tested the concept of adding non-cross-resistant chemotherapy agents and maximizing the dose-intensity of myelosuppressive agents using G-CSF [47]. The BEACOPP and escalated (esc) BEACOPP regimens have now been tested in a number of clinical trials. The initial study was the three-arm GHSG HD9 randomized trial comparing COPP-ABVD, the previous standard, to BEACOPP or escBEACOPP. An interim analysis demonstrated inferior response and time to progression in the COPP-ABVD arm, and this arm was closed. Enrolment continued, randomizing patients to one or the other BEACOPP regimens. At the time of final analysis, patients in both the BEACOPP arms were included in the comparison to COPP-ABVD, although strictly speaking, only those randomized concurrently with the COPP-ABVD patients should have been included for the statistical analysis. The complete response rate, rate of disease progression on therapy, five-year FFTF, and OS all

favor escBEACOPP compared to COPP-ABVD [48] and 10-year follow-up confirms superiority of escBEACOPP over BEACOPP [49]. Although intensification of therapy resulted in improved survival in advanced stage HL, patients in the escBEACOPP arm experienced significantly more acute hematologic toxicity, a greater incidence of gonadal toxicity in both men and women, and, with short follow-up, an increase in risk of secondary acute myeloid leukemia, although the number of cases reported is small. A second randomized trial in advanced stage HL comparing eight cycles of escBEACOPP to four escalated and four standard dose cycles has been reported in abstract form, with no difference in OS; long-term follow-up of this important trial is awaited [50].

Hodgkin lymphoma in persons with human immunodeficiency virus (HIV) infection

Hodgkin lymphoma is not considered an AIDS-defining malignancy in individuals infected with HIV, but the incidence in this population compared to the general population is increased approximately five-fold [51]. Although the incidence of NHLs in those with HIV has declined in recent years, reflecting the effectiveness of antiretroviral therapy in restoring immunity, the relative risk of HL has actually increased in the post-antiretroviral era, with a 60% increase in risk in the years 1996–2002 compared to 1991–1995, according to data from the HIV-AIDS Cancer Match Study [52]. The majority of cases are diagnosed in patients without a prior diagnosis of AIDS. In the Swiss HIV cohort study, HL incidence was higher in men having sex with men compared to intravenous drug users, but did not vary by calendar year or with combination antiretroviral use [53]. HL risk increased with declining CD4 lymphocyte counts, but these trends were not significant. This study showed that the CD4:CD8 ratio was the most important indicator of HL risk, and perhaps reflects the lymphopenia that is often associated with HL. Cases of HL in the setting of HIV infection are more often mixed cellularity or lymphocyte-predominant histology, subtypes which are more strongly associated with EBV-infection [54]. Patients with HIV-related HL more often present with advanced stage disease, often involving extranodal sites, B symptoms, and bone marrow involvement. A number of chemotherapy regimens have been successfully employed for the treatment of HIV-related HL including ABVD, BEACOPP, and Stanford V [55–57], but there have been no direct comparisons to date. Outcome following chemotherapy is improved in patients who receive combination antiretroviral therapy to restore CD4 counts [58]. The use of antiretroviral therapy and concurrent chemotherapy is feasible, with supportive anti-infective agents to prevent opportunistic infection. Recent reports suggest that treatment outcome, at least with short-term follow-up, may be comparable to that achieved with similar regimens in immunocompetent patients, and that the use of high-dose chemotherapy and autologous SCT is appropriate for patients with relapsed HL who are sensitive to second-line chemotherapy [59].

Positron emission tomography (FDG-PET) in staging, response assessment and prognosis

Over the last decade there have been numerous reports of the ability of FDG-PET to potentially contribute to the management of patients with HL (reviewed in [60]). Evaluations of FDG-PET have focused on the ability of this test to improve the accuracy of staging prior to initiation of therapy; to determine prognosis by means of early response assessment; and to more clearly delineate complete response at the end of therapy. Most reports represent single institution retrospective analyses of patient outcomes, although prospective evaluation of the utility of PET has been reported in more recent studies. Studies evaluating the accuracy of FDG-PET scans for staging, either alone or with CT imaging, have determined that the former modality has greater sensitivity that CT scanning, resulting in up-staging of a significant number of patients (20–40%), and down-staging in a smaller percentage (5–10%) [61, 62]. Treatment change in this setting has usually consisted of more prolonged or

intensive courses of chemotherapy. Additional information is required on the impact of staging with FDG-PET, focusing on treatment changes and subsequent long-term outcomes.

Studies of FGD-PET for early response assessment during chemotherapy have recently been the subject of a meta-analysis [63]. Overall, a negative FDG-PET scan, either alone or co-registered with CT images, has a very high negative predictive value for disease recurrence, in the range of 85–95%. A large collaborative effort between centers in Italy and Denmark demonstrated that the prognostic information of an FDG-PET scan after two cycles of chemotherapy was superior to that provided by baseline patient characteristics prior to treatment. In that analysis, patients with a negative PET scan after two cycles of ABVD had a two-year PFS of 95%, while among those with a positive scan only 13% were progression free, regardless of the number of IPS risk factors (0–2 or >3) at baseline [64]. The positive predictive value of early interim PET scanning in this study was 86%. An exception to this may be in the setting of bulky disease at initial presentation: in one recent trial, patients receiving VEBEP chemotherapy for bulky HL >5 cm in diameter had a PET scan performed at the end of treatment, and those with negative scans were randomized to EFRT (extended field radiation therapy) or observation [65]. The relapse rate was 2.5% for those receiving EFRT and 14% on observation (p = 0.03). On the other hand, data from the GHSG HD15 study in advanced HL suggest that not all patients with a positive PET scan at the end of therapy will progress, at least with short follow-up. In that trial, patients with residual masses >2.5 cm on CT scan underwent FDG-PET imaging, and those with a positive scan received 30 Gy IFRT, while those whose scan was negative received no further therapy [66]. Although the PFS at 12 months was 96% for patients with a negative PET scan, it was 86% for those with a positive scan who went on to receive IFRT.

These data are important because, although follow-up is short, they demonstrate that further therapy – in this case, the addition of IFRT – may ameliorate, in part, the prognostic impact of a positive post-treatment scan, and suggests that this imaging technique may be of value in applying risk-adapted therapeutic strategies that both reduce toxicity and maximize long-term disease control. In addition they highlight the need for standardization of interpretation and for further evaluation in carefully designed prospective trials [67]. Examples of such trials are shown in Figure 19.1. In the case of a positive PET scan, biopsy of positive areas on a PET scan remains an important consideration. False-positive scans may be due to rebound thymic hyperplasia in young patients, local inflammation post-chemo or radiotherapy, sarcoidosis or deposition of brown fat. In a recent report that included 57 patients with mediastinal HL, the majority with Stage I or II disease and 25 with bulky mediastinal masses, 21 had a positive FDG-PET scan at the end of treatment or in early follow-up. On biopsy, only 10 had documented relapse; biopsies in the other cases had only fibrosis or other benign etiologies [68]. Patients with a positive post-treatment PET scan should proceed to biopsy whenever this can be done safely, or be reassessed with cross-sectional imaging, before initiating a change in therapy, unless they are enrolled on a prospective clinical trial assessing the outcome of treatment modification based on PET findings [63, 69].

Refractory and recurrent disease: salvage therapy

Second-line therapy for refractory or relapsed HL is required in 10–15% of patients who initially present with localized disease, and in 30–40% of those with advanced stage disease. Factors to be considered in the treatment of refractory or relapsed HL include the interval between initial therapy and relapse, disease stage at the time of recurrence (relapse stage) and the nature of front-line treatment. Patients with limited stage disease who relapse after EFRT or brief chemotherapy and IFRT may be considered for second-line chemotherapy, with or without additional RT if local tissue tolerance allows. Among 422 patients treated on a series of trials from the GHSG, 25% had relapsed following radiation alone for early stage disease, 32% after combined modality therapy for unfavorable early stage disease, and 43% after

chemotherapy with or without radiation for advanced stage HL. The salvage treatment consisted of RT in 13%, chemotherapy in 54% and high-dose chemotherapy with autologous SCT in 33%. The group who relapsed after RT alone had the best outcome following salvage therapy, with FFTF and OS of 81% and 89%, respectively (median follow-up 45 months) [70]. The corresponding FFTF and OS in patients with early relapse (complete remission of 12 months or less, from completion of initial therapy) were 33% and 46%, and for those with late relapse (>12 months), 43% and 71%, respectively. Factors predicting a poor prognosis were: early relapse, Stage III or IV at relapse, and presence of anemia. These three factors were used to construct a prognostic score, where the four-year OS was 83% if no factors were present, and 27% if all three factors were present. Patients who relapse with Stage I or II disease, without any of the above risk factors, may have prolonged disease control with involved field radiation.

Patients with refractory HL (those progressing during or within three months of completion of a complete course of anthracycline-based chemotherapy), have a very poor prognosis. In one recent report, only about 17% of patients with disease refractory to doxorubicin-containing combination chemotherapy were FF2F at five years [71]. OS is significantly better for those receiving salvage chemotherapy and autologous SCT, and approximately one-third of such patients are disease-free three to five years following treatment, while virtually all patients treated with conventional-dose chemotherapy relapse [72].

High-dose chemotherapy and autologous stem cell transplantation

Although there are numerous cohort studies describing the favorable outcome of patients with relapsed or refractory HL following autologous SCT, there are only two small randomized trials that have actually evaluated high-dose compared to standard-dose chemotherapy in this setting. Linch et al. reported the result of a randomized trial of

40 patients, showing an improvement in disease-free survival for patients with refractory or recurrent HL within one year of treatment, using mini-BEAM (carmustine (BCNU), etoposide, cytarabine, melphalan) followed by BEAM supported by bone marrow stem cells, compared to miniBEAM alone [73]. Schmitz et al. randomized 161 patients to a similar salvage regimen, dexaBEAM, for two cycles, followed by either an additional two cycles of salvage chemotherapy or high-dose BEAM

(A) General model of trial design

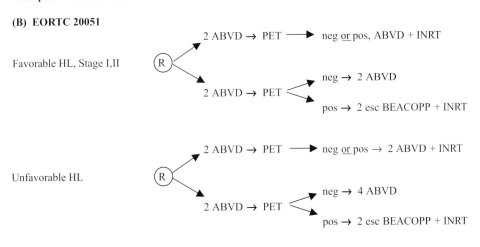

Examples of current trials

(B) EORTC 20051

(C) UK RAPID trial

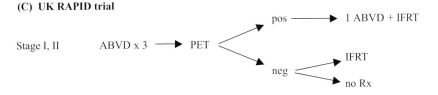

(D) UK RATHL trial Advanced Stage I, II

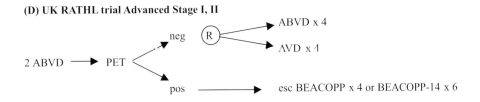

supported by autologous bone marrow or peripheral blood stem cells; patients in both arms received IFRT to areas of residual disease. FFTF at three years was significantly better for those who received autologous SCT compared to standard-dose therapy (55% vs. 34%; p = 0.019), but OS was similar (71% vs. 65%) [74]. Both of these trials are small in comparison to current, large primary treatment studies, and their follow-up is short, which may contribute to the lack of improvement in OS reported. In addition, severe toxicity and mortality from these multi-agent salvage regimens can be substantial: six patients in the German trial died early from treatment-related toxicity (5.6%), a rate that is much higher than currently seen following autologous SCT itself.

Although autologous SCT represents the standard of care for patients with relapsed or refractory HL, improvements in outcome are clearly needed. One potential strategy is to try to improve the complete response rate prior to autologous SCT, one of the most powerful predictors of long-term outcome [75]. Josting and co-workers tested high-dose sequential chemotherapy, in which non-cross-resistant agents are given at maximally tolerated doses over as short an interval as possible [76]. Patients achieving PR or CR after two cycles of DHAP went on to receive high-dose cyclophosphamide ($4 \, g/m^2$) plus G-CSF on day 37, followed by

PBSC harvest, high-dose methotrexate ($8 \, g/m^2$) plus vincristine $1.4 \, mg/m^2$ on day 51, and etoposide $2 \, g/m^2$ plus G-CSF on day 58. Following this, myeloablative treatment was given with BEAM followed by PBSC transplant. The partial and complete response rates to DHAP alone in 102 evaluable patients were 68% and 21%, respectively. After additional high-dose sequential therapy, the complete response rate improved to 72% and overall response to 80%. This concept was tested in a randomized trial recently reported by the GHSG, EORTC, and the European Bone Marrow Transplant Group. Responding patients after two cycles of DHAP were randomized to receive BEAM plus autologous SCT or to high-dose sequential therapy followed by BEAM. Patients in the high-dose sequential arm experienced greater toxicity, but there was no difference in FFTF or OS between the two arms [77].

Intensification of therapy through the addition of a second autologous transplant has been reported by a number of investigators [78], and appears feasible in light of the general good performance status of the patient population and the ability to collect sufficient stem cells for two transplants in most patients. Tandem transplants were used in a prospective evaluation of risk-adapted treatment for recurrent HL, where patients deemed to be at high risk of relapse (defined as those with primary

---

Figure 19.1 Randomized study designs to directly evaluate utility of early/interim FDG-PET on treatment outcomes. (A) In order to evaluate the contribution of interim or end-of-treatment FDG-PET scanning on improved outcome, patients are randomized according to the result obtained; those with a negative scan may be at lower risk of disease recurrence, and therefore may have treatment omitted (e.g., for Stage I and II HL, omission of IFRT); those with a positive scan may be at higher risk of treatment failure and may benefit from therapy augmentation (e.g., escalated prolonged courses of chemotherapy, or extended field radiation (EFRT)). (B) In the EORTC study 20051, all patients with limited stage disease have a PET scan after two cycles of ABVD; the control arm in each stratum consists of continuing with combined modality therapy including involved node radiation (INRT) in both favorable and unfavorable risk patients, the current standard of care. Patients with favorable HL and a negative PET have a low risk of recurrence and may benefit from a strategy that is focused on reduction of long-term effects of treatment, and have radiotherapy omitted; those with unfavorable HL and a positive PET scan are at high risk of disease recurrence and may benefit from more intensive chemotherapy, in addition to INRT. (C) Patients with Stage I/II disease in the UK RAPID trial may be at low risk of recurrence, and the experimental arm of this trial omits radiotherapy after three cycles of ABVD. (D) Patients with Stage III/IV HL in the UK RATHL trial may have a more favorable prognosis and therefore may benefit from efforts to reduce toxicity of chemotherapy, in this case bleomycin pulmonary toxicity; the experimental arm continues for six cycles with bleomycin omitted. Patients with a positive PET scan are assigned to more intensive chemotherapy, with the assumption that their outcome will be improved by therapy augmentation; there is no control arm in this part of the study and the conclusions will be difficult and rest on historical controls.

refractory disease, or those with two of: relapse within 12 months of completion of therapy, Stage III or IV, or in a prior radiation field) were assigned to double ASCT, while those with only one of the above risk factors had a single transplant. Two-thirds of patients were able to proceed to the second transplant, and a CR was obtained in 40% of the former group of patients after the second transplant. Five-year FFTF was 46% for the poor-risk group and OS 57%, which compares favorably to other cohort data in this poor-prognosis subgroup [79]. Those who proceeded to a second transplant, though a selected subset of patients, had FFTF that was similar to those with intermediate-risk relapsed HL (64% versus 73%). A randomized trial of a second round of high-dose chemotherapy and autologous SCT is essential to determine the true utility of this approach.

Functional imaging using FDG-PET or Gallium scintigraphy is also able to identify patients who have a high likelihood of success or failure following autologous SCT [80, 81]. Prospective evaluation of the role of a second transplant or other post-transplant therapy may address whether the results of autologous SCT in these high-risk patients with positive post-salvage chemotherapy functional imaging can be improved. Trials of adjuvant, post-autologous SCT targeted therapies such as the deacetylase inhibitor LBH589 and the antibody-drug conjugate SGN-35 (see below) are currently being carried out.

Investigational agents in relapsed HL post-autologous SCT

A number of new, targeted therapies have been tested or are currently under study. Despite the sound pre-clinical rationale for the use of a proteosome inhibitor in relapsed HL [82], clinical results in the few small studies of bortezomib reported to date have been resoundingly negative [83]. Similarly, response rates reported for monoclonal antibodies to the surface membrane antigen CD30 present on classical HL cells have been very low [84, 85]. However, very

encouraging results have been reported with the use of the SGN30 antibody conjugated to monomethyl auristatin E (MMAE, SGN35), an agent that binds to tubulin and causes cell cycle arrest and apoptosis. In a phase I study in heavily pretreated patients with HL (median of three prior regimens) 15/28 treated at doses >1.2 mg/kg achieved a PR (5) or CR (10) [86]. The deacetylase inhibitor LBH589 [87] and the inhibitor of the mTOR RAD001 (everolimus) [88] have also demonstrated activity in relapsed HL after autologous SCT and continue under active study.

Reduced intensity allogeneic SCT for HL relapsing after autologous SCT

Myeloablative chemoradiotherapy and allogeneic transplantation for relapsed HL after autotransplant previously carried a prohibitively high treatment-related mortality (TRM), and evidence of a graft-versus-tumor effect is sparse. One report from the International Bone Marrow Transplant Registry of 114 patients undergoing myeloablative allogeneic transplants reported a rate of disease progression at three years of 52% and treatment-related mortality of 22% [89]. With further follow-up few patients in this large series were cured, with five-year disease-free survival reported to be only 5% and OS 24%. There was no difference in TRM, PFS, or OS between patients with HL and other lymphoma subtypes. The authors of this multi-institutional study concluded that allogeneic transplant using myeloablative regimens was not curative for most patients with relapsed lymphoma post-autografting.

Significant progress has been made in the application of reduced-intensity conditioning regimens and planned donor leukocyte infusion, to facilitate use of this therapy in high-risk patient populations, in particular those with disease progression after an autologous transplant. Early case series were small, but suggested that such therapy was feasible even in heavily pre-treated recipients, with potentially lower early (day 100) transplant-related mortality (Table 19.5).

Table 19.5 Recent results with reduced intensity allogeneic transplantation for relapsed HL

Lead author	N	Prior ASCT	Prior regimens (median)	Treatment-related mortality	PFS	OS
Peggs [90]	49	44	5	16% (2 y)	32% (4 y)	56% (4 y)
Sureda [92]	89	55	85% ≥3	23% (1 y)	18% (3 y)	35% (3 y)
Alderlini [93]	40	30	5	22% (18 m)	55% (18 m)	61% (18 m)
Armand [94]	36	34	4	15% (3 y)	22% (3 y)	56% (3 y)
Alvarez [95]	40	29	55% ≥3	25% (1 y)	32% (2 y)	48% (2 y)

N: number of allogeneic transplants; ASCT: autologous stem cell transplant; PFS: progression-free survival; OS: overall survival

Renewed interest in exploring RIT in relapsed HL has come from recent reports of graft-versus-tumor effects from related or unrelated donor transplants, as shown by disease response to donor leukocyte infusion for residual masses, mixed (incomplete) chimerism or documented disease regression post-transplant [90]. This anti-tumor affect appears to be related to (and at the cost of) chronic graft-versus-host disease in most but not all cases. A number of patients who have had complete remission following donor leuko-cyte infusions have also had additional chemo-therapy, making the true rate of response to this form of immunotherapy difficult to determine with confidence. Baron et al. [91] recently reported a higher risk of relapse and inferior three-year PFS (8%) for patients with HL com-pared to other hematologic malignancies and for those with lymphoma that was resistant to che-motherapy, indicating the importance of disease biology and chemotherapy sensitivity in outcome of allogeneic SCT after autologous SCT. A number of trials have emphasized the importance of con-tinued sensitivity to chemotherapy prior to RIT, with disease status at transplant (CR or PR) being a very strong predictor of subsequent progression-free and OS (Table 19.5). Larger trials with uni-form eligibility and treatment approaches are needed in order to more clearly define the ben-efits of allogeneic transplantation in this patient population.

Appendix Combination chemotherapy regimens for the treatment of advanced stage Hodgkin lymphoma

Drugs	Recommended dose (mg/m²)	Route	Days
MOPP			
Nitrogen mustard	6	IV	1, 8
Vincristine	1.4	IV	1, 8
Procarbazine	100	PO	1–14
Prednisone	40	PO	1–14
MOPP/ABV			
Nitrogen mustard	6	IV	1
Vincristine	1.4	IV	1
Procarbazine	100	PO	1–7
Prednisone	40	PO	1–14
Doxorubicin	35	IV	8
Bleomycin	10	IV	8
Vinblastine	6	IV	8
COPP/ABVD			
Cyclophosphamide	650	IV	1,8
Vincristine	1.4	IV	1, 8
Procarbazine	100	PO	1–14
Prednisone	40	PO	1–14

(*continued*)

Drugs	Recommended dose (mg/m²)	Route	Days
Doxorubicin	25	IV	29, 43
Bleomycin	10	IV	29, 43
Vinblastine	6	IV	29, 43
Dacarbazine	375	IV	29, 43
BEACOPP Baseline			
Bleomycin	10	IV	8
Etoposide	100	IV	1–3
Doxorubicin	25	IV	1
Cyclophosphamide	650	IV	1
Vincristine	1.4	IV	8
Procarbazine	100	PO	1–7
Prednisone	40	PO	1–14
BEACOPP Escalated			
Bleomycin	10	IV	8
Etoposide	200	IV	1–3
Doxorubicin	35	IV	1
Cyclophosphamide	1200	IV	1
Vincristine	1.4	IV	8
Procarbazine	100	PO	1–7
Prednisone	40	PO	1–14
ABVD			
Doxorubicin	25	IV	1, 15
Bleomycin	5	IV	1, 15
Vinblastine	6	IV	1, 15
Dacarbazine	375	IV	1, 15
Stanford V[a]			
Doxorubicin	25	IV	1, 15
Vinblastine	6	IV	1, 15
Mechlorethamine	6	IV	1
Etoposide	60	IV	15, 16
Vincristine	1.4	IV	8, 22
Bleomycin	5	IV	8, 22
Prednisone	40	PO	every other day

Drugs	Recommended dose (mg/m²)	Route	Days
MOPP-EBV-CAD			
Mechlorethamine	6	IV	1, cycles 1, 3, & 5 only
Lomustine	100	PO	1, cycles 2, 4, & 6 only
Vindesine	3	IV	1
Mephalan	6	PO	1–3
Prednisone	40	PO	1–14
Epidoxorubicin	40	IV	8
Vincristine	1.4	IV	8
Procarbazine	100	PO	8–14
Vinblastine	6	IV	15
Bleomycin	10	IV	15
VEBP			
Epirubicin	70	IV	1
Bleomycin	10	IV/IM	1
Vinblastine	6	IV	1
Prednisone	40	PO	1–5
VEBEP			
Vinblastine	6	IV	1, 15
Etoposide	80	IV	1–3, 15–17
Bleomycin	10	IV	1, 15
Epirubicin	40	IV	1, 15
Prednisone	40	PO	1–5, 15–19
BEAM			
BCNU	300	IV	−6
Etoposide	100–200	IV	−5, −4, −3, −2
Cytosine arabinoside	200–400	IV	−5, −4, −3, −2
Melphalan	140	IV	−1

[a] Followed by radiation administered to initial sites of disease ≥5 cm and macroscopic splenic disease; modified mantle for bulky mediastinal masses

References

1 Morton LM, Wang SS, Devesa SS, et al. (2006) Lymphoma incidence patterns by WHO subtype in the United States, 1992–2001. *Blood* **107**:265–76.

2 Bosetti C, Levi F, Ferlay J, et al. (2009) The recent decline in mortality from Hodgkin lymphomas in central and eastern Europe. *Ann Oncol* **20**:767–74.

3 Favier O, Heutte N, Stamatoullas-Bastard A, et al. (2009) Survival after Hodgkin Lymphoma. *Cancer* **115**:1680–91.

4 Kapatai G, Murray P. (2007) Contribution of the Epstein-Barr virus to the molecular pathogenesis of Hodgkin lymphoma. *J Clin Pathol* **60**:1342–9.

5 Hjalgrim H, Smedby KE, Rostgaard K, et al. (2007) Infectious mononucleosis, childhood social environment, and risk of Hodgkin lymphoma. *Cancer Res* **67**:2382–8.

6 Brennan RM, Burrows Sr., (2008) A mechanism for the HLA-A*01-associated risk for EBV+ Hodgkin lymphoma and infectious mononucleosis. *Blood* **112**:2589.

7 Keegan THM, Glaser SL, Clarke CA, et al. (2005) Epstein-Barr virus as a marker for survival after Hodgkin's lymphoma: A population-based study. *J Clin Oncol* **23**:7604–13.

8 Mack TM, Cozen W, Shibata DK, et al. (1995) Concordance for Hodgkin's disease in identical twins suggesting genetic susceptibility to the young-adult form of the disease. *N Engl J Med* **332**:413–18.

9 Chang ET, Smedby KE, Hjalgrim H, et al. (2005) Family history of hematopoietic malignancy and risk of lymphoma. *J Natl Cancer Inst* **97**:1466–74.

10 Anderson LA, Pfeiffer RM, Rapkin JS, et al. (2008) Survival patterns among lymphoma patients with a family history of lymphoma. *J Clin Oncol* **26**:4958–65.

11 Skibola CF, Curry JD, Nieters A. (2007) Genetic susceptibility to lymphoma. *Haematologica* **92**:960–9.

12 Landgren O, Engels EA, Pfeiffer RM, et al. (2006). Autoimmunity and susceptibility to Hodgkin lymphoma: A population-based case-control study in Scandinavia. *J Natl Cancer Inst* **98**:1321–30.

13 El-Zein R, Monroy CM, Etzel CJ, et al. (2009) Genetic polymorphisms in DNA repair genes as modulators of Hodgkin disease risk. *Cancer* **115**:1651–9.

14 Liang X, Caporaso N, McMaster M, et al. (2009) Common genetic variants in candidate genes and risk of familial lymphoid malignancies. *Br J Haematol* **146**:418–23.

15 Hasenclever D, Diehl V. (1998) A prognostic score for advanced Hodgkin's disease. *N Engl J Med* **339**:1506–14.

16 Franklin J, Paulus U, Lieberz D, et al. for the German Hodgkin Lymphoma Group. (2000) Is the international prognostic score for advanced stage Hodgkin's disease applicable to early stage patients? *Ann Oncol* **11**:617–23.

17 Kaplan HS. (1966) Evidence for a tumoricidal dose level in the radiotherapy of Hodgkin's disease. *Cancer Res* **26**:1221–4.

18 Peters MV. (1966) Prophylactic treatment of adjacent areas in Hodgkin's disease. *Cancer Res* **26**:1232–43.

19 Press OW, LeBlanc M, Lichter AS, et al. (2001) Phase III randomized intergroup trial of subtotal lymphoid irradiation versus doxorubicin, vinblastine, and subtotal lymphoid irradiation for Stage IA to IIA Hodgkin's disease. *J Clin Oncol* **19**:4238–44.

20 Engert A, Franklin J, Eich HT, et al. (2007) Two cycles of doxorubicin, bleomycin, vinblastine and dacarbazine plus extended-field radiotherapy is superior to radiotherapy alone in early favorable Hodgkin's lymphoma: Final results of the GHSG HD7 trial. *J Clin Oncol* **25**:3495–502.

21 Ferme C, Eghbali H, Meerwaldt JH, et al. (2007) Chemotherapy plus involved-field radiation in early-stage Hodgkin's disease. *New Engl J Med* **357**:1916–27.

22 Bonadonna G, Bonfante V, Viviani S, et al. (2004) ABVD plus subtotal nodal versus involved-field radiotherapy in early-stage Hodgkin's disease: long-term results. *J Clin Oncol* **22**:2835–41.

23 Engert A, Schiller P, Josting A, et al. (2003) Involved-field radiotherapy is equally effective and less toxic compared with extended-field radiotherapy after four cycles of chemotherapy in patients with early-stage unfavorable Hodgkin lymphoma: Results of the HD8 trial of the German Hodgkin Lymphoma Study Group. *J Clin Oncol* **21**:3601–8.

24 Girinsky T, van de Maazen R, Specht L, et al., on behalf of the EORTC-GELA Lymphoma Group. (2006) Involved-node radiotherapy (INRT) in patients with early Hodgkin lymphoma: Concepts and guidelines. *Radiother Oncol* **79**:270–7.

25 Campbell BA, Voss N, Pickles T, et al. (2008) Involved-nodal radiation therapy as a component of combination therapy for limited-stage Hodgkin's lymphoma: A question of field size. *J Clin Oncol* **26**:5170–4.

26 Noordijk EM, Carde P, Dupouy N, et al. (2006) Combined-modality therapy for clinical stage I or II Hodgkin's lymphoma: long-term results of the European Organization for Research and Treatment of

Cancer H7 randomized controlled trials. *J Clin Oncol* **24**:3128–35.

27 Carde P, Hagenbeek A, Hayat M, et al. (1993) Clinical staging versus laparotomy and combined modality with MOPP versus ABVD in early-stage Hodgkin's disease: the H6 twin randomized trials from the European Organization for Research and Treatment of Cancer Lymphoma Cooperative Group. *J Clin Oncol* **11**:2258–72.

28 Engert A, Eichenauer DA, Dreyling M,on behalf of the ESMO Guidelines Working Group (2009) Hodgkin's lymphoma: ESMO clinical recommendations for diagnosis, treatment and follow-up. *Ann Oncol* **20**(Suppl 4): iv108–9.

29 Straus DJ, Portlock CS, Qin J, et al. (2004) Results of a prospective randomized clinical trial of doxorubicin, bleomycin, vinblastine and dacarbazine (ABVD) followed by radiation therapy (RT) versus ABVD alone for stages I, II and IIIA non-bulky Hodgkin disease. *Blood* **104**:3483–9.

30 Meyer RM, Gospodarowicz MK, Connors JM,et al: (2005) Randomized comparison of ABVD chemotherapy with a strategy that includes radiation therapy in patients with limited-stage Hodgkin's lymphoma: National Cancer Institute of Canada Clinical Trials Group and the Eastern Cooperative Oncology Group. *J Clin Oncol* **23**:4634–42.

31 Sieniawski M, Franklin J, Nogova L, et al. (2007) Outcome of patients experiencing progression or relapse after primary treatment with two cycles of chemotherapy and radiotherapy for early-stage favorable Hodgkin's lymphoma. *J Clin Oncol* **25**:2000–5.

32 Macdonald DA, Ding K, Gospodarowicz MK, et al. (2007) Patterns of disease progression and outcomes in a randomized trial testing ABVD alone for patients with limited-stage Hodgkin lymphoma. *Ann Oncol* **18**:1680–4.

33 Shahidi M, Kamangari N, Ashley S, et al. (2006) Site of relapse after chemotherapy alone in stage I and II Hodgkin's disease. *Radiother Oncol* **78**:1–5.

34 Goodman KA, Riedel E, Serrano V, et al. (2008) Long-term effects of high-dose chemotherapy and radiation for relapsed and refractory Hodgkin's lymphoma. *J Clin Oncol* **26**:5240–7.

35 DeVita VT, Jr., Chu E. (2008) A history of cancer chemotherapy. *Cancer Res* **68**:8643–53.

36 Longo DL, Young RC, Wesley M, et al. (1986) Twenty years of MOPP therapy for Hodgkin's disease. *J Clin Oncol* **4**:1295–306.

37 Canellos GP, Anderson JR, Propert KJ, et al. (1992) Chemotherapy of advanced Hodgkin's disease with MOPP, ABVD, or MOPP alternating with ABVD. *N Engl J Med* **327**:1478–84.

38 Duggan DB, Petroni GR, Johnson JL, et al. (2003) Randomized comparison of ABVD and MOPP/ABV hybrid for the treatment of advanced Hodgkin's disease: Report of an intergroup trial. *J Clin Oncol* **21**:607–14.

39 Johnson PWM, Radford JA, Cullen MH, et al. (2005) Comparison of ABVD and alternating or hybrid multi-drug regimens for the treatment of advanced Hodgkin's Lymphoma: Results of the United Kingdom Lymphoma Group LY09 Trial (ISRCTN97144519). *J Clin Oncol* **23**:9208–18.

40 Chand VK, Link BK, Ritchie JM, *et al* (2006) Neutropenia and febrile neutropenia in patients with Hodgkin's lymphoma treatment with doxorubicin (Adriamycin), bleomycin, vinblastine and dacarbazine (ABVD) chemotherapy. *Leuk Lymph* **47**:657–63.

41 Evens AM, Cilley J, Ortiz TA, et al. (2007) G-CSF is not necessary to maintain over 99% dose-intensity with ABVD in the treatment of Hodgkin' lymphoma: low toxicity and excellent outcomes in a 10-year analysis. *Br J Haematol* **137**:545–52.

42 Sleijfer S. (2001) Bleomycin-induced pneumonitis. *Chest* **120**:617–24.

43 Horning SJ, Hoppe RT, Breslin S, et al. (2002) Stanford V and radiotherapy for locally extensive and advanced Hodgkin's disease: mature results of a prospective clinical trial. *J Clin Oncol* **20**:630–7.

44 Horning SJ, Williams J, Bartlett NL, et al. (2000) Assessment of the Stanford V regimen and consolidative radiotherapy for bulky and advanced Hodgkin's disease: Eastern Cooperative Oncology Group pilot study E1492. *J Clin Oncol* **18**:972–80.

45 Ferme C, Mounier N, Casasnovas O, et al. (2006) Long-term results and competing risk analysis of the H89 trial in patients with advanced-stage Hodgkin lymphoma: a study by the Groupe d'Etude des Lymphomes de l'Adulte (GELA). *Blood* **107**:4636–42.

46 Gobbi PG, Levis A, Chisesi T, et al. (2005) ABVD versus modified Stanford V versus MOPPEBVCAD with optional and limited radiotherapy in intermediate- and advanced-stage Hodgkin's lymphoma: final results of a multicenter randomized trial by the Intergruppo Italiano Linfomi. *J Clin Oncol* **23**:9198–207.

47 Tesch H, Diehl V, Lathan B, et al. (1998) Moderate dose escalation for advanced stage Hodgkin's disease using the bleomycin, etoposide, adriamycin,

cyclophosphamide, vincristine, procarbazine, and prednisone scheme and adjuvant radiotherapy: A study of the German Hodgkin Lymphoma Study Group. *Blood* **92**:4560–7.

48 Diehl V, Franklin J, Pfreundschuh M, et al. (2003) Standard and increased-dose BEACOPP chemotherapy compared with COPP-ABVD for advanced Hodgkin's disease. *N Engl J Med* **348**:2386–95.

49 Engert A, Diehl V, Franklin J, et al. (2009) Escalated-dose BEACOPP in the treatment of patients with advanced-stage Hodgkin's lymphoma: 10 years of follow-up of the GHSG HD9 study. *J Clin Oncol*, Aug 24 [Epub ahead of print].

50 Diehl V, Haverkamp H, Mueller RP, et al. (2008) Eight cycles of BEACOPP escalated compared with 4 cycles of BEACOPP escalated followed by 4 cycles of BEACOPP baseline with or without radiotherapy in patients in advanced stage Hodgkin lymphoma (HL): Final analysis of the Randomized HD12 Trial of the German Hodgkin Study Group (GHSG). *Blood* **112**:Abstract 1558.

51 Engels EA, Biggar RJ, Hall HI, et al. (2008) Cancer risk in people infected with human immunodeficiency virus in the United States. *Int J Cancer* **123**:187–94.

52 Engels EA, Pfeiffer RM, Goedert JJ, et al. (2006) Trends in cancer risk among people with AIDS in the United States 1980–2002. *AIDS* **20**:1645–54.

53 Clifford GM, Richenbach M, Lise M, et al. (2009) Hodgkin lymphoma in the Swiss HIV Cohort Study. *Blood* **113**:5737–42.

54 Thompson LD, Fisher SI, Chu WS, et al. (2004) HIV-associated Hodgkin lymphoma: a clinicopathologic and immunophenotypic study of 45 cases. *Am J Clin Pathol* **121**:727–38.

55 Spina M, Gabarre J, Rossi G, et al. (2002) Stanford V regimen and concomitant HAART in 59 patients with Hodgkin disease and HIV infection. *Blood* **100**:1984–8.

56 Hartmann P, Rehwald U, Salzberger B, et al. (2003) BEACOPP therapeutic regimen for patients with Hodgkin's disease and HIV infection. *Ann Oncol* **14**:1562–9.

57 Xicoy B, Ribera J-M, Miralles P, et al. (2007) Results of treatment with doxorubicin, bleomycin, vinblastine and dacarbazine and highly active antiretroviral therapy in advanced stage human immunodeficiency virus-related Hodgkin's lymphoma. *Haematologica* **92**:191–8.

58 Hentrich M, Maretta L, Chow KU, et al. (2006) Highly active antiretroviral therapy (HAART) improves survival in HIV-associated Hodgkin's disease: results of a multicenter study. *Ann Oncol* **17**:914–19.

59 Re A, Michieli M, Casari S, et al. (2009) High dose therapy and autologous peripheral blood stem cell transplantation as salvage treatment for AIDS-related lymphoma: long term results of the GICAT study with analysis of prognostic factors. *Blood* **114**:1306–13.

60 Seam P, Juweid ME, Cheson BD. (2007) The role of FDG-PET scans in patients with lymphoma. *Blood* **110**:3507–16.

61 Partridge S, Timothy A, O'Doherty MJ, et al. (2000) 2-Fluorine-18-fluoro-2-deoxy-D glucose positron emission tomography in the pre-treatment staging of Hodgkin's disease: influence on patient management in a single institution. *Ann Oncol* **11**:1273–9.

62 Jerusalem G, Beguin Y, Fassotte MF, et al. (2001) Whole-body positron emission tomography using 18F-fluorodeoxyglucose compared to standard procedures for staging patients with Hodgkin's disease. *Haematologica* **86**:266–73.

63 Terasawa T, Lau J, Bardet S, et al. (2009) Fluorine-18-Fluorodeoxyglucose positron emission tomography for interim response assessment of advanced-stage Hodgkin's lymphoma and diffuse large B-cell lymphoma: A systematic review. *J Clin Oncol* **27**:1906–14.

64 Picardi M, De Renzo A, Pane F, et al. (2007) Randomized comparison of consolidation radiation versus observation in bulky Hodgkin's lymphoma with post-chemotherapy negative positron emission tomography scans. *Leuk Lymphoma* **48**:1721–7.

65 Gallamini A, Hutchings M, Rigacci L, et al. (2007) Early interim 2[^{18}F]Fluoro-2-deoxy-D-glucose positron emission tomography is prognostically superior to international prognostic score in advanced stage Hodgkin's lymphoma: A report from a joint Italian-Danish study. *J Clin Oncol* **25**:3746–52.

66 Kobe C, Dietlein M, Franklin J, et al. (2008) Positron emission tomography has a high negative predictive value for progression or early relapse for patients with residual disease after first-line chemotherapy in advanced stage Hodgkin lymphoma. *Blood* **112**:3989–94.

67 Gallamini A, Fiore F, Sorasio R, Meignan M. (2009) Interim positron emission tomography scan in Hodgkin lymphoma: definitions, interpretation rules, and clinical validation. *Leuk Lymphoma* **50**:1761–4.

68 Zinzani PL, Tani M, Trisolini R, et al. (2007) Histological verification of positive positron emission tomography findings in the follow-up of patients with mediastinal lymphoma. *Haematologia* **92**:771–7.

69 Schaefer NG, Taverna C, Strobel K, et al. (2007) Hodgkin disease: Diagnostic value of FDG PET/CT after first-line therapy – Is biopsy of FDG-avid lesions still needed? *Radiology* **224**:257–62.

70 Josting A, Franklin J, May M, et al. (2002) New prognostic score based on treatment outcome of patients with relapsed Hodgkin's lymphoma registered in the database of the German Hodgkin Lymphoma Study Group. *J Clin Oncol* **20**:221–30.

71 Josting A, Rueffer U, Franklin J, et al. (2000) Prognostic factors and treatment outcome in primary progressive Hodgkin lymphoma: a report from the German Hodgkin Lymphoma Study Group. *Blood* **96**:1280–6.

72 Andre M, Henry-Amar M, Pico JL, et al. (1999) Comparison of high-dose therapy and autologous stem cell transplantation with conventional therapy for Hodgkin's disease induction failure: a case-control study. Société Française de Greffe de Moelle. *J Clin Oncol* **17**:222–9.

73 Linch DC, Winfield D, Goldstone AH, et al. (1993) Dose intensification with autologous bone marrow transplantation in relapsed and resistant Hodgkin's disease: results of a BNLI randomised trial. *Lancet* **341**:1051–4.

74 Schmitz N, Pfistner B, Sextro M, et al. (2002) Aggressive conventional chemotherapy compared with high-dose chemotherapy with autologous hematopoietic stem cell transplantation for relapsed chemosensitive Hodgkin's disease: a randomised trial. *Lancet* **359**:2065–71.

75 Sureda A, Constans M, Iriondo A, et al. (2005) Prognostic factors affecting long-term outcome after stem cell transplantation in Hodgkin's lymphoma autografted after a first relapse. *Ann Oncol* **16**:625–33.

76 Josting A, Rudolph C, Mapara M, et al. (2005) Cologne high-dose sequential chemotherapy in relapsed and refractory Hodgkin lymphoma: results of a large multicenter study of the German Hodgkin Lymphoma Study Group (GHSG). *Ann Oncol* **16**:116–13.

77 Engert M, Haverkamp H, Borchmann P, et al. (2009) Final results of the HDR2 study – A European multicenter trial in patients with relapsed Hodgkin lymphoma. *Hematologica* **94**(Suppl 2): *204* (Abstract 0501).

78 Fung HC, Stiff P, Schriber J, et al. (2007) Tandem autologous stem cell transplantation for patients with primary refractory or poor risk recurrent Hodgkin lymphoma. *Biol Blood Marrow Transplant* **13**:594–600.

79 Morschhauser F, Brice P, Ferme C, et al. (2008) Risk-adapted salvage treatment with single or tandem autologous stem cell transplantation for first relapse/refractory Hodgkin's lymphoma: Results of the prospective multicenter H96 trial by the GELA/SFGM study group. *J Clin Oncol* **26**:5980–7.

80 Spaepen K, Stroobants S, Dupont P, et al. (2003) Prognostic value of pre-transplantation positron emission tomography using fluorine 18-fluorodeoxyglucose in patients with aggressive lymphoma treated with high-dose chemotherapy and stem cell transplantation. *Blood* **102**:53–9.

81 Jabbour E, Hosing C, Ayers G, et al. (2007) Pre-transplant positive positron emission tomography/gallium scans predict poor outcome in patients with recurrent/refractory Hodgkin lymphoma. *Cancer* **109**:2481–9.

82 Jost PJ, Ruland J. (2006) Aberrant NF-kappa B signaling in lymphoma: mechanisms, consequences and therapeutic implications. *Blood* **109**:2700–7.

83 Blum KA, Johnson JL, Niedzwiecki D, et al. (2007) Single agent bortezomib in the treatment of relapsed and refractory Hodgkin lymphoma: Cancer and Leukemia Group B Protocol 50206. *Leuk Lymphoma* **48**:1313–19.

84 Ansell SM, Horwitz SM, Engert A, et al. (2007) Phase I/II study of an anti-CD30 monoclonal antibody (MDX-060) in Hodgkin's lymphoma and anaplastic large-cell lymphoma. *J Clin Oncol* **25**:2764–9.

85 Bartlett NL, Younes A, Carabasi MH, et al. (2008) A phase 1 multidose study of SGN-30 immunotherapy in patients with refractory or recurrent CD30+ hematologic malignancies. *Blood* **111**:1848–54.

86 Younes A, Forero-Torres A, Bartlett NL, et al. (2009) Robust antitumor activity of the antibody-drug conjugate SGN-35 when administered every 3 weeks to patients with relapsed or refractory CD30 positive hematologic malignancies in a phase I study. *Haematologica* **94**(Suppl 2): *205* (Abstract 0503).

87 DeAngelo DJ, Spencer A, Ottmann OG, et al. (2009) Panobinostat has activity in treatment-refractory Hodgkin lymphoma. *Haematologica* **94**(Suppl 2): 205 (Abstract 0505).

88 Johnston PB, Ansell SM, Colgan JP, et al. (2007) mTOR inhibition for relapsed or refractory Hodgkin lymphoma: promising single agent activity with everolimus (RAD001). *Blood* **110**:2555.

89 Freytes CO, Loberiza FR, Rizzo JD, et al. (2004) Myeloablative allogeneic hematopoietic stem cell transplantation in patients who experience relapse after autologous stem cell transplantation for lymphoma: a report of the International Bone Marrow Transplant Registry. *Blood* **104**:3797–803.

90 Peggs KS, Hunter A, Chopra R, et al. (2005) Clinical evidence of a graft-versus-Hodgkin's-lymphoma effect after reduced-intensity allogeneic transplantation. *Lancet* **365**:1934–41.

91 Baron F, Storb R, Storer BE, et al. (2006) Factors associated with outcomes in allogeneic hematopoietic cell transplantation with non-myeloablative conditioning after failed myeloablative hematopoietic cell transplantation. *J Clin Oncol* **24**:4150–7.

92 Sureda A, Robinson S, Canals C, et al. (2008) Reduced-intensity conditioning compared with conventional allogeneic stem cell transplantation in relapsed or refractory Hodgkin's lymphoma: an analysis from the Lymphoma Working Party of the European Group for Blood and Marrow Transplantation. *J Clin Oncol* **26**:455–62.

93 Anderlini P, Saliba R, Acholonu S, et al. (2005) Reduced-intensity allogeneic stem cell transplantation in relapsed and refractory Hodgkin's disease: low transplant-related mortality and impact of intensity of conditioning regimen. *Bone Marrow Transplant* **35**:943–51.

94 Armand P, Kim HT, Ho VT, et al. (2008) Allogeneic transplantation with reduced-intensity conditioning for Hodgkin and non-Hodgkin lymphoma: importance of histology for outcome. *Biol Blood Marrow Transplant* **14**:418–25.

95 Alvarez I, Sureda A, Caballero MD, et al. (2006) Non-myeloablative stem cell transplantation is an effective therapy for refractory or relapsed Hodgkin lymphoma: results of a Spanish prospective cooperative protocol. *Biol Blood Marrow Transplant* **12**:172–83.

96 Federico M, Luminari S, Iannitto E, *et al* (2009) ABVD compared with BEACOPP compared with CEC for the initial treatment of patients with advanced Hodgkin's Lymphoma: Results from the HD2000 Gruppo Italiano per lo Studio dei Linfomi Trial. *J Clin Oncol* **27**:805–11.

97 Hoskin PJ, Lowry L, Horwich A, et al. (2009) Randomized comparison of the Stanford V Regimen and ABVD in the treatment of advanced Hodgkin's lymphoma: United Kingdom National Cancer Research Institute Lymphoma Group Study ISRCTN 64141244. *J Clin Oncol* **27**:5390–6.

98 Engert A, Plütschow A, Eich HT, et al. (2010) Reduced treatment intensity in patients with early-stage Hodgkin's lymphoma. *N Engl J Med* **363**:640–52.

PART 4

Plasma Cell Disorders

CHAPTER 20

Multiple Myeloma: Molecular Biology, Diagnosis and Treatment

Shaji Kumar and S. Vincent Rajkumar

Division of Hematology, Mayo Clinic College of Medicine, Rochester, MN, USA

Background

Multiple myeloma (MM) is a neoplasm of terminally differentiated plasma cells that affects nearly 20 000 individuals each year in the US, leading to over 12 000 deaths annually [1]. The annual incidence of multiple myeloma is 4–5 per 100 000 and constitutes 1% of all malignancies and 10% of all hematological malignancies. While the incidence is similar among the Caucasian population, it is nearly twice as much among the African-American population but is significantly lower among individuals of Asian origin [2, 3]. The median age of the patients at diagnosis is 67 years with a male predominance [4]. While the disease remains incurable with the current approaches, the survival of patients with myeloma appears to have improved over the past decade, likely a reflection of increased use of autologous SCT and the introduction of novel effective therapies (Figure 20.1) [5]. While older studies have suggested a median survival of three to four years, more recent clinical trials have demonstrated three-year survivals exceeding 80% [6]. The mortality rates seem to be higher among the elderly, for men compared to women, and blacks compared to whites [7].

Etiology and risk factors

While various factors have been implicated, including environmental, genetic and infectious, the eti-ology of myeloma remains unknown. Radiation exposure has been implicated based on increased incidence among individuals exposed to radiation (e.g., atomic bomb survivors) as well as those with occupational exposure [8]. However, long-term studies have not consistently validated these findings. Diagnostic radiation exposure has been implicated, but without strong evidence [9, 10]. Chemicals such as benzene, petroleum products, and pesticides have also been associated with myeloma [11–14]. This association has been based on studies in agricultural workers and petroleum industry workers and the strong evidence is lacking [15]. There are also studies linking increased risk of myeloma to hair dye, as well as dietary components, but none appears to be definitive [16, 17].

A clear genetic predisposition is not evident, but family clusters have been reported as has been increased incidence of lymphoid tumors in first-degree relatives [18]. In a family study from Sweden, a two-fold increased risk was seen among first-degree relatives of patients with myeloma [19]. Another prospective family study found that first-degree relatives of patients with MM or monoclonal gammopathy of undetermined significance (MGUS) have a greater than two-fold risk of MGUS compared to the general population, implying underlying genetic predisposition for these diseases [20]. Additional studies are needed to clearly distinguish the impact of inherited predisposition from common

Advances in Malignant Hematology, First Edition. Edited by Hussain I. Saba and Ghulam J. Mufti. © 2011 Blackwell Publishing Ltd. Published 2011 by Blackwell Publishing Ltd.

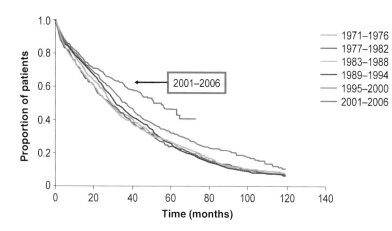

Figure 20.1 Improved survival among patients with multiple myeloma diagnosed in the past decade. (Adapted from Kumar SK et al. (2008) *Blood* **111**:2516–20.)

environmental exposures. An infectious etiology has been hypothesized given the normal plasma cell function, but no definite evidence exists other than a weak link to human herpes virus 8 [21]. Patients with HIV infection appear to be at an increased risk for MM, but this is likely related to the immuno-suppression [22]. Similarly, increased risk has been observed among patients undergoing organ trans-plantation and requiring chronic immunosuppres-sion [23]. Chronic antigenic stimulation has been implicated in the increased incidence of monoclonal gammopathies seen in black people [24].

Pathophysiology

The clonal plasma cells and the secreted monoclonal protein are the hallmarks of a spectrum of plasma cell proliferative disorders that is believed to progress through a multi-step process from the MGUS to early stage asymptomatic or smoldering myeloma (SMM), and finally to symptomatic myeloma requiring ther-apy [25–27]. While the exact sequence of events leading to the initiation of the clonal process and its subsequent progression remains unclear, much has been learned regarding the abnormalities seen in the plasma cells. The malignant plasma cell arises from a post-germinal center cell that has undergone switch recombination. Widespread application of FISH techniques has shed light into the genetic heteroge-neity seen in myeloma, hitherto unappreciated through conventional cytogenetic evaluation [28].

Based on the genetic abnormalities, patients can be broadly separated into hyperdiploid and hypodiploid groups. The hyperdiploid group, which represents roughly half of the patients, is characterized by trisomies of various odd-numbered chromosomes, while the hypodiploid group has translocations and deletions. Translocations involving the immuno-globulin heavy chain (IgH) locus on chromosome 14 can lead to activation of a various oncogenes depending on the partner chromosomes including cyclin D1, cyclin D2, fibroblast growth factor-3, c-maf, and maf-b [28–30]. Deletions involving chro-mosome 13 are frequently seen, especially with FISH techniques, and are often associated with the IgH translocations [31, 32]. Various other cytogenetic abnormalities, thought to be secondary events, can be seen especially in the later stages of the disease and include mutations involving p53 and the reti-noblastoma gene. More recently, there has been increasing appreciation of deletions and duplications involving chromosome 1, which again appear to increase in frequency with increasing duration of disease [33]. Use of more sensitive techniques such as gene expression profiling and comparative genomic hybridization has allowed a better under-standing of the abnormalities at a gene level. Abnor-malities of the myc gene have been implicated in disease progression from MGUS to active mye-loma [34]. It has become increasingly clear that the disease course and eventual outcome is dictated to a large extent by the presence of this genetic heterogeneity [35].

Despite the morphologically similar microscopic appearance of the plasma cells, modern flow cytometric techniques have allowed better appreciation of the phenotypic abnormalities and its heterogeneity among different disease stages [36–42]. The clonal plasma cells typically express CD138 (syndecan) and CD38 on their surface. CD45 is often present on a proportion of the plasma cells, especially in the early stages of the disease and a decrease in the proportion of cells with CD45 expression may signal disease progression and poorer outcome [43]. CD56 (neural cell adhesion molecule, NCAM) is typically present on the myeloma cells seen in the bone marrow and appears to be lost in the later stages of the disease. Aberrant expression of other antigens such as CD117 (c-Kit) and CD200 may be seen in a small proportion of cells, but their significance remains unknown.

There is increasing understanding of the relevance of the bone marrow microenvironment in myeloma, with the cytokine as well as the cellular milieu playing a critical role in its development and progression [44–46]. Interleukin-6 (IL-6) is probably the best studied, and is considered crucial for the plasma cell survival and proliferation [47–49]. It is primarily the surrounding cells in the marrow such as the stromal cells and endothelial cells that secrete IL-6. Other cytokines implicated in myeloma include the vascular endothelial growth factor (VEGF), hepatocyte growth factor (HGF), insulin-like growth factor (IGF-1), stromal-dependent growth factor (SDF), IL-1b and IL-8, among others [50–57]. Many of these cytokines are secreted by the myeloma cells, as well as the surrounding endothelial cells, stromal cells, osteoclasts and osteoblasts, and the myeloma cells themselves setting up complex and redundant autocrine and paracrine loops. These interactions in the marrow microenvironment between the tumor cells and the surrounding cells lead to increased proliferation of the myeloma cells and support their survival. In addition to the cytokines, adhesion molecules on the myeloma cells and their receptors on the surrounding cells also mediate the cross-talk between different cell types [58]. Increased bone marrow angiogenesis has been associated with disease progression and is a powerful prognostic factor [59]. While there are suggestions that there may be primary abnormalities involving the cells in the microenvironment that may predispose to formation of the clonal plasma cells, this is not conclusively proven [60].

These interactions between myeloma cells and the surrounding cells also account for some of the clinical manifestations of the disease. The anemia seen in myeloma is at least partly induced by apoptosis of erythroblasts as a result of interaction between the Fas molecules on the erythroblast and the Fas ligand expressed by myeloma cells [61]. The bone lesions of myeloma are a result of imbalance between the osteoblastic and osteoclastic activity [62]. Different cytokines secreted by myeloma cells, as well as direct interactions, lead to inhibition of osteoblastic activity and stimulation of osteoclastic activity.

Diagnosis and differential diagnosis

Diagnosis of MM rests on the ability to demonstrate a plasma cell clone with or without an accompanying monoclonal protein in the serum or urine and, in those with symptomatic myeloma, evidence of end-organ damage [63, 64]. Clonal plasma cells are typically demonstrated on a bone marrow biopsy, but may also be seen in the biopsy from a plasmacytoma, or in the peripheral blood in more advanced disease. Presence of a monoclonal protein is typically demonstrated by protein electrophoresis of serum or urine or by quantitation of free light chains in the serum. Presence of end-organ damage may be clear from the symptoms or may be detected on more detailed work-up of the patient.

Patients with symptomatic MM typically present with anemia, hypercalcemia, renal failure, and/or bone lesions (Table 20.1), while diagnosis in asymptomatic patients usually results from incidental discovery of a monoclonal protein in the serum or urine [4, 63]. Clinical examination may reveal pallor, tenderness along the spine or other bones, peripheral neuropathy, evidence of cord compression on neurological examination due to vertebral collapse or compression due to plasmacytoma, subcutaneous masses due to extramedullary plasmacytomas, altered mental status related to uremia,

Table 20.1 Symptoms and signs of multiple myeloma (and potential underlying etiology)

• Weakness and fatigue (anemia, hypercalcemia)

• Bone pain (lytic bone lesions with or without fractures, vertebral compression fractures)

• Numbness and tingling (peripheral neuropathy, cord compression, hypercalcemia)

• Confusion, altered mental status (hypercalcemia, hyperviscosity, uremia)

• Paraplegic or quadriplegic symptoms (spinal cord compression due to plasmacytoma or vertebral compression fracture)

• Recurrent infections (hypogammaglobulinemia due to suppression of normal immunoglobulins)

• Peripheral edema (hypoalbuminemia, renal failure)

• Loss of height, kyphosis (vertebral compression fractures)

• Polyuria, polydipsia, constipation (hypercalcemia)

• Increased bleeding and bruising (thrombocytopenia, hyperviscosity, uremia, acquired clotting factor inhibitors, non-specific interference with bleeding cascade by M-protein)

• Skin rash (cryoglobulinemia with vasculitis)

---

hyperviscosity or hypercalcemia, and/or echymoses due to thrombocytopenia or clotting abnormalities. Laboratory evaluation typically demonstrates the presence of monoclonal protein on serum and/or urine protein electrophoresis or immunofixation (Figure 20.2), abnormal serum kappa/lambda free light chain ratio, anemia and thrombocytopenia, or elevated calcium, creatinine or uric acid (Table 20.2). Other laboratory abnormalities typically include hypoalbuminemia, and elevated beta-2 microlobulin (B2M), lactate dehydrogenase (LDH), and C-reactive protein (CRP). Bone marrow examination demonstrates increased numbers of monoclonal plasma cells, which at times may demonstrate a plasmablastic morphology. Radiological evaluation can demonstrate the presence of lytic lesions or evidence of vertebral body compression fractures (Figure 20.3).

Patients with suspected MM should undergo a complete clinical and laboratory evaluation as

detailed in Table 20.3, which will then confirm the diagnosis and lead to therapeutic decisions [25–27, 65]. The most critical step in making a diagnosis of symptomatic MM is distinguishing it from the earlier stages of monoclonal gammopathies, such as MGUS, and asymptomatic or early stage myeloma (smoldering myeloma, SMM). These conditions usually do not require treatment [26, 27, 65]. The diagnostic criteria for myeloma developed by the International Myeloma Working Group is commonly used (Table 20.4) [64]. MGUS is the most common monoclonal gammopathy in the general population, with a prevalence that increases with age, affecting nearly 5–6% of those over 70 years. These individuals typically have a small clonal plasma cell burden without any adverse consequences, but have a lifetime risk of developing myeloma or another related condition that will require therapy. The risk of progression does not appear to change with the duration of the condition, and appears to be approximately 1% per year [66, 67]. A risk stratification system has been developed using the type of involved immunoglobulin, M protein concentration and free light chain measurements, with those having one or more of non-IgG monoclonal protein, M protein >1.5 gm/dL or abnormal free light chain ratio having the maximum risk of progression [68]. Other factors associated with increased risk include presence of significant amounts of urinary M-protein, circulating plasma cells, and increased marrow plasmacytosis. In contrast, patients with SMM have an estimated 5–10% risk of progression each year for the first five years, with the risk decreasing after that to the levels seen in patients with MGUS [69, 70].

Several variants of MM have been described based on clinical and laboratory features. Some patients with clinical features compatible with SMM at times have few small lytic lesions and a slow clinical course, often referred to as indolent myeloma. Occasional patients may present with osteosclerotic bone lesions, in the absence of any of the symptoms of POEMS syndrome (polyneuropathy, organomegaly, endocrinopathy, monoclonal gammopathy, and skin changes), termed as *osteosclerotic myeloma* [71]. While the presence of a monoclonal protein is the hallmark of this condition, 1–2% of patients will have no monoclonal protein detectable

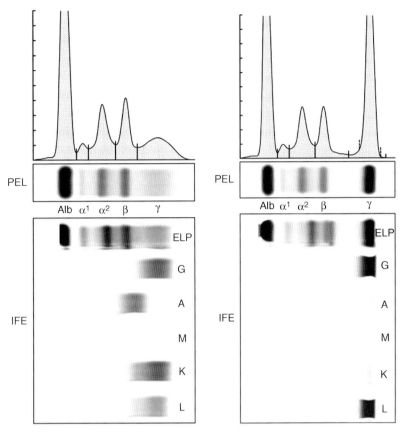

Figure 20.2 Serum electrophoresis demonstrating a monoclonal peak in the gamma region, representing the monoclonal protein and the densitometry tracing above (right panel). The left panel shows a normal tracing for comparison. Immunofixation studies using specific antibodies allow identification of the immunoglobulin type.

on serum or urine electrophoresis. This group of patients, referred to as having *non-secretory myeloma,* have become rare with the introduction of the free light chain assay [72]. In addition, the results of the above work-up should allow us to distinguish MM from other related conditions as further described in Table 20.5.

Staging and prognosis

The Durie-Salmon staging (Table 20.6) has been in use for over two decades and is based on indirect estimate of the tumor burden [73]. It has been shown to correlate with outcome in patients with MM. However, this is increasingly being replaced by the simpler but powerful International Staging System (ISS), that provides a better prognostic assessment [74]. The ISS allows prognostication of patients based on two easily available laboratory tests, namely serum albumin and beta 2 microglobulin (B2M). In addition to the staging system, several prognostic factors have been described in myeloma related to the patient characteristics, laboratory findings, tumor cell morphology, immunophenotype and, most importantly, presence or absence of genetic abnormalities (Table 20.6). Among these, the genetic abnormalities appear to be the primary determinant of outcome in patients with myeloma. Based on these prognostic factors, investigators at the Mayo Clinic have proposed criteria for identification of high-risk patients which, in

Table 20.2 Common laboratory features in patients with multiple myeloma

---

• Monoclonal protein on serum or urine protein electrophoresis or immunofixation

• Elevated immunoglobulin free light chains with abnormal kappa: lambda ratio

• Anemia, thrombocytopenia

• Suppression of uninvolved immunoglobulins

• Circulating clonal plasma cells by flow cytometry

• Hypercalcemia, hyperuricemia

• Elevated creatinine, and blood urea nitrogen (BUN)

• Elevated LDH, β_2 microglobulin, and or C-reactive protein

• Hypoalbuminemia

• Elevated serum viscosity

• Increased proportion of plasma cells in the bone marrow

• Punched out lytic lesions, vertebral compression fractures, pathological fractures or generalized osteopenia on skeletal films

• Vertebral compression fractures, altered bone marrow signal on MRI

---

turn, have implications on the therapeutic decision making (Table 20.7) [75]. In addition to the baseline characteristics at the time of diagnosis, the depth and duration of response to initial therapy are also powerful predictors of eventual outcome [76].

Approach to treatment of newly diagnosed myeloma

Once a diagnosis of myeloma is made, the initial decision is whether the patient needs therapy right away or if a period of careful observation can be appropriate and safe. Given the incurable nature of the disease and the lack of any proven benefit for early therapy, the decision to initiate therapy should be based on evidence of end-organ damage as described previously. Clearly patients with SMM can be carefully observed without treatment and these patients should not be offered therapy outside

of a clinical trial. Once the decision to initiate treatment has been made, the decision on the initial approach to therapy should be based on the eligibility/desire for autologous SCT and the presence or absence of high-risk features. The approach to the treatment of myeloma has undergone a paradigm shift in the last decade with the introduction of thalidomide, its analog lenalidomide and the proteasome inhibitor bortezomib, all very effective agents for treating myeloma. The commonly used drugs for the treatment of myeloma are described in Table 20.8. The current approach to treatment incorporates these new drugs along with the older drugs, and a general approach to initial therapy is outlined in Figure 20.4. This approach has been based on the survival advantage seen with SCT in myeloma compared to conventional alkylator-based therapy in randomized trials, as well as the results obtained with these approaches in patients with high-risk myeloma. Eligibility for SCT has been traditionally based on patient's age, however, evidence point towards selected older patients deriving as much benefit from the procedure [77]. Hence this decision must be based on patient's physiological age and preference.

The response to therapy in MM has traditionally been based on reduction in the serum and urine M-protein measurements and results of bone marrow examinations, along with measurements of other disease-related findings such as bone lesions and soft tissue plasmacytomas. However, these measurements are relatively insensitive with residual tumor even in the absence of detectable disease by these conventional methods. Given the studies demonstrating better outcome among patients in whom presence of residual disease cannot be detected by molecular methods, response criteria were recently revised to incorporate immunophenotypic examination of bone marrow and serum free light chain assay (Table 20.9) [78].

Approach to therapy in transplant eligible patients

Initial therapy in a patient considered eligible for SCT should be able to effectively control the disease,

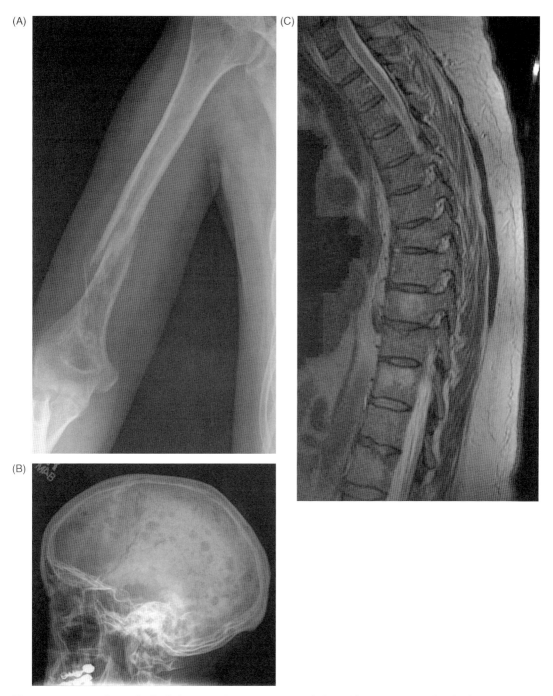

Figure 20.3 (A) Radiograph of right humerus demonstrating a pathological fracture associated with a lytic lesion. (B) Skull radiograph showing diffuse lytic lesions. (C) MRI demonstrating marrow signal changes and vertebral compression fractures.

Table 20.3 Required laboratory evaluation for multiple myeloma

1 Complete blood count and differential peripheral blood smear

2 Chemistry screen including calcium and creatinine

3 $_2$ microglobulin, C-reactive protein, and lactate dehydrogenase

4 Serum protein electrophoresis, immunofixation

5 Nephelometric quantification of immunoglobulins

6 Routine urinalysis, 24 h urine collection for electrophoresis and immunofixation

7 Measurement of free monoclonal light chains in the serum

8 Bone marrow aspirate and trephine biopsy (conventional cytogenetics, immunophenotyping, plasma cell labeling index, and FISH studies)

9 Radiological skeletal bone survey including spine, pelvis, skull, humeri, and femurs (an MRI or a PET scan may be helpful in selected circumstances)

Additional:

• Dental evaluation/dental x-rays should be considered at the time of diagnosis given the risk of ONJ with subsequent bisphosphonate therapy

• Vitamin D levels should be checked and replaced as necessary prior to starting bisphosphonates.

Table 20.4 Diagnostic criteria for MGUS, smoldering myeloma, symptomatic multiple myeloma and plasma cell leukemia [64]

MGUS

Serum M-protein < 3.0 g/dl

and Clonal plasma cells in the bone marrow less than10% (when biopsy is performed)

and No evidence of other lymphoproliferative disorder

and No related organ or tissue impairment (ROTI; see below)

SMM

Serum M-protein ≥ 3.0 g/dl

OR

Clonal plasma cells in the bone marrow $\geq 10\%$

and No related organ or tissue impairment (ROTI; see below)

Symptomatic myeloma

M-protein detectable in serum and/or urine

and Clonal plasma cells in bone marrow or presence of plasmacytoma

and Related organ or tissue impairment (ROTI) (These are often referred to as CRAB)

Calcium levels increased: serum calcium > 0.25 mmol/l above the upper limit of normal or > 2.75 mmol/l

Renal insufficiency: creatinine > 173 mmol/l

Anemia: hemoglobin 2 g/dl below the lower limit of normal or hemoglobin < 10 g/dl

Bone lesions: lytic lesions or osteoporosis with compression fractures (on X-ray, MRI, or CT)

Other: symptomatic hyperviscosity, amyloidosis, recurrent bacterial infections (> 2 episodes in 12 months)

Plasma cell leukemia

Clonal plasma cell proliferation

Absolute plasma cell count > 2000/microL

(Adapted from International Myeloma Working Group [64].)

rapidly reverse disease-related complications and minimize risk of early death. Early mortality has been a significant problem in myeloma with a number of deaths related to infections, poor control of complications (such as renal failure, as well as treatment-related complications), with 10–15% of patients failing to reach SCT in earlier studies [79]. The therapy chosen should be well tolerated with manageable toxicity and least impact on the quality of life. Finally, it is imperative that the initial therapy should not interfere with the ability to collect adequate numbers of stem cells for one or more SCT. With clinical trials demonstrating equivalent efficacy for SCT used as first line or second line of treatment, the ability to continue on the induction therapy among those deciding to delay transplantation should also be factored in when initiating ther-

apy [80]. Traditionally, this has included four to six months of therapy with the chosen regimen, followed by stem cell collection and high-dose therapy [81, 82]. The long-term impact of the initial

Table 20.5 Differential diagnosis of monoclonal gammopathies

Diagnosis	Disease characteristics
Solitary plasmacytoma	• Presence of an isolated plasmacytoma in the absence of any bony lytic lesions, no monoclonal plasma cells in the bone marrow, or other features of myeloma.
	• Nearly half of these patients will eventually develop myeloma, with increased risk among those with persistent monoclonal protein after treatment of the solitary plasmacytoma, those with axial skeletal involvement and those with abnormal free light chain ratio.
	• Tissue deposition of light chain-derived amyloid fibrils (beta pleated sheets), apple green birefringence on polarizing microscopy, tissue deposits stain for kappa or lambda light chain and tandem mass spectrometry-based methods confirming light chain origin of amyloid.
Primary systemic amyloidosis	• May present as cardiomyopathy, nephrotic syndrome, malabsorption, hepatic failure, peripheral neuropathy or other symptoms based on organ involvement.
	• Typically, associated with <10% plasma cells in the bone marrow and no lytic lesions and hypercalcemia. Rarely, a diagnosis of myeloma may be made simultaneously or myeloma may develop subsequently.
POEMS syndrome (*polyneuropathy, organomegaly, endocrinopathy, monoclonal protein, skin changes*)	• *Major criteria*: polyneuropathy, monoclonal plasma cell disorder.
	• *Minor criteria*: sclerotic bone lesions, Castleman's disease, organomegaly (spleen, liver, or lymph nodes), volume overload (peripheral edema, pleural effusion, ascites), endocrinopathy (adrenal, thyroid, pituitary, gonadal, parathyroid, pancreatic), skin changes (hyperpigmentation, hypertrichosis, plethora, hemangiomata, white nails), papilledema.
	• Two major criteria plus at least one minor criterion required for diagnosis.
Waldenström's macroglobulinemia[a]	• Typically associated with IgM monoclonal gammopathy regardless of the size of the M protein
	• Ten percent or greater bone marrow infiltration by lymphoplasmacytic cells.
	• Typical immunophenotype (surface IgM+, CD5+/−, CD10−, CD19+, CD20+, CD22+, CD23−)
	• Often associated with lymphadenopathy and hepatoslenomegaly.
Cryoglobulinemia	• Cryoglobulins are either immunoglobulins or a mixture of immunoglobulins and complement components that precipitate out of blood at temperatures lower than 37 °C.
	• *Type I* (5–25%) Isolated monoclonal Ig (typically IgG or IgM, less commonly IgA or free immunoglobulin light chains) typically Waldenström's macroglobulinemia or multiple myeloma.
	• *Type II* (essential mixed cryoglobulinemia; 40–60%) Mixture of polyclonal Ig along with a monoclonal Ig, typically IgM or IgA, with rheumatoid factor activity, often related to infections.

(continued)

Table 20.5 (*Continued*)

Diagnosis	Disease characteristics
	• *Type III* (40–50%) Mixed cryoglobulins consisting of polyclonal immunoglobulins, often secondary to connective tissue diseases.
Light chain deposition disease(LCDD)	• Granular deposits of monoclonal light chains that can affect kidneys, heart, or liver. • Deposits do not have the fibrillar ultra-structure of amyloid deposits on electron microscopy. • Associated with elevated free light chains, kappa more common than lambda (compared to amyloidosis, where lambda is more common).
Heavy chain deposition disease(HCDD)	• Rare condition associated with non-amyloid deposits arising from immunoglobulin light chains as well as fragments of heavy chains.

[a] Patients with serum IgM concentration < 3.0 g/dL, in the absence of anemia, hepatosplenomegaly, lymphadenopathy, and systemic symptoms and minimal or no lymphoplasmacytic infiltration of the bone marrow (<10 %) is considered to have an IgM MGUS rather than Waldenström's macroglobulinemia.

therapy on the outcome of autologous SCT remains undefined, with individuals refractory to initial therapy obtaining as much benefit from autologous SCT as those who have responded to initial therapy [83]. Also, the impact of obtaining a deep response with initial therapy prior to SCT remains unclear, and more recent trials of novel agent combinations used as initial therapy will help us answer this question.

Until the introduction of newer agents during the past few years, the most commonly used initial regimen has either been single-agent dexamethasone or a combination of vincristine, doxorubicin, and dexamethasone (VAD) [84–87]. The current approach to initial therapy outside of a clinical trial should be an immunomodulatory drug (IMiD) or bortezomib-based regimen: typically the combination of lenalidomide (Revlimid, Celgene) and low-dose dexamethasone; thalidomide and dexamethasone; or bortezomib (Velcade, Millennium Pharmaceuticals) and dexamethasone. While trials have demonstrated that the efficacy of three and four drug regimens incorporating one or more of the newer drugs along with older drugs such as alkylating agents or anthracycline is higher compared to these two drug regimens, there is no data to support better long-term outcome for the more intense regimens.

Results of multiple clinical trials in the setting of newly diagnosed myeloma provide the rationale for this approach. In two phase III trials, the combination of thalidomide (200–400 mg daily) and dexamethasone (40 mg days 1–4, 9–12, 17–20 of a 28-day cycle) was associated with increased response rates and longer time to progression (TTP), when compared with dexamethasone alone. However, toxicities, especially thrombotic events, were higher with the addition of thalidomide in the combination [88, 89]. The combination has also been compared with the VAD regimen and found to have superior response rates and improved PFS [90]. The combination of lenalidomide (25 mg daily days 1–21 of a 28-day cycle) and dexamethasone as above was examined in a phase II study, with high response rates including high rates of complete response which continued to improve with increasing duration of therapy [91]. Long-term follow-up has demonstrated a two-year survival rate greater than 90% for patients undergoing initial therapy with this combination. In a phase III trial comparing the combination to dexamethasone alone, the combination was associated with a higher response rate and longer PFS [92]. Another phase III trial compared lenalidomide and high-dose dexamethasone (as above) with lenalidomide and low-dose (40 mg weekly) dexamethasone. This study demon-

Table 20.6 Staging systems in myeloma

Durie Salmon Staging [73]	
Stage I	All of the following: • Hemoglobin value >10 g/dL • Serum calcium value normal or ≤12 mg/dL • Normal bone X-rays solitary bone plasmacytoma only • Low M-component production rate IgG value <5 g/dL; IgA value <3 g/dL Bence Jones protein <4 g/24 h
Stage II	Neither Stage I nor Stage III
Stage III	One or more of the following: • Hemoglobin value <8.5 g/dL • Serum calcium value >12 mg/dL • Advanced lytic bone lesions (scale 3) • High M-component production rate IgG value >7 g/dL; IgA value >5 g/dL Bence Jones protein >12 g/24 h

International Staging System [74]		
Stage	Definition	Median survival
I	Serum B2M <3.5 mg/L Serum Albumin >=3.5 gm/dL	62 months
II	Serum β_2-microglobulin <3.5 mg/L and serum albumin <3.5 g/dL **OR** Serum β_2-microglobulin 3.5 to <5.5 mg/L irrespective of the serum albumin level	44 months
III	Serum B2M >5.5 mg/L	29 months

Table 20.7 Prognostic factors in multiple myeloma

Prognostic factors

International Staging System (ISS) stage [74]

Age [133]

Performance status

Metaphase cytogenetics on marrow aspirate [28]

  Chromosome 13 monosomy or deletions

  Hypodiploidy

FISH examination of plasma cells [28]

  Translocations t(4;14), t(14;16)

  Deletion 17p (p53 abnormalities)

Plasma cell labeling index (PCLI) ≥1% [134]

High LDH

Circulating plasma cells [135]

Abnormal serum free light chain ratio [136]

Plasmablastic morphology [137]

Increased bone marrow microvessel density [138]

High-risk myeloma [139]

Del 17p-, t(4;14), or t(14;16) on FISH

Deletion 13 or hypodiploidy on cytogenetics

PCLI >3%

β_2 microglobulin >5.5 mcg/dL (in the absence of renal failure)

---

tively eliminated high-dose dexamethasone treatment from the setting of newly diagnosed disease [93]. The bortezomib-dexamethasone combination has been examined in the setting of newly diagnosed MM in several clinical trials, with high response rates and excellent safety [94, 95]. This combination has been compared with VAD as induction therapy prior to SCT in a phase III trial, with deeper responses and reduced need for tandem autologous SCT, as well as improved PFS post-SCT [96].

The exciting results seen with the novel agents raised the question whether these agents in combination among themselves or with previously available drugs can further enhance the initial therapy of

strated improved survival despite a lower response rate, with lower toxicity for patients treated with weekly dexamethasone. The results of this study have effec-

Table 20.8 Commonly used drugs for treatment of myeloma

Drug	Usual dose	Route	Mechanism	Common/serious side effects
Melphalan	Various	PO or IV	Alkylating agent, causes DNA damage.	Leukopenia, anemia, thrombocytopenia, mucositis, long-term risk of leukemia.
Cyclophosphamide	Various	PO or IV	Alkylating agent, causes DNA damage.	Leukopenia, anemia, thrombocytopenia, mucositis, hemorrhagic cystitis, skin rash, nausea, cardiomyopathy.
Glucocorticoids (prednisone, dexamethasone)	Various	PO or IV	Various mechanisms proposed.	Hyperglycemia, infections, osteoporosis, mood disturbances, edema, hypertension, adrenal insufficiency, cataracts.
Doxorubicin/ pegylated doxorubicin	Various	IV	Anthracycline, DNA damage.	Leukopenia, anemia, thrombocytopenia, mucositis, long-term risk of leukemia.
Thalidomide	200–400 mg daily	PO	Various mechanisms proposed, down regulates TNF, anti-angiogenic, modifies microenvironment.	Neuropathy, skin rash, constipation, somnolence, edema, hepatitis, venous thromboembolism, teratogenesis.
Lenalidomide	25 mg days 1–21 every 28 days	PO	Immunomodulatory analog of thalidomide, more potent inhibitor of cytokines like TNF, likely multiple mechanisms.	Leukopenia, anemia, thrombocytopenia, skin rash, muscle cramps, constipation, fatigue, venous thromboembolism.
Bortezomib	$1.3\,mg/m^2$ Days, 1, 4, 8, 11 of a 21-day cycle	IV	Inhibits proteasome-mediated degradation of proteins, NFkB inhibition believed to play a major role in its anti-myeloma activity.	Thrombocytopenia, peripheral neuropathy, fatigue, myalgias, constipation or diarrhea, nausea, herpes zoster reactivation.

myeloma. The combination of bortezomib (Velcade), thalidomide and dexamethasone (VTD) was compared to vincristine, adriamycin (doxorubicin) and dezamethasone (VAD) in a phase III trial, with VTD leading to significantly higher response rates and deeper responses, resulting in improved PFS post-SCT [97]. Subsequently, lenalidomide has been combined with bortezomib and dexamethasone, resulting in a 100% response rate with very good partial response (VGPR) or better in nearly two-thirds of the patients [98]. In an attempt at maximizing the initial treatment, another trial added cyclophosphamide to the VRD combination and reported a 100% response rate with high VGPR rates after a median of four cycles of therapy [99]. Other phase II trials have examined the combination of pegylated doxorubicin with lenalidomide and dexamethasone or bortezomib and dexamethasone. The long-term impact of these highly active regimens is not clear, and longer follow-up will be required to delineate their effect on the natural history of the disease.

There is increasing appreciation of the impact of high-risk features, especially genetic factors, on the outcome of patients with myeloma and the need to

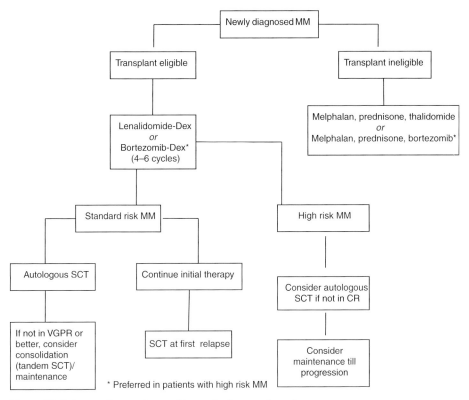

Figure 20.4 Approach to patients with newly diagnosed myeloma.

develop a risk-adapted approach to treatment. Patients with cytogenetic deletion 13; Del 17p-, t(4;14) or t(14;16) on fluorescence in situ hybridization tests; cytogenetic hypodiploidy, plasma cell labeling index greater than 3%; and B2M greater than 5.5 tend to have poor outcome with current treatments including SCT. There is emerging data on the effect of newer agents such as bortezomib and lenalidomide in patients with these poor prognostic features [94, 100–102]. Based on analysis of some of the recent trials, it appears that bortezomib can overcome the increased risk associated with del 13 and t(4;14) and should be integrated into the initial therapy of high-risk patients [94, 102].

Autologous stem cell transplantation in myeloma

Several randomized clinical trials have indicated that SCT improves outcome of patients with MM compared to conventional therapy, whereas others have suggested no benefit for SCT, especially in patients responsive to initial therapy. In the IFM94 and Myeloma VII trials, previously untreated patients younger than age 65 were randomly assigned to receive either conventional chemotherapy (CCT) or SCT [81, 82]. In both these trials, patients receiving SCT had a superior response rate, EFS, and OS compared with those receiving CCT. In contrast, the MAG91 trial, which also randomized patient to SCT or CCT, only demonstrated improved EFS and time without symptoms, treatment, and toxicity (TWiSTT) with SCT with no improvement in OS, in similar patients [103]. In the Intergroup Study S9321 patients with untreated MM were randomly assigned to either SCT or CCT, with further randomization of responding patients to interferon maintenance or no maintenance. This study also failed to reveal any OS benefit [104]. The Spanish cooperative group PETHEMA conducted a randomized trial

Table 20.9 Response criteria for multiple myeloma

Response subcategory	Response criteria
CR	• Negative immunofixation on the serum and urine and
	• Disappearance of any soft tissue plasmacytomas and
	• ≤ 5% plasma cells in bone marrow
stringent CR (CR as above plus)	• Normal FLC ratio and
	• Absence of clonal cells in bone marrow by immunohistochemistry or immunoflourescence
	• Serum and urine M-component detectable by immunofixation but not on electrophoresis or
VGPR	• ≥90% or greater reduction in serum M-component plus urine M-component <100 mg per 24 h
	• ≥50% reduction of serum M-protein and reduction in 24-h urinary M-protein by ≥90% or to <200 mg per 24 h
PR	• If the serum and urine M-protein are unmeasurable a ≥ 50% decrease in the difference between involved and uninvolved FLC levels is required in place of the M-protein criteria
	• If serum and urine M-protein are unmeasurable, and serum free light assay is also unmeasurable, ≥50% reduction in bone marrow plasma cells is required in place of M-protein, provided baseline percentage was ≥30%
	• In addition to the above criteria, if present at baseline, ≥50% reduction in the size of soft tissue plasmacytomas is also required
SD	• Not meeting criteria for CR, VGPR, PR or progressive disease
	• Increase of 25% from baseline in
	• Serum M-component (absolute increase must be ≥0.5 g/dl) and/or
	• Urine M-component (absolute increase must be ≥200 mg/24 h) and/or
PD	• Only in patients without measurable serum and urine M-protein levels: the difference between involved and uninvolved FLC levels(absolute increase must be >10 mg/dl)
	• Bone marrow plasma cell percentage (absolute % must be 10%)
	• Definite development of new bone lesions or soft tissue plasmacytomas or definite increase in the size of existing bone lesions or soft tissue plasmacytomas
	• Development of hypercalcemia (corrected serum calcium >11.5 mg/dl) that can be attributed solely to the plasma cell proliferative disorder
	Any one of the following:
	• Reappearance of serum or urine M-protein by immunofixation or electrophoresis
Relapse from CR	• Development of ≥5% plasma cells in the bone marrow
	• Appearance of any other sign of progression (i.e., new plasmacytoma, lytic bone lesion, or hypercalcemia as defined in the PD category above)

comparing SCT with CCT in patients who responded to initial therapy and demonstrated higher CR rates with autologous SCT but no difference in PFS or OS [105]. In the MAG90 trial, patients were randomly assigned to receive SCT after three to four cycles of initial therapy or to continue CCT, with SCT done at time of first relapse or if the patient became refractory to initial therapy [80]. Although the OS was similar in this study confirming equivalent efficacy for SCT applied as first- or second-line therapy, TWiSTT was significantly better for the early SCT group.

SCT in myeloma involves collection of peripheral blood stem cells, using either granulocyte stimulating factors (G-CSF or GM-CSF) alone or by using these growth factors following initial priming with cyclophosphamide and collecting stem cells during recovery of the blood counts. Purging of tumor cells from the stem cell collection, using various selection methods, has not translated into any improvement, likely a reflection of the inability of the conditioning regimens to completely eradicate the tumor clone from the marrow. The most widely used conditioning regimen is that of melphalan (200 mg/m^2), based on results of the IFM95-02 trial, in which patients were randomly assigned to receive either 8 Gy total body irradiation (TBI) plus 140 or 200 mg/m^2 melphalan [106]. Patients receiving the melphalan-only regimen had a faster recovery of neutrophils and platelets, and milder mucositis, without any effect on EFS or OS. Ongoing trials are trying to improve melphalan conditioning by increasing the melphalan dose (alone or in combination with cytoprotectants such as amifostine), adding skeletal targeted radioisotopes such as Samarium or Holmium, using skeletal targeted TBI, or adding novel agents such as bortezomib to the melphalan.

Tandem autologous stem cell transplantation

The concept of a second transplant arose from the desire to provide additional consolidation therapy and the potential to obtain deeper responses with transplant, given that all patients eventually relapse. Several randomized clinical trials have been done to examine the role tandem SCT compared to a single SCT or to allogeneic SCT [107–110]. The IFM94 trial showed a slight improvement in the combined CR and VGPR rate with double transplant (50% vs. 42%) but, at seven years, EFS (20% vs. 10%) and OS (42% vs. 21%) doubled with the second SCT [108]. The benefit of second transplant was mostly seen among patients failing to achieve a VGPR after first transplant (OS at seven years of 43% vs. 11%). In the Bologna 96 trial, the addition of a second SCT prolonged EFS by 12 months and TTP by 17 months, with a projected OS at six years of 44% for single transplant and 63% for double transplant [109]. Similar to the findings from the French trial, patients who failed to achieve a CR or near complete response after the first SCT obtained the maximum benefit from the tandem approach. In the MAG95 clinical trial, patients were randomly assigned to receive one or two SCTs and then further randomized to selected or unselected CD34-positive cells [111]. The study again confirmed an OS advantage for this approach. A second transplant may also be entertained as salvage therapy after failure of the first SCT. This approach clearly has a merit among patients obtaining a prolonged response to the first SCT and those who tolerated the procedure well.

Post-transplant therapy

SCT clearly improves response rates in patients with newly diagnosed MM compared with conventional therapy, but patients invariably relapse. Attempts have been made to maintain the response through maintenance approaches applied in the post-transplant setting. In a small randomized clinical trial, interferon alfa (3×10^6 units/m^2) administered subcutaneously three times weekly following initial SCT, suggested a modest improvement in EFS [112]. Similarly, maintenance therapy with prednisone has been associated with a longer time to progression. In the IFM99-02 clinical trial, patients with standard-risk MM (B2M <3 mg/L, no deletion of chromosome 13 by FISH), were randomly assigned to receive no maintenance, pamidronate, or pamidronate plus thalidomide two months after tandem SCT [113]. The response rates were significantly higher for the thalidomide arm; this translated into improved EFS of 52%, compared with 36% with no maintenance, and 37% with pamidronate alone. The four-year estimated survival from diagnosis was higher with thalidomide (87%) compared with no maintenance (77%). There have been additional studies examining the role of thalidomide maintenance and a PFS advantage has been noted for thalidomide post-SCT in all studies, with OS advantage seen in some [114, 115]. A large ongoing study (CALGB) is evaluating lenalidomide as maintenance after single SCT. Long-term results of these trials should be evaluated before these approaches can be adopted into routine practice. Immunotherapeutic strategies using dendritic cell vaccines are also currently undergoing trials in this setting.

Clearly, the role of SCT in the treatment of MM continues to be redefined in the context of novel agents. The high response rates seen with the new combination regimens that include the novel agents have encouraged a new debate on the role of SCT in myeloma. Recent studies have shown that even with the high response rates obtained with the novel agent combinations, SCT provides additional tumor reduction following the initial therapy. However, myeloma remains an incurable disease and in the absence of randomized trials demonstrating that the new therapies can substitute for SCT, it should be still considered a part of the therapeutic line-up for myeloma. Ongoing trials are trying to understand the best way to integrate these treatment modalities to provide the best outcome for the patients.

Allogeneic stem cell transplantation in myeloma

Allogeneic SCT has been used for the treatment of myeloma for over two decades. Its introduction was based on the potential to obtain a clean graft and the presence of a graft myeloma effect that could eliminate the tumor cells and possibly cure the disease [116–118]. However, more widespread adoption of this modality has been hampered by the high treatment-related mortality and failure to demonstrate a long-term survival advantage. Most of the existing data on the utility of allogeneic approaches

have come from small single institution studies or from analyses from transplant registries. In a retrospective case-matched analysis from the European Blood and Marrow Transplant Registry, patients treated with allogeneic bone marrow transplant (BMT) were compared with a similar group of patients who received SCT [117]. The OS was significantly better for the SCT arm than for the allogeneic BMT arm, with median survival of 34 and 18 months, respectively. The poorer survival in allogeneic BMT patients could be attributed mostly to the higher treatment-related mortality (41% vs. 13%). Among patients surviving the first year, there was a trend for better OS and EFS for allogeneic BMT. Several other comparisons have been done, with no definite benefit seen with allogeneic approaches [119, 120].

The high treatment-related mortality seen with conventional allogeneic SCT, even though it appears to have improved recently, led to increased use of non-myeloablative SCT [121]. This approach relies more on the antitumor effect of the graft than on the initial cyto-reduction achieved by the conditioning regimen. The IFM99-03/99-04 trials included patients with high-risk myeloma (B2M level >3 mg/L and chromosome 13 deletion at diagnosis) [51]. In IFM99-03, 65 patients with an HLA-identical sibling donor were randomized to receive reduced-intensity conditioning (RIC) allogeneic SCT; in IFM99-04, 219 patients without an HLA-identical sibling donor were randomized to undergo a second SCT. The investigators found that RIC-allogeneic-SCT was associated with an inferior outcome compared to tandem SCT. In an Italian trial, 108 patients younger than 65 years of age with newly diagnosed MM were randomized to receive either standard SCT, followed by low-dose TBI conditioning and HLA-matched sibling peripheral blood SCT (median of two to four months from SCT), or a second autologous SCT [52]. At a median follow-up of three years, treatment-related mortality was 11% for the allogeneic SCT group versus 4% for the double SCT group; CR rate was 46% versus 16%; OS was 84% versus 62% ($P = 0.003$); and PFS was 75% versus 41% ($P = 0.00008$). However, this trial had several shortcomings and the results cannot be generalized. Large ongoing trials have been completed and the results are awaited.

Approach to therapy in non-transplant eligible patients

Given the median age at onset of myeloma, over half of the patients with newly diagnosed myeloma may not be able to undergo STC. For decades, the combination of melphalan and prednisone (MP) had been the mainstay of therapy for these patients. A meta-analysis of multiple randomized trials failed to demonstrate any benefit for combination regimens compared to MP [122]. In a phase III clinical trial, Palumbo et al. randomized patients older than 65 years of age with newly diagnosed MM, or younger than 65 and ineligible for SCT, to receive MP (melphalan $4\,mg/m^2$, days 1–7, and prednisone $40\,mg/m^2$, days 1–7) or MPT (MP plus thalidomide $100\,mg$ daily) for six cycles [123]. Patients in the MPT arm continued on maintenance thalidomide after the six cycles until relapse. At six months from initiation of therapy, 76% of patients in the MPT arm had a response (CR or partial), compared with 47.6% in the MP arm. With comparable follow-up, the EFS at two years doubled with the addition of thalidomide to MP (54% vs. 27%), with those older than 70 years deriving similar benefit as the younger patients. Grade 3 and 4 adverse events, however, nearly doubled with the addition of thalidomide (48% for MPT vs. 25% for MP), and 11 patients had toxicity-related deaths in the MPT group compared with six patients in the MP group. Deep vein thrombosis (DVT) was the most common grade 3/4 adverse event in the MPT group, with 13 of the first 65 patients developing DVT. After introduction of enoxaparin prophylaxis, however, two of the remaining 64 patients developed thrombosis. Another phase III trial (IFM99-06) randomly assigned patients aged 65 to 75 years to receive MP (12 cycles at six-week intervals), MPT (maximum tolerated thalidomide dose, up to $400\,mg$ per day), or MEL100 (induction therapy with VADx2, cyclophosphamide $3\,g/m^2$-based mobilization, and two courses of melphalan $100\,mg/m^2$ with stem cell support) [124]. A CR or VGPR was seen in 9%, 64%, and 58% of patients in the MP, MPT, and MEL100 groups, respectively; at a median follow-up of 32.2 months, the corresponding PFS rates were 17.2, 29.5, and 19 months. The median OS rates were 30.3 months, not reached at 56 months, and 38.6 months in the MP, MPT, and MEL100 groups, respectively. There have been several other trials examining the role of thalidomide in combination with melphalan and prednisone in the setting of newly diagnosed myeloma, for individuals not considered eligible for an SCT. The trials have consistently demonstrated a PFS advantage for addition of thalidomide with two of the five showing an improvement in OS as well. One commonly used approach is to add $100\,mg$ daily of thalidomide to the MP regimen and limit the therapy to 12 months for patients ineligible for SCT. Patients should be given daily aspirin for thromboprophylaxis, with low-molecular-weight heparin used for patients at higher risk of thrombosis.

The utility of adding bortezomib to MP was examined in the large Phase III VISTA trial, in which patients with previously untreated MM who were not candidates for SCT were randomly assigned to receive bortezomib plus MP (VMP) or MP alone [102]. Patients in the VMP arm received IV bortezomib ($1.3\,mg/m^2$ twice per week, weeks 1, 2, 4, 5) for four cycles of six weeks (eight doses per cycle), followed by once per week (weeks 1, 2, 4, 5) for five cycles of six weeks (four doses per cycle) in combination with oral melphalan ($9\,mg/m^2$) and prednisone ($60\,mg/m^2$) once daily on days 1 to 4 of each cycle. Patients in the MP arm received MP once daily on days 1 through 4 for nine cycles of six weeks. Both the median TTP and OS at two years were significantly better in the VMP group: TTP, 24 months with VMP versus 16.6 months with MP; OS at two years, 82.6% with VMP versus 69.5% with MP. MP also has been studied in combination with lenalidomide. Phase II results are promising and a phase III trial comparing this regimen to MPT is ongoing [125].

Management of relapsed MM

Several factors including type of previous therapy, duration of response to previous therapy, tolerance to different agents, and presence of high-risk cytogenetic features should be taken into account when making decisions regarding management of relapsed disease. Patients relapsing on initial therapy or within 12 months of an SCT used as first line of treatment, and those with the high-risk genetic abnormalities especially p53 abnormalities should be considered as having high-risk disease. SCT remains an option for those with a previous SCT who had more than 12 months of response duration from the first one, as well as for those who had no previous SCT as long as they are considered eligible for transplant. Non-transplant approaches can involve the use of a single active agent or combinations of active agents that have been studied in different clinical trials. A summary of the regimens that have been evaluated in different clinical trials is presented in Table 20.10. Studies into the natural history of MM point toward decreasing response duration, with each relapse reflecting increasingly acquired drug resistance [126].

Two of the most promising drugs undergoing clinical trials in this setting include the IMiD CC4047, and the proteasome inhibitor carfilzomib. The phase II trial of CC4047 and dexamethasone enrolled 60 patients with relapsed MM who had had one to three prior regimens [127]. The overall response rate was 58%, including a 25% VGPR, and the regimen was very well tolerated with manage-

Table 20.10 Commonly used treatments for relapsed multiple myeloma

---

- Dexamethasone (pulse dose)

- Melphalan, prednisone (± thalidomide, lenalidomide or bortezomib)

- Cyclophosphamide, prednisone

- Vincristine, Adriamycin, dexamethasone

- Thalidomide, dexamethasone (± cyclophosphamide or doxorubicin)

- Lenalidomide, dexamethasone (± cyclophosphamide, or doxorubicin)

- Bortezomib, dexamethasone (± cyclophosphamide)

- Bortezomib, Doxil (± dexamethasone)

- Bortezomib, thalidomide, dexamethasone

- DT-PACE (±bortezomib)

---

able toxicity profile. The response rate among patients who were previously refractory to lenalidomide was 29%, demonstrating non-overlapping mechanisms of action. The phase II trial of carfilzomib, a proteasome inhibitor, enrolled 31 patients with relapsed myeloma, who had had three or less prior therapies [128, 129]. The responses were relatively rapid and occurred within two cycles with an overall response rate of 36%, and were higher among those without previous exposure to bortezomib. Several other drugs are being evaluated in ongoing clinical trials including the HDAC inhibitors, various cyclin D inhibitors, heat shock protein inhibitors, and inhibitors of the bcl2 family proteins.

Supportive care

Bone disease and resultant fractures contribute significantly to the morbidity and mortality related to this disease. Bisphosphonates have been used extensively to prevent these complications. However, recent reports of increasing recognition of osteonecrosis of the jaw (ONJ) as a complication of the therapy has led to reassessment of the duration of therapy and the frequency of administration. Although zoledronic acid has been associated with a higher risk of ONJ, pamidronate can also lead to this side effect, with the risk related mostly to the duration of therapy. Guidelines have been developed recommending monthly use of bisphosphonates for the first 12–18 months following diagnosis with less frequent use after that guided by disease activity [130, 131].

Anemia is a common finding and is multifactorial in origin. Effective control of underlying disease is associated with improvement in hemoglobin. Given the recent concern regarding the use of erythropoietic agents in the cancer in general and the increased risk of thrombosis seen with concurrent use of erythropoietin in patients taking lenalidomide or thalidomide has led to recommendations regarding limiting the use of these agents in myeloma.

Renal impairment of varying degree is present in over 20% of patients at the time of diagnosis of MM. Renal insufficiency in MM is often multifactorial in etiology and may be due to cast nephropathy, hypercalcemia, hyperuricemia, dehydration, hyper-viscosity, medications such as non-steroidal anti-inflammatory drugs or, rarely, coexistent amyloidosis or light chain deposition disease. Renal insufficiency in MM should be managed aggressively because renal function can improve significantly. This includes aggressive hydration as well as management of hypercalcemia and hyperuricemia. The role of plasmapheresis is controversial and this procedure is more likely to benefit patients with high levels of free light chains [132]. Prompt institution of antimyeloma therapy is important to prevent further deterioration of, and possibly ensure improvement of, renal function. Patients with advanced renal failure will require dialysis support.

References

1 Jemal A, Siegel R, Ward E, et al. (2009) Cancer statistics, 2009. *CA Cancer J Clin* **59**:225–49.

2 Landgren O, Katzmann JA, Hsing AW, et al. (2007) Prevalence of monoclonal gammopathy of undetermined significance among men in Ghana. *Mayo Clin Proc* **82**:1468–73.

3 Landgren O, Gridley G, Turesson I, et al. (2006) Risk of monoclonal gammopathy of undetermined significance (MGUS) and subsequent multiple myeloma among African American and white veterans in the United States. *Blood* **107**:904–6.

4 Kyle RA, Gertz MA, Witzig TE, et al. (2003) Review of 1027 patients with newly diagnosed multiple myeloma. *Mayo Clin Proc* **78**:21–33.

5 Kristinsson SY, Landgren O, Dickman PW, Derolf AR, Bjorkholm M. (2007) Patterns of survival in multiple myeloma: a population-based study of patients diagnosed in Sweden from 1973 to 2003. *J Clin Oncol* **25**:1993–9.

6 Rajkumar SV. (2008) Treatment of myeloma: cure vs control. *Mayo Clin Proc* **83**:1142–5.

7 Brenner H, Gondos A, Pulte D. (2008) Recent major improvement in long-term survival of younger patients with multiple myeloma. *Blood* **111**:2521–6.

8 Neriishi K, Nakashima E, Suzuki G. (2003) Monoclonal gammopathy of undetermined significance in atomic bomb survivors: incidence and transformation to multiple myeloma. *Br J Haematol* **121**:405–10.

9 Hatcher JL, Baris D, Olshan AF, et al. (2001) Diagnostic radiation and the risk of multiple myeloma (United States). *Cancer Causes Control* **12**:755–61.

10 Darby SC, Nakashima E, Kato H. (1985) A parallel analysis of cancer mortality among atomic bomb survivors and patients with ankylosing spondylitis given X-ray therapy. *J Natl Cancer Inst* **75**:1–21.

11 Sonoda T, Nagata Y, Mori M, Ishida T, Imai K. (2001) Meta-analysis of multiple myeloma and benzene exposure. *J Epidemiol* **11**:249–54.

12 Baris D, Silverman DT, Brown LM, et al. (2004) Occupation, pesticide exposure and risk of multiple myeloma. *Scand J Work Environ Health* **30**:215–22.

13 Cuzick J, De Stavola B. (1988) Multiple myeloma – a case-control study. *Br J Cancer* **57**:516–20.

14 Landgren O, Kyle RA, Hoppin JA, et al. (2009) Pesticide exposure and risk of monoclonal gammopathy of undetermined significance (MGUS) in the Agricultural Health Study. *Blood* **113**:6386–91.

15 Khuder SA, Mutgi AB. (1997) Meta-analyses of multiple myeloma and farming. *Am J Ind Med* **32**:510–6.

16 Brown LM, Everett GD, Burmeister LF, Blair A. (1992) Hair dye use and multiple myeloma in white men. *Am J Public Health* **82**:1673–4.

17 Brown LM, Gridley G, Pottern LM, et al. (2001) Diet and nutrition as risk factors for multiple myeloma among blacks and whites in the United States. *Cancer Causes Control* **12**:117–25.

18 Lynch HT, Ferrara K, Barlogie B, et al. (2008) Familial myeloma. *N Engl J Med* **359**:152–7.

19 Landgren O, Linet MS, McMaster ML, et al. (2006) Familial characteristics of autoimmune and hematologic disorders in 8406 multiple myeloma patients: a population-based case-control study. *Int J Cancer* **118**:3095–8.

20 Vachon CM, Kyle RA, Therneau TM, et al. (2009) Increased risk of monoclonal gammopathy in first-degree relatives of patients with multiple myeloma or monoclonal gammopathy of undetermined significance. *Blood* **114**:785–90.

21 Berenson JR, Vescio RA. (1999) HHV-8 and multiple myeloma. *Pathol Biol (Paris)* **47**:115–8.

22 Dezube BJ, Aboulafia DM, Pantanowitz L. (2004) Plasma cell disorders in HIV-infected patients: from benign gammopathy to multiple myeloma. *AIDS Read* **14**:372–4, 377–9.

23 Sun X, Peterson LC, Gong Y, Traynor AE, Nelson BP. (2004) Post-transplant plasma cell myeloma and

polymorphic lymphoproliferative disorder with monoclonal serum protein occurring in solid organ transplant recipients. *Mod Pathol* **17**:389-94.

24 Lewis DR, Pottern LM, Brown LM, et al. (1994) Multiple myeloma among blacks and whites in the United States: the role of chronic antigenic stimulation. *Cancer Causes Control.* **5**:529-39.

25 Kyle RA, Rajkumar SV. (2004) Multiple myeloma. *N Engl J Med* **351**:1860-73.

26 Kyle RA, Remstein ED, Therneau TM, et al. (2007) Clinical course and prognosis of smoldering (asymptomatic) multiple myeloma. *N Engl J Med* **356**: 2582-90.

27 Kyle RA, Therneau TM, Rajkumar SV, et al. (2002) A long-term study of prognosis in monoclonal gammopathy of undetermined significance. *N Engl J Med* **346**:564-9.

28 Fonseca R, Barlogie B, Bataille R, et al. (2004) Genetics and cytogenetics of multiple myeloma: a workshop report. *Cancer Res* **64**:1546-58.

29 Bergsagel PL, Kuehl WM. (2005) Molecular pathogenesis and a consequent classification of multiple myeloma. *J Clin Oncol* **23**:6333-8.

30 Bergsagel PL, Kuehl WM, Zhan F, et al. (2005) Cyclin D dysregulation: an early and unifying pathogenic event in multiple myeloma. *Blood* **106**:296-303.

31 Fonseca R, Harrington D, Oken MM, et al. (2002) Biological and prognostic significance of interphase fluorescence in situ hybridization detection of chromosome 13 abnormalities (delta13) in multiple myeloma: an Eastern Cooperative Oncology Group Study. *Cancer Res* **62**:715-20.

32 Avet-Loiseau H, Attal M, Moreau P, et al. (2007) Genetic abnormalities and survival in multiple myeloma: the experience of the Intergroupe Francophone du Myelome. *Blood* **109**:3489-95.

33 Chang H, Ning Y, Qi X, Yeung J, Xu W. (2007) Chromosome 1p21 deletion is a novel prognostic marker in patients with multiple myeloma. *Br J Haematol* **139**:51-4.

34 Chesi M, Robbiani DF, Sebag M, et al. (2008) AID-dependent activation of a MYC transgene induces multiple myeloma in a conditional mouse model of post-germinal center malignancies. *Cancer Cell* **13**:167-80.

35 Shaughnessy JD, Jr., Zhan F, Burington BE, et al. (2007) A validated gene expression model of high-risk multiple myeloma is defined by deregulated expression of genes mapping to chromosome 1. *Blood* **109**:2276-84.

36 Ohwada C, Nakaseko C, Koizumi M, et al. (2008) CD44 and hyaluronan engagement promotes dexamethasone resistance in human myeloma cells. *Eur J Haematol* **80**:245-50.

37 Bataille R, Pellat-Deceunynck C, Robillard N, et al. (2008) CD117 (c-kit) is aberrantly expressed in a subset of MGUS and multiple myeloma with unexpectedly good prognosis. *Leuk Res* **32**:379-82.

38 Ise T, Nagata S, Kreitman RJ, et al. (2007) Elevation of soluble CD307 (IRTA2/FcRH5) protein in the blood and expression on malignant cells of patients with multiple myeloma, chronic lymphocytic leukemia, and mantle cell lymphoma. *Leukemia* **21**:169-74.

39 Hundemer M, Klein U, Hose D, et al. (2007) Lack of CD56 expression on myeloma cells is not a marker for poor prognosis in patients treated by high-dose chemotherapy and is associated with translocation t (11;14). *Bone Marrow Transplant* **40**:1033-7.

40 Ng AP, Wei A, Bhurani D, et al. (2006) The sensitivity of CD138 immunostaining of bone marrow trephine specimens for quantifying marrow involvement in MGUS and myeloma, including samples with a low percentage of plasma cells. *Haematologica* **91**:972-5.

41 Moreaux J, Hose D, Reme T, et al. (2006) CD200 is a new prognostic factor in multiple myeloma. *Blood* **108**:4194-7.

42 Moreau P, Robillard N, Jego G, et al. (2006) Lack of CD27 in myeloma delineates different presentation and outcome. *Br J Haematol* **132**:168-70.

43 Kumar S, Rajkumar SV, Kimlinger T, Greipp PR, Witzig TE. (2005) CD45 expression by bone marrow plasma cells in multiple myeloma: clinical and biological correlations. *Leukemia* **19**:1466-70.

44 Hideshima T, Mitsiades C, Tonon G, Richardson PG, Anderson KC. (2007) Understanding multiple myeloma pathogenesis in the bone marrow to identify new therapeutic targets. *Nat Rev Cancer* **7**:585-98.

45 Podar K, Chauhan D, Anderson KC. (2009) Bone marrow microenvironment and the identification of new targets for myeloma therapy. *Leukemia* **23**:10-24.

46 Roodman GD. (2002) Role of the bone marrow microenvironment in multiple myeloma. *J Bone Miner Res* **17**:1921-5.

47 Chatterjee M, Honemann D, Lentzsch S, et al. (2002) In the presence of bone marrow stromal cells human multiple myeloma cells become independent of the IL-6/gp130/STAT3 pathway. *Blood* **100**:3311-8.

48 Papadaki H, Kyriakou D, Foudoulakis A, et al. (1997) Serum levels of soluble IL-6 receptor in multiple myeloma as indicator of disease activity. *Acta Haematol* **97**:191–5.

49 Klein B, Lu ZY, Gaillard JP, Harousseau JL, Bataille R. (1992) Inhibiting IL-6 in human multiple myeloma. *Curr Top Microbiol Immunol* **182**:237–44.

50 Kumar S, Witzig TE, Timm M, et al. (2003) Expression of VEGF and its receptors by myeloma cells. *Leukemia* **17**:2025–31.

51 Bellamy WT. (2001) Expression of vascular endothelial growth factor and its receptors in multiple myeloma and other hematopoietic malignancies. *Semin Oncol* **28**:551–9.

52 Seidel C, Borset M, Turesson I, et al. (1998) Elevated serum concentrations of hepatocyte growth factor in patients with multiple myeloma. *The Nordic Myeloma Study Group. Blood* **91**:806–12.

53 Borset M, Hjorth-Hansen H, Seidel C, Sundan A, Waage A. (1996) Hepatocyte growth factor and its receptor c-met in multiple myeloma. *Blood* **88**: 3998–4004.

54 Hideshima T, Chauhan D, Hayashi T, et al. (2002) The biological sequelae of stromal cell-derived factor-1alpha in multiple myeloma. *Mol Cancer Ther* **1**:539–44.

55 Chng WJ, Gualberto A, Fonseca R. (2006) IGF-1R is overexpressed in poor-prognostic subtypes of multiple myeloma. *Leukemia* **20**:174–6.

56 Kline M, Donovan K, Wellik L, et al. (2007) Cytokine and chemokine profiles in multiple myeloma; significance of stromal interaction and correlation of IL-8 production with disease progression. *Leuk Res* **31**:591–8.

57 Lacy MQ, Donovan KA, Heimbach JK, Ahmann GJ, Lust JA. (1999) Comparison of interleukin-1 beta expression by in situ hybridization in monoclonal gammopathy of undetermined significance and multiple myeloma. *Blood* **93**:300–5.

58 Mitsiades CS, Mitsiades NS, Munshi NC, Richardson PG, Anderson KC. (2006) The role of the bone microenvironment in the pathophysiology and therapeutic management of multiple myeloma: interplay of growth factors, their receptors and stromal interactions *Eur J Cancer* **42**:1564–73.

59 Kumar S, Gertz MA, Dispenzieri A, et al. (2004) Prognostic value of bone marrow angiogenesis in patients with multiple myeloma undergoing high-dose therapy. *Bone Marrow Transplant* **34**:235–9.

60 Rigolin GM, Fraulini C, Ciccone M, et al. (2006) Neoplastic circulating endothelial cells in multiple myeloma with 13q14 deletion. *Blood* **107**:2531–5.

61 Silvestris F, Tucci M, Cafforio P, Dammacco F. (2001) Fas-L up-regulation by highly malignant myeloma plasma cells: role in the pathogenesis of anemia and disease progression. *Blood* **97**:1155–64.

62 Roodman GD. (2009) Pathogenesis of myeloma bone disease. *Leukemia* **23**:435–41.

63 Kyle RA, Rajkumar SV. (2009) Criteria for diagnosis, staging, risk stratification and response assessment of multiple myeloma. *Leukemia* **23**:3–9.

64 International Myeloma Working Group (2003) Criteria for the classification of monoclonal gammopathies, multiple myeloma and related disorders: a report of the International Myeloma Working Group. *Br J Haematol* **121**:749–57.

65 Kyle RA, Therneau TM, Rajkumar SV, et al. (2006) Prevalence of monoclonal gammopathy of undetermined significance. *N Engl J Med* **354**:1362–9.

66 Cesana C, Klersy C, Barbarano L, et al. (2002) Prognostic factors for malignant transformation in monoclonal gammopathy of undetermined significance and smoldering multiple myeloma. *J Clin Oncol* **20**: 1625–34.

67 Kyle RA, Therneau TM, Rajkumar SV, et al. (2006) Prevalence of monoclonal gammopathy of undetermined significance. *N Engl J Med* **354**:1362–9.

68 Rajkumar SV, Kyle RA, Therneau TM, et al. (2005) Serum free light chain ratio is an independent risk factor for progression in monoclonal gammopathy of undetermined significance. *Blood* **106**:812–7.

69 Kyle RA, Remstein ED, Therneau TM, et al. (2007) Clinical course and prognosis of smoldering (asymptomatic) multiple myeloma. *New Engl J Med* **356**: 2582–90.

70 Dispenzieri A, Kyle RA, Katzmann JA, et al. (2008) Immunoglobulin free light chain ratio is an independent risk factor for progression of smoldering (asymptomatic) multiple myeloma. *Blood* **111**:785–9.

71 Lacy MQ, Gertz MA, Hanson CA, Inwards DJ, Kyle RA. (1997) Multiple myeloma associated with diffuse osteosclerotic bone lesions: a clinical entity distinct from osteosclerotic myeloma (POEMS syndrome). *Am J Hematol* **56**:288–93.

72 Drayson M, Begum G, Basu S, et al. (2006) Effects of paraprotein heavy and light chain types and free light chain load on survival in myeloma: an analysis of patients receiving conventional-dose chemotherapy

in Medical Research Council UK multiple myeloma trials. *Blood* **108**:2013–9.

73 Durie BG, Salmon SE. (1975) A clinical staging system for multiple myeloma. Correlation of measured myeloma cell mass with presenting clinical features, response to treatment, and survival. *Cancer* **36**:842–54.

74 Greipp PR, San Miguel J, Durie BG, et al. (2005) International staging system for multiple myeloma. *J Clin Oncol* **23**:3412–20.

75 Dispenzieri A, Rajkumar SV, Gertz MA, et al. (2007) Treatment of newly diagnosed multiple myeloma based on Mayo Stratification of Myeloma and Risk-adapted Therapy (mSMART): consensus statement. *Mayo Clinic Proc* **82**:323–41.

76 Kumar S, Mahmood ST, Lacy MQ, et al. (2008) Impact of early relapse after auto-SCT for multiple myeloma. *Bone Marrow Transplant* **42**:413–20.

77 Siegel DS, Desikan KR, Mehta J, et al. (1999) Age is not a prognostic variable with autotransplants for multiple myeloma. *Blood* **93**:51–4.

78 Durie BG, Harousseau JL, Miguel JS, et al. (2006) International uniform response criteria for multiple myeloma. *Leukemia* **20**:1467–73.

79 Augustson BM, Begum G, Dunn JA, et al. (2005) Early mortality after diagnosis of multiple myeloma: analysis of patients entered onto the United Kingdom Medical Research Council trials between 1980 and 2002 – Medical Research Council Adult Leukaemia Working Party. *J Clin Oncol* **23**:9219–26.

80 Fermand JP, Ravaud P, Chevret S, et al. (1998) High-dose therapy and autologous peripheral blood stem cell transplantation in multiple myeloma: up-front or rescue treatment? Results of a multicenter sequential randomized clinical trial. *Blood* **92**:3131–6.

81 Attal M, Harousseau JL, Stoppa AM, et al. (1996) A prospective, randomized trial of autologous bone marrow transplantation and chemotherapy in multiple myeloma. Intergroupe Français du Myelome. *N Engl J Med* **335**:91–7.

82 Child JA, Morgan GJ, Davies FE, et al. (2003) High-dose chemotherapy with hematopoietic stem-cell rescue for multiple myeloma. *N Engl J Med* **348**: 1875–83.

83 Kumar S, Lacy MQ, Dispenzieri A, et al. (2004) High-dose therapy and autologous stem cell transplantation for multiple myeloma poorly responsive to initial therapy. *Bone Marrow Transplant* **34**:161–7.

84 Barlogie B, Smith L, Alexanian R. (1984) Effective treatment of advanced multiple myeloma refractory to alkylating agents. *N Engl J Med* **310**:1353–6.

85 Alexanian R, Barlogie B, Tucker S. (1990) VAD-based regimens as primary treatment for multiple myeloma. *Am J Hematol* **33**:86–9.

86 Alexanian R, Dimopoulos MA, Delasalle K, Barlogie B. (1992) Primary dexamethasone treatment of multiple myeloma. *Blood* **80**:887–90.

87 Kumar S, Lacy MQ, Dispenzieri A, et al. (2004) Single agent dexamethasone for pre-stem cell transplant induction therapy for multiple myeloma. *Bone Marrow Transplant* **34**:485–90.

88 Rajkumar SV, Rosinol L, Hussein M, et al. (2008) Multicenter, randomized, double-blind, placebo-controlled study of thalidomide plus dexamethasone compared with dexamethasone as initial therapy for newly diagnosed multiple myeloma. *J Clin Oncol* **26**:2171–7.

89 Rajkumar SV, Blood E, Vesole D, et al. and Eastern Cooperative Oncology Group (2006) Phase III clinical trial of thalidomide plus dexamethasone compared with dexamethasone alone in newly diagnosed multiple myeloma: a clinical trial coordinated by the Eastern Cooperative Oncology Group. *J Clin Oncol* **24**:431–6.

90 Cavo M, Zamagni E, Tosi P, et al. (2005) Superiority of thalidomide and dexamethasone over vincristine-doxorubicindexamethasone (VAD) as primary therapy in preparation for autologous transplantation for multiple myeloma. *Blood* **106**:35–9.

91 Lacy MQ, Gertz MA, Dispenzieri A, et al. (2007) Long-term results of response to therapy, time to progression, and survival with lenalidomide plus dexamethasone in newly diagnosed myeloma. *Mayo Clin Proc* **82**:1179–84.

92 Zonder JA, Crowley J, Hussein MA, et al. (2007) Superiority of lenalidomide (Len) plus high-dose dexamethasone (HD) compared to HD alone as treatment of newly-diagnosed multiple myeloma (NDMM): Results of the randomized, double-blinded, placebo-controlled SWOG Trial S0232. *Blood (ASH Annual Meeting Abstracts)* **110**:77.

93 Rajkumar SV, Jacobus S, Callander N, et al. (2007) A randomized trial of lenalidomide plus high-dose dexamethasone (RD) versus lenalidomide plus low-dose dexamethasone (Rd) in newly diagnosed multiple myeloma (E4A03): A trial coordinated by the Eastern Cooperative Oncology Group. Blood *(ASH Annual Meeting Abstracts)* **110**:74.

94 Jagannath S, Durie BG, Wolf J, et al. (2005) Bortezomib therapy alone and in combination with

dexamethasone for previously untreated symptomatic multiple myeloma. *Br J Haematol* **129**:776–83.

95 Richardson PG, Xie W, Mitsiades C, et al. (2009) Single-agent bortezomib in previously untreated multiple myeloma: efficacy, characterization of peripheral neuropathy, and molecular correlations with response and neuropathy. *J Clin Oncol* **27**:3518–25.

96 Harousseau JL, Mathiot C, Attal M, et al. (2007) VELCADE/dexamethasone (Vel/D) versus VAD as induction treatment prior to autologous stem cell transplantion (ASCT) in newly diagnosed multiple myeloma (MM): Updated results of the IFM 2005/01 Trial. *Blood (ASH Annual Meeting Abstracts)* **110**:450.

97 Cavo M, Testoni N, Terragna C, et al. (2008) Superior rate of complete response with up-front velcade-thalidomide-dexamethasone versus thalidomide-dexamethasone in newly diagnosed multiple myeloma is not affected by adverse prognostic factors, including high-risk cytogenetic abnormalities. *Blood (ASH Annual Meeting Abstracts)* **112**:1662.

98 Richardson P, Lonial S, Jakubowiak A, et al. (2008) Lenalidomide, bortezomib, and dexamethasone in patients with newly diagnosed multiple myeloma: encouraging efficacy in high risk groups with updated results of a Phase I/II study. *Blood (ASH Annual Meeting Abstracts)* **112**:92.

99 Kumar S, Flinn IW, Noga SJ, et al. (2008) Safety and efficacy of novel combination therapy with bortezomib, dexamethasone, cyclophosphamide, and lenalidomide in newly diagnosed multiple myeloma: initial results from the Phase I/II Multi-Center EVOLUTION Study. *Blood (ASH Annual Meeting Abstracts)* **112**:93.

100 Kapoor P, Kumar S, Fonseca R, et al. (2009) Impact of risk stratification on outcome among patients with multiple myeloma receiving initial therapy with lenalidomide and dexamethasone. *Blood* **114**:518–21.

101 Reece D, Song KW, Fu T, et al. (2009) Influence of cytogenetics in patients with relapsed or refractory multiple myeloma treated with lenalidomide plus dexamethasone: adverse effect of deletion 17p13. *Blood* **114**:522–5.

102 San Miguel JF, Schlag R, Khuageva NK, et al. (2008) Bortezomib plus melphalan and prednisone for initial treatment of multiple myeloma. *N Engl J Med* **359**:906–17.

103 Fermand JP, Katsahian S, Divine M, et al. (2005) High-dose therapy and autologous blood stem-cell transplantation compared with conventional treatment in myeloma patients aged 55 to 65 years: long-term

results of a randomized control trial from the Group Myelome-Autogreffe. *J Clin Oncol* **23**:9227–33.

104 Barlogie B, Kyle RA, Anderson KC, et al. (2006) Standard chemotherapy compared with high-dose chemoradiotherapy for multiple myeloma: final results of Phase III US Intergroup Trial S9321. *J Clin Oncol* **24**:929–36.

105 Blade J, Rosinol L, Sureda A, et al. (2005) High-dose therapy intensification compared with continued standard chemotherapy in multiple myeloma patients responding to the initial chemotherapy: long-term results from a prospective randomized trial from the Spanish cooperative group PETHEMA. *Blood* **106**:3755–9.

106 Moreau P, Facon T, Attal M, et al. (2002) Comparison of 200 mg/m(2) melphalan and 8 Gy total body irradiation plus 140 mg/m(2) melphalan as conditioning regimens for peripheral blood stem cell transplantation in patients with newly diagnosed multiple myeloma: final analysis of the Intergroupe Francophone du Myelome 9502 randomized trial. *Blood* **99**:731–5.

107 Barlogie B, Jagannath S, Vesole DH, et al. (1997) Superiority of tandem autologous transplantation over standard therapy for previously untreated multiple myeloma. *Blood* **89**:789–93.

108 Attal M, Harousseau JL, Facon T, et al. (2003) Single versus double autologous stem-cell transplantation for multiple myeloma. *N Engl J Med* **349**:2495–502.

109 Cavo M, Tosi P, Zamagni E, et al. (2007) Prospective, randomized study of single compared with double autologous stem-cell transplantation for multiple myeloma: Bologna 96 clinical study. *J Clin Oncol* **25**:2434–41.

110 Sonneveld P, van der Holt B, Vellenga E, et al. (2005) Intensive versus double intensive therapy in untreated multiple myeloma: Final analysis of the HOVON 24 Trial. *Blood (ASH Annual Meeting Abstracts)* **106**:2545.

111 Fermand JP, Alberti C, Marolleau JP. (2003) Single versus tandem high dose therapy (HDT) supported with autologous blood stem cell (ABSC) transplantation using unselected or CD34-enriched ABSC: results of a two by two designed randomized trial in 230 young patients with multiple myeloma (MM). *Hematol J* **4**:S59.

112 Cunningham D, Powles R, Malpas J, et al. (1998) A randomized trial of maintenance interferon following high-dose chemotherapy in multiple myeloma: long-term follow-up results. *Br J Haematol* **102**:495–502.

113 Attal M, Harousseau JL, Leyvraz S, et al. (2006) Maintenance therapy with thalidomide improves survival in patients with multiple myeloma. *Blood* **108**:3289–94.

114 Barlogie B, Tricot G, Anaissie E, et al. (2006) Thalidomide and hematopoietic-cell transplantation for multiple myeloma. *N Engl J Med* **354**:1021–30.

115 Spencer A, Prince HM, Roberts AW, et al. (2009) Consolidation therapy with low-dose thalidomide and prednisolone prolongs the survival of multiple myeloma patients undergoing a single autologous stem-cell transplantation procedure. *J Clin Oncol* **27**: 1788–93.

116 Tricot G, Vesole DH, Jagannath S, et al. (1996) Graft-versus-myeloma effect: proof of principle. *Blood* **87**:1196–8.

117 Bjorkstrand BB, Ljungman P, Svensson H, et al. (1996) Allogeneic bone marrow transplantation versus autologous stem cell transplantation in multiple myeloma: a retrospective case-matched study from the European Group for Blood and Marrow Transplantation. *Blood* **88**:4711–8.

118 Gahrton G, Bjorkstrand B. (2008) Allogeneic transplantation in multiple myeloma. *Haematologica* **93**:1295–300.

119 Alyea E, Weller E, Schlossman R, et al. (2003) Outcome after autologous and allogeneic stem cell transplantation for patients with multiple myeloma: impact of graft-versus-myeloma effect. *Bone Marrow Transplant* **32**:1145–51.

120 Kuruvilla J, Shepherd JD, Sutherland HJ, et al. (2007) Long-term outcome of myeloablative allogeneic stem cell transplantation for multiple myeloma. *Biol Blood Marrow Transplant* **13**:925–31.

121 Gahrton G, Svensson H, Cavo M, et al. (2001) Progress in allogenic bone marrow and peripheral blood stem cell transplantation for multiple myeloma: a comparison between transplants performed 1983-93 and 1994-8 at European Group for Blood and Marrow Transplantation centres. *Br J Haematol* **113**:209–16.

122 Myeloma Trialists' Collaborative Group (1998) Combination chemotherapy versus melphalan plus prednisone as treatment for multiple myeloma: an overview of 6,633 patients from 27 randomized trials. *J Clin Oncol* **16**:3832–42.

123 Palumbo A, Bringhen S, Caravita T, et al. (2006) Oral melphalan and prednisone chemotherapy plus thalidomide compared with melphalan and prednisone

alone in elderly patients with multiple myeloma: randomised controlled trial. *Lancet* **367**:825–31.

124 Facon T, Mary JY, Hulin C, et al. (2007) Melphalan and prednisone plus thalidomide versus melphalan and prednisone alone or reduced-intensity autologous stem cell transplantation in elderly patients with multiple myeloma (IFM 99-06): a randomised trial. *Lancet* **370**:1209–18.

125 Palumbo A, Falco P, Corradini P, et al. (2007) Melphalan, prednisone, and lenalidomide treatment for newly diagnosed myeloma: a report from the GIMEMA – Italian Multiple Myeloma Network. *J Clin Oncol* **25**:4459–65.

126 Kumar SK, Therneau TM, Gertz MA, et al. (2004) Clinical course of patients with relapsed multiple myeloma. *Mayo Clin Proc* **79**:867–74.

127 Lacy MQ, Hayman SR, Gertz MA, et al. (2008) Pomalidomide (CC4047) plus low-dose dexamethasone (pom/dex) is highly effective therapy in relapsed multiple myeloma. *Blood (ASH Annual Meeting Abstracts)* **112**:866.

128 Vij R, Wang M, Orlowski R, et al. (2008) Initial results of PX-171-004, an open-label, single-arm, Phase II study of carfilzomib (CFZ) in patients with relapsed myeloma (MM). *Blood (ASH Annual Meeting Abstracts)* **112**:865.

129 Jagannath S, Vij R, Stewart AK, et al. (2008) Initial results of PX-171-003, an open-label, single-arm, Phase II study of carfilzomib (CFZ) in patients with relapsed and refractory multiple myeloma (MM). *Blood (ASH Annual Meeting Abstracts)* **112**:864.

130 Lacy MQ, Dispenzieri A, Gertz MA, et al. (2006) Mayo clinic consensus statement for the use of bisphosphonates in multiple myeloma. *Mayo Clin Proc* **81**: 1047–53.

131 Kyle RA, Yee GC, Somerfield MR, et al. (2007) American Society of Clinical Oncology 2007 clinical practice guideline update on the role of bisphosphonates in multiple myeloma. *J Clin Oncol* **25**:2464–72.

132 Leung N. (2006) Plasma exchange in multiple myeloma. *Ann Intern Med* **144**:455 [author reply].

133 Ludwig H, Durie BG, Bolejack V, et al. (2008) Myeloma in patients younger than age 50 years presents with more favorable features and shows better survival: an analysis of 10 549 patients from the International Myeloma Working Group. *Blood* **111**: 4039–47.

134 Greipp PR, Lust JA, O'Fallon WM, et al. (1993) Plasma cell labeling index and beta 2-microglobulin predict survival independent of thymidine kinase

and C-reactive protein in multiple myeloma. *Blood* **81**:3382–7.

135 Nowakowski GS, Witzig TE, Dingli D, et al. (2005) Circulating plasma cells detected by flow cytometry as a predictor of survival in 302 patients with newly diagnosed multiple myeloma. *Blood* **106**:2276–9.

136 Snozek CL, Katzmann JA, Kyle RA, et al. (2008) Prognostic value of the serum free light chain ratio in newly diagnosed myeloma: proposed incorporation into the international staging system. *Leukemia* **22**:1933–7.

137 Greipp PR, Leong T, Bennett JM, et al. (1998) Plasma-blastic morphology – an independent prognostic factor with clinical and laboratory correlates: Eastern Cooperative Oncology Group (ECOG) myeloma trial E9486 report by the ECOG Myeloma Laboratory Group. *Blood* **91**:2501–7.

138 Rajkumar SV, Leong T, Roche PC, et al. (2000) Prognostic value of bone marrow angiogenesis in multiple myeloma. *Clin Cancer Res* **6**:3111–6.

139 Dispenzieri A, Rajkumar SV, Gertz MA, et al. (2007) Treatment of newly diagnosed multiple myeloma based on Mayo stratification of myeloma and risk-adapted therapy (mSMART): Consensus statement. *Mayo Clin Proc* **82**:323–41.

CHAPTER 21
Waldenström's Macroglobulinemia

Robert A. Kyle and Suzanne Hayman
Laboratory Medicine and Pathology, College of Medicine, Mayo Clinic, Rochester, MN, USA

Introduction

Two patients with oronasal bleeding, thrombocytopenia, normochromic anemia, elevated erythrocyte sedimentation rate, lymphadenopathy, and low serum fibrinogen were reported by Jan Waldenström in 1944 [1]. Both patients had a large homogeneous gamma globulin component with a sedimentation coefficient of 19S to 20S, and a molecular weight of approximately 1 000 000. The serum viscosity was elevated. The serum of one patient precipitated at low temperatures (cryoglobulinemia). The serum globulin was subsequently identified as an immunoglobulin and was later designated IgM. The basic abnormality in Waldenström's macroglobulinemia (WM) is the proliferation of clonal cells with lymphocyte and plasma cell characteristics producing an IgM monoclonal protein. It must be differentiated from monoclonal gammopathy of undetermined significance (MGUS), other low-grade lymphomas, and primary systemic (AL) amyloidosis. An excellent review of WM has been published [2].

Diagnosis

The diagnosis of WM depends upon the presence of an IgM monoclonal protein of any size in the serum and 10% or more infiltration of the bone marrow aspirate or biopsy by clonal small lymphocytes and/ or plasma cells (lymphoplasmacytic lymphoma) with an intertrabecular pattern. The diagnosis and

management of WM has been reviewed by Dimopoulous et al. [3].

Epidemiology

The incidence of WM is 0.3 per 100 000 white men and 0.17 per 100 000 white women, resulting in approximately 1400 new cases in the US each year. The incidence in black males is 0.17 per 100 000 and 0.13 per 100 000 in black females [4].

Waldenström's macroglobulinemia is one-seventh as common as multiple myeloma (MM) in our practice. The incidence increases markedly with age, from 0.1 at <45 years of age, to 36.3 per 100 000 at age ≥75 years for males. Data from the South Thames Hematology Registry recorded 152 new cases of WM between 1999 and 2001. The age standardized rate was 5.5 per million European standard population. The median age at diagnosis is approximately 65 years; fewer than 1% are under 40 years of age. Approximately 60% of patients are male [5].

The etiology of WM is unknown. In a case control study of 65 patients with WM compared to 213 hospital control subjects, there were no differences in socio-demographic features, prior medical conditions, medication use, cigarette smoking, alcohol consumption, occupational exposures, or familial cancer history [6]. Hepatitis C viral infections were associated with a three-fold higher risk of WM in US veterans [7]. Chronic immune stimulation and autoimmune disorders have also been associated with WM [8].

Waldenström's macroglobulinemia and related abnormalities are generally considered to be sporadic diseases, but have been reported in several families. Blattner et al. [9] described a father and two children with an IgM monoclonal protein and a lymphoproliferative process and a third child with WM. Four brothers, all with a serum IgM monoclonal protein, had WM, MGUS, MGUS with a peripheral neuropathy, or AL amyloidosis. Five of 12 family members had increased serum immunoglobulin levels; two were IgM [10]. Another report of three WM families with at least two members with WM have been described [11]. Five of 27 first-degree relatives had an IgM MGUS, while four others had a polyclonal IgM gammopathy. During follow-up, the five patients with IgM monoclonal gammopathy persisted or progressed, with three evolving into WM. IgM monoclonal gammopathy developed in two of the four patients with a polyclonal gammopathy.

In a large study of 2749 patients with WM or lymphoplasmacytic lymphoma (LPL) and 8279 controls, the 24 609 first-degree relatives had a 20-fold increased risk of developing WM or LPL. First-degree relatives also had an increased risk of developing non-Hodgkin lymphoma, chronic lymphocytic leukemia (CLL), and MGUS [12].

Pathogenesis

The normal counterpart of the WM clonal cell has not been definitively identified, although it is believed that the cells most resemble post-germinal center memory B-cells. In the vast majority of cases, the WM cells do not undergo isotype class switch recombination. There are no chromosomal abnormalities specific for WM, but the most common chromosomal abnormality seen is deletion of 6q21, which was found in 42% of patients [13]. Schop et al. [14] also reported that more than 50% of patients had chromosome 6q deletions when using interphase fluorescence in situ hybridization (FISH). These deletions usually involved 6q21-q23 when utilizing a high-resolution array-based comparative genomic hybridization approach. Braggio et al. [15] reported chromosomal abnormalities in 83% of 42

WM patients. They also noted an association of TRAF-3 inactivation with increased transcriptional activity of NF–kappa B [15]. Upregulation of IL-6 has also been reported [16]. Unlike MM, translocations involving the IgH locus are uncommon and do not appear to play a major role in the pathogenesis of WM. A human cell line (BCWM.1) has been established from a culture of CD19$^+$ bone marrow lymphoplasmacytic cells from a patient with WM. The cells are CD5$^-$, CD10$^-$, CD19$^+$, CD20$^+$, CD23$^+$, CD38$^+$, CD40$^+$, CD138$^+$, and express monoclonal IgM. No cytogenetic abnormalities were demonstrated. Inoculation of the BCWM.1 cells in human bone marrow chips implanted in immunodeficient mice resulted in rapid engraftment of tumor cells and production of IgM [17].

Clinical features

The disease onset is usually insidious and characterized by weakness and fatigue. Chronic oozing of blood from the nose and gums and skin pallor may be seen. Fever, night sweats, and weight loss may also occur. The clinical features of WM relate to the organs involved. Hepatomegaly occurs in approximately one quarter of patients at diagnosis, while splenomegaly and generalized lymphadenopathy are slightly less frequent. It is useful to make a distinction between symptoms and signs caused by the clonal neoplastic cells themselves and the rheologic consequences of the monoclonal IgM protein they produce.

Neurologic/ophthalmologic
Approximately 25% of patients with WM have neurologic abnormalities [18]. In one series of 217 patients with WM, neurologic symptoms occurred in 22% [19]. Peripheral neuropathy is not uncommon and is usually a distal, symmetric, and slowly progressive sensorimotor process, with the lower extremities usually more involved than the upper extremities. The frequency of a peripheral neuropathy is higher if one relies on electrophysiologic tests rather than clinical examination. Anti-myelin associated glycoprotein (anti-MAG) activity is found in approximately half of patients with a sensorimotor

peripheral neuropathy. Cranial nerve palsies, mono-neuropathy, and mononeuritis multiplex may result from infiltration of the nerves by tumor cells, hyper-viscosity, or a bleeding diathesis [20]. IgM deposits are frequently seen in the myelin sheath. However, it is impossible to determine whether the presence of IgM on the biopsy specimen is a causative factor or whether it represents passive deposition of IgM in an already damaged nerve [21, 22]. In most cases, biopsy of the sural nerve reveals myelin degeneration, but no sig-nificant infiltration by lymphocytes or plasma cells.

We have described 50 patients with an IgM monoclonal protein with peripheral neuropathies and AL amyloidosis [23]. In the eight patients with a peripheral neuropathy in which the type of amyloid was determined, the amyloidosis was of the AL type. In a recent series of 64 patients with an IgM-related systemic AL amyloidosis, 83% had a prior diagnosis of WM or LPL [24]. The median duration between diagnosis of the IgM-related disorder and amyloid-osis was eight months.

The central nervous system may also be affected. Infiltration of the meninges by plasmacytoid lym-phocytes has been noted. Lower extremity sensori-motor neuropathy developed in four patients with WM from leptomeningeal and nerve root lympho-plasmacytic infiltration [25]. Multifocal leukoence-phalopathy is rare [26]. Hearing loss may be a presenting symptom of WM [27]. Hyperviscosity syndrome may produce headache, blurred vision, dizziness, vertigo, ataxia, diplopia, seizures, altered consciousness, or coma. Cerebral hemorrhage has been seen. Retinal vein engorgement with vascular segmentation (sausaging), flame-shaped hemor-rhages, and exudates are common with hypervis-cosity, while papilledema is rare.

Infections

Recurrent infections are less common than in MM, but approximately twice as common compared to normal individuals.

Renal involvement

Although deposits of monoclonal IgM on the endo-thelial aspect of the basement membrane are com-mon, renal insufficiency is uncommon in WM. Infiltration of lymphocytes or plasmacytoid cells

identical to those found in the bone marrow is frequent. Nephrotic syndrome is rare, but when present, is usually due to systemic amyloidosis. However, non-amyloid nephrotic syndrome has been reported [28].

Pulmonary involvement

Occasionally, diffuse pulmonary infiltrates, isolated masses, or pleural effusion may be seen in WM. In a review of 20 patients, Winterbauer et al. [29] found five with pulmonary involvement. The major symptoms were cough and dyspnea. The chest radiograph revealed multiple nodular infiltrates in both lungs in four patients and unilateral pleural effusion in one.

Gastrointestinal tract

Diarrhea and steatorrhea are uncommon features of WM. Rarely, deposition of the IgM protein itself produces an amorphous hyaline-like material in the small intestine. Infiltration of lymphocytes and plasma cells may also be responsible for diarrhea and malabsorption. Portal hypertension has been reported. Retroperitoneal and/or mesenteric lymph nodes may be prominent [30].

Dermatologic involvement

The presence of an IgM monoclonal protein and erythematous urticarial skin lesions (Schnitzler's syndrome) have been described [31]. Lymphoplas-macytic cells may also infiltrate the dermis and produce macular or papulonodular lesions. Rarely, the IgM monoclonal protein itself may be deposited in the skin and produce macular or papulonodular lesions. Occasionally, the monoclonal IgM acts as a type I cryoglobulin and precipitates at >22° C, pro-ducing Raynaud's phenomenon, urticaria, purpura, acral cyanosis, or tissue necrosis upon exposure to cold [32].

Bleeding diathesis

A bleeding diathesis is common in WM and results from interference of the IgM protein with clotting factors and platelet function, as well as from hyper-viscosity. Purpura and gross bleeding, especially from the gastrointestinal tract, may be seen in addition to epistaxis and gingival oozing.

In one report, bleeding occurred in 5 of 14 patients with WM due to prolongation of the bleeding time, abnormalities in platelet adhesiveness, prothrombin time, and thromboplastin generation, as well as reduced levels of factor VIII [33]. Thrombocytopenia from marrow infiltration, chemotherapy, splenomegaly, or Idiopathic thrombocytopenic purpura (ITP) may be a contributing factor.

Bone involvement

Bone lesions are rare in WM, unlike in MM. No osteolytic lesions were found at presentation in a series of 217 patients with WM [19].

Laboratory findings

Anemia is present in the majority of patients with symptomatic WM. It is caused by inadequate red cell synthesis, decreased erythrocyte survival, or blood loss. In one series, the Coombs test was positive in 10% of patients, but only 3% developed significant hemolysis [19]. Increased plasma volume is frequent and is responsible for spuriously low hemoglobin and hematocrit levels. Rouleaux formation is striking and the erythrocyte sedimentation rate is usually markedly increased. Neutropenia and thrombocytopenia are uncommon. Lymphocytosis or monocytosis may be seen.

The IgM protein may interfere with various laboratory tests by specific binding properties or precipitation during analysis. Low values for cholesterol, high values for bilirubin, as well as abnormal inorganic phosphate levels may be seen. Measurements of C-reactive protein, antistreptolysin-O, creatinine, glucose, urea nitrogen, iron, and inorganic calcium may all be inaccurate. Hyperuricemia may be present, but the serum creatinine value is usually normal. The beta-2-microglobulin value is elevated in about half of patients with WM and is an important prognostic feature.

Serum and urine protein abnormalities

Serum protein electrophoresis always shows a sharp, narrow, spike or dense band, usually migrating in the gamma area. Serum immunofixation must then be performed in order to confirm the presence of a monoclonal protein and to determine its type (Figure 21.1). Seventy-five percent of IgM proteins have kappa light chains. The quantitation of IgM obtained by nephelometry may be 2–3 g/dl more than that found by the densitometric measurement of the electrophoretic spike [34]. The Workshop Consensus Panel recommended that the use of densitometry should be used to measure IgM levels, rather than nephelometry [35]. It is essential that one measures the protein abnormality by the same technique during follow-up. The IgG level is reduced in approximately 60% of patients, while the IgA value is below normal in approximately 20% [36]. Macroglobulins may precipitate in the cold (cryoglobulins), but are almost always asymptomatic. Bence Jones proteinuria (monoclonal light chains) is found in 70 to 80% of patients with WM, but the level is usually low [36].

Serum viscosity

Although hyperviscosity syndrome was noted in 1929 [37], it was little appreciated until the review by Fahey et al. [38] in 1965. Serum viscosity should be determined when the serum M spike is more than 4 g/dL or in any patient with oronasal bleeding, blurred vision, or neurologic symptoms suggestive of hyperviscosity. The Ostwald-100 viscometer is a satisfactory instrument for measurement of serum viscosity, but one may use a Wells-Brookfield or Sonoclot viscometer. It must be emphasized that there is a poor correlation between the serum viscosity value and clinical symptoms. In general, most patients with symptoms have a relative viscosity more than 4 centipoise (cP). An occasional patient will have symptoms when the viscosity is <4 cP, and some patients have no symptoms when the relative viscosity is 6 to 8 cP. However, the level of relative viscosity producing symptoms in an individual patient is usually the same; a patient having hyperviscosity symptoms at the relative viscosity of 5 cP will usually have symptoms when the patient

Immunofixation
Serum

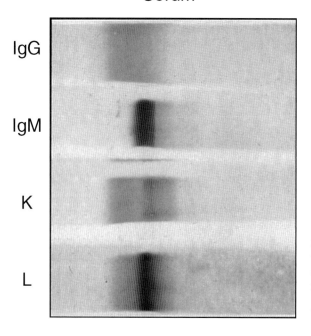

IgG

IgM

K

L

Figure 21.1 Serum immunofixation. Top: dense, localized band with IgM (μ) antiserum. Middle: no band with κ antiserum. Bottom: dense band with λ antiserum corresponding to IgM band. Patient has IgM λ monoclonal protein. (Reproduced from Kyle RA et al. (1986) *Semin Oncol* **13**:310–17, with permission from WB Saunders.)

reaches that level at a subsequent time. The viscosity-protein concentration curve of IgM is nonlinear. At low serum IgM levels, an increase of 1 to 2 g/dL produces little or no increase in the serum viscosity, but if the IgM is 4 to 5 g/dL, an increment of 1 to 2 g/dL greatly increases the relative viscosity. The level at which clinical symptoms occur is due not only to the absolute serum protein concentration, but to the molecular characteristics and aggregation of the proteins, microvasculature changes, hematocrit level, and cardiac status of the patient [39].

Bone marrow examination

The bone marrow aspirate is often hypocellular, but the biopsy specimen is usually hypercellular and reveals extensive infiltration with clonal lymphoid or plasmacytoid cells. Dutcher bodies (intranuclear vacuoles containing IgM protein) are common. Mast cells (nonclonal) are frequently increased and may help differentiate WM from other lymphomas or myeloma. The pattern of marrow involvement may be diffuse (45%), nodular-interstitial (22%), mixed paratrabecular-nodular (20%), or paratrabecular

(13%) [40]. Bone marrow involvement can also be detected by magnetic resonance imaging [30]. The cells in WM are B-cells with a low proliferative rate, and typically have the following phenotype: IgM$^+$, CD5$^{+/-}$, CD10$^-$, CD19$^+$, CD20$^+$, CD22$^+$, CD23$^-$, CD 25$^+$, CD 27$^+$, FMC 7$^+$, CD103$^-$, and CD138$^-$. The plasmacytic component may express CD138$^+$, CD38$^+$, and CD45$^-$ or dim. They express only one type of light chain (kappa or lambda). CD5 is expressed in 10%, while CD9 and CD10 expression are infrequent.

Differential diagnosis

Waldenström's macroglobulinemia must be differentiated from IgM MGUS, smoldering WM (SWM), CLL, mantle cell lymphoma (MCL), marginal zone lymphoma (MZL), and MM.

IgM MGUS is characterized by an IgM monoclonal protein <3.0 g/dL, bone marrow containing <10% lymphoplasmacytic cells, absence of symptomatic anemia, lymphadenopathy, hepatosplenomegaly or hyperviscosity, and no constitutional symptoms. In a long-term follow-up of 213 patients with IgM MGUS from Southeastern Minnesota, 29 developed lymphoma (n = 17), WM (n = 6), AL amyloidosis (n = 3), or CLL (n = 3) [41]. The relative risk of progression was 15.9-fold higher than that expected, and amounted to 1.5% per year. The size of the serum M protein, serum albumin, and hemoglobin values were the major risk factors for progression.

Smoldering WM is characterized by the presence of a serum IgM monoclonal protein $\geq 3.0\,g/dL$ and/or $\geq 10\%$ lymphoplasmacytic infiltration of the bone marrow. There must be no evidence of symptomatic anemia, hyperviscosity, constitutional symptoms or symptomatic lymphadenopathy or hepatosplenomegaly. Forty-eight persons with SWM were identified at Mayo Clinic and followed for 292 person-years. The median duration at follow-up was 13.9 years. During that time, 33 patients progressed to symptomatic WM, when only 0.004 were expected in a normal population. Risk factors for progression included the size of the serum M protein, degree of bone marrow lymphoplasmacytic infiltration, hemoglobin value, and reduced levels of the uninvolved immunoglobulins. The risk of progression was 55% at five years (11% per year).

The abnormal B-cells in CLL are $CD5^+$, $CD23^+$, and $FMC7^-$. Mantle cell lymphoma is characterized by nuclear staining for Cyclin-D (BCL-1), which is present in more than 70% of cases. In addition, more than two-thirds of patients with MCL have t(11;14) (q13;q32) [42]. IgM-MM frequently has t(11;14), while WM does not. In addition, patients with IgM myeloma frequently have lytic bone lesions and the bone marrow contains more plasma cells. Patients with WM must also be differentiated from patients with an IgG or IgA-MM who have many lymphocytoid cells in the bone marrow and no lytic lesions [43].

Treatment

Patients with SWM should not be treated until symptoms develop as these patients may remain stable for long periods of time [35]. Indications for therapy include constitutional symptoms consisting of weakness, fatigue, night sweats, fever, or weight loss. The presence of progressive symptomatic lymphadenopathy or splenomegaly, anemia with a hemoglobin value $\leq 10\,g/dL$ or a platelet count $<100 \times 10^9/L$ due to bone marrow infiltration also justify therapy. Hyperviscosity syndrome demands urgent treatment. Acute therapy for hyperviscosity syndrome consists of plasmapheresis. However, plasmapheresis is a temporizing measure to avoid the acute complications of hyperviscosity, so therapy against the lymphoplasmacytic proliferative process is also indicated [35]. It should be emphasized that the size of the M protein per se or the beta-2-microglobulin level are not indications to begin chemotherapy in the absence of the previously mentioned indications for therapy.

There is no standard therapy for the treatment of symptomatic WM. Although several prospective trials have demonstrated the efficacy of various drugs or combination of agents, it is difficult to compare these agents on the basis of response rates. Few prospective randomized studies have been performed. An update on the treatment of WM has been published following the Fourth International Workshop on Waldenström's Macroglobulinemia [44]. A review on the diagnosis and management of WM has been published recently [45].

Rituximab

Rituximab, an anti-CD20 monoclonal antibody that is directed against an antigenic determinate (CD20) on the surface of lymphoid cells, was introduced over a decade ago [46]. Most physicians have incorporated rituximab as a single agent or combined with other agents in the initial treatment of WM. The toxicity profile is modest and it can be given in the presence of cytopenias. A transient increase in serum IgM level (IgM flare) occurs in about half of patients one to eight weeks following initiation of treatment. Delayed responses for six months or more may occur in patients treated with rituximab. Consequently, one should not re-institute additional therapy for at least six months. The standard dose of rituximab is $375\,mg/m^2$ weekly for four infusions (one cycle). Some physicians recommend plasmapheresis prior to institution of rituximab if the initial IgM value is high. Patients with minimal symptoms and a low tumor burden are reasonable candidates for single agent rituximab. There is no evidence that maintenance with rituximab is beneficial. Sixteen cases of rituximab-induced interstitial lung disease have been reported in the literature [47].

Rituximab plus other agents

Although higher response rates have been reported when rituximab has been combined with other agents, there are no solid data to support this approach. Outcomes of cyclophosphamide and prednisone; cyclophosphamide, vincristine, and prednisone; or cyclophosphamide, doxorubicin, vincristine, and prednisone (CHOP) combined with rituximab have been summarized [48]. No phase III studies comparing combinations of rituximab and other agents have been reported.

Seventy-two symptomatic WM patients were treated with dexamethasone (20 mg) intravenously, followed by rituximab (375 mg/m^2 IV on day 1) and cyclophosphamide (100 mg/m^2 orally bid. on days 1 to 5). This regimen was repeated every 21 days for six months. This resulted in a partial response in 67% and complete response in 7%. The two-year overall survival (OS) was 90% [49]. In a prospective randomized trial utilizing CHOP, with or without rituximab in 69 previously untreated patients with LPL, 48 fulfilled the criteria for WM. Rituximab plus CHOP produced an overall response of 94%, compared to 67% for CHOP only. Toxicities were similar in the two treatment groups [50].

Nucleoside analogs

Fludarabine: Fludarabine, a nucleoside analog, was first reported by Dimopoulous et al. [51] to be active in WM and produced responses in 8 of 26 patients (31%) who were resistant to prior therapy. The median duration of response in the absence of maintenance therapy was 38 months. In a group of 78 patients with low-grade lymphomas, including patients with WM and LPL, fludarabine produced a complete response in 15% and a median duration of response of 2.5 years [52]. Dhodapkar et al. [53] reported a complete response in 2% and a partial response in 34% of 182 patients treated with

fludarabine (30 mg/m^2 intravenously daily for five days) every four weeks for four cycles. The estimated five-year survival was 62% for previously untreated patients and 32% for previously treated patients. Leblond et al. [54] reported that 92 patients with primary resistant or relapsed WM after alkylating agent therapy were randomized to either 25 mg/m^2 fludarabine intravenously on days 1 through 5, or a combination of cyclophosphamide, doxorubicin (adriamycin), and prednisone (CAP) every four weeks for six cycles. Partial responses were obtained in 30% of patients receiving fludarabine and 11% receiving CAP, but OS was not different. There were no differences in the hematologic or infectious toxicities between the two regimens, but patients receiving CAP had more mucositis and alopecia. In a separate analysis of the study, the quality-adjusted time without symptoms or toxicity was 5.9 months longer with the fludarabine regimen than with the CAP group [55]. Fludarabine-based combination therapies for WM have been reviewed [56].

Cladribine: Cladribine produced a response in 22 (85%) of 26 patients with previously untreated, symptomatic WM [57]. Five patients relapsed during a median follow-up of 13 months, but all again responded to cladribine. Dimopoulous et al. [58] reported that 20 of 46 patients resistant to an alkylating agent and a glucocorticoid responded to cladribine. The median survival after treatment was 28 months. Only 22% of patients with refractory disease late in their course responded to cladribine. Liu et al. [59] reported that complete responses were obtained in 5% and partial responses in 50% of 20 patients with previously treated or untreated WM when given cladribine. Survival at a median follow-up of 1.7 years was 85%. The major toxicity was myelosuppression; 16% of patients had grade 3 or 4 neutropenia.

Cladribine also may be given subcutaneously. Forty-five patients with previously treated symptomatic WM received subcutaneous cladribine producing an overall response rate, including disease stabilization, in 68% [60]. Cladribine has also been given in combination with cyclophosphamide and prednisone for low-grade lymphoproliferative disorders. A complete response was achieved in 21%, and the overall response rate was 88% [61].

The main toxicities of fludarabine and cladribine are myelosuppression and immunosuppression resulting in an increased risk of infections. Thus, these agents should be avoided in patients who are potential candidates for stem cell transplant (SCT). The mortality rate may be as high as 5%. There is also a risk of transformation to more aggressive disease. A retrospective analysis of 439 patients with WM who had received a nucleoside analog (193) and 136 patients who did not receive nucleoside analogs or 110 patients who were observed without therapy revealed that 6.2% of patients receiving a nucleoside analog had a rate of transformation to an aggressive lymphoma, myelodysplasia or acute leukemia, compared to 0.4% of those not receiving a nucleoside analog after a median follow-up of five years [62].

Alkylating agents

Chlorambucil: Chlorambucil given continuously was reported as beneficial in four patients with WM 50 years ago [63]. In another report, 46 patients with symptomatic WM were randomized to receive 0.1 mg/kg chlorambucil daily or 0.3 mg/kg chlorambucil daily orally for seven days every six weeks. The criteria for response included ≥50% reduction of the serum M protein, increase in hemoglobin of 2 g/dL without transfusion, ≥50% decrease of urine M protein, or a reduction in size of the liver, spleen, or lymph nodes of 2 cm or more. Continuous chlorambucil therapy produced an objective response in 79%, by either reduction of serum M protein or increase in hemoglobin, while 68% given chlorambucil intermittently had a similar objective response. The size of the liver decreased by 2 cm or more in 55% of patients and the size of the spleen decreased 2 cm or more in 67%, while lymphadenopathy decreased in 71%. Acute leukemia or refractory anemia developed in four patients. Median survival was 5.4 years, but there was no difference between the two regimens [64]. In another study, intermittent oral chlorambucil therapy in 50 patients with WM produced a 92% response [65]. The dosage of chlorambucil must be altered depending on the leukocyte and platelet counts, which should be measured every two weeks. Treatment should be continued until the patient reaches a plateau state and then discontinued. If relapse occurs greater than six months after reaching a plateau state chlorambucil should be re-instituted.

Combinations of alkylating agents have also been reported as beneficial. In one study, responses to the combination of BCNU, cyclophosphamide, vincristine, melphalan, and prednisone (M2 protocol) were achieved in 27 of 33 symptomatic WM patients. Fifty-eight percent of patients were projected to be alive at 10 years. Annibali et al. [66] reported that melphalan, cyclophosphamide, and prednisone given daily on days 1 to 7 every 4 to 6 weeks for a maximum of 12 cycles, followed by chlorambucil and prednisone, produced response in 77% of 71 evaluable patients. Median OS was 5.5 years.

The use of alkylating agents may be associated with the development of myelodysplasia or acute leukemia. Rosner et al. [67] described 10 patients with WM in whom acute leukemia developed. Alkylating agents should also be avoided until stem cells have been collected in patients who are potential candidates for hematopoietic SCT.

Novel agents

Thalidomide produced a partial response in 3 of 10 patients with previously untreated WM and in 2 of 10 patients with previously treated WM. Only low doses of thalidomide were tolerated because of adverse side effects [68]. Thalidomide plus rituximab produced an overall response rate of 72% in 35 patients with symptomatic WM [69]. Eleven patients developed ≥grade 2 sensorimotor peripheral neuropathy. Bortezomib produced some response in 85% of 27 patients with relapsed or refractory symptomatic WM. The median time to progression was eight months [70]. A grade 3/4 sensory neuropathy occurred in 22%, but resolved in the majority after discontinuation of bortezomib. In another report, bortezomib produced a partial response in 26% of 27 patients [71]. Lenalidomide has been combined with rituximab, but the study was discontinued because of a fall in hemoglobin levels in the first week of therapy [72].

Autologous stem cell transplantation

There is limited experience with autologous or allogeneic SCT for symptomatic WM. Dreger et al. [73] reported that all seven patients with WM responded to an autologous SCT but immunofixation revealed a persistent M protein in five patients. There was no evidence of progression at 3 to 30 months. In another series of six patients with previously treated WM, an autologous SCT revealed a complete response in one and a partial response in the remainder. Four patients were event-free at 52, 15, 12, and 2 months after transplantation [74]. In another report of 10 patients receiving an autologous SCT, the three-year OS was 70% [75].

Allogenic SCT in 26 patients with WM resulted in an OS of only 45% at three years [75]. In a review of allogenic transplantation for WM, the treatment-related mortality was 27% [76].

Other therapy

Alpha-2 interferon has also been reported to be of benefit. In one study, 2 of 41 evaluable patients had a major response and six others had a minor response [77]. Pentostatin (2′-deoxycoformycin) has shown some activity in WM [78]. Splenectomy produced a complete response in two patients who were refractory to chemotherapy. Both were disease-free at 12 and 13 years after splenectomy [79]. Sildenafil [80] and Oblimersen, a BCL-2 antagonist [81] have shown some clinical activity, but further studies are needed. Perifosine is an oral alkyl phospholipid which produced a partial response in 2 of 21 patients with relapsed/refractory WM. A minimal response occurred in five (24%) additional patients [82]. RAD-001 (everolimus), an mTOR inhibitor, also shows activity in WM [83].

Course and prognosis

The median survival of 74 patients with WM from Sweden was seven years [84]. In our group of 71 patients, the median survival of WM was five years [36].

In a series of 167 patients with WM from a single institution, Facon et al. [85] reported a median survival of 60 months. Using multivariate regression analysis, a neutrophil value $<1.7 \times 10^9/L$, age >60 years, and hemoglobin $<10\,g/dL$ were the most important adverse prognostic factors for survival. In another report of prognostic factors in WM requiring therapy, multivariate analysis revealed that age >70 years, hemoglobin $<9\,g/dL$, and the presence or absence of weight loss or cryoglobulinemia were the most significant prognostic factors [86]. In a series of 232 French patients with WM ≥65 years, albumin $<4\,g/dL$ and the presence of one or more cytopenias were the major factors adversely affecting survival. The five-year OS was 87% in patients at low risk (≤1 adverse factor), 62% in those at intermediate risk (two adverse factors) and 25% in those at high risk (≥3 adverse factors) [87].

Dhodapkar et al. [88] developed a staging system for WM using serum beta-2-microglobulin level, hemoglobin value, and serum IgM concentration: Stage A (low risk) beta-2-microglobulin $<3\,mg/L$ and Hb $\geq12\,g/dL$; Stage B (medium risk) beta-2-microglobulin $<3\,mg/L$ and Hb $<12\,g/dL$; Stage C (medium risk) beta-2-microglobulin $\geq3\,mg/L$ and serum IgM $\geq4\,g/dL$; and Stage D (high risk) beta-2-microglobulin $\geq3\,mg/L$ and IgM $\geq4\,g/dL$ [88]. The five-year OS rates with Stage A, B, C, or D were 87, 63, 53, and 21%, respectively (Table 21.1). This cohort has been followed up at 10 years and an elevated serum lactate dehydrogenase (LDH) level has now been identified as an additional poor prognostic factor [88].

Ghobrial et al. [89] reported that age >65 years and organomegaly were associated with a poor

Table 21.1 Staging system for Waldenström's macroglobulinemia

Stage	Risk	Hgb, g/dL	β_2M	IgM, g/dL	5-year overall survival, %
A	Low	≥12	<3		87
B	Medium	<12	<3		63
C	Medium		≥3	≥4	53
D	High		≥3	≥4	21

prognosis in 337 symptomatic patients with WM. Patients with neither, one, or both of these adverse factors had 10-year estimated survival rates of 57, 16, and 5%, respectively. A beta-2-microglobulin level $\geq$4 mg/L, when added to this model, was associated with a three-fold increase in the risk of death.

The International Prognostic Staging System for WM (IPSS WM) was developed by Morel et al. [90] and based on 587 patients from seven international institutions. The significant adverse features were age >65 years, hemoglobin $\leq$11.5 g/dL, platelets $\leq$100 000 $\times$ 10^9/L, beta-2-microglobulin >3 mg/L, and serum IgM >7.0 g/dL. Low-risk patients were defined as being <65 years of age and having 0 or 1 risk factors. High-risk patients (35%) were those who had more than two risk factors, while intermediate-risk patients (38%) were those with two risk factors or those >age 65. Five-year OS rates for patients in the low-, intermediate-, and high-risk groups were 87, 68, and 36%, respectively (P<0.001).

Acknowledgment

This work was supported in part by Research Grant CA62242 and CA10747603 from the National Institutes of Health.

References

1 Waldenström J. (1944) Incipient myelomatosis or "essential" hyperglobulinemia with fibrinogenopenia: A new syndrome? *Acta Med Scand* **216**:433–4.

2 Fonseca R, Hayman S. (2007) Waldenström macroglobulinaemia. *Br J Haematol* **138**:700–20.

3 Dimopoulos MA, Kyle RA, Anagnostopoulos A, Treon SP. (2005) Diagnosis and management of Waldenström's macroglobulinemia. *J Clin Oncol* **23**:1564–77.

4 Groves FD, Travis LB, Devesa SS, Ries LA, Fraumeni JF, Jr., (1998) Waldenström's macroglobulinemia: incidence patterns in the United States, 1988–1994. *Cancer* **82**:1078–81.

5 Phekoo KJ, Jack RH, Davies E, Moller H, Schey SA. (2008) The incidence and survival of Waldenström's macroglobulinaemia in South East England. *Leuk Res* **32**:55–9.

6 Linet MS, Humphrey RL, Mehl ES, et al. (1993) A case-control and family study of Waldenström's macroglobulinemia. *Leukemia* **7**:1363–9.

7 Giordano TP, Henderson L, Landgren O, et al. (2007) Risk of non-Hodgkin lymphoma and lymphoproliferative precursor diseases in US veterans with hepatitis C virus. *JAMA* **297**:2010–7.

8 Koshiol J, Gridley G, Engels EA, McMaster ML, Landgren O. (2008) Chronic immune stimulation and subsequent Waldenström macroglobulinemia. *Arch Intern Med* **168**:1903–9.

9 Blattner WA, Garber JE, Mann DL, et al. (1980) Waldenström's macroglobulinemia and autoimmune disease in a family. *Ann Intern Med* **93**:830–2.

10 Renier G, Ifrah N, Chevailler A, et al. (1989) Four brothers with Waldenström's macroglobulinemia. *Cancer* **64**:1554–9.

11 McMaster ML, Csako G, Giambarresi TR, et al. (2007) Long-term evaluation of three multiple-case Waldenström macroglobulinemia families. *Clin Cancer Res* **13**:5063–9.

12 Kristinsson SY, Bjorkholm M, Goldin LR, et al. (2008) Risk of lymphoproliferative disorders among first-degree relatives of lymphoplasmacytic lymphoma/Waldenström macroglobulinemia patients: a population-based study in Sweden. *Blood* **112**:3052–6.

13 Schop RF, Jalal SM, Van Wier SA, et al. (2002) Deletions of 17p13.1 and 13q14 are uncommon in Waldenström macroglobulinemia clonal cells and mostly seen at the time of disease progression. *Cancer Genet Cytogenet* **132**:55–60.

14 Schop RF, Kuehl WM, Van Wier SA, et al. (2002) Waldenström macroglobulinemia neoplastic cells lack immunoglobulin heavy chain locus translocations but have frequent 6q deletions. *Blood* **100**:2996–3001.

15 Braggio E, Keats JJ, Leleu X, et al. (2009) Identification of copy number abnormalities and inactivating mutations in two negative regulators of nuclear factor-kappaB signaling pathways in Waldenström's macroglobulinemia. *Cancer Res* **69**:3579–88.

16 Gutierrez NC, Ocio EM, de Las Rivas J, et al. (2007) Gene expression profiling of B lymphocytes and plasma cells from Waldenström's macroglobulinemia: comparison with expression patterns of the same cell counterparts from chronic lymphocytic leukemia, multiple myeloma and normal individuals. *Leukemia* **21**:541–9.

17 Ditzel Santos D, Ho AW, Tournilhac O, et al. (2007) Establishment of BCWM.1 cell line for Waldenström's macroglobulinemia with productive in vivo engraftment in SCID-hu mice. *Exp Hematol* **35**:1366–75.

18 Logothetis J, Silverstein P, Coe J. (1960) Neurologic aspects of Waldenström's macroglobulinemia: report of a case. *Arch Neurol* **3**:564–73.

19 Garcia-Sanz R, Montoto S, Torrequebrada A, et al. (2001) Waldenström's macroglobulinaemia: presenting features and outcome in a series with 217 cases. *Br J Haematol* **115**:575–82.

20 Kelly JJ, Kyle RA, Latov N. (1987) *Polyneuropathies associated with plasma cell dyscrasias.* Boston: Martinus Nijhoff.

21 Nobile-Orazio E, Marmiroli P, Baldini L, et al. (1987) Peripheral neuropathy in macroglobulinemia: incidence and antigen-specificity of M proteins. *Neurology* **37**:1506–14.

22 Dalakas MC, Flaum MA, Rick M, Engel WK, Gralnick HR. (1983) Treatment of polyneuropathy in Waldenström's macroglobulinemia: role of paraproteinemia and immunologic studies. *Neurology* **33**:1406–10.

23 Gertz MA, Kyle RA, Noel P. (1993) Primary systemic amyloidosis: a rare complication of immunoglobulin M monoclonal gammopathies and Waldenström's macroglobulinemia. *J Clin Oncol* **11**:914–20.

24 Terrier B, Jaccard A, Harousseau JL, et al. (2008) The clinical spectrum of IgM-related amyloidosis: a French nationwide retrospective study of 72 patients. *Medicine (Baltimore)* **87**:99–109.

25 Abad S, Zagdanski AM, Brechignac S, et al. (1999) Neurolymphomatosis in Waldenström's macroglobulinaemia. *Br J Haematol* **106**:100–3.

26 Scheithauer BW, Rubinstein LJ, Herman MM. (1984) Leukoencephalopathy in Waldenström's macroglobulinemia: immunohistochemical and electron microscopic observations. *J Neuropath Exp Neur* **43**:408–25.

27 Syms MJ, Arcila ME, Holtel MR. (2001) Waldenström's macroglobulinemia and sensorineural hearing loss. *Am J Otolaryngol* **22**:349–53.

28 Tsuji M, Ochiai S, Taka T, et al. (1990) Nonamyloidotic nephrotic syndrome in Waldenström's macroglobulinemia. *Nephron* **54**:176–8.

29 Winterbauer RH, Riggins RC, Griesman FA, Bauermeister DE. (1974) Pleuropulmonary manifestations of Waldenström's macroglobulinemia. *Chest* **66**:368–75.

30 Moulopoulos LA, Dimopoulos MA, Varma DG, et al. (1993) Waldenström macroglobulinemia: MR imaging of the spine and CT of the abdomen and pelvis. *Radiology* **188**:669–73.

31 Schnitzler L, Schubert B, Boasson M, Gardais J, Tourmen A. (1974) Urticaire chronique, lésions osseuses, macroglobulinémie IgM: Maladie de Waldenström? *Bulletin de la Socíefe Française de Dermatologie et de Syphiligraphie* **81**:363.

32 Letendre L, Kyle RA. (1982) Monoclonal cryoglobulinemia with high thermal insolubility. *Mayo Clin Proc* **57**:629–33.

33 Perkins HA, MacKenzie MR, Fudenberg HH. (1970) Hemostatic defects in dysproteinemias. *Blood* **35**:695–707.

34 Riches PG, Sheldon J, Smith AM, Hobbs JR. (1991) Overestimation of monoclonal immunoglobulin by immunochemical methods. *Ann Clin Biochem* **28**:253–9.

35 Kyle RA, Treon SP, Alexanian R, et al. (2003) Prognostic markers and criteria to initiate therapy in Waldenström's macroglobulinemia: consensus panel recommendations from the Second International Workshop on Waldenström's Macroglobulinemia. [Review] [17 refs]. *Semin Oncol* **30**:116–20.

36 Kyle RA, Garton JP. (1987) The spectrum of IgM monoclonal gammopathy in 430 cases. *Mayo Clin Proc* **62**:719–31.

37 Bannick EG, Greene CH. (1929) Renal insufficiency associated with Bence-Jones proteinuria: report of thirteen cases with a note on the changes in the serum proteins. *Arch Intern Med* **44**:486–501.

38 Fahey JL, Barth WF, Solomon A. (1965) Serum hyperviscosity syndrome. *JAMA* **192**:464–7.

39 Gertz MA, Kyle RA. (1995) Hyperviscosity syndrome. [Review] [138 refs]. *J Intensive Care Med* **10**:128–41.

40 Andriko JA, Aguilera NS, Chu WS, Nandedkar MA, Cotelingam JD. (1997) Waldenström's macroglobulinemia: a clinicopathologic study of 22 cases. *Cancer* **80**:1926–35.

41 Kyle RA, Therneau TM, Rajkumar SV, et al. (2003) Long-term follow-up of IgM monoclonal gammopathy of undetermined significance. *Blood* **102**:3759–64.

42 Avet-Loiseau H, Garand R, Lode L, Harousseau JL, Bataille R. (2003) Translocation t(11;14)(q13;q32) is the hallmark of IgM, IgE, and nonsecretory multiple myeloma variants. *Blood* **101**:1570–1.

43 Maldonado JE, Kyle RA, Brown AL, Jr., Bayrd ED. (1966) "Intermediate" cell types and mixed cell proliferation in multiple myeloma: electron microscopic observations. *Blood* **27**:212–26.

44 Dimopoulos MA, Gertz MA, Kastritis E, et al. (2009) Update on treatment recommendations from the Fourth International Workshop on Waldenström's Macroglobulinemia. *J Clin Oncol* **27**:120–6.

45 Ansell SM, Kyle RA, Reeder CB, et al. (2010) Diagnosis and management of Waldenström's macroglobulinemia: Mayo stratification of macroglobulinemia and risk-adapted therapy (mSMART) guidelines. *Mayo Clin Proc* **85**:824–33.

46 Byrd JC, White CA,Link B, et al. Rituximab therapy in Waldenström's macroglobulinemia: preliminary evidence in clinical activity. *Ann Oncol* **10**:1525–7, 1999.

47 Wagner SA, Mehta AC, Laber DA. (2007) Rituximab-induced interstitial lung disease. *Am J Hematol* **82**:916–9.

48 Ioakimidis L, Patterson CJ, Hunter ZR, et al. (2009) Comparative outcomes following CP-R, CVP-R, and CHOP-R in Waldenström's macroglobulinemia. *Clin Lymphoma Myeloma* **9**:62–6.

49 Dimopoulos MA, Anagnostopoulos A, Kyrtsonis MC, et al. (2007) Primary treatment of Waldenström's macroglobulinemia with dexamethasone, rituximab, and cyclophosphamide. *J Clin Oncol* **25**:3344–9.

50 Buske C, Hoster E, Dreyling M, et al. (2009) The addition of rituximab to front-line therapy with CHOP (R-CHOP) results in a higher response rate and longer time to treatment failure in patients with lymphoplasmacytic lymphoma: results of a randomized trial of the German Low-Grade Lymphoma Study Group (GLSG). *Leukemia* **23**:153–61.

51 Dimopoulos MA, O'Brien S, Kantarjian H, et al. (1993) Fludarabine therapy in Waldenström's macroglobulinemia. *Am J Med* **95**:49–52.

52 Foran JM, Rohatiner AZ, Coiffier B, et al. (1999) Multicenter phase II study of fludarabine phosphate for patients with newly diagnosed lymphoplasmacytoid lymphoma, Waldenström's macroglobulinemia, and mantle-cell lymphoma. *J Clin Oncol* **17**:546–53.

53 Dhodapkar MV, Jacobson JL, Gertz MA, et al. (2001) Prognostic factors and response to fludarabine therapy in patients with Waldenström macroglobulinemia: results of United States intergroup trial (Southwest Oncology Group S9003). *Blood* **98**:41–8.

54 Leblond V, Levy V, Maloisel F, et al. (2001) Multicenter, randomized comparative trial of fludarabine and the combination of cyclophosphamide-doxorubicin-

prednisone in 92 patients with Waldenström macroglobulinemia in first relapse or with primary refractory disease. *Blood* **98**:2640–4.

55 Levy V, Porcher R, Leblond V, et al. (2001) Evaluating treatment strategies in advanced Waldenström macroglobulinemia: use of quality-adjusted survival analysis. *Leukemia* **15**:1466–70.

56 Tedeschi A, Alamos SM, Ricci F, Greco A, Morra E. (2009) Fludarabine-based combination therapies for Waldenström's macroglobulinemia. *Clin Lymphoma Myeloma* **9**:67–70.

57 Dimopoulos MA, Kantarjian H, Weber D, et al. (1994) Primary therapy of Waldenström's macroglobulinemia with 2-chlorodeoxyadenosine. *J Clin Oncol* **12**:2694–8.

58 Dimopoulos MA, Weber D, Delasalle KB, Keating M, Alexanian R. (1995) Treatment of Waldenström's macroglobulinemia resistant to standard therapy with 2-chlorodeoxyadenosine: identification of prognostic factors. *Ann Oncol* **6**:49–52.

59 Liu ES, Burian C, Miller WE, Saven A. (1998) Bolus administration of cladribine in the treatment of Waldenström macroglobulinaemia. *Br J Haematol* **103**:690–5.

60 Betticher DC, Hsu Schmitz SF, Ratschiller D, et al. (1997) Cladribine (2-CDA) given as subcutaneous bolus injections is active in pretreated Waldenström's macroglobulinaemia. Swiss Group for Clinical Cancer Research (SAKK). *Br J Haematol* **99**:358–63.

61 Laurencet FM, Zulian GB, Guetty-Alberto M, et al. (1999) Cladribine with cyclophosphamide and prednisone in the management of low-grade lymphoproliferative malignancies. *Br J Cancer* **79**:1215–9.

62 Leleu X, Soumerai J, Roccaro A, et al. (2009) Increased incidence of transformation and myelodysplasia/acute leukemia in patients with Waldenström macroglobulinemia treated with nucleoside analogs. *J Clin Oncol* **27**:250–5.

63 Bayrd ED. (1961) Continuous chlorambucil therapy in primary macroglobulinemia of Waldenström: report of four cases. *Proc Staff Meet Mayo Clin* **36**:135–47.

64 Kyle RA, Greipp PR, Gertz MA, et al. (2000) Waldenström's macroglobulinaemia: a prospective study comparing daily with intermittent oral chlorambucil. *Br J Haematol* **108**:737–42.

65 Kyrtsonis MC, Vassilakopoulos TP, Angelopoulou MK, et al. (2001) Waldenström's macroglobulinemia: clinical course and prognostic factors in 60 patients: experience from a single hematology unit. *Ann Hematol* **80**:722–7.

66 Annibali O, Petrucci MT, Martini V, et al. (2005) Treatment of 72 newly diagnosed Waldenström macroglobulinemia cases with oral melphalan, cyclophosphamide, and prednisone: results and cost analysis. *Cancer* **103**:582–7.

67 Rosner F, Grunwald HW. (1980) Multiple myeloma and Waldenström's macroglobulinemia terminating in acute leukemia: review with emphasis on karyotypic and ultrastructural abnormalities. *NY State J Med* **80**:558–70.

68 Dimopoulos MA, Zomas A, Viniou NA, et al. (2001) Treatment of Waldenström's macroglobulinemia with thalidomide. *J Clin Oncol* **19**:3596–601.

69 Treon SP, Soumerai JD, Branagan AR, et al. (2008) Thalidomide and rituximab in Waldenström macroglobulinemia. *Blood* **112**:4452–7.

70 Treon SP, Hunter ZR, Matous J, et al. (2007) Multicenter clinical trial of bortezomib in relapsed/refractory Waldenström's macroglobulinemia: results of WMCTG Trial 03-248. *Clin Cancer Res* **13**:3320–5.

71 Chen CI, Kouroukis CT, White D, et al. (2007) Bortezomib is active in patients with untreated or relapsed Waldenström's macroglobulinemia: a phase II study of the National Cancer Institute of Canada Clinical Trials Group. *J Clin Oncol* **25**:1570–5.

72 Treon SP, Soumerai JD, Branagan AR, et al. (2009) Lenalidomide and rituximab in Waldenström's macroglobulinemia. *Clin Cancer Res* **15**:355–60.

73 Dreger P, Glass B, Kuse R, et al. (1999) Myeloablative radiochemotherapy followed by reinfusion of purged autologous stem cells for Waldenström's macroglobulinaemia. *Br J Haematol* **106**:115–8.

74 Desikan R, Dhodapkar M, Siegel D, et al. (1999) High-dose therapy with autologous haemopoietic stem cell support for Waldenström's macroglobulinaemia. *Br J Haematol* **105**:993–6.

75 Anagnostopoulos A, Hari PN, Perez WS, et al. (2006) Autologous or allogeneic stem cell transplantation in patients with Waldenström's macroglobulinemia. *Biol Blood Marrow Transplant* **12**:845–54.

76 Kyriakou C, Canals C, Taghipour G, et al. (2007) Allogeneic stem cell transplantation in Waldenström's macroglobulinemia: an analysis of 106 cases from the European Bone Marrow Registry. *Haematologica* **92**:WM3.9.

77 Rotoli B, De Renzo A, Frigeri F, et al. (1994) A phase II trial on alpha-interferon (alpha IFN) effect in patients with monoclonal IgM gammopathy. *Leuk Lymphoma* **13**:463–9.

78 Riddell S, Johnston JB, Rayner HL, Israels LG. (1986) Response of Waldenström's macroglobulinemia to pentostatin (2′-deoxycoformycin). *Cancer Treat Rep* **70**:546–8.

79 Humphrey JS, Conley CL. (1995) Durable complete remission of macroglobulinemia after splenectomy: a report of two cases and review of the literature. *Am J Hematol* **48**:262–6.

80 Treon SP, Tournilhac O, Branagan AR, et al. (2004) Clinical responses to sildenafil in Waldenström's macroglobulinemia. *Clin Lymphoma* **5**:205–7.

81 Gertz MA, Geyer SM, Badros A, Kahl BS, Erlichman C. (2005) Early results of a phase I trial of oblimersen sodium for relapsed or refractory Waldenström's macroglobulinemia. *Clin Lymphoma* **5**:282–4.

82 Ghobrial I, Leleu X, Rubin N, et al. (2007) Phase II trial of perifosine (KRX-0401) in relapsed and/or refractory Waldenström macroglobulinemia: preliminary results. *Blood* **110**:Abstract 4493.

83 Ghobrial I, Leduc R, Nelson M, et al. (2007) Phase II trial of the oral mTOR inhibitor RAD001 (Everolimus) in relapsed and/or refractory Waldenström macroglobulinemia: preliminary results. *Blood* **110**:Abstract 4496.

84 Waldenström JG. (1980) The prognosis of myeloma and macroglobulinemia. *Ann Life Insurance Med* **6**:93–8.

85 Facon T, Brouillard M, Duhamel A, et al. (1993) Prognostic factors in Waldenström's macroglobulinemia: a report of 167 cases. *J Clin Oncol* **11**:1553–8.

86 Gobbi PG, Bettini R, Montecucco C, et al. (1994) Study of prognosis in Waldenström's macroglobulinemia: a proposal for a simple binary classification with clinical and investigational utility. *Blood* **83**:2939–45.

87 Morel P, Monconduit M, Jacomy D, et al. (2000) Prognostic factors in Waldenström macroglobulinemia: a report on 232 patients with the description of a new scoring system and its validation on 253 other patients. *Blood* **96**:852–8.

88 Dhodapkar MV, Hoering A, Gertz MA, et al. (2009) Long-term survival in Waldenström macroglobulinemia: 10-year follow-up of Southwest Oncology Group-directed intergroup trial S9003. *Blood* **113**:793–6.

89 Ghobrial IM, Fonseca R, Gertz MA, et al. (2006) Prognostic model for disease-specific and overall mortality in newly diagnosed symptomatic patients with Waldenström macroglobulinaemia. *Br J Haematol* **133**:158–64.

90 Morel P, Duhamel A, Gobbi P, et al. (2009) International prognostic scoring system for Waldenström macroglobulinemia. *Blood* **113**:4163–70.

CHAPTER 22
Primary Systemic Amyloidosis (AL)

Efstathios Kastritis and Meletios Athanasios Dimopoulos
Department of Clinical Therapeutics, University of Athens School of Medicine, Athens, Greece

Introduction

The term amyloidosis encompasses a spectrum of diseases caused by the extracellular accumulation of insoluble amyloid fibrils that are formed by "misfolded" proteins or protein residues. These "amyloidogenic" proteins tend to acquire a specific 3D conformation that facilitates their polymerization and fibril formation. At least 24 different proteins have been shown to form amyloid deposits, but with different patterns of organ involvement and clinical background. In primary systemic (AL) amyloidosis, the amyloid fibrils are composed of the N-terminal of a monoclonal immunoglobulin light chain that is produced by a plasma cell clone; rarely a fragment of an immunoglobulin heavy chain may also form amyloid fibrils [1, 2]. Organ dysfunction results from the accumulation of amyloid fibrils that disrupt tissue architecture and organ function; every organ except CNS can be affected. Although AL amyloidosis is the most common form of amyloidosis in the Western world, it is a rare disorder with an incidence of about 8–12 per million persons per year, about five times less common than multiple myeloma. Up to 25% of myeloma patients can also have identifiable immunoglobulin light chain amyloid in tissue biopsies.

Pathophysiology

Amyloid fibrils are non-branching polypeptide strands, where the precursor protein (the N-fragment of a monoclonal light chain, which includes the variable region of the immunoglobulin) is in a predominantly antiparallel b-sheet secondary structure. In the b-sheet structure, amino acid residues are connected laterally by hydrogen bonds forming a Z-like pleated sheet that facilitates their segregation and formation of polymers. Secreted amyloidogenic light chains escape the cell's mechanism of "quality" control, undergo limited proteolysis, initially form oligomers and finally fibrils that are deposited in the microcirculation. The most important determinant of proteins' conformation is their amino acid sequence, but post-translational modifications (glycosylation etc.) may alter the final three-dimensional structure of a protein. Local concentrations of the amyloidogenic proteins, local environmental factors (such as pH, oxidation, temperature, ions, osmolytes) and extracellular matrix also play a critical role in amyloid formation. Not all light chains have the same ability to form amyloid. Unlike myeloma, lambda light chains are more common ($\varkappa/\lambda$ ratio is 1:3). Specific V_L genes (coding the variable region of the immunoglobulin) are significantly more commonly used in amyloidogenic light chains than other V_L genes. Organ specificity has also been suggested for certain V_L genes [3]. Some Light Chain dimers (more commonly by lambda light chains) can have some antibody-binding activity and may recognize specific epitopes, playing a role in tissue specificity. A direct cytotoxic effect has also been suggested for some immunoglobulin light chains [4].

Advances in Malignant Hematology, First Edition. Edited by Hussain I. Saba and Ghulam J. Mufti. © 2011 Blackwell Publishing Ltd.
Published 2011 by Blackwell Publishing Ltd.

Clinical presentation

The spectrum of the disease's presentation is related to the pattern of amyloid organ involvement. Patients may present with symptoms and signs from one or several organ systems; non-specific symptoms (such as fatigue, breathlessness, weight loss) can sometimes be the only initial symptoms [1, 5] (Table 22.1). Kidneys (in about 75%) and heart (in about 50–70%) are most commonly involved, followed by liver and peripheral nervous system [1, 5]. Patients with nephrotic range proteinuria may present with peripheral edema, weight gain and, less often, with rapidly deteriorating renal function. Patients with symptomatic cardiac involvement usually present due to fatigue and exertional dyspnea or peripheral edema. Liver involvement may manifest as right upper quadrant fullness, sometimes accompanied by early satiation due to compression of the stomach by a massively enlarged liver. Peripheral neuropathy is common, usually symmetric, sensory and often painful; patients complain of numbness, tingling, burning or pain of the legs. Orthostatic hypotension may be due to congestive heart failure (CHF) or concomitant autonomic neuropathy. Other manifestations

Table 22.1 Organ involvement and clinical syndromes in patients with AL amyloidosis

Involved organ	Clinical syndrome	Symptoms
Heart	Congestive heart failure/ restrictive cardiomyopathy	Dyspnea on exercise, peripheral edema, fatigue, hypotension.
Kidneys	Nephrotic syndrome	Peripheral edema, anasarca, hypotension.
Liver	Liver enlargement, liver failure (uncommon)	Upper-right quadrant fullness, palpable liver, early satiety.
Peripheral nerve	Peripheral sensory neuropathy, CIDP[a]-like syndrome	Paresthesias, numbness, tingling, pain.
Autonomic neuropathy	Dysautonomia	Blurred vision, dry eyes/mouth, sweating, heat intolerance, cold hands and feet with discoloration, light-headedness, dizziness, shoulder aching resulting from orthostatic hypotension, nausea, vomiting, bloating, early satiety, abdominal colic, incontinence, or alternating diarrhea and constipation, voiding dysfunction, sexual dysfunction.
Soft tissue	Macroglossia	Hoarseness, voice change, submandibular swelling.
	Salivary gland infiltration	Xerostomia.
	Articular enlargement	Carpal tunnel syndrome, "shoulder pad" sign.
	Lymph node enlargement	
	Vascular amyloid	
	Muscle pseudohypertrophy	May manifest as claudication of the limbs or jaw.
GI	Altered bowel movement, malabsorption	Diarrhea, steatorrhea, bleeding due to "fragile mucosa".

[a] CIDP: chronic inflammatory demyelinating polyneuropathy

of autonomic neuropathy may include diarrhea or constipation, bladder or erectile dysfunction. Involvement of the GI tract may be associated with symptoms of malabsorption such as diarrhea, weight loss, or signs and symptoms of vitamin deprivation. Specific signs are not very common (10–15% of patients), however when present they greatly increase the suspicion of the disease. Macroglossia, usually documented by the dental prints on the side of the tongue, may be massive. Amyloid purpura around the orbits (raccoon eyes) is characteristic but can also found in other sites such as the neck, hands, and feet. Shoulder joint enlargement due to amyloid deposition upon articular cartilages (shoulder pad sign) is quite specific but rather rare. Lymph nodes or salivary glands may also be enlarged by amyloid infiltration. Nail changes, alopecia, and skin amyloidomas are rare manifestations.

Laboratory and imaging features

A monoclonal immunoglobulin, which in about 40–50% of cases is only a monoclonal light chain, is almost always found when all assays (electrophoresis and immunofixation electrophoresis of serum, urine, and serum-free light chains (FLC)) are performed [5]. Typical AL patients do not have features of symptomatic myeloma, such as bone osteolysis, and hypercalcemia. Anemia is uncommon and, if present, an etiology different to that of AL amyloidosis should be investigated, such as concurrent myeloma, renal disease-associated anemia, or GI hemorrhage. Howell-Jolly bodies may be found in the peripheral blood in patients with extensive amyloidosis. Renal failure is not common at initial presentation; however, in about 20% of patients with renal involvement, renal function may rapidly deteriorate due to involvement of renal vessels by amyloid [6]. The hallmark of renal amyloidosis is non-selective proteinuria that can sometimes reach up to 20–30 g/day; massive proteinuria in a middle-aged non-diabetic patient should always raise suspicions of amyloidosis. In urine electrophoresis, albumin dominates with a usually small spike in the gamma region where monoclonal light chains run. Renal ultrasonography may reveal kidneys of increased size even in patients with end-stage renal disease (ESRD). Liver involvement is predominantly associated with elevation of alkaline phosphatase and γGT and only in late stages may AST and ALT be increased. Bilirubin is usually normal; a bilirubin above 2.5 mg/dL in a patient with liver involvement is associated with an extremely poor outcome [7]. Other laboratory abnormalities include low ferritin, B12, serum iron, vitamin D, etc. which may be associated with malabsorption. Levels of factor X may be low due to its trapping within the amyloid deposits. In patients with cardiac involvement, serum NT-proBNP or BNP and cardiac troponins (troponin-T or –I) are usually elevated (either or both). Their levels are influenced by renal function but, in general, NT-proBNP above 332 ng/ml and troponin-T above 0.035 ng/ml are associated with poor outcome, especially for patients in whom both cardiobiomarkers are elevated [8]. The most common ECG abnormality is low-voltage (<5 mm) QRS complexes in the limb leads with signs of hypertrophy in precordial leads with ST abnormalities that may include ST elevation or depression, even mimicking ischemia. Typical echocardiographic findings are of a restrictive cardiomyopathy pattern. Usually a thickened intraventricular septum and posterior wall of the left ventricle, right ventricular free wall thickening and diastolic dysfunction are found. Reduction of the ejection fraction is a late event. However, several conditions, especially age and hypertension, may be associated with cardiac hypertrophy and diastolic dysfunction, and the interpretation of echocardiography should be made carefully [9]. Twenty-four hour Holter monitoring may reveal rhythm and conduction abnormalities and should be performed in all patients with heart involvement [9, 10]. In advanced cardiac amyloidosis, cardiac MRI typically shows global subendocardial late gadolinium enhancement and associated abnormal myocardial and blood-pool gadolinium kinetics that may occasionally be confused as "artifact". In cardiac catheterization, a restrictive pattern of impaired ventricular filling with elevated left ventricular end-diastolic pressure and a "dip-and-plateau" waveform may be seen in advanced cardiac amyloidosis [9] (Table 22.2).

Table 22.2 Initial diagnostic work up and risk stratification procedures

		Test	Comments
Hematologic assessment		Serum and urine electrophoresis and immunofixation electrophoresis, serum-free light chains (FLCs-Freelite assay)	Serial assessment during treatment and post-treatment follow-up. Assessment of response by electrophoresis is often difficult due to the small size of M-spike in most AL patients. FLCs can be used for the response assessment in patients without measurable disease by electrophoresis.
Assessment of organ involvement	Kidney	24h urine protein, serum creatinine, serum urea, serum albumin	Kidney involvement is defined as proteinuria of at least 0.5 g/day, which should be predominantly albumin. Other causes of proteinuria should be excluded.
			24h urine protein should be followed during treatment and follow-up. At least 50% decrease (of at least 0.5 g/day) is considered a renal response while creatinine and creatinine clearance must not worsen by 25% over baseline.
	Cardiac	Echocardiography with Doppler studies and strain echo	Inter-observer variability is a significant issue in echocardiography – a decrease of at least 2 mm in mean left ventricular wall thickness or symptomatic improvement of two New York Heart Association classes without increase in diuretics, if wall thickness has not increased are considered as cardiac responses.
		ECG	
		24-hour Holter study	
		Cardiac troponins (−T or −I)	Cardiac biomarkers accompany hematologic response and correlate with functional status, especially in patients with normal renal function.
		NT-proBNP (or BNP) Assessment of functional status (NYHA class, cardiopulmonary studies)	
	Liver	Abdominal ultrasound (or CT/MRI)	Liver enlargement may be due to CHF and right-sided stasis.
		Alkaline phosphatase, gGT, AST, ALT, total and direct bilirubin, prothrombin time	
	GI tract	Serum albumin, serum B12, ferritin, folic acid, lipid profile	Patients with symptomatic GI tract involvement will have diarrhea, motility disturbances, and weight loss that strongly resemble autonomic failure. Nearly 80% of patients who undergo an endoscopic biopsy will demonstrate vascular only amyloid deposits biopsy. These deposits are asymptomatic and should not be considered evidence of intestinal organ involvement for the purpose of counting the number of organs involved.

ECG: electrocardiography; NT-proBNP: N-terminal of the Brain Natriuretic Peptide; NYHA: New York Heart Association functional class; CHF: congestive heart failure; GI: gastro-intestinal; CT: computed tomography; MRI: magnetic resonance imaging

Diagnosis

The identification of a monoclonal protein in the serum and/or urine of a patient with symptoms and signs as above should raise the suspicion of AL amyloidosis. A correct diagnosis may be difficult and cannot be based only on clinical findings. AL amyloidosis must always be confirmed with a Congo red positive-stained biopsy specimen and a monoclonal light chain should be identified as the amyloidogenic protein. Imaging with technetium-labeled aprotinin or iodinated serum amyloid P (SAP) do not provide diagnosis but only estimates of amyloid deposits. Fat aspiration for Congo red staining is an easy, risk-free procedure with sensitivity of about 70–80% in patients with high suspicion for AL amyloidosis. Other sites such as the rectum or gum are also easily accessible. A bone marrow biopsy may be helpful by establishing the presence of a monoclonal plasma cell dyscrasia, while the presence of amyloid within the bone marrow greatly increases the possibility that it is of the AL type [11]. The plasma cell clone is usually small (median being 7% of monoclonal plasma cells). Biopsy of involved organs such as kidneys, liver or heart is highly sensitive, however not always necessary. Consideration of increased risk of bleeding in AL patients undergoing renal biopsy has not been confirmed, in retrospective study at highly experienced centers [12].

Almost all patients have a demonstrable clonal plasma cell dyscrasia but most AL patients produce rather small amounts of monoclonal proteins, thus routine serum or urine electrophoresis may not show a monoclonal protein. Therefore, an immunofixation electrophoresis (IFE) is required in all cases (the sensitivity of serum IFE is 70–75% and urine IFE is 75–85%). In patients with initially negative results and strong suspicion for AL, a repeat immunofixation may also be required with undiluted antisera or with high-resolution IFE [13]. All patients should also have an immunonephelometric immunoglobulin serum-FLC assay which quantitates free light chains and identifies an abnormal kappa:lambda ratio in 76–92% of patients [13]. When all three assays (serum and urine IFE, and serum-FLCs) are performed, sensitivity for the documentation of a monoclonal protein is 99% [13]. Although

immunohistochemistry for κ and λ immunoglobulin light chains in amyloid deposits is specific, it is not as sensitive. Antisera to amyloid A (AA), and anti-transthyretin are quite specific and sensitive and, when combined with light chain immunohistochemistry, can recognize most types of amyloid. Electron and immunoelectron microscopy and mass spectrometry have been used successfully but are not widely available. Genetic studies may be used to exclude the presence of a known amyloidogenic genetic mutation in transthyretin, apolipoprotein A-I (APOA1), apolipoprotein A-II (APOA2), lysozyme, fibrinogen, etc. as the cause of amyloidosis.

Cytogenetics/chromosomal abnormalities

Plasma cell dyscrasias are characterized by non-random chromosomal abnormalities involving numerical and structural changes, such as deletions, duplications and translocations (specifically involving chromosome 14q), and are better identified by interphase FISH. Numerical and structural abnormalities are common in AL and are probably found in a similar frequency to those of MGUS. At least one chromosomal abnormality can be detected in up to 95% of AL patients when studied with FISH [14]. Translocation t(11;14) is the most common in AL (in 39–47%) and, although it is considered prognostically "neutral" in myeloma, may be associated with poor outcome in AL patients [15]. Other frequent aberrations include deletion of *13q14*, gain of *1q21* while translocations t(4;14) (in 0–14%), t(14;16) (in 0–4%) and deletion 17p (p53), which are associated with poor outcome in myeloma, are rarely found in AL [14–17]. There is no evidence of correlation of cytogenetic abnormalities with any clinical characteristics or the pattern of organ involvement in AL [14]. Gene expression studies have revealed that plasma cells from AL patients have a significantly different molecular profile than those of MM patients [18].

Differential diagnosis

The symptoms of amyloidosis are multisystemic and often vague; formulation of the correct differential diagnosis may be difficult and requires a certain degree of suspicion. Patients with localized AL amyloidosis, usually found accidentally after biopsy for a tumor-like finding, should not be treated for systemic AL amyloidosis. Correctly classifying the amyloid as being of AL type is critical [1, 5]. All forms of amyloid are Congo red-positive but not all patients with amyloidosis and a plasma cell disorder have AL amyloidosis. Some patients with an intact serum monoclonal immunoglobulin molecule without evidence of circulating FLCs in the serum (normal levels of FLCs and normal ratio) or in the urine may actually have another type of amyloidosis (such as familial, AA, or senile) and a coexistent MGUS (about 3% of individuals over the age of 60 have MGUS). Patients with myeloma usually present with bone lesions, hypercalcemia, anemia, and acute renal impairment while the plasma cell clone is more extensive. Identification of myeloma patients who have symptomatic amyloid organ involvement may help these patients to avoid excess toxicity associated with aggressive antimyeloma treatments. For example, a cardiac ultrasound and cardiobiomarkers can be helpful in a patient suspected of having cardiac involvement, while a simple abdominal fat aspirate can confirm the diagnosis of amyloidosis. In patients presenting with nephrotic range proteinuria, in which a monoclonal light chain is identified, light chain deposition disease (LCDD) should also be considered. In this plasma cell dyscrasia, light chains form glomerular non-amyloid (thus Congo red-negative) granular deposits. These patients usually present with more elevated serum creatinine and hypertension but heart and liver may also be involved. A Congo red-positive fat aspiration would confirm amyloidosis, but in the case of Congo red negativity, a renal biopsy may be indicated for the correct diagnosis. In patients presenting with peripheral neuropathy in whom a monoclonal gammopathy is found, amyloid should be excluded before they are diagnosed as having MGUS-associated neuropathy.

Treatment

As there is no proven effective therapy that acts directly on amyloid fibrils, treatment is directed at the plasma cell clone; supportive therapy for AL patients is also as important (Table 22.3). The aim of treatment is the reduction or the elimination of the production of amyloidogenic light chains. Even a partial decrease of the amount of light chains may lead to improvement in organ function and prolong survival. Some therapies may be too toxic for patients with cardiac or multiorgan involvement, thus, it is essential to thoroughly assess organ involvement and a patient's functional status before choosing the appropriate treatment strategy. Cardiobiomarkers may help identify patients at high risk. In general, younger patients (<65–70 years) without cardiac involvement and with normal cardiobiomarkers are candidates for high-dose melphalan with autologous transplantation (HDM-ASCT) [19]. In contrast, for patients in whom aggressive treatments are associated with substantial mortality (such as those with multiorgan or cardiac involvement, symptomatic heart failure, and/or elevated cardiobiomarkers), conventional chemotherapy, low-dose regimens or novel agent-based therapies are preferred. Alkylating agents (melphalan) can improve the outcome of AL patients, especially in those who achieve a hematologic response. Melphalan with prednisone (MP) [20–22] is equally effective as combination chemotherapy regimens [23] and was the standard treatment for several years. However, MP is associated with a delayed hematologic response, a low probability of complete responses, and an overall hematologic response rate of about 50% with only 20% organ responses, mainly in patients with nephrotic syndrome or liver amyloidosis [22]. Substitution of prednisone with dexamethasone resulted in more rapid and higher response rates. Melphalan with dexamethasone (MDex) results in response rates of 67–74% within two to three months, complete responses in about one-third and improvement in at least one affected organ in almost half of the responding patients [24, 25] (Table 22.4). High-dose dexamethasone may cause fluid accumulation and arrhythmias especially in patients with cardiac amyloidosis, while MDex is not very effective for patients with cardiac involvement [26]. Prolonged use of alkylating agents may increase the risk of myelodysplasia, especially in patients with favorable outcome who are expected to have a long survival [27].

Table 22.3 Supportive care in patients with AL amyloidosis

Symptoms (Syndrome)	Drugs/measures	Comments
Symptomatic heart failure (dyspnea, edema)	Diuretics	Often complicated by orthostatic hypotension, aggravated by autonomic neuropathy or volume contraction due to nephrotic syndrome and resultant hypoalbuminemia.
	β-blockers, calcium channel blockers	Narrow therapeutic window/may worsen congestive heart failure (CHF), hypotension, AV block.
	Angiotensin-converting enzyme inhibitors	May cause hypotension/their use is challenging, even at low doses.
	Digitalis	Relatively contraindicated; is trapped within amyloid deposits and may have unpredictable toxicity [9], needs adjustment in renal impairment, is moderately affected by hypoalbuminemia.
Conduction abnormalities (AV block)	Permanent pacemaker [42]	Common in patients with advanced cardiac amyloidosis.
Ventricular arrhythmias	Amiodarone	Toxicity with long-term use. Preemptive therapy with amiodarone may be helpful in patients with ventricular arrhythmias in 24-Holter monitoring [10] – limited data.
	Implantable cardioverter-defibrillator (ICD)	May have a role in some selected high-risk patients [43] – limited data.
Edema due to nephrotic syndrome	Diuretics	May cause postural hypotension, especially in patients with autonomic neuropathy or CHF.
	Salt restriction	
End-stage renal disease	Dialysis	Frequent episodes of hypotension, may be difficult to construct an arteriovenous fistula due to hypotension and vascular amyloid infiltration.
Diarrhea	Loperamide, diphenoxylate, tincture of opium	May be either due to autonomic neuropathy or amyloid infiltration of the submucosa.
	Octreotide	For difficult to control cases.
Constipation	Metoclopramide	Intestinal hypokinesia may cause pseudo-obstruction.
	High dose erythromycin	
	Cisapride	Contraindicated due to risk for cardiac arrhythmias.
Bleeding abnormalities	Plasma, coagulation factors	May be due to acquired factor X deficiency, endothelial dysfunction, capillary infiltration by amyloid or reduced synthesis of procoagulant factors.
Thromboembolism	Heparin/LMWH Coumadin	Intracardiac thrombi are a common finding in patients with advanced cardiac amyloid.
	Thrombin inhibitors	Limited data in AL patients.

(*continued*)

Table 22.3 (*Continued*)

Symptoms (Syndrome)	Drugs/measures	Comments
		Prophylaxis should be given in patients who are treated with combinations of thalidomide or lenalidomide with dexamethasone and/or chemotherapy.
Orthostatic hypotension	Elastic stockings	Common and often difficult to manage complication.
	Fluorocortisone	Associated with fluid retention and supine hypertension, edema, and hypokalemia.
	Midodrine	Can cause tachycardia, supine hypertension, restlessness; needs dose adjustment in renal impairment. Initiating at low doses and titration over days to weeks may be helpful.

LMWH: low molecular weight heparin; CHF: congestive heart failure

HDM with autologous SCT is associated with a significant probability of long-lasting complete hematologic responses and organ function improvement [28]. However, this is at the cost of significant treatment-related mortality [19, 24]. Despite advances in supportive care and stringent patient selection, there is an 11% risk of death even in highly specialized centers. Appropriate patient selection is mandatory; younger patients with normal cardiobiomarkers and with adequate renal function are the best candidates for the procedure [19]. For sicker or older patients, attenuated doses of melphalan conditioning (100 to 140 mg/m^2) have been used with acceptable toxicity [19], but hematologic and organ response rates as well as OS may not be as favorable [29]. Tandem HDM with autologous SCT has also given encouraging results in selected patients [30]. In unselected patients, HDM with autologous SCT may be inferior to MDex, primarily due to high treatment-related mortality with HDM [24]. This procedure should be performed in carefully selected patients in centers with experience in performing autologous SCT in amyloidosis patients.

Thalidomide, lenalidomide, and bortezomib are very effective in myeloma and have recently been introduced to the treatment of AL patients. Thalidomide-based combinations have been studied more extensively (Table 22.4). Thalidomide is associated with neuropathy, arrhythmias, somnolence, constipation, thrombotic events, and may be toxic for many AL patients [31]. A combination of low-dose thalidomide and low-dose cyclophosphamide and dexamethasone has been shown to be well tolerated and associated with significant response rates [32], although results were poor in patients with cardiac amyloid [33].

Lenalidomide, a thalidomide derivative, has increased immunomodulatory activity over thalidomide, does not cause significant neuropathy, constipation or somnolence but is associated with hematologic toxicity and thrombotic complications. As a single agent it has modest activity in previously treated patients, but when combined with dexamethasone it is associated with significant response rates. However, lenalidomide should be used in lower doses than in myeloma patients due to toxicity, with careful follow-up and as-needed dose reductions [34, 35].

Bortezomib is a selective proteasome inhibitor, and preclinical data have shown that plasma cells producing amyloidogenic light chains may be very sensitive to proteasome inhibition. In two small series, bortezomib with or without dexamethasone, was associated with high response rates and complete responses, both in previously treated or refractory patients and in previously untreated patients [36, 37].

Table 22.4 Non-transplant regimens for patients with AL amyloidosis

Regimen	Dosing	
Melphalan/Prednisone	Melphalan 0.15 mg/kg and	For up to two years or indications of toxicity.
	Prednisone 0.8 mg/kg days 1–7 q6 weeks. Melphalan increased by 2 mg until mid-cycle leukopenia or thrombocytopenia develops [22]	
Melphalan/ Dexamethasone	Melphalan 0.22 mg/kg and Dexamethasone 40 mg PO days 1–4 q28 days [25]	For 9 cycles or CR.
	Melphalan 10 mg/m^2 and Dexamethasone 40 mg PO days 1–4 [24]	For up to 18 cycles unless toxicity occurs.
Cyclophosphamide/ Dexamethasone/ Thalidomide	PO Cyclophosphamide 500 mg once weekly, Thalidomide 200 mg/day, and Dexamethasone 40 mg days 1–4 and 9–12 q21 days	Thalidomide starting at 100 mg/day, increased after 4 weeks if tolerated.
	Attenuated PO Cyclophosphamide 500 mg days 1, 8, and 15; Thalidomide 200 mg/day; and Dexamethasone 20 mg days 1–4 and days 15–18 q28days [37]	For elderly (≥70 years) or those with CHF NYHA>II, significant fluid overload, etc. Thalidomide starting at 50 mg/day, increased by 50 mg at 4-week intervals as tolerated.
Melphalan/ Thalidomide/ Dexamethasone	PO Melphalan 0.22 mg/kg	Poor results in patients with advanced cardiac amyloidosis.
	days 1–4, Dexamethasone 20 mg on days 1–4, Thalidomide 100 mg/day, q28 days [33]	
Lenalidomide/ Dexamethasone	Lenalidomide 5–15 mg/day for 21 days q28 days +/− Dexamethasone 20–40 mg days 1–4 [34, 35]	Doses of 25 mg poorly tolerated/dose adjustment for renal impairment. May be toxic in patients with renal impairment.
Bortezomib/ Dexamethasone	Bortezomib 1–1.3 mg/m2 IV days 1,4,8,11 +/− Dexamethasone 20–40 mg days 1–4, q21 days [36, 37]	Significant activity even in refractory patients. Safe in patients with renal impairment or undergoing dialysis.

NYHA: New York Heart Association functional class; CHF: congestive heart failure

Bortezomib is safe in patients with renal impairment and is probably the fastest acting agent in AL amyloidosis, especially in combination with dexamethasone (Table 22.4). Bortezomib-based treatment is promising; however, toxicity such as neuropathy, orthostatic hypotension, constipation or diarrhea, may cause significant complications in AL patients.

Organ transplantation may be an option for some selected patients with end-stage renal disease or with severe amyloid cardiomyopathy. Relapse of organ amyloid infiltration is common, especially in patients with residual light chain production. Sequential autologous SCT and organ transplantation have also been used.

Course and prognosis

The major prognostic factor is the extent of cardiac involvement: more than two-thirds of patients die of cardiac amyloidosis due to progressive deterioration of congestive cardiomyopathy or die suddenly due to malignant arrhythmias or asystole/electromechanic dissociation [5, 38]. Patients presenting with heart failure and elevated cardiobiomarkers have a median survival of about six months or less. In contrast, patients with only renal involvement can enjoy a long survival, even if they do not achieve a complete response to treatment. Response to treatment is associated with significant improvement in survival and quality of life [1, 5]. Improvement of organ function may be delayed; it may take more than 12 months after autologous SCT for patients with nephrotic syndrome to have a significant reduction of proteinuria, the median being nine months [39]. Patients with persisting proteinuria may have progressive renal function deterioration due to tubular damage by the urinary protein. About one-third of patients with AL-related nephrotic syndrome respond to therapy and their renal function stabilizes, another third will receive dialysis after a median of one to two years, but most die due to extrarenal (mainly cardiac) complications of AL [6, 40]. Regression of cardiac amyloid is not commonly documented – reduction in wall thickness may take several months or years. However, a significant functional improvement and reduction of cardiobiomarkers may be seen in responding patients. Follow-up of cardiobiomarkers can help in the assessment of cardiac injury and are sensitive prognostic indicators [8]. Patients with myeloma-related amyloidosis tend to have worse outcome than patients with myeloma and without amyloidosis, or AL patients without myeloma [1, 5, 41].

References

1 Merlini G, Stone MJ. (2006) Dangerous small B-cell clones. *Blood* **108**:2520–30.

2 Merlini G, Bellotti V. (2003) Molecular mechanisms of amyloidosis. *N Engl J Med* **349**:583–96.

3 Comenzo RL, Zhang Y, Martinez C, et al. (2001) The tropism of organ involvement in primary systemic amyloidosis: contributions of Ig V(L) germ line gene use and clonal plasma cell burden. *Blood* **98**:714–20.

4 Brenner DA, Jain M, Pimentel DR, et al. (2004) Human amyloidogenic light chains directly impair cardiomyocyte function through an increase in cellular oxidant stress. *Circ Res* **94**:1008–10.

5 Gertz MA, Merlini G, Treon SP. (2004) Amyloidosis and Waldenström's macroglobulinemia. *Hematology (Am Soc Hematol Educ Program)* **2004**:257–82.

6 Gertz MA, Leung N, Lacy MQ, et al. (2009) Clinical outcome of immunoglobulin light chain amyloidosis affecting the kidney. *Nephrol Dial Transplant* [Epub ahead of print http://ndt.oxfordjournals.org/cgi/reprint/gfp201v1]

7 Park MA, Mueller PS, Kyle RA, et al. (2003) Primary (AL) hepatic amyloidosis: clinical features and natural history in 98 patients. *Medicine (Baltimore)* **82**:291–8.

8 Dispenzieri A, Gertz MA, Kyle RA, et al. (2004) Serum cardiac troponins and N-terminal pro-brain natriuretic peptide: a staging system for primary systemic amyloidosis. *J Clin Oncol* **22**:3751–7.

9 Falk RH. (2005) Diagnosis and management of the cardiac amyloidoses. *Circulation* **112**:2047–60.

10 Palladini G, Malamani G, Co F, et al. (2001) Holter monitoring in AL amyloidosis: prognostic implications. *Pacing Clin Electrophysiol* **24**:1228–33.

11 Swan N, Skinner M, O'Hara CJ. (2003) Bone marrow core biopsy specimens in AL (primary) amyloidosis. A morphologic and immunohistochemical study of 100 cases. *Am J Clin Pathol* **120**:610–6.

12 Soares SM, Fervenza FC, Lager DJ, et al. (2008) Bleeding complications after transcutaneous kidney biopsy in patients with systemic amyloidosis: single-center experience in 101 patients. *Am J Kidney Dis* **52**:1079–83.

13 Palladini G, Russo P, Bosoni T, et al. (2009) Identification of amyloidogenic light chains requires the combination of serum-free light chain assay with immunofixation of serum and urine. *Clin Chem* **55**:499–504.

14 Bochtler T, Hegenbart U, Cremer FW, et al. (2008) Evaluation of the cytogenetic aberration pattern in amyloid light chain amyloidosis as compared with monoclonal gammopathy of undetermined significance reveals common pathways of karyotypic instability. *Blood* **111**:4700–5.

15 Bryce AH, Ketterling RP, Gertz MA, et al. (2009) Translocation t(11;14) and survival of patients with light chain (AL) amyloidosis. *Haematologica* **94**:380–6.

16 Fonseca R, Ahmann GJ, Jalal SM, et al. (1998) Chromosomal abnormalities in systemic amyloidosis. *Br J Haematol* **103**:704–10.

17 Perfetti V, Coluccia AM, Intini D, et al. (2001) Translocation T(4;14)(p16.3;q32) is a recurrent genetic lesion in primary amyloidosis. *Am J Pathol* **158**:1599–603.

18 Abraham RS, Ballman KV, Dispenzieri A, et al. (2005) Functional gene expression analysis of clonal plasma cells identifies a unique molecular profile for light chain amyloidosis. *Blood* **105**:794–803.

19 Comenzo RL, Gertz MA. (2002) Autologous stem cell transplantation for primary systemic amyloidosis. *Blood* **99**:4276–82.

20 Kyle RA, Greipp PR. (1978) Primary systemic amyloidosis: comparison of melphalan and prednisone versus placebo. *Blood* **52**:818–27.

21 Skinner M, Anderson J, Simms R, et al. (1996) Treatment of 100 patients with primary amyloidosis: a randomized trial of melphalan, prednisone, and colchicine versus colchicine only. *Am J Med* **100**:290–8.

22 Kyle RA, Gertz MA, Greipp PR, et al. (1997) A trial of three regimens for primary amyloidosis: colchicine alone, melphalan and prednisone, and melphalan, prednisone, and colchicine. *N Engl J Med* **336**:1202–7.

23 Gertz MA, Lacy MQ, Lust JA, et al. (1999) Prospective randomized trial of melphalan and prednisone versus vincristine, carmustine, melphalan, cyclophosphamide, and prednisone in the treatment of primary systemic amyloidosis. *J Clin Oncol* **17**:262–7.

24 Jaccard A, Moreau P, Leblond V, et al. (2007) High-dose melphalan versus melphalan plus dexamethasone for AL amyloidosis. *N Engl J Med* **357**:1083–93.

25 Palladini G, Perfetti V, Obici L, et al. (2004) Association of melphalan and high-dose dexamethasone is effective and well tolerated in patients with AL (primary) amyloidosis who are ineligible for stem cell transplantation. *Blood* **103**:2936–8.

26 Lebovic D, Hoffman J, Levine BM, et al. (2008) Predictors of survival in patients with systemic light-chain amyloidosis and cardiac involvement initially ineligible for stem cell transplantation and treated with oral melphalan and dexamethasone. *Br J Haematol* **143**:369–73.

27 Gertz MA, Lacy MQ, Lust JA, et al. (2008) Long-term risk of myelodysplasia in melphalan-treated patients with immunoglobulin light-chain amyloidosis. *Haematologica* **93**:1402–6.

28 Sanchorawala V, Skinner M, Quillen K, et al. (2007) Long-term outcome of patients with AL amyloidosis treated with high-dose melphalan and stem-cell transplantation. *Blood* **110**:3561–3.

29 Gertz MA, Lacy MQ, Dispenzieri A, et al. (2004) Risk-adjusted manipulation of melphalan dose before stem cell transplantation in patients with amyloidosis is associated with a lower response rate. *Bone Marrow Transplant* **34**:1025–31.

30 Sanchorawala V, Wright DG, Quillen K, et al. (2007) Tandem cycles of high-dose melphalan and autologous stem cell transplantation increases the response rate in AL amyloidosis. *Bone Marrow Transplant* **40**:557–62.

31 Palladini G, Perfetti V, Perlini S, et al. (2005) The combination of thalidomide and intermediate-dose dexamethasone is an effective but toxic treatment for patients with primary amyloidosis (AL). *Blood* **105**:2949–51.

32 Wechalekar AD, Goodman HJ, Lachmann HJ, et al. (2007) Safety and efficacy of risk-adapted cyclophosphamide, thalidomide, and dexamethasone in systemic AL amyloidosis. *Blood* **109**:457–64.

33 Palladini G, Russo P, Lavatelli F, et al. (2008) Treatment of patients with advanced cardiac AL amyloidosis with oral melphalan, dexamethasone, and thalidomide. *Ann Hematol* **88**:347–50.

34 Dispenzieri A, Lacy MQ, Zeldenrust SR, et al. (2007) The activity of lenalidomide with or without dexamethasone in patients with primary systemic amyloidosis. *Blood* **109**:465–70.

35 Sanchorawala V, Wright DG, Rosenzweig M, et al. (2007) Lenalidomide and dexamethasone in the treatment of AL amyloidosis: results of a phase 2 trial. *Blood* **109**:492–6.

36 Kastritis E, Anagnostopoulos A, Roussou M, et al. (2007) Treatment of light chain (AL) amyloidosis with the combination of bortezomib and dexamethasone. *Haematologica* **92**:1351–8.

37 Wechalekar AD, Lachmann HJ, Offer M, et al. (2008) Efficacy of bortezomib in systemic AL amyloidosis with relapsed/refractory clonal disease. *Haematologica* **93**:295–8.

38 Palladini G, Kyle RA, Larson DR, et al. (2005) Multicentre versus single centre approach to rare diseases: the model of systemic light chain amyloidosis. *Amyloid* **12**:120–6.

39 Gertz MA, Leung N, Lacy MQ, et al. (2005) Myeloablative chemotherapy and stem cell transplantation in myeloma or primary amyloidosis with renal involvement. *Kidney Int* **68**:1464–71.

40 Gertz MA, Lacy MQ, Dispenzieri A. (2002) Immuno-globulin light chain amyloidosis and the kidney. *Kidney Int* **61**:1–9.

41 Leung N, Gunderson HD, Tan TS, et al. (2008) Mel-phalan and dexamethasone is less effective for patients with immunoglobulin light chain amyloidosis (AL) with high bone marrow plasmacytosis. *ASH Annual Meeting Abstracts* **112**:1735.

42 Mathew V, Olson LJ, Gertz MA, et al. (1997) Symp-tomatic conduction system disease in cardiac amyloid-osis. *Am J Cardiol* **80**:1491–2.

43 Kristen AV, Dengler TJ, Hegenbart U, et al. (2008) Prophylactic implantation of cardioverter-defibrilla-tor in patients with severe cardiac amyloidosis and high risk for sudden cardiac death. *Heart Rhythm* **5**:235–40.

PART 5

Bone Marrow Transplantation and Quality of Life

Advances in Allogeneic Hematopoietic Cell Transplantation: Progress in Transplantation Technology and Disease-Specific Outcomes

Joseph Pidala and Claudio Anasetti
Department of Blood and Marrow Transplantation, H. Lee Moffitt Cancer Center, and
University of South Florida, Tampa, FL, USA

Introduction

While allogeneic hematopoietic cell transplantation (HCT) provides effective control and often cure of hematopoietic malignancies, donor availability and limitations in resolution of HLA typing, transplant regimen-related toxicity, morbidity and mortality from graft-versus-host disease, infectious complications, and relapse of the original disease have circumscribed its overall success. While several challenges remain, major advances in transplantation technology, as well as novel approaches in disease-specific investigation have improved outcomes, thereby increasing the overall benefit realized with this therapy. The aim of this chapter is to examine major developments in transplantation technology, and to review results of current transplantation approaches in disease-specific outcomes.

Advances in transplantation technology

Donor selection

The human leukocyte antigen (HLA) system, a complex of genes on chromosome 6, encodes the polymorphic polypeptide chains that comprise Class I and II major histocompatibility complex (MHC) molecules. As critical determinants of the adaptive immune response, MHC molecules present antigenic peptides to T-cell receptors and provide a stimulatory signal for T-cell effector functions. Disparity at MHC loci serves as the major determinant of alloimmune donor/host reactions, consisting of graft rejection and graft-versus-host disease [1, 2]. Accordingly, optimal MHC matching of donor and host is of vital importance in successful transplantation outcome. As the majority of prospective HCT recipients will not have an HLA-matched sibling donor, many will require a search for an unrelated donor. The US National Marrow Donor Program (NMDP), established in 1986, serves as a repository of volunteer donor HLA typing information. Over seven million potential donors are registered in the NMDP registry; most donors have molecular typing performed at low to intermediate level for HLA-A, -B, and many also at -C and -DRB1, while a minority only have serological level typing. The likelihood of finding a fully matched unrelated donor is 60% in Caucasians, but is as low as 15% for ethnic/racial minorities

Advances in Malignant Hematology, First Edition. Edited by Hussain I. Saba and Ghulam J. Mufti. © 2011 Blackwell Publishing Ltd.
Published 2011 by Blackwell Publishing Ltd.

due to under-representation of potential donors and, in some instances, increased genetic polymorphism of the population [3]. This and other international registries have facilitated the identification of unrelated stem cell donors and cord blood units for thousands of patients.

Molecular HLA typing, made possible after the sequencing of the HLA complex, represents a major breakthrough in the accuracy of HLA typing methods. Historically, serologic methods, including microcytotoxicity assay and mixed lymphocyte reaction, suffered from several technical limitations, but chiefly those of poor accuracy and limited resolution: With the use of molecular typing methods, greater than 50% of pairs considered matched by serologic methods were found to have HLA allelic differences between donor and recipient. In several series of unrelated donor/recipient pairs matched by serologic methods, those with allelic disparity by molecular methods have suffered significantly worse acute graft-versus-host disease, non-relapse mortality (NRM), and inferior OS [4, 5]. Further, large retrospective analyses from the NMDP have clarified the prognostic impact of disparity at specific HLA alleles: In a study of 1874 donor/recipient pairs, mismatch at HLA-A, -B, -C, and -DRB1 had a similar adverse impact on mortality. Importantly, this analysis demonstrated that mismatch at the HLA-DQ or -DP locus did not adversely affect transplantation outcome [6]. In an analysis extended to 3857 donor/recipient pairs from NMDP data ranging from 1988 to 2003, high resolution matching at HLA-A, -B, -C and -DRB1 was associated with optimal survival, while a single or greater mismatch was associated with increased mortality. This analysis similarly demonstrated that HLA-DP or DQ locus mismatch did not adversely affect survival [7]. Advances in molecular HLA-typing technology have allowed for more accurate donor/recipient matching, selection of optimal donors, and enhanced prognostic information for counsel of prospective HCT recipients. In those without a suitable related or unrelated donor, ongoing research aims to define the role of alternative stem cell sources including umbilical cord blood and the use of related donors incompatible for one HLA haplotype.

Acute graft-versus-host disease

Acute graft-versus-host disease (aGVHD) is the major determinant of early transplant-related morbidity and mortality following allogeneic HCT. The underlying pathophysiology is complex, and consists of several cellular and molecular processes, characterized as inter-related phases. The syndrome is initiated when host dendritic cells process and then present antigens to alloreactive donor T-cells, which in turn produce cytokines including IL-2 and TNF-α, thereby driving T-cell activation and expansion. Activated T-cells produce inflammatory cytokines, and mediate cytotoxicity, as do key mediators of the innate immune system [8–11].

Clinically, the syndrome manifests with target organ damage primarily including skin rash, cholestatic hepatitis, nausea and vomiting, and diarrhea either combined or in isolation. The cumulative incidence of aGVHD following HCT varies across studies, and particularly according to patient, source of stem cells, donor relation, HLA disparity, and aGVHD prophylaxis conditions, but has generally been reported in the range of 30–50%. Risk factors for the development of aGVHD have been examined in several large retrospective series to date. These analyses have most consistently implicated older age of the recipient and HLA disparity between donor and recipient as determinants of aGVHD risk; other reported factors include male recipient/female donor pairs, conditioning regimen employed, condition requiring HCT, race, use of peripheral blood stem cells, reduced performance status, and CMV serostatus of donor and recipient [10, 12–15].

While seminal advances have been made, the incomplete protection provided by aGVHD prophylaxis and the inadequacy of both primary and salvage therapy clearly demonstrate the need for novel approaches. Successive generations of aGVHD prophylaxis pharmacologic regimens have evolved from the original approach of single agent methotrexate; these later generation regimens have proved more effective, and methotrexate (MTX)/tacrolimus (TAC) currently is supported by the best quality evidence as the most effective regimen: two large randomized controlled trials have demonstrated that grade II–IV aGVHD was significantly lower with

MTX/TAC compared to MTX/cyclosporine (CSA) in both sibling donor (32% vs. 44%; p = 0.01), and unrelated donor (56% vs. 74%; p = 0.0002) allografts [16, 17]. Novel approaches, including the regimen of sirolimus (SIR)/TAC [18, 19], have produced encouraging results in early phase trials; a phase III randomized controlled trial of MTX/TAC versus SIR/TAC is currently underway through the Blood and Marrow Transplant Clinical Trials Network (BMT CTN). Alternatively, the strategy of donor T-cell depletion has resulted in improved aGVHD prophylaxis. However, this approach has been complicated by increased risk of infectious complications, graft rejection, and primary disease relapse [20]. Other emerging approaches, including a regimen of total lymphoid irradiation and antithymocyte globulin (ATG) [21], and other combination immunosuppressive regimens are the subject of ongoing investigation. There is also great enthusiasm for the potential use of regulatory T-cells (Tregs) for the prevention and/or treatment of aGVHD. Preclinical evidence in murine HLA mismatched models demonstrates that Tregs can prevent otherwise lethal aGVHD, and may not affect the beneficial tumor control provided by alloreactive T-cells. Further, early clinical evidence has demonstrated the reciprocal relationship between Tregs and the occurrence and severity of acute and chronic GVHD in humans. Early phase trials utilizing *ex vivo* expanded polyclonal Tregs for aGVHD prevention either with or without concurrent immunosuppressive agents are underway both in the US and in Europe, and early reported results suggest the feasibility of this approach.

Several challenges remain in the primary therapy of established aGVHD, as complete response rates to the historical standard of ≥1 mg/kg of glucocorticoids only approach 20–50% in multiple series. Additionally, the treatment of aGVHD is empiric, and the largest series to date examining primary therapy with glucocorticoids have not produced consistent predictors of response [13, 22]. However, most data suggest decreasing likelihood of complete response to primary therapy with increasing aGVHD grade, as well as with increasing number of organs involved. Several investigators have attempted to improve response to first-line therapy by utilizing combined

therapy with glucocorticoids and additional immunosuppressive agents, including daclizumab as well as etanercept, with mixed success [23, 24]. However, a recent phase II BMT CTN trial provides early evidence that the combination of mycophenolate mofetil (MMF) and glucocorticoids may provide more effective primary therapy for aGVHD compared to other combination regimens [25]. This regimen of glucocorticoids and MMF is now the subject of an ongoing phase III trial through the CTN.

Multiple challenges remain in the management of those patients with aGVHD who fail first-line treatment with glucocorticoids. While there has been heterogeneity in definitions of refractoriness to primary therapy with glucocorticoids, relative consensus provides the following definition: progression of at least one overall grade within three days, failure to demonstrate any overall grade improvement over five to seven days, or incomplete response by 14 days of 1–2 mg/kg/day of glucocorticoids. In the treatment of glucocorticoid-refractory aGVHD, several salvage immunosuppressive agents have been demonstrated to have activity. However, response to individual salvage agents is modest, and survival is significantly worse compared to those with glucocorticoid-responsive aGVHD, largely due to refractory aGVHD and opportunistic infections [26]. Further, the literature suffers from methodological concerns, most notably the near absence of comparative efficacy data to guide the rational selection of one salvage agent over another. In total, aGVHD remains a significant obstacle to successful HCT, and ongoing efforts to improve primary prophylaxis, initial therapy, and salvage therapy for glucocorticoid-refractory aGVHD are of vital importance.

Chronic graft-versus-host disease

Chronic graft-versus-host disease (cGVHD) is an immune-mediated complication of allogeneic HCT, and is the greatest source of late transplant-related morbidity and mortality. It is also a major determinant of post-HCT QOL. The development of cGVHD also portends prolonged treatment with immunosuppressive therapy: Stewart et al. reported a median duration of immunosuppressive treatment (IS) of 23 months in 274 of 751 patients with cGVHD who were able to liberate from IS before recurrent malignancy or death. Of the entire cohort, 47% were alive in remission seven years after diagnosis of cGVHD, 7% remained on IS medications, and 40% were alive off IS; importantly, as the majority of HCT now utilize peripheral blood stem cells, recipients of peripheral blood stem cells were less likely to liberate from IS compared to those who received bone marrow stem cells, with HR 0.5 (0.3–0.7), p <0.0001 [27].

Chronic GVHD affects up to 70% of those living past 100 days post-HCT, and is characterized by protean manifestations. Importantly, major re-classification has taken place in the diagnosis and grading of cGVHD, as described in the series of manuscripts originating from the US National Institutes of Health (NIH) consensus conference on cGVHD that occurred in 2004. Among other important conclusions, consensus definitions of cGVHD have resulted, and have distinguished the syndrome of cGVHD from that of acute GVHD based on its distinct manifestations, rather than purely based on the commonly accepted convention dependent on time after HCT. This has important ramifications for interpretation of historical literature on cGVHD. On review of cases previously considered cGVHD, evaluation according to these NIH consensus criteria has resulted in re-classification of cGVHD to persistent, recurrent, or late aGVHD in approximately 40% of cases [28]. Further, uniform grading schemes, and response criteria have been proposed, which will help standardize reporting and allow improved comparisons across studies. While these represent significant progress in this field, a number of therapeutic challenges remain.

According to the NIH consensus recommendations, overall mild cGVHD manifestations can be treated with local or topical measures, while moderate to severe disease warrants systemic therapy. The current accepted systemic primary therapy remains glucocorticoids at 1 mg/kg body weight. Investigation into combined primary therapy has not demonstrated a clear benefit to this approach: For example, combination therapy with cyclosporine, thalidomide, or hydroxychloroquine has not demonstrated benefit over glucocorticoid monotherapy. Martin et al. conducted a randomized multicenter trial to determine if the addition of MMF improved the efficacy of primary glucocorticoid systemic therapy for cGVHD; the primary end point of the study was withdrawal of all systemic therapy within two years. This study was closed after four years as an interim analysis demonstrated low likelihood for positive results for this primary end point. There was no benefit observed in secondary end points, and there actually was an increased hazard of death observed (HR 1.99, 95% CI 0.9–4.3) in the MMF arm versus control [29]. As primary therapy with glucocorticoids only promises an overall response rate of near 60% and complete response of approximately 20%, there is a clear ongoing need for improvement in cGVHD therapy. Importantly, the limited complete response rates achieved with primary glucocorticoid therapy engender a burden of glucocorticoid refractory cGVHD.

While the criteria for steroid-refractoriness have varied in the literature, a relative consensus provides the following definition: Baseline manifestations of cGVHD either do not improve after at least two months, or demonstrate progression in severity after one month of standard glucocorticoid-based immunosuppressive therapy. There are a number of immunosuppressive agents with reported activity in phase I–II trials for the salvage of glucocorticoid-refractory cGVHD. Overall response rates for these various salvage agents have included the following: mycophenolate mofetil 46–75%; high-dose glucocorticoids 48%; extracorporeal photopheresis 61%; sirolimus 63– 94%; pentostatin 53%; tacrolimus 35%; rituximab 65–70%; and thalidomide 20–38% [28]. Given the lack of comparative, randomized, prospective trial data in the salvage therapy of refractory cGVHD, there is no salvage therapy with proven superiority, and practice patterns vary.

Ongoing challenges in the field of cGVHD include the following: further work remains to define the cellular and molecular basis of the disease; insight into the prevention of cGVHD is needed; novel approaches at primary therapy are needed to improve upon the current modest complete response rate achieved with glucocorticoid therapy; in addition, further investigation, and in particular comparative studies of salvage agents, are needed to better inform the current practice of salvage therapy for glucocorticoid-refractory cGVHD.

Hematopoietic stem cell source

Hematopoietic stem cells have been increasingly obtained for transplantation by mobilization and collection from peripheral blood, rather than bone marrow harvest, with the majority of allogeneic HCT currently utilizing peripheral blood stem cells (PBSC). As the cell composition, most notably the CD34+ cell and T-cell numbers, differ across these products, there is rationale that transplantation outcomes including graft-versus-host disease, engraftment kinetics, and disease control could vary according to stem cell source. Accordingly, a number of randomized controlled trials have examined the impact of stem cell source on outcomes in the setting of myeloablative conditioning and entirely with related donor allografts; the impact of stem cell source in the setting of unrelated donors is the focus of an ongoing trial under the BMT CTN.

As these individual trials have reached in part disparate conclusions, and individually represent relatively small patient samples, a systematic review and individual patient data meta-analysis was performed and reported by a group of investigators, the Stem Cell Trialists. Data was obtained from nine randomized trials, encompassing a total of 1111 adult patients. The use of PBSC was significantly associated with a number of important transplantation outcomes: First, compared with bone marrow stem cells (BMSC), the use of PBSC resulted in faster neutrophil and platelet engraftment. Further, the use of PBSC was associated with a significant increase in severe (grade III–IV) acute graft-versus-host disease, and overall and extensive stage chronic graft-versus-host disease. PBSC also resulted in decreased incidence of primary disease relapse in both early and late stage disease. There was no significant difference in NRM between the two stem cell sources. Finally, the use of PBSC was associated with a significant benefit in overall and disease-free survival in those with late stage disease [15]. These therapeutic alternatives have also been recently addressed in a decision analysis, which demonstrates the superiority of PBSC in both

overall life expectancy and quality-adjusted life expectancy [30].

Infectious complications

Infectious complications are a nearly universal concern after allogeneic HCT. Major developments in the prevention, early diagnosis and preemptive therapy, and breadth of effective primary and secondary treatment options have reduced the burden of morbidity and mortality resultant from infectious complications of HCT. Two major areas of ongoing investigation center on cytomegalovirus (CMV), and invasive fungal infections.

CMV infection remains a threat after HCT despite advances in surveillance and preemptive therapy as well as primary prophylaxis. However, the risk of CMV disease has decreased from up to 35% to now 10% in sero-positive recipients in the era of ganciclovir [31]. The recommended approach to CMV prevention begins prior to HCT in determining the CMV sero-status of the recipient, and in identifying appropriate recipient/donor CMV sero-matching. Sero-negative donors are preferred for sero-negative recipients, as the risk of CMV transmission is 20–30% in sero-negative recipients with a sero-positive donor. There is conflicting evidence on the impact of donor CMV sero-status in sero-positive recipients. Further, the use of leukocyte-reduced, filtered blood products nearly obviates the risk of CMV acquisition through transfusion of platelet and red cell products, although this does not apply to hematopoietic cells that should not be filtered. Important work has demonstrated the activity of several antimicrobial agents in the primary prophylaxis of CMV: Existing evidence demonstrates a reduction in CMV infection and disease with the use of either high-dose acyclovir or valacyclovir, and better still with ganciclovir or valganciclovir after HCT [32]. Additionally, a strategy of CMV surveillance by either detection of pp65 antigenemia or CMV DNA by polymerase chain reaction (PCR) has allowed early identification of CMV viremia and institution of pre-emptive antiviral therapy. The PCR method confers greater sensitivity. However, the lack of validated threshold values for the initiation of preemptive therapy is reflected in institutional practice variation. Importantly, a randomized trial of valganciclovir prophylaxis versus placebo with initiation of preemptive valganciclovir therapy upon detection of CMV DNA >1000 copies/mL by PCR failed to show significant advantage in prevention of CMV disease or survival with prophylaxis [33]. In total, advances in CMV prophylaxis have allowed a reduction in the burden of CMV infection and disease, and methods aimed at early detection have allowed successful preemptive therapy.

Invasive fungal infections are an important source of infectious morbidity and mortality following HCT. HCT recipients are at particular risk on account of granulocytopenia, compounded by ongoing immunosuppressive agents to prevent GVHD, and commonly prolonged glucocorticoid treatment. While disseminated fungal infection increases mortality [34], new developments, including second generation broad-spectrum triazoles including posaconazole and voriconazole, as well as echinocandins including caspofungin and micafungin, have expanded the repertoire of available antifungal agents. Seminal trials have demonstrated the efficacy of fluconazole as primary fungal prophylaxis [35], but have not shown a significant advantage of prophylaxis with voriconazole over fluconazole after allogeneic HCT. [36] One additional trial has established the comparable efficacy of micafungin [37] in primary fungal prophylaxis compared to fluconazole. A trial of posaconazole in patients with GVHD treated with glucocorticoids showed improvement in invasive fungal infections but same survival [38]. Aditionally, two randomized trials have demonstrated comparable efficacy, but reduced toxicity in the setting of empiric antifungal therapy with caspofungin or voriconazole, respectively, as compared with liposomal amphotericin [39, 40]. Early detection of invasive fungal infection has been facilitated by sensitive culture methods, antigenic assays including galactomannan and beta-D-glucan, and high-resolution diagnostic imaging. Available evidence supports caspofungin, micafungin, liposomal amphotericin (or fluconazole for fluconazole-sensitive species) as effective therapy for invasive Candida infections. In the treatment of invasive Aspergillus infections, voriconazole and liposomal amphotericin are indicated; in this setting, voriconazole has been demonstrated to have superior antifungal efficacy and survival compared to conventional amphotericin B [41]. Ongoing challenges in the management of invasive fungal infections include the relative increase in the incidence of other serious invasive fungal infections, including yeast-like pathogens, filamentous fungi including *Fusarium* and *Scedosporium* species, and the zygomycetes.

Disease-specific regimens with reduced toxicity

Acute myelogenous leukemia and myelodysplastic syndrome

Major randomized trials as well as meta-analyses have demonstrated that allogeneic HCT from an HLA-identical sibling provides superior outcomes for AML in first complete remission (CR1) with intermediate- or high-risk cytogenetics, and offers the greatest likelihood of long-term disease-free survival in those with more advanced disease [42, 43]. However, while the median age at diagnosis of AML is 68, the superior disease control provided by HCT utilizing myeloablative conditioning with cyclophosphamide (CY) and total body irradiation (TBI) or busulfan (BU) is offset by prohibitive NRM in those over age 30–35 [44, 45]. Non-transplantation treatment approaches for older adults >age 60 produce disappointing results, with less than 10% achieving long-term disease-free survival.

Based on this background, there is rationale to pursue approaches at transplantation with reduced toxicity in older adults. Several investigators have reported outcomes in the treatment of myelodysplastic syndrome (MDS) and AML utilizing novel less toxic conditioning regimens that range in intensity from non-myeloablative with fludarabine (FLU) plus low-dose TBI to ablative with reduced toxicity using FLU with standard doses of BU. Early evidence demonstrates encouraging long-term disease-free survival with NRM that compares favorably to historical rates resulting from myeloablative conditioning. These studies, however, have been characterized by great heterogeneity of patient populations, thereby limiting conclusions of comparative efficacy of the different regimens: First, the disease risk characteristics differ with respect to remission status at time of transplant, relative contributions from MDS versus AML, and the relative composition of primary AML versus AML secondary to antecedent hematologic disorder or prior therapy. As well, the patient age, comorbidity, and candidacy for traditional myeloablative conditioning have differed. Accordingly, comparisons across studies are limited by these factors.

Hegenbart et al. has reported their results of a non-myeloablative approach with 2 Gy TBI with or without FLU [46]. In this series of 122 AML patients with median age of 58, this regimen produced little toxicity, with a NRM of only 16% at two years. Further, relapse rate was 39% overall; this differed according to donor relation, with relapse for those in CR1 with a sibling donor of 50% versus 16% for those with an unrelated donor. OS for the total patient sample was 48% at two years.

Several groups have reported outcomes after a reduced intensity approach of FLU/melphalan (MEL) with or without alemtuzumab [47–49]. In these studies, median age ranged from 52 to 58, variable proportion of MDS and AML largely with advanced disease, and 12–39% in CR1. One year NRM ranged from 19–33%, relapse ranged from 32–40%, and OS was 34–41% at three years.

Others have studied a regimen of FLU given in concert with reduced dose BU with or without antithymocyte globulin [50–55]. Results have markedly differed according to patient, disease risk, and transplantation conditions: In a series entirely consisting of AML in CR1 with 100% matched sibling donors, NRM was low at 9%, relapse only reached 18%, and OS at 18 months was 79% [50]. Conversely, in a series with only 22% in CR1 and 44% with matched sibling donors, NRM was 53% at two years, and OS was 32% at two years [51].

An approach of induction chemotherapy followed by 4Gy TBI/CY/ATG with prophylactic DLI has been pioneered by Schmid et al. [56, 57]. NRM was 23% for sibling donors and 50% for unrelated donors. Utilizing this combined approach, a group of advanced AML (only 11% in CR1) achieved an OS of 42% at two years [56].

In total, the available literature to date suggests that reduced-intensity conditioning (RIC) followed by allogeneic HCT is a promising strategy to limit NRM, but complicated by increased risk of primary disease relapse [58, 59]. There is also evidence among RIC regimens that relative dose intensity is important for primary disease control after transplant [47, 52, 60]. Further conclusions regarding the relative efficacy of reduced intensity approaches will require comparative clinical trials of myeloablative versus reduced intensity conditioning regimens in a homogeneous patient sample.

Chronic myelogenous leukemia

While CML historically was a leading indication for allogeneic HCT, insights into the molecular biology of CML, and the resultant development and success of tyrosine kinase inhibitors, have resulted in a marked decrease in the number of allogeneic transplants performed for CML, as well as a shift in the landscape of disease stage transplanted. Center for International Blood and Marrow Transplant Research (CIBMTR) data indicate that the number of allogeneic transplants performed annually has declined from 574 in 1999 to 223 in 2003, and the proportion who had been treated pre-HCT with imatinib increased from 1% in 1999 to 77% in 2003. Current consensus indications for HCT include those who are refractory to or intolerant of TKIs.

Given these trends, the bulk of transplantation outcome data reflects the use of myeloablative conditioning, wherein five-year OS for chronic phase CML with HLA-matched sibling donor reaches 60–70%, and rather 57% in the setting of unrelated donors [61]. However, emerging data demonstrates the efficacy of reduced intensity conditioning followed by HCT: In a series of 24 CML patients in first chronic phase, a regimen of FLU (150 mg/m^2), BU (8 mg/kg), and ATG (40 mg) was employed for HCT conditioning; the regimen was associated with minimal toxicity, and five-year OS was 85% [62]. Investigators at Fred Hutchinson Cancer Research Center utilized a regimen of 2 Gy TBI with or without FLU (90 mg/m^2) in 24 CML patients (including first and second chronic phase, and accelerated phase) who were not deemed candidates for conventional myeloablative therapy. The two-year OS for those transplanted in first chronic phase was 70%, and rather 56% for those with disease stage beyond first chronic phase [63]. In a large retrospective series from the European Group for Blood and Marrow Transplantation registry, 211 reduced intensity transplants were examined from 1994 to 2002. Conditioning regimens employed were diverse, but FLU (30 mg/m^2/day × 5 days), BU (8 mg/kg) and antithymocyte globulin were utilized in 40% of patients. In the overall sample, TRM was only 4% at 100 days, and 13% at one year. As well, OS at three years was 69% for first chronic phase, 57% for second chronic phase, 24% for accelerated phase, and only 8% for blast phase at two years [64]. These data, as well as the success of donor lymphocyte infusion (DLI) in the setting of relapsed CML after transplant, demonstrate the efficacy of the immunologic graft-versus-leukemia effect in this condition.

Although the paradigm of CML therapy continues to evolve, and second-generation TKIs can offer effective therapy for those who fail imatinib, a current approach for timing of referral for allogeneic HCT consultation includes failure to achieve the following response milestones during therapy with TKIs: failure to achieve complete hematologic response by three months; failure to achieve cytogenetic response by six months; failure to achieve major cytogenetic response by 12 months; failure to achieve complete cytogenetic response by 18 months; and finally, disease progression on therapy.

Acute lymphoblastic leukemia

Success seen in the treatment of childhood ALL has not been realized in adult ALL; while comparable remission rates are achieved with multi-agent induction chemotherapy, relapse incurred during or after consolidation and maintenance chemotherapy compromises the efficacy of this approach. Multiple adult ALL treatment protocols have employed allogeneic HCT as post-remission therapy, resulting in OS of 28–48% at five years. However, several trials, most notably the recent MRC UKALL XII/ECOG E2993 trial, have demonstrated the prohibitive NRM realized with myeloablative conditioning regimens in adults age >35 [65]. This is particularly

relevant in the application of HCT to adult ALL, as the median age of diagnosis is 60 years. While control of ALL has been considered to be dependent on the intensity of myeloablative conditioning therapy, several investigators have challenged this paradigm through demonstrating encouraging outcomes following reduced intensity conditioning and allogeneic HCT.

In a series of 97 adult ALL patients (29% in CR1, and the remainder with more advanced disease) from the EBMT Registry, Mohty et al. reported outcomes utilizing reduced intensity conditioning consisting of either ATG- or TBI-based regimens. In those patients transplanted in CR1, NRM was only 18%, and two-year OS was 52% [66]. In those with more advanced stage disease, outcomes were significantly worse on account of increased NRM and ALL relapse. Remission status and chronic GVHD predicted OS on multivariable analysis. Martino et al. reported the outcomes of reduced intensity conditioning (primarily FLU and MEL with or without Campath) for a series of 27 adult ALL patients (median age 50) with largely advanced disease; 85% were advanced beyond CR1, 44% were refractory to chemotherapy, and 41% were Philadelphia chromosome positive. Here, the two-year NRM was 23%, two-year incidence of disease progression was 49%, and two-year OS was 31%. Those with chronic GVHD had a lower incidence of disease progression [67]. Hamaki et al. examined a series of 33 adult ALL patients with median age of 55 years conditioned with a heterogeneous mixture of conditioning regimens (primarily BU/FLU or FLU/MEL), of a heterogeneous mix of remission status. With a median follow-up of 11.6 months, the projected one-year OS was 39.6% and relapse-free survival 29.8%. The three-year progression-free mortality was estimated at 30.4% [68]. Finally, Bachanova et al. reported the outcomes of 22 high-risk adult ALL patients in CR treated with FLU (40 mg/m^2 × 5), CY (50 mg/kg), and 200 cGy TBI, followed by matched related or umbilical cord blood grafts. NRM was 27%, and OS was 50%. Those in CR1 had significantly less NRM and improved OS [69]. In total, the evidence to date for RIC followed by HCT in adult ALL supports lower NRM in adults compared to historical rates seen after myeloablative conditioning. However, heterogeneity in the patient (age, prior myeloablative HCT), disease (disease risk, remission status, Philadelphia chromosome positivity), and transplantation source are such variables across these studies as to limit the ability to compare regimens. Future work, including comparative trials of RIC versus myeloablative conditioning, is needed to clarify the role of RIC and HCT in adults with ALL.

Chronic lymphocytic leukemia

Significant progress has been made in biologic insights, prognostic markers, and effective therapy for CLL, including transplantation approaches. Disease risk markers, including common cytogenetic abnormalities, immunoglobulin mutation status, surface expression of CD38, and zeta-associated protein 70 (ZAP-70), have provided additional prognostic information to guide initial therapy. Failure to response to initial FLU-based therapy has helped to define those who may benefit from a more intensive treatment approach including transplantation. Consensus recommendations for consideration of allogeneic HCT include 17p deletion, or relapsed or fludarabine-refractory CLL. While autologous HCT produces encouraging responses with low NRM (reported less than 10%), this modality fails in many cases to produce durable remissions. Further, therapy-related myelodysplasia and acute leukemia after high-dose therapy and autologous HCT, reported as high as 8–9% in several series, adds an additional late burden to this therapy. Conversely, multiple lines of pre-clinical and clinical evidence demonstrate an immunologic graft-versus-leukemia effect after allogeneic HCT, resulting in superior disease control. The major obstacle to successful allogeneic HCT in adults with CLL has been prohibitive NRM: In several series examining primarily TBI- or BU-based myeloablative conditioning regimens, adults (median age ranging from 41 to 49) with CLL have suffered NRM as high as 48%, with reported five-year OS ranging from 33–62% [70]. Given the older age and potential comorbid conditions present in adults with CLL, investigators have aimed to study RIC regimens to

reduce toxicity and exploit the beneficial graft-versus-leukemia effect.

Investigators have examined several reduced-intensity approaches in adults with CLL. Schetelig et al. conducted a prospective trial in 30 adult CLL patients (median age of 50) utilizing a conditioning regimen of FLU/BU/ATG. NRM was only 15% at two years, and OS at two years was 72% [71]. Also utilizing a regimen of BU/FLU, Brown et al. reported in a trial of 46 patients (median age 53) low TRM, only 17% at two years, and OS of 54% at two years [72]. Sorror et al. reported the results of low-dose TBI with or without FLU in 64 CLL patients with a median age of 56. TRM was 22% at two years, and OS was 60% at two years [73]. Further, Caballero et al. reported a TRM of 20% and six-year OS of 70% following reduced-intensity conditioning, primarily consisting of FLU/MEL [74]. In total, the results from these trials suggest that RIC and allogeneic HCT can be performed in adults with CLL, with TRM as well as long-term disease control that compare favorably with myeloablative conditioning regimens. While a trial directly comparing these strategies has not been performed, retrospective analysis of outcomes suggests a significant increase in relapse and decrease in TRM after reduced-intensity versus myeloablative conditioning therapy [75]. The hurdle for CLL therapy remains debulking fludarabine-resistant disease before transplantation.

Non-Hodgkin lymphoma

Therapy for NHL including multi-agent chemotherapy regimens, and importantly the use of rituximab for CD20 positive malignancies has resulted in a large proportion of affected individuals achieving long-term disease control or cure. However, high-dose therapy and autologous or allogeneic transplantation continue to play a vital role in the management of relapsed or refractory disease. While high-dose therapy and autologous SCT can result in impressive results with up to 60% of those with chemotherapy-sensitive relapsed diffuse large B-cell lymphoma achieving eradication of the disease, allogeneic HCT remains the only curative therapeutic modality for many other lymphomas, particularly in the setting of prior failed autologous transplantation. As with other disease entities, the success of allogeneic HCT in the management of relapsed/refractory NHL has been limited by excess NRM, an issue which may be circumvented with the adoption of RIC.

Several investigators have examined RIC and HCT for relapsed/refractory aggressive NHL, largely represented by diffuse large B-cell lymphoma. The bulk of subjects in these series have failed a prior autologous transplant for the management of relapsed disease. Conditioning regimens employed have included the Seattle regimen of 90 mg/m^2 FLU and 2 Gy TBI, the regimen of FLU/MEL/alemtuzumab, as well as that of FLU (30 mg/m^2 daily × 3 days)/CY (750 mg/m^2 daily x 3 days)/rituximab per the M.D. Anderson experience. In total, these regimens result in NRM that compares favorably to that incurred with myeloablative regimens, have activity in relapsed/refractory disease, and have resulted in OS of approximately 50% by two years. It is clear, however, that the success of this approach varies according to salvage chemotherapy responsiveness prior to HCT; those with disease refractory to salvage chemotherapy suffer inferior response and worse overall and progression-free survival [76].

Allogeneic HCT also plays an important role in the management of relapsed/refractory follicular lymphoma, as salvage chemo- or radioimmunotherapy approaches and autologous transplantation do not result in durable eradication of the disease in most cases. As reviewed by van Besien, myeloablative conditioning consisting primarily of CY/TBI or BU/CY followed by allogeneic HCT has resulted in remarkable disease control for relapsed/refractory follicular lymphoma, but with an associated burden of NRM that reaches >40–50%. Based on the mature results of multiple studies utilizing RIC and HCT for relapsed/refractory follicular lymphoma, it appears that NRM is largely reduced (reported in most series in the range of 15–30%), disease control is comparable (with relapse rates largely in the range of 10–20%), and encouraging long-term outcomes are achieved, with OS reported at approximately 60–80% [77]. Again, those with chemotherapy refractory relapsed disease suffer worse outcomes, with increased NRM, increased risk of relapse, and worse OS.

Several advances in the therapy of mantle cell lymphoma (MCL) have led to improved outcomes: Aggressive multi-agent rituximab-containing regimens have led to impressive CR rates and OS. The approach of high-dose therapy and autologous SCT after achieving CR1 may also produce long-term disease control for some. In a recent trial from the Nordic group, 160 patients treated with rituximab-maxi-CHOP alternating with high-dose ara-C were then treated with high-dose BEAM or BEAC therapy and *in vivo* rituximab-purged autologous SCT. Impressively, the projected six-year event-free survival was 56%, and no further relapses occurred after five years [78]. However, the burden of relapsed disease remains. Several investigators have demonstrated the potentially curative potential of allogeneic HCT in those with relapsed/refractory MCL. In these series, patients have failed several prior chemotherapy regimens, and a large proportion has failed to achieve sustained remission after a prior autologous HCT, thus representing advanced, refractory disease. In this setting, RIC with FLU/CY/rituximab or FLU/2 Gy TBI has resulted in low NRM, and OS of >60% [79]. This evidence shows the feasibility and efficacy of this approach, and demonstrates the important role of allogeneic HCT in relapsed/refractory MCL, for which there are no other curative options.

Multiple myeloma

Recent advances have resulted in both biologic insights and improvements in the treatment of MM, a clonal plasma cell dyscrasia. Successive trials have demonstrated the activity of novel agents in both *de novo* and relapsed/refractory disease including thalidomide, lenalidomide, and bortezomib, and have demonstrated improved overall and complete response rates with combination regimens including these novel agents. As well, several large, prospective trials, including the French Intergroup study and the MRC Myeloma VII trial, have demonstrated a significant advantage in response, progression-free, and OS with high-dose therapy and autologous SCT compared to conventional chemotherapy. It has also been demonstrated that tandem autologous transplantation provides additional benefit in those with less than a very good partial response (VGPR) after initial autologous SCT. While direct randomized trials comparing novel regimens with high-dose therapy and autologous transplantation have not been performed, the proportion achieving CR with combination regimens including novel agents has brought into question the relative importance of high-dose therapy and autologous transplantation. However, despite improvements in response with combination regimens including novel agents, as well as the prolongation in survival provided by high-dose therapy and autologous transplantation, the condition remains incurable with these therapeutic modalities. Allied efforts aimed at improving these outcomes, including purging of autologous stem cell products to remove contaminating myeloma cells, post-autologous maintenance therapy with interferon or thalidomide, and post-autologous transplantation vaccines to restore antimyeloma immunity have also not resulted in durable eradication of the disease. These shortcomings suggest the need for alternative therapeutic strategies.

High-dose therapy and allogeneic HCT offer potential to circumvent these issues. First, high-dose conditioning therapy may provide more effective eradication of the disease. Second, available evidence supports an immunologic graft-versus-myeloma effect: relapse rates are reduced after allogeneic HCT compared to other therapeutic modalities, including autologous HCT; and DLI upon relapse of myeloma after HCT can restore remission in some patients. However, the benefit of allogeneic HCT has been limited by excessive morbidity and NRM, which has been reported as high as 50% after myeloablative conditioning. Accordingly, several investigators have pursued an approach of RIC followed by allogeneic HCT. While randomized trial evidence comparing myeloablative conditioning with RIC is lacking, one EBMT registry analysis has retrospectively examined the outcomes of 320 reduced-intensity and 196 myeloablative allogeneic transplants performed from 1998 to 2002. The reduced-intensity HCT group consisted of older subjects, and had a significantly greater proportion with prior transplants. For reduced-intensity and myeloablative groups respectively, two-year NRM (24 vs. 37%; p = 0.002) was reduced, and OS was not significantly different at

38.1% and 50.8%. On multivariable analysis, RIC was associated with decreased NRM, but increased risk of relapse [80].

Several groups have examined RIC and allogeneic HCT, and have reported durable eradication of the disease, with two-year OS approaching 50%. An alternative approach has been to perform planned tandem autologous transplant followed by RIC with HCT. Several trials of this tandem autologous-reduced-intensity allogeneic HCT approach have been published, with allogeneic HCT regimens consisting primarily of MEL ($100–140 \text{ mg/m}^2$) plus FLU or 2Gy TBI or CY plus FLU. These studies demonstrate a more acceptable NRM of 18–24%, and OS ranging from 58–74% at two years [81]. Prospective trials have also compared tandem autologous transplantation to tandem autologous-reduced-intensity allogeneic HCT: a French trial compared these approaches in 284 high-risk (defined by elevated beta-2-microglobulin and deletion of chromosome 13) myeloma patients with randomization based on the availability of a matched sibling donor. For tandem autologous and auto-allogeneic HCT respectively, NRM was 5% and 11%, and two-year OS was not significantly different at 35 and 41% [82]. In an Italian trial of 162 myeloma patients, investigators examined an approach of tandem autologous transplant versus autologous transplant followed by reduced-intensity allogeneic HCT with assignment based on the presence of a matched sibling donor. In an intention to treat analysis for these approaches respectively, complete response rate was 26% versus 55% (p = 0.004), NRM was 2% versus 10% (p = ns), and median OS was 54 months and 80 months (p = 0.01) [83].

These results demonstrate the feasibility and limited NRM following this approach of tandem autologous transplant-reduced intensity allogeneic HCT, and suggest that it provides durable eradication of the disease and benefit over that seen with tandem autologous HCT. Further conclusions will require longer follow-up, additional evidence to corroborate this benefit, as well as further investigation to discern the optimal therapeutic approach utilizing the available modalities in the treatment of myeloma.

References

1 Klein J, Sato A. (2000) The HLA system. First of two parts. *N Engl J Med* **343**:702–9.

2 Klein J, Sato A. (2000) The HLA system. Second of two parts. *N Engl J Med* **343**:782–6.

3 Beatty PG, Mori M, Milford E. (1995) Impact of racial genetic polymorphism on the probability of finding an HLA-matched donor. *Transplantation* **60**:778–83.

4 Speiser DE, Tiercy JM, Rufer N, et al. (1996) High resolution HLA matching associated with decreased mortality after unrelated bone marrow transplantation. *Blood* **87**:4455–62.

5 Sasazuki T, Juji T, Morishima Y, et al. (1998) Effect of matching of class I HLA alleles on clinical outcome after transplantation of hematopoietic stem cells from an unrelated donor. Japan Marrow Donor Program. *N Engl J Med* **339**:1177–85.

6 Petersdorf EW, Longton GM, Anasetti C, et al. (1997) Association of HLA-C disparity with graft failure after marrow transplantation from unrelated donors. *Blood* **89**:1818–23.

7 Lee SJ, Klein J, Haagenson M, et al. (2007) High-resolution donor-recipient HLA matching contributes to the success of unrelated donor marrow transplantation. *Blood* **110**:4576–83.

8 Ferrara JL, Levine JE, Reddy P, Holler E. (2009) Graft-versus-host disease. *Lancet* **373**:1550–61.

9 Ferrara JL, Levy R, Chao NJ. (1999) Pathophysiologic mechanisms of acute graft-vs. -host disease. *Biol Blood Marrow Transplant* **5**:347–56.

10 Ferrara JL, Reddy P. (2006) Pathophysiology of graft-versus-host disease. *Semin Hematol* **43**:3–10.

11 Copelan EA. (2006) Hematopoietic stem-cell transplantation. *N Engl J Med* **354**:1813–26.

12 Hahn T, McCarthy PL, Jr., Zhang MJ, et al. (2008) Risk factors for acute graft-versus-host disease after human leukocyte antigen-identical sibling transplants for adults with leukemia. *J Clin Oncol* **26**:5728–34.

13 Anasetti C, Beatty PG, Storb R, et al. (1990) Effect of HLA incompatibility on graft-versus-host disease, relapse, and survival after marrow transplantation for patients with leukemia or lymphoma. *Hum Immunol* **29**:79–91.

14 Weisdorf D, Hakke R, Blazar B, et al. (1991) Risk factors for acute graft-versus-host disease in histocompatible donor bone marrow transplantation. *Transplantation* **51**:1197–203.

15 Stem Cell Trialists' Collaborative Group (2005) Allogeneic peripheral blood stem-cell compared with bone marrow transplantation in the management of hematologic malignancies: an individual patient data meta-analysis of nine randomized trials. *J Clin Oncol* **23**:5074–87.

16 Ratanatharathorn V, Nash RA, Przepiorka D, et al. (1998) Phase III study comparing methotrexate and tacrolimus (prograf, FK506) with methotrexate and cyclosporine for graft-versus-host disease prophylaxis after HLA-identical sibling bone marrow transplantation. *Blood* **92**:2303–14.

17 Nash RA, Antin JH, Karanes C, et al. (2000) Phase 3 study comparing methotrexate and tacrolimus with methotrexate and cyclosporine for prophylaxis of acute graft-versus-host disease after marrow transplantation from unrelated donors. *Blood* **96**:2062–8.

18 Cutler C, Kim HT, Hochberg E, et al. (2004) Sirolimus and tacrolimus without methotrexate as graft-versus-host disease prophylaxis after matched related donor peripheral blood stem cell transplantation. *Biol Blood Marrow Transplant* **10**:328–36.

19 Cutler C, Li S, Ho VT, et al. (2007) Extended follow-up of methotrexate-free immunosuppression using sirolimus and tacrolimus in related and unrelated donor peripheral blood stem cell transplantation. *Blood* **109**:3108–14.

20 Ho VT, Soiffer RJ. (2001) The history and future of T-cell depletion as graft-versus-host disease prophylaxis for allogeneic hematopoietic stem cell transplantation. *Blood* **98**:3192–204.

21 Kohrt HE, Turnbull BB, Heydari K, et al. (2009) TLI and ATG conditioning with low risk of graft-versus-host disease retains antitumor reactions after allogeneic hematopoietic cell transplantation from related and unrelated donors. *Blood* **114**:1099–109.

22 MacMillan ML, Weisdorf DJ, Davies SM, et al. (2002) Early antithymocyte globulin therapy improves survival in patients with steroid-resistant acute graft-versus-host disease. *Biol Blood Marrow Transplant* **8**:40–6.

23 Lee SJ, Zahrieh D, Agura E, et al. (2004) Effect of up-front daclizumab when combined with steroids for the treatment of acute graft-versus-host disease: results of a randomized trial. *Blood* **104**:1559–64.

24 Levine JE, Paczesny S, Mineishi S, et al. (2008) Etanercept plus methylprednisolone as initial therapy for acute graft-versus-host disease. *Blood* **111**:2470–5.

25 Alousi AM, Weisdorf DJ, Logan BR, et al. (2009) Etanercept, mycophenolate, denileukin, or pentostatin

plus corticosteroids for acute graft-versus-host disease: a randomized phase 2 trial from the Blood and Marrow Transplant Clinical Trials Network. *Blood* **114**:511–7.

26 Deeg HJ. (2007) How I treat refractory acute GVHD. *Blood* **109**:4119–26.

27 Stewart BL, Storer B, Storek J, et al. (2004) Duration of immunosuppressive treatment for chronic graft-versus-host disease. *Blood* **104**:3501–6.

28 Lee SJ, Flowers ME. (2008) Recognizing and managing chronic graft-versus-host disease. *Hematol (Am Soc Hematol Educ Program)* **2008**:134–41.

29 Martin PJ, Storer BE, Rowley SD, et al. (2009) Evaluation of mycophenolate mofetil for initial treatment of chronic graft-versus-host disease. *Blood* **113**:5074–82.

30 Pidala J, Anasetti C, Kharfan-Dabaja MA, et al. (2009) Decision analysis of peripheral blood versus bone marrow hematopoietic stem cells for allogeneic hematopoietic cell transplantation. *Biol Blood Marrow Transplant* **15**:1415–21.

31 Boeckh M, Nichols WG, Papanicolaou G, et al. (2003) Cytomegalovirus in hematopoietic stem cell transplant recipients: Current status, known challenges, and future strategies. *Biol Blood Marrow Transplant* **9**:543–58.

32 Boeckh M, Ljungman P. (2009) How we treat cytomegalovirus in hematopoietic cell transplant recipients. *Blood* **113**:5711–9.

33 Boeckh M, Nichols W, Chemaly R, et al. (2008) Prevention of late CMV disease after HCT: A randomized double-blind multicenter trial of valganciclovir [VGCV] prophylaxis versus PCR-guided GCV/VGCV preemptive therapy. *Biol Blood Marrow Transplant* **14**:30 [Abstract 75].

34 Groll AH, Tragiannidis A. (2009) Recent advances in antifungal prevention and treatment. *Semin Hematol* **46**:212–29.

35 Slavin MA, Osborne B, Adams R, et al. (1995) Efficacy and safety of fluconazole prophylaxis for fungal infections after marrow transplantation – a prospective, randomized, double-blind study. *J Infect Dis* **171**:1545–52.

36 Wingard J. (2007) Results of a randomized, double-blind trial of fluconazole [FLU] vs. voriconazole [VORI] for the prevention of invasive fungal infections [IFI] in 600 allogeneic blood and marrow transplant [BMT] patients. *Blood* **110**:[Abstract].

37 van Burik JA, Ratanatharathorn V, Stepan DE, et al. (2004) Micafungin versus fluconazole for prophylaxis against invasive fungal infections during neutropenia in patients undergoing hematopoietic stem cell transplantation. *Clin Infect Dis* **39**:1407–16.

38 Ullmann AJ, Lipton JH, Vesole DH, et al. (2007) Posaconazole or fluconazole for prophylaxis in severe graft-versus-host disease. *N Engl J Med* **356**:335–47.

39 Walsh TJ, Pappas P, Winston DJ, et al. (2002) Voriconazole compared with liposomal amphotericin B for empirical antifungal therapy in patients with neutropenia and persistent fever. *N Engl J Med* **346**:225–34.

40 Walsh TJ, Teppler H, Donowitz GR, et al. (2004) Caspofungin versus liposomal amphotericin B for empirical antifungal therapy in patients with persistent fever and neutropenia. *N Engl J Med* **351**:1391–402.

41 Herbrecht R, Denning DW, Patterson TF, et al. (2002) Voriconazole versus amphotericin B for primary therapy of invasive aspergillosis. *N Engl J Med* **347**: 408–15.

42 Cornelissen JJ, van Putten WL, Verdonck LF, et al. (2007) Results of a HOVON/SAKK donor versus no-donor analysis of myeloablative HLA-identical sibling stem cell transplantation in first remission acute myeloid leukemia in young and middle-aged adults: benefits for whom? *Blood* **109**:3658–66.

43 Koreth J, Schlenk R, Kopecky KJ, et al. (2009) Allogeneic stem cell transplantation for acute myeloid leukemia in first complete remission: systematic review and meta-analysis of prospective clinical trials. *JAMA* **301**:2349–61.

44 Ringden O, Horowitz MM, Gale RP, et al. (1993) Outcome after allogeneic bone marrow transplant for leukemia in older adults. *JAMA* **270**:57–60.

45 Appelbaum FR. (2008) What is the impact of hematopoietic cell transplantation [HCT] for older adults with acute myeloid leukemia [AML]? *Best Pract Res Clin Haematol* **21**:667–75.

46 Hegenbart U, Niederwieser D, Sandmaier BM, et al. (2006) Treatment for acute myelogenous leukemia by low-dose, total-body, irradiation-based conditioning and hematopoietic cell transplantation from related and unrelated donors. *J Clin Oncol* **24**:444–53.

47 de Lima M, Anagnostopoulos A, Munsell M, et al. (2004) Nonablative versus reduced-intensity conditioning regimens in the treatment of acute myeloid leukemia and high-risk myelodysplastic syndrome: dose is relevant for long-term disease control after allogeneic hematopoietic stem cell transplantation. *Blood* **104**:865–72.

48 Tauro S, Craddock C, Peggs K, et al. (2005) Allogeneic stem-cell transplantation using a reduced-intensity conditioning regimen has the capacity to produce durable remissions and long-term disease-free survival in

patients with high-risk acute myeloid leukemia and myelodysplasia. *J Clin Oncol* **23**:9387–93.

49 van Besien K, Artz A, Smith S, et al. (2005) Fludarabine, melphalan, and alemtuzumab conditioning in adults with standard-risk advanced acute myeloid leukemia and myelodysplastic syndrome. *J Clin Oncol* **23**:5728–38.

50 Blaise DP, Michel Boiron J, Faucher C, et al. (2005) Reduced intensity conditioning prior to allogeneic stem cell transplantation for patients with acute myeloblastic leukemia as a first-line treatment. *Cancer* **104**:1931–8.

51 Sayer HG, Kroger M, Beyer J, et al. (2003) Reduced intensity conditioning for allogeneic hematopoietic stem cell transplantation in patients with acute myeloid leukemia: disease status by marrow blasts is the strongest prognostic factor. *Bone Marrow Transplant* **31**:1089–95.

52 Shimoni A, Hardan I, Shem-Tov N, et al. (2006) Allogeneic hematopoietic stem-cell transplantation in AML and MDS using myeloablative versus reduced-intensity conditioning: the role of dose intensity. *Leukemia* **20**:322–8.

53 Valcarcel D, Martino R, Caballero D, et al. (2008) Sustained remissions of high-risk acute myeloid leukemia and myelodysplastic syndrome after reduced-intensity conditioning allogeneic hematopoietic transplantation: chronic graft-versus-host disease is the strongest factor improving survival. *J Clin Oncol* **26**:577–84.

54 de Lima M, Couriel D, Thall PF, et al. (2004) Once-daily intravenous busulfan and fludarabine: clinical and pharmacokinetic results of a myeloablative, reduced-toxicity conditioning regimen for allogeneic stem cell transplantation in AML and MDS. *Blood* **104**:857–64.

55 Bornhauser M, Storer B, Slattery JT, et al. (2003) Conditioning with fludarabine and targeted busulfan for transplantation of allogeneic hematopoietic stem cells. *Blood* **102**:820–6.

56 Schmid C, Schleuning M, Ledderose G, Tischer J, Kolb HJ. (2005) Sequential regimen of chemotherapy, reduced-intensity conditioning for allogeneic stem-cell transplantation, and prophylactic donor lymphocyte transfusion in high-risk acute myeloid leukemia and myelodysplastic syndrome. *J Clin Oncol* **23**:5675–87.

57 Schmid C, Schleuning M, Hentrich M, et al. (2008) High antileukemic efficacy of an intermediate intensity conditioning regimen for allogeneic stem cell transplantation in patients with high-risk acute myeloid leukemia in first complete remission. *Bone Marrow Transplant* **41**:721–7.

58 Aoudjhane M, Labopin M, Gorin NC, et al. (2005) Comparative outcome of reduced intensity and myeloablative conditioning regimen in HLA identical sibling allogeneic haematopoietic stem cell transplantation for patients older than 50 years of age with acute myeloblastic leukaemia: a retrospective survey from the Acute Leukemia Working Party (ALWP) of the European group for Blood and Marrow Transplantation (EBMT). *Leukemia* **19**:2304–12.

59 Alyea EP, Kim HT, Ho V, et al. (2005) Comparative outcome of nonmyeloablative and myeloablative allogeneic hematopoietic cell transplantation for patients older than 50 years of age. *Blood* **105**:1810–4.

60 Feinstein LC, Sandmaier BM, Hegenbart U, et al. (2003) Non-myeloablative allografting from human leucocyte antigen-identical sibling donors for treatment of acute myeloid leukaemia in first complete remission. *Br J Haematol* **120**:281–8.

61 Hansen JA, Gooley TA, Martin PJ, et al. (1998) Bone marrow transplants from unrelated donors for patients with chronic myeloid leukemia. *N Engl J Med* **338**:962–8.

62 Or R, Shapira MY, Resnick I, et al. (2003) Nonmyeloablative allogeneic stem cell transplantation for the treatment of chronic myeloid leukemia in first chronic phase. *Blood* **101**:441–5.

63 Kerbauy FR, Storb R, Hegenbart U, et al. (2005) Hematopoietic cell transplantation from HLA-identical sibling donors after low-dose radiation-based conditioning for treatment of CML. *Leukemia* **19**:990–7.

64 Crawley C, Szydlo R, Lalancette M, et al. (2005) Outcomes of reduced-intensity transplantation for chronic myeloid leukemia: an analysis of prognostic factors from the Chronic Leukemia Working Party of the EBMT. *Blood* **106**:2969–76.

65 Goldstone AH, Richards SM, Lazarus HM, et al. (2008) In adults with standard-risk acute lymphoblastic leukemia, the greatest benefit is achieved from a matched sibling allogeneic transplantation in first complete remission, and an autologous transplantation is less effective than conventional consolidation/maintenance chemotherapy in all patients: final results of the International ALL Trial (MRC UKALL XII/ECOG E2993). *Blood* **111**:1827–33.

66 Mohty M, Labopin M, Tabrizzi R, et al. (2008) Reduced intensity conditioning allogeneic stem cell transplantation for adult patients with acute lymphoblastic leukemia: a retrospective study from the European Group

for Blood and Marrow Transplantation. *Haematologica* **93**:303–6.

67 Martino R, Giralt S, Caballero MD, et al. (2003) Allogeneic hematopoietic stem cell transplantation with reduced-intensity conditioning in acute lymphoblastic leukemia: a feasibility study. *Haematologica* **88**: 555–60.

68 Hamaki T, Kami M, Kanda Y, et al. (2005) Reduced-intensity stem-cell transplantation for adult acute lymphoblastic leukemia: a retrospective study of 33 patients. *Bone Marrow Transplant* **35**:549–56.

69 Bachanova V, Verneris MR, DeFor T, Brunstein CG, Weisdorf DJ. (2009) Prolonged survival in adults with acute lymphoblastic leukemia after reduced-intensity conditioning with cord blood or sibling donor transplantation. *Blood* **113**:2902–5.

70 Kharfan-Dabaja MA, Anasetti C, Santos ES. (2007) Hematopoietic cell transplantation for chronic lymphocytic leukemia: an evolving concept. *Biol Blood Marrow Transplant* **13**:373–85.

71 Schetelig J, Thiede C, Bornhauser M, et al. (2003) Evidence of a graft-versus-leukemia effect in chronic lymphocytic leukemia after reduced-intensity conditioning and allogeneic stem-cell transplantation: the Cooperative German Transplant Study Group. *J Clin Oncol* **21**:2747–53.

72 Brown JR, Kim HT, Li S, et al. (2006) Predictors of improved progression-free survival after nonmyeloablative allogeneic stem cell transplantation for advanced chronic lymphocytic leukemia. *Biol Blood Marrow Transplant* **12**:1056–64.

73 Sorror ML, Maris MB, Sandmaier BM, et al. (2005) Hematopoietic cell transplantation after nonmyeloablative conditioning for advanced chronic lymphocytic leukemia. *J Clin Oncol* **23**:3819–29.

74 Caballero D, Garcia-Marco JA, Martino R, et al. (2005) Allogeneic transplant with reduced intensity conditioning regimens may overcome the poor prognosis of B-cell chronic lymphocytic leukemia with unmutated immunoglobulin variable heavy-chain gene and chromosomal abnormalities (11q- and 17p-). *Clin Cancer Res* **11**:7757–63.

75 Dreger P, Brand R, Milligan D, et al. (2005) Reduced-intensity conditioning lowers treatment-related mortality of allogeneic stem cell transplantation for chronic lymphocytic leukemia: a population-matched analysis. *Leukemia* **19**:1029–33.

76 Khouri IF. (2006) Reduced-intensity regimens in allogeneic stem-cell transplantation for non-Hodgkin lymphoma and chronic lymphocytic leukemia. *Hematology (Am Soc Hematol Educ Program)* **2006**:390–7.

77 van Besien K. (2009) Allogeneic stem cell transplantation in follicular lymphoma: recent progress and controversy. *Hematology (Am Soc Hematol Educ Program)* **2009**:610–8.

78 Geisler CH, Kolstad A, Laurell A, et al. (2008) Long-term progression-free survival of mantle cell lymphoma after intensive front-line immunochemotherapy with in vivo-purged stem cell rescue: a nonrandomized phase 2 multicenter study by the Nordic Lymphoma Group. *Blood* **112**:2687–93.

79 Ghielmini M, Zucca E. (2009) How I treat mantle cell lymphoma. *Blood* **114**:1469–76.

80 Crawley C, Iacobelli S, Bjorkstrand B, et al. (2007) Reduced-intensity conditioning for myeloma: lower nonrelapse mortality but higher relapse rates compared with myeloablative conditioning. *Blood* **109**: 3588–94.

81 Bensinger WI. (2009) Role of autologous and allogeneic stem cell transplantation in myeloma. *Leukemia* **23**:442–8.

82 Garban F, Attal M, Michallet M, et al. (2006) Prospective comparison of autologous stem cell transplantation followed by dose-reduced allograft (IFM99-03 trial) with tandem autologous stem cell transplantation (IFM99-04 trial) in high-risk de novo multiple myeloma. *Blood* **107**:3474–80.

83 Bruno B, Rotta M, Patriarca F, et al. (2007) A comparison of allografting with autografting for newly diagnosed myeloma. *N Engl J Med* **356**:1110–20.

CHAPTER 24

Quality of Life after the Diagnosis of Hematologic Malignancies

Mohamed Sorror, MD, MSc

Fred Hutchinson Cancer Research Center and University of Washington, Seattle, WA, USA

Introduction

Definition

Health-related quality of life (QOL) has an inherent meaning to most people. It is comprised of broad concepts that affect global life satisfaction, including good health, adequate housing, employment, personal and family safety, education, and leisure pursuits. QOL can be more formally defined as: "The extents to which one's usual or expected physical, emotional and social well-being are affected by a medical condition or its treatment" [1]. It is a multidimensional construct comprising physical and functional well-being, psychological function, social role function, family well-being, sexuality/ intimacy, and disease or treatment symptoms (e.g., pain and nausea) [2, 3].

The evolution of importance of QOL assessment

Advances in the conventional chemo-immunotherapy for hematologic malignancies (HM) and the success of hematopoietic cell transplantation (HCT) have resulted in a large number of long-term surviving patients, bringing the issue of QOL to the forefront [4, 5]. Therefore, improvements in QOL have become one of two potential benefits that are considered by the US FDA for the approval of new anticancer drugs [6]. Incorporating QOL in traditional clinical outcome assessment can provide valuable information to better guide clinical decision making. The availability of different treatment modalities with similar effectiveness for disease control and survival has made differences in patients' health status during the survival period as critical variables in making final and individualized treatment choices. QOL could be used to delineate differences among treatments with regard to toxicity and quality of survival.

Types of measures

QOL must be measured from the individual's viewpoint rather than that of outside observers. This is because QOL represents a subjective appraisal of the impact of illness or its treatment to the extent that individual patients with the same objective health status can report different QOL due to differences in expectations and coping abilities [7]. Several validated and reliable questionnaires are available for assessment of QOL [8]. They could be generally classified into general health status instruments, general illness instruments, and disease-specific instruments. General health status instruments are applicable to all populations and can be completed by individuals both with and without medical illness. They are ideal for comparison across diverse groups, such as healthy and ill populations. Examples include the Nottingham Health Profile (NHP) [9] and the Short Form-36 (SF-36) from the Medical Outcomes Study [10, 11]. General illness instruments are applicable to populations with any medical illness, and can be used to compare different illnesses, levels of disease severity, or types of interventions. Examples include the Sickness Impact Profile (SIP) [12] and the Functional Assessment of Chronic Illness Therapy (FACIT) [13]. Disease-specific instruments are designed to assess the QOL of individuals with specific illnesses, specific types of treatment, or specific symptoms; such as the Functional Living Index – Cancer (FLIC). These instruments are likely to be more sensitive to specific treatment-related changes in QOL [14]. It is not uncommon to combine general and disease-specific instruments to fully assess QOL.

Limited information on QOL for patients with HM

While the impact of QOL for patients with solid tumors has been well studied and incorporated as end points for clinical trials, only scarce data are available to date for HM [15]. QOL was rarely tested as an end point in randomized clinical trials for HM and attempts to assess QOL were based only on indirect measures, such as days of hospitalization or clinician-reported observations. This has been due to: (1) historical poor prognosis or acute course of some HM; and (2) the possible general perception that seriously compromising a patient's QOL was an indispensable step towards cure of HM. Nevertheless, a few recent studies have systematically assessed QOL after either conventional treatment or HCT, which will be reviewed here.

Impact of conventional treatments of HM on QOL aspects

Childhood HM survivors have provided unique opportunities for studying QOL outcomes, as diagnosis and treatment take place during formative development of organ systems, cognition, emotions, and life experiences. Further, factors that impact educational attainment, employment, marriage and intimacy, fertility, and other life values differ in the emerging young adult compared with the older adult [16]. Varied, and sometimes contradictory, results are reported due to small sample sizes, dif-

ferent QOL measures, and selection of population norms for the comparison group. Siblings of long-term survivors constitute a better comparison group for QOL outcomes, particularly given the similarities in ethnicity, culture, community, socioeconomic status, genetics, and family environment.

Acute leukemia

Studies of childhood cancer survivors have shown that long-term leukemia survivors demonstrate elevated rates of psychological distress compared with their siblings [17]. During patient adolescence, parents report that leukemia survivors experience increased rates of depression, anxiety, and social-skills deficits when compared with sibling controls [18]. Those given CNS irradiation report no differences in fatigue, sleep disruption, or daytime sleepiness from survivors not given CNS irradiation [19], although the former ones are reported to have more functional limitations [20]. Chemotherapy exposures, including alkylating agents and anthracyclines, are associated with an increase in physical impairment and psychological distress, including anxiety [21]. Survivors exposed to intensive chemotherapy report more psychological distress, including depression and somatization [22].

With regard to neurocognitive outcomes, childhood leukemia survivors were reported with attention problems when compared to siblings. Attention problems were even higher among patients given cranial radiation $\pm$ intrathecal methotrexate [18]. Survivors who received high-dose cranial radiation to frontal area of their brains ($\geq$35 Gy) had significantly higher problems with attention and processing speed, memory, and emotional regulation [23].

Impaired neurocognitive functioning is an increasingly recognized long-term consequence of acute lymphocytic leukemia (ALL) treatment. Declines in overall intellectual ability [24], academic performance [25], memory and learning [26], attention and concentration [27], information-processing speed [28], visuospatial skill [29], psychomotor functioning [30], and executive functioning [31] are among the adverse neurocognitive outcomes reported in the literature. A recent meta-analysis quantitatively estimated the magnitude of both general and specific neurocognitive sequelae of treatment for childhood ALL. The meta-analysis included 28 empirical studies that reported sufficient data to calculate effect sizes for comparisons with control groups of healthy peers or siblings and groups of children treated for solid tumors or other chronic illnesses without CNS prophylaxis. All 13 mean effect sizes that extracted across the nine evaluated neurocognitive domains were in the negative direction ($g = -0.34$ to -0.71) demonstrating that children treated for ALL experienced consistent clinically significant deficits in overall cognitive or intellectual functioning, academic achievement, and specific neurocognitive abilities when compared to healthy or illness control groups. The authors suggested that declines in multiple areas of neurocognitive functioning occurred as a result of contemporary ALL treatment. It is likely that failure to properly assess and address treatment-related learning problems in school leads to inadequate preparation for higher education or the workforce. The meta-analysis also revealed clinically significant deficits in specific neurocognitive abilities, such as attention and speed of information processing, and also in areas of executive functioning, which have implications beyond school, to areas such as occupational functioning, social relationships, emotion regulation, coping skills, and general QOL. The use of the psychostimulant methylphenidate has been shown to reduce deficits in attention and social skills problems in some survivors of childhood cancer [32].

Approximately two-thirds of the studies measuring global intellectual abilities, neuropsychological, and/or academic achievement performance of ALL survivors given CNS chemotherapy documented declines in cognitive functioning. *All* of the studies enlisting a sibling control group, and all but one study enlisting a non-CNS-treated cancer group documented declines in one or more aspect of cognitive functioning among ALL survivors. Taken together, it may be concluded that CNS chemotherapy for ALL is not a benign form of treatment. Furthermore, long-term deficits in attention and non-verbal memory have also been reported. In addition, the acute effects of CNS-directed chemotherapy on fine-motor and perceptual-motor skills are documented. Significant declines in academic achievement have been found in mathematics,

reading, and spelling, with approximately twice as many studies finding significant decreases in mathematics than in reading or spelling [33].

Campbell et al. examined associations among several domains of executive function (EF), coping with stress, and emotional/behavioral problems in childhood ALL survivors and a matched healthy control cohort. ALL survivors had significantly lower composite working memory scores when compared to the control group. However, these scores, as well as those for the other EF domains, fell within the average range for both groups. This suggests that despite the differences in working memory, childhood ALL survivors generally demonstrate intact EF abilities [34].

Chronic leukemia

Although chronic lymphocytic leukemia (CLL) accounts for 25–30% of leukemia cases, there has been only limited psychosocial research in the field of CLL. Holzner et al., in a one-year prospective study, reported that 76 patients with CLL had a lower QOL compared with age-matched controls, which was more pronounced on physical than cognitive functioning domains. (ES $= -0.43$; $P < 0.01$ and ES $= -0.27$; $P < 0.1$, respectively) [35]. There was no statistical difference between patients given chemotherapy versus "watch and wait", suggesting well-tolerated chemotherapy with no substantial long-term effects. Younger males were found to have a higher QOL while females, irrespective of age, had in general, reported a lower QOL. Over the course of one year, QOL remained remarkably stable compared to baseline.

QOL was improved when anemia in CLL was treated with erythropoietin [36]. Another study found a similar QOL among CLL conventionally treated patients and bone marrow transplant patients, despite the younger age of the transplant group (mean age, 34 years). The only difference between the two groups was seen in the emotional well-being domain – the bone marrow transplant group had a lower score (ES $= 0.787$), reflecting a worse emotional QOL [37]. Levin et al. assessed 105 CLL patients who completed a mail-in battery of depression, anxiety, and QOL measures. No statistical difference was shown between depression, anxiety, and physical/mental QOL in "watch and wait" versus active-treatment groups. Among, the "watch and wait" group, patients ≤60 years reported more depression and worse emotional and social QOL. They also had more "watch and wait" anxiety. Social and emotional QOL were similar in both newly diagnosed patients and those diagnosed more than six years ago, although physical QOL worsens with time [38].

Data on impacts of conventional treatment on QOL of patients with chronic myeloid leukemia (CML) are rare. In one study [39], investigators from the US and Europe analyzed QOL outcomes in patients with chronic phase CML, who were randomly assigned to imatinib or interferon alfa plus subcutaneous low-dose cytarabine (IFN + LDAC). Patients completed cancer-specific QOL (Functional Assessment of Cancer Therapy-Biologic Response Modifiers) and utility (Euro QoL-5D) questionnaires at baseline and during treatment (n = 1049). Patients receiving IFN + LDAC experienced a significant decline in the trial outcome index (TOI), whereas those receiving imatinib maintained their baseline level. Treatment differences at each visit were significant (P <0.001) and clinically relevant in favor of imatinib. Mean social and family well-being (SFWB), emotional well-being (EWB), and utility scores were also significantly better for those patients taking imatinib. Patients who crossed over to imatinib experienced a significant increase in TOI (P <0.001). The authors concluded that imatinib offers advantages in QOL compared with IFN + LDAC as first-line treatment of chronic phase CML [39].

Lymphoma

A recent update from the Childhood Cancer Survivor Study [40] has shown childhood lymphoma survivors to have higher rates of psychological distress, including anxiety and somatization compared with siblings and population norms [17]. More specifically, survivors of Hodgkin lymphoma (HL) reported increases in physical health impairment compared with leukemia survivors [21] and more symptoms of somatization compared with leukemia and non-Hodgkin lymphoma (NHL) survivors [22], in addition to higher rates of clinically significant somatization compared with

siblings [17]. They also endorsed more complaints of fatigue, sleep disruption, and daytime sleepiness compared with siblings [19]. In the large comparison study between leukemia and lymphoma survivors (n = 5736) versus sibling controls (n = 2565), intensive chemotherapy added to the risk of depression and somatic distress among leukemia/lymphoma survivors. Gender and socioeconomic status predicted depression and somatic distress equally in both cohorts NHL survivors reported [22]. NHL survivors also reported lower vitality in assessment of their QOL scores compared with siblings and norms, which demonstrated the largest effect size with respect to impaired vitality.

The European Organization for Research and Treatment of Cancer (EORTC) Lymphoma Group and the Groupe d'Études des Lymphomes de l'Adulte (GELA) assessed QOL among patients with HL treated on the EORTC and GELA H8 trials [41]. Patients received QOL questionnaires at the end of primary therapy and during follow-up. The EORTC QLQ-C30 was used to assess QOL, and the Multidimensional Fatigue Inventory (MFI-20) was used to assess fatigue. Mean follow-up was 90 months (range 52–118). Age affected all functioning and symptom scores except emotional functioning, with younger age associated with higher functioning and lower severity of symptoms; improvement with time showed similar patterns between age groups. Women reported lower QOL and higher symptom scores than men. Key findings included a significant improvement in most QOL domains within 18 months of the end of treatments, except for cognitive functioning and reduced motivation, suggesting that neither the treatment nor the disease affect these two dimensions. By contrast, very few (<10%) patients showed QOL impairment. Scores were similar to those of long-term survivors of HL or healthy controls from the general population matched for age and sex. Fatigue (MFI-20 scores) at the end of treatment was the only predictive variable for persistent fatigue.

Kornblith et al. compared the long-term psychosocial adaptation of 273 HL and 206 adult acute leukemia survivors. Patients were interviewed by telephone and were evaluated using identical research procedures and a common set of instruments [42]. All participants had been treated on one of nine Hodgkin's disease or 13 acute leukemia CALGB clinical trials from 1966–1988, and had been off treatment for one year or more. HL survivors' risk of having a high distress score was almost twice that found for leukemia survivors (odds ratio = 1.90), with 21% of HL versus 14% of leukemia survivors (P <0.05) having scores that were 1.5 standard deviations above the norm. HL survivors reported greater fatigue, greater conditioned nausea, and greater impact of cancer on their family life and poorer sexual function than leukemia survivors.

In Norway, 610 HL survivors were assessed for total (TF) and chronic fatigue (CF) eight years after treatment using a fatigue questionnaire [43]. Mean TF scores were elevated in HL survivors compared with the general population (mean score, 14.6 vs. 12.1, respectively; P <0.001), as was the proportion of persons with CF (30% vs. 11%, respectively; odds ratio = 3.6; P <0.001). The 70 patients with CF eight years earlier still reported higher TF at follow-up than the 210 patients without CF at the previous assessment (mean score, 17.0 vs. 13.1, respectively; P <0.001). There was a positive association between age and TF (P <0.05), whereas presence of B symptoms (fever, drenching night sweats, and/or weight loss) at diagnosis and treatment before 1980 were associated with CF. Significantly more patients with persisting CF had B symptoms at diagnosis compared with patients who had recovered (P = 0.05). No significant association with treatment modality and intensity was found [44].

The sexual functioning of male lymphoma survivors has rarely been studied. In a survey of 459 HL survivors, transient or long-term reduction of sexual interest and activity was reported by 28% [45]. Similarly, in another study, 24% reported at least one sexual problem [46]. Sexual interest and sexual activity had decreased compared with before treatment in approximately 20% of men with a median of nine years after treatment for HL [47]. When using a standard questionnaire on erectile function, however, 36 of 59 (61%) lymphoma survivors aged between 18 to 55 years reported reduced erectile function [48]. Thus, the prevalence of self-reported reduced sexual function may be higher when more detailed questionnaires are used. Both chemotherapy and radiotherapy can damage Leydig cell and/or pituitary function [49, 50], resulting in subnormal testosterone levels that could potentially lead to sexual problems [51]. In a follow-up survey, 246 male lymphoma survivors having low testosterone and/or elevated luteinizing hormone (LH) had lower Brief Sexual Function Inventory (BSFI) scores than survivors with normal gonadal hormones. Multivariate analyses showed that increasing age, more emotional distress, poor physical health, and low testosterone and/or elevated LH were significantly associated with reduced sexual function within the lymphoma group. Lymphoma survivors had significantly lower BSFI domain scores than did controls on erection, ejaculation, and sexual satisfaction [52].

QOL after HCT for patients with HM

HCT has been used as potentially curative or consolidation treatment option for a variety of HM. HCT is usually followed by acute morbidity, which is commonly associated with various distressing physical symptoms. Recent literature has begun to explore the impact of this procedure on QOL and psychosocial issues. While HCT survivors often report highly rated global QOL, a number of patients suffer from psychosocial difficulties that could persist for years.

Autologous HCT
QOL among patients given autologous HCT is generally excellent. This is mainly due to lack of graft-versus-host disease (GVHD) and the high frequency of post-HCT relapse as the major cause of morbidity and mortality.

Among patients who were alive and free of disease for at least one year, 88% reported QOL of above average or excellent and 78% were employed [53]. Three months post-HCT, a significant proportion of patients reported a number of concerns, including employment, appearance, and sexual functioning. However, most of these concerns had resolved by one year following autologous HCT [53]. Patients with acute leukemia had prolonged transfusion requirements, especially for platelets. In another study, 82 patients who had survived for one or more years following autologous HCT were surveyed for QOL issues by written questionnaire and telephone interview [54]. The most commonly reported symptoms were insomnia, fatigue, and pain. Sexual interest and sexual activity were more frequent after versus before HCT. The majority of patients who were employed prior to HCT returned to work, with a median time away from work of 48 weeks.

Whedon et al. reported on QOL of 29 patients with lymphoma, leukemia, or breast cancer given autologous HCT. They used the City of Hope QOL-BMT instrument. Global QOL was high (mean = 8.17 on a 1–10 scale). Moderate-severe fatigue was reported by 50%, while 93% reported moderate-severe distress over illness' effect on family. Lowest score was found on sexual functioning subscale. Most respondents experienced few long-term physical disruptions and had only mild psychological distress, and 66% had returned to work [55].

The remaining literature on QOL after autologous HCT either were devoted to breast cancer (which is beyond the scope of this review), or incorporated data on allogeneic HCT for comparison (will be discussed later).

Allogeneic HCT

Allogeneic HCT is a potentially curative treatment for many patients with HM. However, this treatment modality carries risks of significant acute complications and late effects including chronic GVHD, infections, organ toxicity, osteoporosis, cataracts, secondary cancers, and infertility, as well as decrements in QOL [56–58].

Overall QOL

The first study evaluating survivors of allogeneic HCT revealed that the majority of patients were employed and in reasonably good health, with acceptable objective and subjective function. However, about a quarter of the subjects reported ongoing medical problems. Also, 15–25% reported significant emotional distress, low self-esteem, and less-than-optimal life satisfaction [59]. A subsequent study done in patients given allogeneic HCT for acute or chronic leukemia revealed direct correlation between dose of TBI and cognitive dysfunction. Furthermore, this relationship remained even after the impact of psychological distress upon cog-

nitive functioning was accounted for. TBI-related cognitive impairment primarily involved slowed reaction time, reduced attention and concentration, and difficulties in reasoning and problem solving [60]. Several other reports have confirmed that the QOL of long-term survivors following HCT is generally excellent, with >90% of patients enjoying Karnofsky performance scores of 80% or higher [61–63].

Syrjala et al. evaluated 67 HCT recipients at baseline, 90 days, 1 year and 4.5 years after transplantation [64]. Physical functioning was found to be most impaired at the 90-day time point. Most HCT patients had returned to pre-transplant levels of function at the one-year time point, and they continued at the same level beyond five years after HCT. Duell et al. found that 93% of patients were in good health and 89% had returned to full-time work or school [56]. However, when compared with their siblings, long-term allogeneic HCT survivors were more likely to report difficulty in holding jobs and in obtaining life or health insurance [65].

When adult survivors of allogeneic HCT were surveyed with a mailed questionnaire 6 to 149 months after HCT, over 170 patients were eligible and 86% responded. Survivors showed a high degree of overall satisfaction with major life domains but were least satisfied with their bodies, level of physical strength, and ability to attain sexual satisfaction. Positive and negative affect were higher than general population samples and less tension, fatigue, confusion, and depression were displayed than comparison groups. Multiple regression analyses showed that self-esteem and level of current physical functioning made significant contributions on predicting multiple QOL outcomes [66]. Sexual problems were also identified as a concern for allogeneic HCT survivors [67].

Physical functioning

Physical functioning tended to decline immediately after allogeneic HCT [58, 68]. While Syrjala et al. reported on improvement in physical functioning in the year after HCT [58], Bush et al. found out that over four years are required for the gradual improvement [69]. Fluctuation in physical functioning could be seen over time, with 25% of patients reporting major physical limitations at baseline; 44%, at 90 days; 12%, at one year; 22%, at three years; and 18%, at five years [58].

Emotional functioning

Emotional functioning appears to be most affected both immediately prior to and after allogeneic HCT due to high levels of distress at these times [68, 70]. Significant improvements in emotional functioning were reported early after HCT. McQuellon et al. found that 43% of HCT recipients reported depressive symptoms at one or more points through the first year after HCT. Some studies showed stable emotional function findings at later time points thereafter [64, 68], while others demonstrated ongoing improvement two to four years after HCT [69, 71]. Nevertheless, significant impairments in emotional functioning in HCT survivors have been observed compared to healthy controls 5–10 years after HCT [72].

Social functioning

Impairments in social functioning were reported in the first 100 days after allogeneic HCT [64]. Social functioning similar to or better than baseline could be noted 12 months after HCT [64, 68]. As high as 84% of HCT survivors were found to be fairly socializing with family and friends by two years [69]. Long-term follow-up has shown persistent small decrements in social functioning among HCT survivors compared to healthy controls [73].

Role functioning

Even though an immediate decline in home management and return to work or school is noted after HCT, gradual improvements occur with time. About 60–70% of HCT survivors were found to return to work, school, or homemaking by one year [74, 75], while up to 80% were found to regain role function at or beyond two years after allogeneic HCT [58, 69].

Risk factors

QOL was found to be good, intermediate, or poor among 25%, 44%, and 31% of 244 survivors five years after HCT [76]. Sexual and psychological domains were more impaired among female versus male survivors. In multivariate analysis, poor QOL was predicted by age, long-term sequelae, chronic GVHD, and duration after HCT.

Long-term problems and QOL issues after HCT may be due to pre-HCT comorbid conditions. Only humble studies are available for impacts of pre-transplant physical and psychosocial status on post-HCT QOL. The physical and psychosocial status of 28 adult BMT recipients was assessed prior to BMT and 12–16 months after BMT. Analysis of group means indicated few significant differences between pre- and post-BMT assessments. However, inspection of residual change scores suggested that physical and psychosocial status improved following BMT for some individuals, while that of others declined. Analysis of residual change scores indicated that males and older patients at time of BMT reported the largest declines in physical and psychosocial status [77].

To date, no studies have been performed on impacts of pre-HCT medical comorbidities on post-HCT QOL. The HCT-comorbidity index has been recently developed to appropriately capture medical comorbidities [78], and has show good prediction for post-HCT mortalities [79–81]. Systemic assessment of the impacts of medical comorbidities on QOL is greatly warranted.

Chronic GVHD

Chronic GVHD has been defined as the major factor limiting QOL in recipients of allogeneic HCT [76, 82–84]. Fraser et al. assessed 584 survivors ≥2 years following allogeneic HCT. Incidence of cGVHD was 54%; 46% of those had active disease at the time of the survey [85]. In multivariable analyses, subjects with active cGVHD were more likely to report adverse general health, mental health, functional impairments, activity limitation, and pain than were those with no history of cGVHD. However, health status did not differ between those with resolved cGVHD and those who had never had cGVHD. In another study, 96 survivors prospectively completed self-assessment surveys (including the Medical Outcomes Study Short Form 12 (SF12) and the Functional Assessment of Cancer Therapy-Bone Marrow Transplant scale) before HCT, and at 6 and/or 12 months post-HCT [83]. Eighty-three percent of survivors responded at 6 and 12 months. Physical and mental functioning assessed by SF12 was not associated with either acute or chronic GVHD. In contrast, the TOI of the Functional Assessment of Cancer Therapy-Bone Marrow Transplant was sensitive to occurrence of either acute or chronic GVHD. Investigators found that GVHD was a major determinant of the long-term QOL of survivors. The adverse effects of acute GVHD were detectable with TOI at six months post-HCT after which development of cGVHD was the one most strongly correlated with worse QOL [83].

Unrelated donor HCT

Studies describing QOL issues in recipients of unrelated donor HCT have shown good QOL, with 75% of patients returning to full- or part-time work In another study, impairments were most noticed in the areas of sexual relationships, vocational and social adjustment, and psychological distress; and were more pronounced in females and older adults. Fatigue, present in almost 80% of patients, was the most common symptom interfering with daily life; this symptom was associated with the presence of anxiety, pain, infection, and weight loss [86].

Reduced-intensity conditioning for allogeneic HCT

Reduced-intensity conditioning regimens have been increasingly used to enable allogeneic HCT with lessened regimen-related morbidity and mortality than conventional myeloablative allogeneic HCT. As a result, the HCT eligibility criteria have been expanded to include elderly and comorbid patients who were usually excluded from allogeneic HCT. While the lessened toxicities could theoretically result in improved QOL, this advantage might be offset by the inclusion of high-risk patients. At least one study compared both conditioning modalities pre-transplant (baseline), and at days 0, 30, 100, one and two years following HCT. QOL was found to progressively improve (P<0.01) in both groups with higher scores at day 100 compared to days 0 and 30; there was no difference between groups during early recovery. At two years, all survivors (n = 43) reported QOL similar or better than baseline, with the exception of worse physical health among myeloablative patients [71].

Comparison studies

Autologous versus allogeneic HCT

Multiple confounders exist among recipients of autologous and allogeneic HCT, mainly including age, comorbidities, disease status, more relapse after autologous HCT, and GVHD after allogeneic HCT. Comparison studies have rarely adjusted for these confounders.

Andrykowski et al. compared the two modalities among 200 patients who were alive and disease-free at 12 months post-HCT. Allogeneic recipients reported poorer QOL than autologous recipients. Older age, lower level of education, and more advanced disease at BMT were consistent risk factors for poorer QOL [77].

No differences in QOL could be found between autologous and allogeneic HCT recipients at 90 days and 1, 3, and 5 years after controlling for a variety of medical and sociodemographic variables, with the exception of slower recovery of HCT-related distress found among allogeneic HCT recipients [58]. In contrast, other data suggest that allogeneic patients recover more slowly from transplantation [75, 87]. Long-term QOL has been generally found to be poorer after allogeneic versus autologous HCT [88, 89].

Peripheral blood mononuclear cells versus marrow grafts

In the autologous HCT setting, significant differences in QOL, as assessed by the Rotterdam Symptom Checklist, were found in favor of PBMC, both at 14 days post-HCT and at three months after discharge [90, 91]. In contrast, the global QOL, assessed by the EORTC QOL Questionnaire C30, did not differ between 150 recipients of PBMC or marrow allogeneic grafts. It was thought that higher incidence of acute and chronic GVHD in patients given PBMC was responsible for increasing impairments of role and social functioning in this group [92].

HCT versus conventional chemotherapy

Ninety-one and 73 patients given HCT and chemotherapy, respectively, were compared for QOL. Both cohorts were matched for age, post-treatment duration, sociodemographic and disease characteristics [93]. The HCT patients reported good to excellent QOL and in some domains even better QOL than that reported by the chemotherapy patients. However, approximately 20% of the HCT patients had lingering problems, including failure to return to work or school, symptoms of anxiety and depression, as well as decreased sexual and body image satisfaction.

Patients (n = 479) with acute myeloid leukemia (AML) in first remission, randomized between allogeneic and autologous HCT, and intensive consolidation chemotherapy, were assessed for differences in sexual function and fertility [94]. HCT recipients had severe, highly significant impairment of sexual health. HCT recipients reported more significant decrease in interest in sex, sexual activity, pleasure from sex, and ability to have sex compared to chemotherapy recipients (P<0.001 in each case). Hormonal disorders and infertility were also more common in HCT than in chemotherapy patients. These differences were more apparent in women and remained after adjustment for age.

QOL issues were evaluated at one year in patients treated on a UK MRC AML10 trial comparing HCT with chemotherapy in AML [95]. Mouth dryness problems and worse sexual and social relationships, professional, and leisure activities were more frequent among HCT versus chemotherapy recipients. Allogeneic HCT had a more adverse impact on most QOL issues than either autologous HCT or chemotherapy.

Summary, remaining problems, and potential interventions

For years, the main goal of investigators and clinicians has been to achieve cure of HM. On the other hand, our patients hoped for both cure and QOL that is better than what they had with their malignancy. Great advances have been made in creating new agents for conventional treatment of HM and in designing novel conditioning regimens essential for successful and almost uneventful HCT. With these advances, excellence in QOL is becoming one of the goals of treatment. QOL impairments among ALL survivors have been found mainly due to CNS treatments and to less extent, due to systemic chemotherapy. Most QOL studies in AML were done in correlation with autologous or allogeneic HCT, given the short interval between induction chemotherapy and the need for HCT. The "watch and wait" approach for patients with CLL does not seem to improve QOL over conventional interventions, suggesting the need for continuing exploration of novel treatments for this disease. Some of the new agents have insignificant differences in efficacies. Therefore, differences in QOL might improve the risk-benefit ratio assessment of these treatment modalities. The introduction of tyrosine kinase inhibitors for treatment of CML has improved not only prognosis but also QOL over traditional approaches. Imatinib has delayed the need for allogeneic HCT for CML, but there is no data on comparison of QOL between the two approaches. Survivors of HL reported the greatest impairments in QOL after conventional chemo-radiotherapy, mainly due to younger age at diagnosis, a trend for aggressive initial intervention, and a longer duration between diagnosis and the need for HCT compared to other HM. Lack of sufficient data on QOL among multiple myeloma (MM) patients could be due to the nature of the disease, which imposes several adverse effects on QOL that are hard to delineate from the effects of chemotherapy.

QOL was found only mildly affected after autologous HCT, given absence of GVHD and the occurrence of only mild and transient regimen-related toxicities. Allogeneic HCT is always followed by acute deterioration in QOL domains till day 100. Different profiles of recovery have been reported after allogeneic HCT. While some patients might regain reasonable QOL after day 100, others could suffer beyond four years after HCT. The presence or absence of cGVHD and the duration of immunosuppressive treatment, but not the type of conditioning regimen, play the most crucial roles in determining the profile of recovery. Multiple confounders limited the comparison studies between autologous and allogeneic HCT, and between HCT and conventional chemotherapy. Nevertheless, it seemed that specific groups of patients might benefit from HCT over conventional chemotherapy in improving the disease-related impairments in QOL. Also, in carefully selected low-risk patients, QOL after allogeneic HCT could be similar to that after autologous HCT.

Clearly, measuring QOL can be of help in guiding decisions on treatment preference when survival, as an end point, fails to do so. Three areas remain to be addressed. One is how to increase our knowledge about the role of QOL next to survival in treatment decision making. This will require routine incorporation of QOL into end points of prospective trials, good sample size, multi-institutional studies, adjusting for confounders, and introducing new concepts to differentiate disease-related from intervention-related QOL impairments. Second is how to improve QOL assessments. A large number of different scales has been used to cover a wide variety of QOL domains. For clinical investigators, a simplified and unified single instrument that covers the most important domains would be crucial for future trials. Such a tool should also have the ability to discriminate between the actual causes of QOL impairments. Finally, ways are needed to be able to integrate the knowledge gained from longitudinal information on QOL assessed before treatment, after conventional treatments, and after HCT. This would require national prospective longitudinal studies operated by registry organizations, such as the Childhood Cancer Survivor Group, the Center of International Blood and Marrow Transplantation Research, or perhaps a new multi-institutional collaboration devoted to HM survivors. Such longitudinal trials could provide crucial information that would aid in decisions on the timing of conventional chemotherapy versus HCT.

Interventions to improve QOL should be considered as a research and clinical goal. Interventions could include but should not be limited to: (1) lessening the burden of organ toxicities by scientifically opting for the least toxic conventional agents, conditioning regimens for HCT, and immunosuppressive combinations; (2) the use of different exercise programs during and after treatment [96, 97]; (3) psychosocial interventions including stress management and coping skills for pain, gastrointestinal and psychological symptoms [98–101]; (4) the use of specialized cognitive, educational, and vocational services for survivors with poor school attendance or with cognitive and emotional disabilities [102];

(5) using the ideal tools for communication with survivors, including telephone, Internet, DVD, or other delivery methods; and (6) the possible use of drugs like psycho-stimulants to reduce attention deficits [32].

References

1 Cella DF. (1995) Measuring quality of life in palliative care. *Semin Oncol* **22**:73–81.

2 de Haes JC. (1988) Quality of life: conceptual and theoretical considerations. In Watson M, Greer S, Thomas C (eds.) *Psychosocial Oncology: Proceedings of the Second and Third Meetings of the British Psychosocial Oncology Group, London and Leicester, 1985 and 1986*, pp. 61–70. Oxford, UK: Pergamon Press.

3 Kornblith AB, Holland JC. (1994) *Handbook of Measures for Psychological, Social, and Physical Function in Cancer*. New York, NY: Memorial Sloan Kettering Cancer Center.

4 Pidala J, Anasetti C, Jim H. (2009) Quality of life after allogeneic hematopoietic cell transplantation (Review). *Blood* **114**:7–19.

5 Lee SJ, Joffe S, Haesook TK, et al. (2004) Physicians' attitudes about quality-of-life issues in hematopoietic stem cell transplantation. *Blood* **104**:2194–200.

6 Johnson JR, Temple R. (1985) Food and Drug Administration requirements for approval of new anticancer drugs. *Cancer Treat Rep* **69**:1155–9.

7 Testa MA, Simonson DC. (1996) Assessment of quality-of-life outcomes. *N Engl J Med* **334**:835–40.

8 Kirkova J, Davis MP, Walsh D, et al. (2006) Cancer symptom assessment instruments: a systematic review (Review). *J Clin Oncol* **24**:1459–73.

9 Hunt SM, McEwen J, McKenna SP. (1985) Measuring health status: a new tool for clinicians and epidemiologists. *J R Coll Gen Pract* **35**:185–8.

10 Ware JE, Jr., Sherbourne CD. (1992) The MOS 36-item short-form health survey (SF-36). I. Conceptual framework and item selection. *Med Care* **30**:473–83.

11 Reeve BB, Potosky AL, Smith AW, et al. (2009) Impact of cancer on health-related quality of life of older Americans. *J Natl Cancer Inst* **101**:860–8.

12 Bergner M, Bobbitt RA, Carter WB, Gilson BS. (1981) The Sickness Impact Profile: development and final revision of a health status measure. *Med Care* **19**:787–805.

13 Cella D. (1997) The Functional Assessment of Cancer Therapy-Anemia (FACT-An) Scale: a new tool for the assessment of outcomes in cancer anemia and fatigue. *Semin Hematol* **34**:13–19.

14 Schipper H, Clinch J, McMurray A, Levitt M. (1984) Measuring the quality of life of cancer patients: the Functional Living Index-Cancer: development and validation. *J Clin Oncol* **2**:472–83.

15 Molica S. (2005) Quality of life in chronic lymphocytic leukemia: a neglected issue (Review). *Leuk Lymphoma* **46**:1709–14.

16 Zebrack BJ, Zeltzer LK. (2003) Quality of life issues and cancer survivorship (Review). *Curr Probl Cancer* **27**:198–11.

17 Zeltzer LK, Lu Q, Leisenring W, et al. (2008) Psychosocial outcomes and health-related quality of life in adult childhood cancer survivors: a report from the Childhood Cancer Survivor Study. *Cancer Epidemiol Biomarkers Prev* **17**:435–46.

18 Schultz KA, Ness KK, Whitton J, et al. (2007) Behavioral and social outcomes in adolescent survivors of childhood cancer: a report from the Childhood Cancer Survivor Study. *J Clin Oncol* **25**:3649–56.

19 Mulrooney DA, Ness KK, Neglia JP, et al. (2008) Fatigue and sleep disturbance in adult survivors of childhood cancer: a report from the Childhood Cancer Survivor Study (CCSS). *Sleep* **31**:271–81.

20 Thornton KE, Carmody DP. (2005) Electroencephalogram biofeedback for reading disability and traumatic brain injury (Review). *Child Adolesc Psychiatric Clin N Am* **14**:137–62.

21 Hudson MM, Mertens AC, Yasui Y, et al. (2003) Health status of adult long-term survivors of childhood cancer: a report from the Childhood Cancer Survivor Study. *JAMA* **290**:1583–92.

22 Zebrack BJ, Zeltzer LK, Whitton J, et al. (2002) Psychological outcomes in long-term survivors of childhood leukemia, Hodgkin's disease, and non-Hodgkin's lymphoma: a report from the Childhood Cancer Survivor Study. *Pediatrics* **110**:42–52.

23 Krull KR, Gioia G, Ness KK, et al. (2008) Reliability and validity of the Childhood Cancer Survivor Study neurocognitive questionnaire. *Cancer* **113**:2188–97.

24 Mulhern RK, Ochs J, Fairclough D. (1992) Deterioration of intellect among children surviving leukemia: IQ test changes modify estimates of treatment toxicity. *J Consult Clin Psychol* **60**:477–80.

25 Anderson VA, Godber T, Smibert E, et al. (2000) Cognitive and academic outcome following cranial irradiation and chemotherapy in children: a longitudinal study. *Br J Cancer* **82**:255–62.

26 Hill DE, Ciesielski KT, Sethre-Hofstad L, et al. (1997) Visual and verbal short-term memory deficits in childhood leukemia survivors after intrathecal chemotherapy. *J Pediatr Psychol* **22**:861–70.

27 Lockwood KA, Bell TS, Colegrove RW, Jr., (1999) Long-term effects of cranial radiation therapy on attention functioning in survivors of childhood leukemia. *J Pediatr Psychol* **24**:55–66.

28 Cousens P, Ungerer JA, Crawford JA, Stevens MM. (1991) Cognitive effects of childhood leukemia therapy: a case for four specific deficits. *J Pediatr Psychol* **16**:475–88.

29 Espy KA, Moore IM, Kaufmann PM, et al. (2001) Chemotherapeutic CNS prophylaxis and neuropsychologic change in children with acute lymphoblastic leukemia: a prospective study. *J Pediatr Psychol* **26**:1–9.

30 Kaleita TA, Reaman GH, MacLean WE, et al. (1999) Neurodevelopmental outcome of infants with acute lymphoblastic leukemia: a Children's Cancer Group report. *Cancer* **85**:1859–65.

31 Anderson V, Godber T, Smibert E, Ekert H. (1997) Neurobehavioural sequelae following cranial irradiation and chemotherapy in children: an analysis of risk factors. *Pediatr Rehabil* **1**:63–76.

32 Mulhern RK, Khan RB, Kaplan S, et al. (2004) Short-term efficacy of methylphenidate: a randomized, double-blind, placebo-controlled trial among survivors of childhood cancer. *J Clin Oncol* **22**:4795–803.

33 Moleski M. (2000) Neuropsychological, neuroanatomical, and neurophysiological consequences of CNS chemotherapy for acute lymphoblastic leukemia. *Arch Clin Neuropsychol* **15**:603–30.

34 Campbell LK, Scaduto M, Van Slyke D, et al. (2009) Executive function, coping, and behavior in survivors of childhood acute lymphocytic leukemia. *J Pediatr Psychol* **34**:317–27.

35 Holzner B, Kemmler G, Kopp M, et al. (2004) Quality of life of patients with chronic lymphocytic leukemia: results of a longitudinal investigation over one year. *Eur J Haematol* **72**:381–9.

36 Osterborg A, Brandberg Y, Molostova V, et al. (2002) Randomized, double-blind, placebo-controlled trial of recombinant human erythropoietin, epoetin beta, in hematologic malignancies. *J Clin Oncol* **20**:2486–94.

37 Holzner B, Kemmler G, Sperner-Unterweger B, et al. (2001) Quality of life measurement in oncology – a matter of the assessment instrument? *Eur J Cancer* **37**:2349–56.

38 Levin TT, Li Y, Riskind J, Rai K. (2007) Depression, anxiety and quality of life in a chronic lymphocytic leukemia cohort. *Gen Hosp Psychiatry* **29**:251–6.

39 Hahn EA, Glendenning GA, Sorensen MV, et al. (2003) Quality of life in patients with newly diagnosed chronic phase chronic myeloid leukemia on imatinib versus interferon alfa plus low-dose cytarabine: results from the IRIS Study. *J Clin Oncol* **21**:2138–2146.

40 Zeltzer LK, Recklitis C, Buchbinder D, et al. (2009) Psychological status in childhood cancer survivors: a report from the Childhood Cancer Survivor Study (Review). *J Clin Oncol* **27**:2396–404.

41 Ferme C, Eghbali H, Meerwaldt JH, et al. (2007) Chemotherapy plus involved-field radiation in early-stage Hodgkin's disease. *N Engl J Med* **357**:1916–27.

42 Kornblith AB, Herndon JE, Zuckerman E, et al. (1998) Comparison of psychosocial adaptation of advanced stage Hodgkin's disease and acute leukemia survivors. Cancer and Leukemia Group B. *Ann Oncol* **9**:297–306.

43 Chalder T, Berelowitz G, Pawlikowska T, et al. (1993) Development of a fatigue scale. *J Psychosom Res* **37**:147–53.

44 Hjermstad MJ, Fossa SD, Oldervoll L, et al. (2005) Fatigue in long-term Hodgkin's disease survivors: a follow-up study. *J Clin Oncol* **23**:6587–95.

45 Abrahamsen AF, Loge JH, Hannisdal E, et al. (1998) Socio-medical situation for long-term survivors of Hodgkin's disease: a survey of 459 patients treated at one institution. *Eur J Cancer* **34**:1865–70.

46 Kornblith AB, Anderson J, Cella DF, et al. (1992) Comparison of psychosocial adaptation and sexual function of survivors of advanced Hodgkin's disease treated by MOPP, ABVD, or MOPP alternating with ABVD. *Cancer* **70**:2508–16.

47 Fobair P, Hoppe RT, Bloom J, et al. (1986) Psychosocial problems among survivors of Hodgkin's disease. *J Clin Oncol* **4**:805–14.

48 Aksoy S, Harputluoglu H, Kilickap S, et al. (2008) Erectile dysfunction in successfully treated lymphoma patients. *Support Care Cancer* **16**:291–7.

49 Howell SJ, Shalet SM. (2001) Testicular function following chemotherapy (Review). *Hum Reprod Update* **7**:363–9.

50 Lee SJ, Schover LR, Partridge AH, et al. (2006) American Society of Clinical Oncology recommendations on fertility preservation in cancer patients. *J Clin Oncol* **24**:2917–31.

51 Howell SJ, Radford JA, Smets EM, Shalet SM. (2000) Fatigue, sexual function and mood following treatment for haematological malignancy: the impact of mild Leydig cell dysfunction. *Br J Cancer* **82**:789–93.

52 Kiserud CE, Schover LR, Dahl AA, et al. (2009) Do male lymphoma survivors have impaired sexual function? *J Clin Oncol* **27**:6019–26.

53 Chao NJ, Tierney DK, Bloom JR, et al. (1992) Dynamic assessment of quality of life after autologous bone marrow transplantation. *Blood* **80**:825–30.

54 Winer EP, Lindley C, Hardee M, et al. (1999) Quality of life in patients surviving at least 12 months following high dose chemotherapy with autologous bone marrow support. *Psycho-Oncology* **8**:167–76.

55 Whedon M, Stearns D, Mills LE. (1995) Quality of life of long-term adult survivors of autologous bone marrow transplantation. *Oncol Nurs Forum* **22**:1527–35.

56 Duell T, van Lint MT, Ljungman P, et al. (1997) Health and functional status of long-term survivors of bone marrow transplantation. EBMT Working Party on Late Effects and EULEP Study Group on Late Effects. *Ann Intern Med* **126**:184–92.

57 Socie G, Stone JV, Wingard JR, et al. (1999) Long-term survival and late deaths after allogeneic bone marrow transplantation. Late Effects Working Committee of the International Bone Marrow Transplant Registry. *N Engl J Med* **341**:14–21.

58 Syrjala KL, Langer SL, Abrams JR, et al. (2004) Recovery and long-term function after hematopoietic cell transplantation for leukemia or lymphoma. *JAMA* **291**:2335–43.

59 Wolcott DL, Wellisch DK, Fawzy FI, Landsverk J. (1986) Psychological adjustment of adult bone marrow transplant donors whose recipient survives. *Transplantation* **41**:484–8.

60 Andrykowski MA, Altmaier EM, Barnett RL, et al. (1990) Cognitive dysfunction in adult survivors of allogeneic marrow transplantation: relationship to dose of total body irradiation. *Bone Marrow Transplant* **6**:269–76.

61 Wingard JR, Curbow B, Baker F, Piantadosi S. (1991) Health, functional status, and employment of adult survivors of bone marrow transplantation. *Ann Intern Med* **114**:113–18.

62 Schmidt GM, Niland JC, Forman SJ, et al. (1993) Extended follow-up in 212 long-term allogeneic bone marrow transplant survivors. *Transplantation* **55**:551–7.

63 Harder H, Cornelissen JJ, Van Gool AR, et al. (2002) Cognitive functioning and quality of life in long-term adult survivors of bone marrow transplantation. *Cancer* **95**:183–92.

64 Syrjala KL, Chapko MK, Vitaliano PP, et al. (1993) Recovery after allogeneic marrow transplantation: prospective study of predictors of long-term physical and psychosocial functioning. *Bone Marrow Transplant* **11**:319–27.

65 Bhatia S, Francisco L, Carter A, et al. (2007) Late mortality after allogeneic hematopoietic cell transplantation and functional status of long-term survivors: report from the Bone Marrow Transplant Survivor Study. *Blood* **110**:3784–92.

66 Baker F, Wingard JR, Curbow B, et al. (1994) Quality of life of bone marrow transplant long-term survivors. *Bone Marrow Transplant* **13**:589–96.

67 Altmaier EM, Gingrich RD, Fyfe MA. (1991) Two-year adjustment of bone marrow transplant survivors. *Bone Marrow Transplant* **7**:311–16.

68 McQuellon RP, Russell GB, Rambo TD, et al. (1998) Quality of life and psychological distress of bone marrow transplant recipients: the "time trajectory" to recovery over the first year. *Bone Marrow Transplant* **21**:477–86.

69 Bush NE, Donaldson GW, Haberman MH, et al. (2000) Conditional and unconditional estimation of multidimensional quality of life after hematopoietic stem cell transplantation: a longitudinal follow-up of 415 patients. *Biol Blood Marrow Transplant* **6**:576–91.

70 Hjermstad MJ, Loge JH, Evensen SA, et al. (1999) The course of anxiety and depression during the first year after allogeneic or autologous stem cell transplantation. *Bone Marrow Transplant* **24**:1219–28.

71 Bevans MF, Marden S, Leidy NK, et al. (2006) Health-related quality of life in patients receiving reduced-intensity conditioning allogeneic hematopoietic stem cell transplantation. *Bone Marrow Transplant* **38**:101–9.

72 Andrykowski MA, Bishop MM, Hahn EA, et al. (2005) Long-term health-related quality of life, growth, and spiritual well-being after hematopoietic stem-cell transplantation. *J Clin Oncol* **23**:599–608.

73 Sutherland HJ, Fyles GM, Adams G, et al. (1997) Quality of life following bone marrow transplantation:
a comparison of patient reports with population norms. *Bone Marrow Transplant* **19**:1129–36.

74 Hjermstad MJ, Evensen SA, Kvaloy SO, et al. (1999) Health-related quality of life 1 year after allogeneic or autologous stem-cell transplantation: a prospective study. *J Clin Oncol* **17**:706–18.

75 Lee SJ, Fairclough D, Parsons SK, et al. (2001) Recovery after stem-cell transplantation for hematologic diseases. *J Clin Oncol* **19**:242–52.

76 Chiodi S, Spinelli S, Ravera G, et al. (2000) Quality of life in 244 recipients of allogeneic bone marrow transplantation. *Br J Haematol* **110**:614–19.

77 Andrykowski MA, Greiner CB, Altmaier EM, et al. (1995) Quality of life following bone marrow transplantation: findings from a multicentre study. *Br J Cancer* **71**:1322–9.

78 Sorror ML, Maris MB, Storb R, et al. (2005) Hematopoietic cell transplantation (HCT)-specific comorbidity index: a new tool for risk assessment before allogeneic HCT. *Blood* **106**:2912–19.

79 Sorror ML, Sandmaier BM, Storer BE, et al. (2007) Comorbidity and disease status-based risk stratification of outcomes among patients with acute myeloid leukemia or myelodysplasia receiving allogeneic hematopoietic cell transplantation. *J Clin Oncol* **25**:4246–54.

80 Sorror ML, Giralt S, Sandmaier BM, et al. (2007) Hematopoietic cell transplantation-specific comorbidity index as an outcome predictor for patients with acute myeloid leukemia in first remission: Combined FHCRC and MDACC experiences. *Blood* **110**:4608–13.

81 Sorror ML, Storer BE, Maloney DG, et al. (2008) Outcomes after allogeneic hematopoietic cell transplantation with nonmyeloablative or myeloablative regimens for treatment of lymphoma and chronic lymphocytic leukemia. *Blood* **111**:446–52.

82 Baker KS, Gurney JG, Ness KK, et al. (2004) Late effects in survivors of chronic myeloid leukemia treated with hematopoietic cell transplantation: results from the Bone Marrow Transplant Survivor Study. *Blood* **104**:1898–906.

83 Lee SJ, Kim HT, Ho VT, et al. (2006) Quality of life associated with acute and chronic graft-versus-host disease. *Bone Marrow Transplant* **38**:305–10.

84 Kiss TL, Abdolell M, Jamal N, et al. (2002) Long-term medical outcomes and quality-of-life assessment of patients with chronic myeloid leukemia followed at least 10 years after allogeneic bone marrow transplantation. *J Clin Oncol* **20**:2334–43.

85 Fraser CJ, Bhatia S, Ness K, et al. (2006) Impact of chronic graft–versus-host disease on the health status of hematopoietic cell transplantation survivors: a report from the Bone Marrow Transplant Survivor Study. *Blood* **108**:2867–73.

86 Marks DI, Gale DJ, Vedhara K, Bird JM. (1999) A quality of life study in 20 adult long-term survivors of unrelated donor bone marrow transplantation. *Bone Marrow Transplant* **24**:191–195.

87 Hjermstad MJ, Knobel H, Brinch L, et al. (2004) A prospective study of health-related quality of life, fatigue, anxiety and depression 3–5 years after stem cell transplantation. *Bone Marrow Transplant* **34**:257–66.

88 Zittoun R, Suciu S, Watson M, et al. (1997) Quality of life in patients with acute myelogenous leukemia in prolonged first complete remission after bone marrow transplantation (allogeneic or autologous) or chemotherapy: a cross-sectional study of the EORTC-GIMEMA AML 8A trial. *Bone Marrow Transplant* **20**:307–15.

89 Molassiotis A, van den Akker OBA, Milligan DW, et al. (1992) Quality of life in long-term survivors of marrow transplantation: comparison with a matched group receiving maintenance chemotherapy. *Bone Marrow Transplant* **17**:249–58.

90 Vellenga E, van Agthoven M, Croockewit AJ, et al. (2001) Autologous peripheral blood stem cell transplantation in patients with relapsed lymphoma results in accelerated haematopoietic reconstitution, improved quality of life and cost reduction compared with bone marrow transplantation: the HOVON 22 study. *Br J Haematol* **114**:319–26.

91 van Agthoven M, Vellenga E, Fibbe WE, et al. (2001) Cost analysis and quality of life assessment comparing patients undergoing autologous peripheral blood stem cell transplantation or autologous bone marrow transplantation for refractory or relapsed non-Hodgkin's lymphoma or Hodgkin's disease. A prospective randomised trial. *Eur J Cancer* **37**:1781–9.

92 Gallardo D, De la Camara R, Nieto JB, et al. (2009) Is mobilized peripheral blood comparable with bone marrow as a source of hematopoietic stem cells for allogeneic transplantation from HLA-identical sibling donors? A case-control study. *Haematologica* **94**:1282–8.

93 Molassiotis A, van den Akker OB, Milligan DW, et al. (1996) Quality of life in long-term survivors of marrow transplantation: comparison with a matched group receiving maintenance chemotherapy. *Bone Marrow Transplant* **17**:249–58.

94 Watson M, Wheatley K, Harrison GA, et al. (1999) Severe adverse impact on sexual functioning and fertility of bone marrow transplantation, either allogeneic or autologous, compared with consolidation chemotherapy alone: analysis of the MRC AML 10 trial. *Cancer* **86**:1231–9.

95 Watson L, Vestbo J, Postma DS, et al. (2004) Gender differences in the management and experience of chronic obstructive pulmonary disease. *Respir Med* **98**:1207–13.

96 Mello M, Tanaka C, Dulley FL. (2003) Effects of an exercise program on muscle performance in patients undergoing allogeneic bone marrow transplantation. *Bone Marrow Transplant* **32**:723–8.

97 Defor TE, Burns LJ, Gold EM, Weisdorf DJ. (2007) A randomized trial of the effect of a walking regimen on the functional status of 100 adult allogeneic donor hematopoietic cell transplant patients. *Biol Blood Marrow Transplant* **13**:948–55.

98 Syrjala KL, AbramsJr., (1996) Hypnosis and imagery in the treatment of pain. In Gatchel RJ, Turk DC (eds.) *Psychological Approaches to Pain Management: A Practitioner's Handbook*, pp. 231–58. New York: Guilford Press.

99 Syrjala KL, Cummings C, Donaldson GW. (1992) Hypnosis or cognitive behavioral training for the reduction of pain and nausea during cancer treatment: a controlled clinical trial. *Pain* **48**:137–46.

100 Syrjala KL, Donaldson GW, Davis MW, et al. (1995) Relaxation and imagery and cognitive-behavioral training reduce pain during cancer treatment: a controlled clinical trial. *Pain* **63**:189–98.

101 Donnelly JM, Kornblith AB, Fleishman S, et al. (2000) A pilot study of interpersonal psychotherapy by telephone with cancer patients and their partners. *Psycho-Oncology* **9**:44–56.

102 Butler RW, Copeland DR, Fairclough DL, et al. (2008) A multicenter, randomized clinical trial of a cognitive remediation program for childhood survivors of a pediatric malignancy. *J Consult Clin Psychol* **76**:367–78.

Index

Note: page numbers in *italics* refer to figures, those in **bold** refer to tables

Advances in Malignant Hematology, First Edition. Edited by Hussain I. Saba and Ghulam J. Mufti. © 2011 Blackwell Publishing Ltd.
Published 2011 by Blackwell Publishing Ltd.